ENCYCLOPEDIA OF

GLOBAL HEALTH

ENCYCLOPEDIA OF
GLOBAL HEALTH

YAWEI ZHANG
GENERAL EDITOR

VOLUME 2

A SAGE Reference Publication

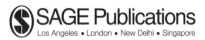

SAGE Publications

Los Angeles • London • New Delhi • Singapore

For information:

SAGE Publications, Inc.
2455 Teller Road
Thousand Oaks, California 91320
E-mail: order@sagepub.com

SAGE Publications Ltd.
1 Oliver's Yard
55 City Road
London EC1Y 1SP
United Kingdom

SAGE Publications India Pvt. Ltd.
B 1/I 1 Mohan Cooperative Industrial Area
Mathura Road, New Delhi 110 044
India

SAGE Publications Asia-Pacific Pte. Ltd.
33 Pekin Street #02-01
Far East Square
Singapore 048763

Library of Congress Cataloging-in-Publication Data

Encyclopedia of global health / Yawei Zhang, general editor.
    p. ; cm.
Includes bibliographical references and index.
ISBN 978-1-4129-4186-0 (cloth : alk. paper)
  1. World health—Encyclopedias. 2. Public health—Encyclopedias. 3. Medicine—Encyclopedias. I. Zhang, Yawei.
  [DNLM: 1. World Health—Encyclopedias—English. 2. Medicine—Encyclopedias—English. WA 13 E5566 2008]

RA441.E53 2008
362.103—dc22   2007037954

This book is printed on acid-free paper.
08 09 10 11 12 10 9 8 7 6 5 4 3 2 1

Photo credits are on page I–64

GOLSON BOOKS, LTD.

President and Editor	J. Geoffrey Golson
Creative Director	Mary Jo Scibetta
Managing Editor	Susan Moskowitz
Copyeditor	Joyce Li
Layout Editors	Chad Brobst
	Susan Honeywell
	Julie Murphy
	Oona Patrick
Proofreader	Joan K. Griffitts
Indexer	J S Editorial

SAGE REFERENCE

Vice President and Publisher	Rolf Janke
Project Editor	Tracy Buyan
Cover Production	Janet Foulger
Marketing Manager	Amberlyn Erzinger
Editorial Assistant	Michele Thompson

ENCYCLOPEDIA OF

GLOBAL HEALTH

CONTENTS

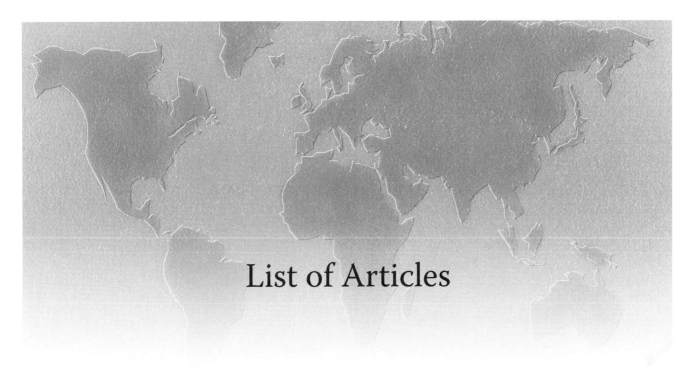

List of Articles

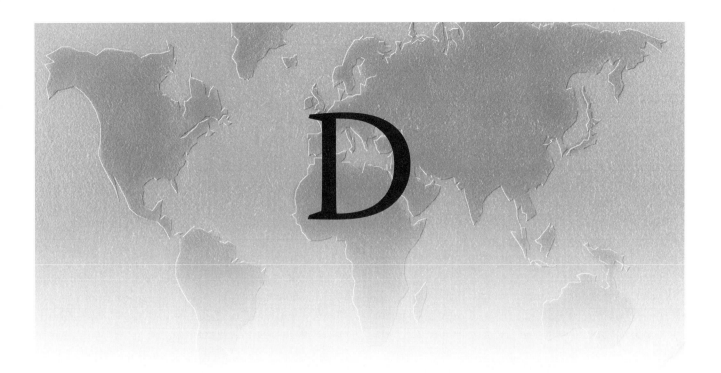

Daily Reference Values (DRVs)

The daily reference value (DRV) is a number of statistics assigned by the U.S. Department of Agriculture for the optimum diet, both in overall amount and in type. The DRV for adults and children over the age of 4, based on a diet of 2,000 calories a day suggests that about 30 percent of all calories can be fat (about 65 g), of which just a bit less than a third of it (20 g) should be saturated fat. Some 60 percent of the diet should consist of carbohydrates (300 g), with 10 percent consisting of protein (50 g). The diet should also contain 300 mg of cholesterol, 25 g of fiber, some 2,400 mg of sodium, and 3,500 mg of potassium.

DRVs have been important in food labeling, although many people only study them from the information on cereal packets, even though it appears on many other items of food. In Australia and New Zealand, DRVs are known as recommended dietary intake, although the U.S. Department of Agriculture does state categorically that DRVs are not the recommended amounts of nutrients that people should eat in one day but more the balance of the diet they should aim to have over a period of time.

Most of the nutritional information figures printed on food labels include the average size of servings, the number of servings in a particular package, and the nutritional information in regard to the quantity per serving, the percentage of the suggested daily intake per serving, and the quantity per 100 g, which may be larger or smaller than the serving size. For some foods that are generally eaten with something else, such as most people eating cereal with milk, figures are also given for the overall level of nutrients when the two are combined.

The use of DRVs allow people to assess whether their diet exceeds the amount of fat, saturated fat, cholesterol, or carbohydrates that they should be eating, and serve as an important reference point for people dealing with dietary problems. In particular, most people play close attention to the fat level of products such as cookies, peanut butter, and potato chips, which vary considerably from brand to brand.

SEE ALSO: Dieting.

BIBLIOGRAPHY. Paula Kurtzwell, "Daily Values Encourage Healthy Diet," http://www.fda.gov/FDAC/special/foodlabel/dvs.html (cited August 2007).

JUSTIN CORFIELD
GEELONG GRAMMAR SCHOOL, AUSTRALIA

Darwin, Charles (1809–82)

The naturalist and evolutionary biologist Charles Darwin was born in Shrewsbury, England, on February 12, 1809. A polymath, Darwin was also educated in theology, chemistry, medicine, and geology. Extensive field research, comparative study and reflection on the writings of other natural scientists led him to infer that natural selection explained how species differentiated from one another, including species whose only trace was found in ancient fossil records.

During 1831–36, Darwin sailed along the coast of the Atlantic and Pacific coasts of South America in the British naval vessel *HMS Beagle*. Periodically, Darwin went ashore for weeks and months at a time. During those five years, his analytic methods consisted almost entirely of making extensive observations, recording his findings systematically, and making comparative and inductive generalizations. During that period, Darwin spent a crucial three months doing field research on the isolated Galapagos Islands where species varied astonishingly from one island to another.

Darwin first thought of natural selection as early as 1838. More than 20 years later, the first edition of Darwin's *The Origin of Species* was published in 1859. This underwent six editions. As Darwin concisely summarized his theory of evolution through natural selection in the final edition, "Species have been modified through a long course of descent. This has been effected chiefly through the natural selection of numerous successive, slight, favourable variations." Darwin acknowledged intellectual debts to 20 others who had written about evolution, including Erasmus Darwin, Jean-Baptiste Lamarck, Charles Lyell, and Alfred Russel Wallace.

Darwin died in Downe, England, in 1882. As a result of a petition in Parliament, he was buried in Westminster Abbey. Subsequent discoveries have validated and elaborated many of Darwin's claims. Others used Darwin's work to support political arguments that he might have rejected. For example, Social Darwinism crudely asserted racist claims that the predominance of the strongest nations over weaker societies justified imperialists' right to rule over vast colonies in Africa, the Americas, Asia, and the Pacific.

Despite corroborating evidence, Darwin's theory of gradual, incremental change over millions of years has been contentious. Controversially, humans are part of nature—not separate from it. In reaction, opponents of Darwin on state and local U.S. public school boards have attempted to relegate Darwin's theory of evolution in the curriculum to a theory competing with theological explanations like creationism or intelligent design.

SEE ALSO: Acquired Mutation; DNA; Watson, James.

BIBLIOGRAPHY. Charles Darwin, *The Voyage of the Beagle* (First published, 1839; P. F. Collier & Son, 1909); Charles Darwin, *On the Origin of Species*, 6th ed., The Harvard Classics, vol. 29 (First published, 1872; Franklin Center, Franklin Library, 1975); Frank. J. Sulloway, "Why Darwin Rejected Intelligent Design," in *Intelligent Thought: Science versus the Intelligent Design Movement*, ed. John Brockman (Vintage Books, 2005).

VINCENT KELLY POLLARD
UNIVERSITY OF HAWAII AT MANOA

Date Rape

Date rape is a term used largely in industrialized countries to describe what a victim experiences when he or she is forced or coerced into unwanted sexual activity by a friend, romantic suitor, or peer through violence, verbal pressure, misuse of authority, or threat of violence. While some prefer the more inclusive term *acquaintance rape*, which does not imply any sort of romantic relationship between the rapist and the victim, both terms acknowledge the fact that the majority of women (and men) who are raped know their attackers, and that the victim did not consent to sexual activity.

Both terms were originally introduced into public health parlance in the 1980s in an attempt to dispel the myth that the majority of rapes occurred due to random attacks by strangers, and to give voice to sexual experiences many women believed had been nonconsensual, but were not criminal in nature as they occurred in the context of a romantic relationship. Advocates for the rights of rape victims emphasized the concept of date rape to promote awareness that all sexual activity requires explicit consent from both parties; a new, prior,

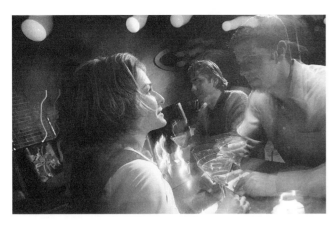

A recent concern is the use of "date rape drugs" such as rohypnol, which can be slipped into alcoholic or other drinks.

or ongoing dating or intimate relationship does not necessarily imply that either party has a "'right" to sexual relations. This new awareness of date rape has led to legal changes in the United States that make it easier for victims to prosecute attackers, although much discussion remains about the legal standards of consent.

While it is hard to determine the rates of date rape in the United States, even less is known regarding rates of date rape worldwide, especially in cultures where dating and premarital romantic and sexual relationships either do not occur, or in very different contexts. The related concept of marital rape has recently been utilized in developing countries to describe unwanted sexual contact by a spouse, particularly in regards to increasing women's sexual rights as a means of preventing HIV infection.

A recent concern, particularly among young people, is the use of "date rape drugs" such as rohypnol, GHB, and ketamine, which can be slipped into alcoholic or other drinks when a victim is not looking. These drugs are odorless, colorless, and produce paralysis, blackouts, and memory loss, making victims vulnerable to attackers. Intoxication due to alcohol or other drugs is often associated with date rape.

SEE ALSO: Club Drugs; Sexually Transmitted Diseases.

BIBLIOGRAPHY. William A. Bridges, and James Hale, eds., *Date Rape* (Thomson Gale, 2004).

ANNIE DUDE
UNIVERSITY OF CHICAGO

Da Vinci, Leonardo (1452–1519)

Leonardo da Vinci was one of history's great polymaths, a supremely talented artist, sculptor, inventor, architect, and engineer. He was also the most gifted anatomist of the Renaissance era.

Born in April 1452 in the town of Anchiano and raised in Vinci, 50 miles west of Florence, Leonardo di ser Piero da Vinci was an illegitimate child, and thus blocked from most professions of the time. Noting his son's skill for drawing, around 1468 Leonardo's father sent him to apprentice with famed artist Andrea del Verrocchio in Florence. In Verrocchio's workshop, da Vinci would study alongside a generation of famous artists, including Sandro Botticelli, Cosimo Rosselli, Piero Perugino, and Domenico Ghirlandaio.

Anatomy was part of the training for any budding young apprentice painter, and one that da Vinci approached with great interest. Most painters would have confined themselves to external observation, but da Vinci was driven by a desire to understand the inner workings of man, and eventually, the skills he honed dissecting frogs, cows, birds, and bears gave way to the desire to dissect a human body.

Exactly when he began this work is not clear, but it was probably in the early 1500s. In 1507, while living in or near a hospital in Florence, he gave this account: "An old man a few hours before his death told me that he had passed a hundred years, and that he did not feel any bodily deficiency other than weakness. And thus while sitting on a bed in the hospital of Santa Maria Nuova in Florence, without any movement or sign of distress he passed away from his life. And I made an anatomy of him in order to see the cause of so sweet a death." Inside the old man's heart, da Vinci observed thick deposits within the aorta and surrounding veins—the first observation of atherosclerosis, or hardening of the arteries—centuries before the medical profession had a name for it.

Estimates of how many autopsies da Vinci performed vary, with most scholars putting the count at 30; the majority of them were conducted between 1510 and 1513. It was challenging work for the artist, and conditions were far from pleasant. There was always the chance of contracting disease or infection, and without benefit of embalming, bodies decomposed rapidly. However, he persevered in the work and rendered his observations in almost 1,000 exquisitely detailed drawings.

One of his great innovations was the cross-sectional view of anatomy. " ... [To] give knowledge of the true form of any member of man . . . I shall observe this rule, making of each member four representations from the four sides. And in the case of the bones, I shall make five, cutting them through the middle and showing the cavity of each of them ... ," he once wrote of his technique. One of his more famous sketches showed a fetus in the cross-section of a womb. He was the first to accurately show the S-curve of the human spine and the first to depict an appendix.

Human dissection was rare outside medical schools, and religious and social taboos abounded. The artist was eventually accused of necromancy, or communicating with the spirits of the dead. When he moved to Rome in 1513, he had to worry about running afoul of the Church; Pope Leo X did eventually prohibit him from conducting more autopsies.

Da Vinci had always intended to publish his anatomical work, perhaps as an encyclopedia or atlas of the body, but like so many projects he had planned, he never had the time to see it through to fruition. He died in May 1519. Over 150 years later, in 1680, many of his drawings were finally put in book form, not as a work on anatomy, but in a work entitled *Treatise on Painting*.

SEE ALSO: Heart Diseases (General); Italy.

BIBLIOGRAPHY. Martin Kemp, *Leonardo da Vinci: The Marvellous Works of Nature and Man* (Oxford University Press, 2007); Charles Nicholl, *Leonardo da Vinci: Flights of the Mind* (Viking Adult, 2004).

HEATHER K. MICHON
INDEPENDENT SCHOLAR

Deafness

Deafness refers to the loss of a portion or all of the sense of hearing. This is the pathological definition and should not be confused with the term "Deaf" which is always capitalized and defines the culture of persons who cannot fully hear, do not view their deafness as a pathological or medical condition, and whose choice of communication is typically Sign Language. The term "deaf" (with a small "d") refers to persons who have a hearing loss, and who do not consider themselves as culturally Deaf and frequently prefer spoken or manually coded language (i.e., Signed Exact English) and if they had no hearing loss they would be a part of the hearing world.

In general, there are three types of hearing loss: conductive, sensorineural, and mixed. Because of the development of the fetus and the young child, there are different subtypes or etiologies when considering pediatric and adult deafness. Conductive hearing loss is caused by any obstruction that limits external sound from traversing the external auditory canal, the tympanic membrane, the ossicles, and into the inner ear. Common acquired conductive obstacles of the external auditory canal encountered in clinical practice in adults include excessive buildup of cerumen (ear wax), external auditory canal infection with swelling and debris (otitis externa), fluid in the middle ear (both sterile and infected), and a loss of the ossicular mobility so that vibrations are not completely carried to the inner ear. Less commonly, tumors of the external auditory canal can cause conductive hearing loss. The most common cancerous tumor is squamous cell carcinoma, followed by basal cell carcinoma and melanoma. Tumors of bony origin include osteomata and exostoses and limit hearing by blocking sounds from reaching the tympanic membrane. Conductive hearing losses due to middle ear pathology include Eustachian tube dysfunction, development of a cholesteatoma; infection and fluid buildup with or without tympanic membrane perforation. Congenital malformations of the external auditory canal, tympanic membrane, and ossicles are also causes of conductive hearing loss.

In the pediatric population, congenital atresia (lack of development) of the external auricle, external canal, tympanic membranes, ossicles, and or the cochlea are causes of conductive hearing loss. Also, suppurative otitis media (infected) and otitis externa; dysfunctional tympanic membranes with or without perforation; and cholesteatoma all cause conductive hearing loss. A cholesteatoma is a growth of epithelium from the external canal migrating into the middle ear and causing a buildup of sloughed surface cells and chemicals which both block the hearing and destroy the inner ear. Malformations caused by trauma can cause any degree of conductive hearing loss depending on the obstructive sequelae.

Sensorineural hearing loss is caused by a deficient functioning of the inner ear cochlea and eighth cranial nerve (Vestibulocochlear nerve). Presbycussis (hearing loss of old age) is multifactorial and probably is caused by lifelong noise exposure, medications, and familial tendencies. In one series screening over 2,000 Medicare recipients, nearly 60 percent qualified as having sensorineural hearing loss. Another cause of sensorineural hearing loss is ototoxicity from multiple drugs, representative of which are the aminoglycosides (gentamicin, etc.); cancer chemotherapeutic agents (the worst being cisplatinum, then 5-FU and nitrogen mustard and bleomycin); aspirin; and antimalarial medications (chloroquine).

Degenerative and destructive causes of sensorineural hearing loss include multiple sclerosis, diabetes, cerebrovascular insufficiency, and cholesteatoma, while compressive causes include Arnold-Chiari malformations (downward traction of the base of the brain, thus stretching the acoustic nerve) and acoustic neuroma. This is a non-cancerous tumor arising from the eighth cranial nerve, which can destroy the hearing in that ear.

Perilymphatic fistula (caused generally by congenital malformations or mechanical trauma or barotraumas [excessive positive or negative air pressure exposure] to the inner ear) causes the internal fluid from the cochlea to leak out, thus distorting the sound/fluid wave mechanism of the inner ear, which causes a sensorineural hearing loss. This requires surgery to repair the round or oval window of the cochlea.

Congenital sensorineural hearing loss can be caused by intrauterine exposure to viral infections such as HIV, syphllis, cytomegalovirus, hepatitis, rubella, and toxoplasmosis. Inherited forms of sensorineural hearing loss follow both autosomal dominant and autosomal recessive patterns yielding all combinations of hearing/deaf parents and children.

EVALUATION OF DEAFNESS

The evaluation of deafness in the adult begins with a complete history and physical examination. The history should be complete as to the patient's mother's prenatal course, including establishment of the maternal immunity to rubella and lack of exposure to other ototoxic viruses (see above). Patient-specific questions should focus on the onset, severity, associated symptoms (dysequilibrium, tinnitus, etc.), history of recurrent infections, mechanical and barotraumas, previous otologic surgery, otalgia, and otorrhea (ear pain and drainage from the external auditory canal). Besides routine blood work (a complete blood count, chemistry panel, and TSH to evaluate the thyroid function), an office-based tuning fork examination is a high-yield screening test to help differentiate between conductive and sensorineural hearing. Tuning forks of 256 and 512 Hz are used to estimate the amount of hearing loss present. If a person cannot hear the 256 Hz tuning fork and can hear the 512 Hz tuning fork, then a 10-15 dB loss is present. If the person cannot hear the 512 Hz tuning fork, then the loss is estimated at 20 to 30 dB.

Air conduction should produce a louder sound than bone conduction and is tested by striking the tuning fork and holding it near the external canal opening. Bone conduction is then tested by placing the vibrating tuning fork on the mastoid process and the patient reports which of the two tones seemed the loudest, which should be the air conduction in the normal ear. This is the Rinne test. The Weber test is performed by placing the vibrating tuning fork on a midline osseous facial structure (bridge of the nose, between the upper central incisors, etc.) and asking the patient which ear perceives the louder sound. In the normal ear exam, the sound is heard equally well bilaterally. If the patient reports that the tone lateralizes to one ear, this indicates a conductive hearing loss to that ear or a sensorineural hearing loss to the contralateral ear.

Direct otoscopy should be performed and pathological changes such as cerumen impaction, infections, tumors, tympanic membrane abnormalities and middle ear fluid or ossicular abnormalities can be visualized. As a part of the workup of hearing loss, pneumoscopy should be performed. The size of the otoscope speculum is chosen to create an air tight chamber of the external auditory canal and with direct visualization of the tympanic membrane (TM) a small amount of air is insufflated. A nonmobile TM indicates a middle ear effusion, tumor, or a sclerosis (scarring). A hypermobile TM is seen with disruption of the ossicles.

Formal audiometric evaluation in a soundproof room is indicated in conditions of sudden hearing loss, sensorineural loss, and as a part of the workup for possible hearing amplification and or cochlear implant consideration.

Otoacoustic emissions (OAE) testing is now required in over 30 states as a hearing screening test in the newborn nursery. The basis of the test is that when the cochlea is presented with certain sounds, the outer hair cells can respond with sound production which is then measured by a sound emitting and receiving probe placed in the external ear canal.

TREATMENT OF HEARING LOSS

The treatment of hearing loss should be directed at the source of the deficit. Obviously, the treatment would be indicated for infections, TM perforations, ossicular abnormalities, tumors, and trauma. If, however, the reason for the hearing loss is sensorineural, hearing amplification (hearing aids) might be indicated. Hearing aids increase the volume of the external sounds and may help the patient hear better. Problems encountered include impacted cerumen buildup, otalgia, and the increased volume of background noises as well as the desired speech and sound. Cochlear implant surgery might be indicated in adults who have attempted hearing aids, and still have less than 50 percent recognition of spoken sentences, and have no medical contraindications to surgery. The cochlear implant is a medical apparatus that perceives sound, changes the sound to digital format, sends these signals to the cochlea, where electrodes bypass the damaged hair cells and stimulate the acoustic nerve which sends impulses to the brain for processing. This requires a surgery and follow-up visits for programming the speech processor for the appropriate level of electrode stimulation. An accommodation period is required for the brain to "learn" to process these new signals and recognize them as spoken language.

Statistics on the numbers of deaf and hard-of-hearing are difficult to identify because many people are hesitant to acknowledge the condition. Estimates of 20 to 30 million Americans have deafness and public awareness programs are certainly indicated. Education is essential about hearing screening in the schools and newborn nursery to identify problems with learning and appropriate speech formation. Warning the population about noise pollution is becoming more of an issue with the popularity of the digitalized pocket personal music systems. Environmental noises such as a lawn mower can easily emit sounds greater than the 80 dB limit, which is considered potentially hazardous, while jet plane takeoffs, rock band practice at four to six feet, and jack-hammers can surpass 120 dB. Hearing protection can certainly offer hearing perpetuation.

SEE ALSO: Ear Disorders; Hearing Problems in Children.

BIBLIOGRAPHY. John C. O'Handley, Evan Tobin, and Bryan Tagge, *Textbook of Family Practice 6th Edition: Otolaryngology* (Saunders, 2002); Betsy Sanford, and Peter C. Weber, "Etiology of Hearing Impairment in Children," UpToDate, www.uptodate.com (cited March 29, 2006);Peter C. Weber, "Etiology of Hearing Loss in Adults," UpToDate, www.uptodate.com (cited April 20, 2006); Peter C. Weber, "Evaluation of Hearing Loss in Adults," UpToDate, www.uptodate.com (cited January 6, 2005); Peter C Weber, "Hearing Amplification in Adults," UpToDate, www.uptodate.com (cited April 20, 2006).

RICHARD K. OGDEN, D.O., FACOFP, FAAFP
KANSAS CITY UNIVERSITY OF MEDICINE
AND BIOSCIENCES

Death and Dying

Death has always fascinated humankind. The interest on death and in the process of dying is more ancient than civilization itself. In fact, archaeological findings of burial sites and evidences of ritual funerals attest to this interest. Its inexorability and the unknown associated with it have long been focus of conjectures. The process of dying has always been a source of fear, not only due to its ultimate result, but also because of the suffering usually associated with it.

While many fields of knowledge have been dedicated to the study of death throughout human history, the recent progresses of science and medicine have brought into discussion many issues regarding death and dying, such as palliative care and euthanasia or one's right to dignity during the process of dying. The important aging of the world's population, in action in the last decades, has put death and dying into the forefront of societal attention. Extremely medicalized all over the world until recently, death is currently being more regarded as a natural and expected part of life—and the quest for a peaceful death—as a natural human right.

HISTORIC PERSPECTIVES

The reality and ubiquity of death has had a profound impact in human psyche and civilization. The personalization of death as a figure or character has been present in the mythologies of many different cultures. The black-dressed skeleton with a scythe, well known in the United States, is only one of several images that came to use in different times and places, often reflecting popular values and beliefs toward death.

The beliefs and attitudes concerning death have varied a great deal: The Latin term *memento mori*, first evoked in Roman antiquity and translated as *remember that you are mortal*, was popular for centuries, but its meanings varied in the course of the years. Originally associated with the ideal of carpe diem (seize the day), memento mori was an advice toward hedonism. The idea is present even in the Bible: "Eat and drink, for tomorrow we die!" (*Isaiah* 22:13), but as Christian theology developed and brought death and dying to the forefront of religious life, the idea that was to influence the whole Western civilization was the moralizing role of death. In a system of belief with emphasis on the afterlife where a soul could either be sent to heaven or hell, depending on the Christian success on avoiding sin. Memento mori became a warning advice: By remembering one's own mortality, one would have it easier to uphold a pious life.

In the mid-14th century's Europe, the Black Death, a devastating pandemic, changed peoples' views on life and death, with long-lasting effects. During the Black Death, anyone who seemed perfectly well could quickly die without apparent causes. In fact, the pandemia killed nearly two-thirds of the European population and virtually everyone was acquainted with victims of the disease, leading to deep cultural impacts. The uncertainty of life and the ubiquity of death came to populate the minds of medieval Europeans; as an example, the *danse macabre*, the dance of death, a popular allegory in which a personified Death danced with representatives of each segment of society of those times (typically an emperor, a king, a monk, a pope, a young

boy, and a beautiful girl) was a popular remembrance of death not distinguishing between its victims.

In the following years, the perceived need for spiritual comfort and a Christian death and the lack of sufficient Church personnel (the Church itself having suffered huge losses during the Black Death) resulted in the appearance of the *Ars Moriendi* (the art of dying), a book of rules and procedures to ensure a good death and on how to "die well," i.e., according to the Christian principles and to reassure the entrance into Heaven. Apart from the solely religious issues, the book stated that people did not need to be afraid of death: As a pathway to Heaven, it was a good thing. The book oriented dying people on how to avoid different temptations common to the dying process and addressed friends and relatives on how to behave at deathbed. The *Ars Moriendi* became very popular and was the first of a series of guides to death and dying that were to influence Western culture toward a natural view of the process.

Until a century ago, most Americans died at home in a process that was considered a normal event of life. With the relatively recent progresses of science, medicine, and sanitation, humanity became as capable as ever of prolonging life and avoiding death in many cases. The limit between a mild and a mortal disease became blunted when many severe diseases and conditions gained a perspective of cure, as it was the case for cancer.

The same progress, nevertheless, has also contributed to important changes on how society views and deals with death. Once much more common in all age groups, death was viewed as a proper part of life: as mentioned above, a terminally sick person would often die at home, surrounded by family and friends.

With death reduced to a medical event and more avoidable than ever, it progressively ceased to be considered such a normal part of life. Avoiding death became a medical challenge—not succeeding became almost a defeat.

Today more than 80 percent of American deaths occur at a healthcare facility. Dying at a hospital, alone or surrounded by unknown, professionally acting people, became almost the rule. Death became a distant event, something most people may never expect to witness. This social distance led to a lack of knowledge of people in general about death and dying, which further contributes to the maintenance of such distance.

Finally, a considerable amount of health resources is spent during the final weeks of life—frequently with curative intentions toward an incurable disease, which do not enhance quality of life—sometimes actually reducing it. This phenomenon that has been called therapeutic futility, diverts financial and human resources from uses that could benefit society. In the last few decades, this practice has started to be recognized as a menace to a person's right to a peaceful death and a misuse of social resources. The perspective of prioritizing quality of life and suffering relief in terminal diseases is leading a worldwide discussion on what is to be considered a good death and what is the role of health professionals.

RECOGNIZING DEATH

Recognizing the exact moment of death has always been difficult. For a long time, death was defined as the cessation of breathing and heartbeats, but these may be quite difficult to detect in severely ill patients due to superficial breathing or an extremely slow heart frequency, which led to a myriad of tests used to diagnose recent death.

Difficulties diagnosing cardiorespiratory arrest were overcome in the last century with the advent of the electrocardiograph, capable of accurately detecting the heart's electrical activity or its absence. However, the recent use of cardiopulmonary resuscitation (CPR) and prompt defibrillation made cardiorespiratory arrest potentially reversible and thus not synonymous with death. Cardiorespiratory arrest then became known as clinical death.

The quest for an early diagnosis of death, essential in many cases (e.g., the need for early removal of organs from donor in organ transplantation) led to the concept of brain death. With the recognition that the source of consciousness is the brain, this organ is considered the only part of the human body that is essential for what is called one's self or individuality. Brain death is synonymous with death even with other organs still functioning.

Diagnosing brain death, nonetheless, is often not trivial: With other organs functioning, the sole source of definite information concerns the brain itself and the physician has to demonstrate a state of permanent lack of brain activity.

Many exam protocols are precise but not always present on site, especially in developing countries. In such cases, the delay in the diagnosis of death may harm or prevent transplantation.

CARING FOR A DYING PERSON

A patient without perspectives of cure may be cared for and die at home, and more people are choosing this alternative. In this case, and to assure a peaceful death, it is of utmost importance that family and caregivers (who may be the relatives of the patient) be fully informed on the process of dying and the actions they will likely have to do during this time. Many times the problems leading to the failure of home care and dying at home lie in the lack of knowledge of the caregivers, that either may interpret expected events as unexpected or attribute a nonexisting suffering to them. Another common factor of failure lies in the difficulties in reacting to common situations, for example, the caregiver may take the patient to the hospital without real need.

The medical estimation of the time of death is important for the patient and family to prepare for the process, but it is important to stress that there is no precise way to predict survival, because it varies in different individuals and in different diseases.

The dying patient may experience different symptoms, because these depend on the cause underlying the process. Receiving information from the health team on those symptoms and the problematic situations likely to occur in a specific case is important for planning the home care and how to behave in both the expected and the troublesome events.

During the process of dying, two kinds of events are distinguished: the physical phenomena linked to death and the psychological phases the terminally ill patient experiences.

Although death assumes many forms, some physical features are common to anyone experiencing death from a chronic condition. As a person at the end stage of life becomes weaker, their appetite decreases and swallowing may be very difficult. As the time of death approaches, people may not be able to feed anymore and offering food may increase the patient's distress with no benefit: At this stage, feeding will not do any good because the body is not able to process nutrients any longer.

Consciousness variations are not always present. While some people early in the stage of dying become and remain unconscious until they die, other people may sleep and wake alternately and some retain consciousness until just before dying. Visions or hallucinations are common and normally not distressful, when there is no need for medication. In either condition, they may still hear and listening to their loved ones may be a relief.

Breathing changes are a common potential source of discomfort both for the patient and caregivers and range from none at all to severe shortness of breath; the breathing rate may be decreased or increased and breathing can be regular or irregular. When breathing discomfort is present, physicians usually have medications to alleviate them. Noisy breathing, also known as the death rattle, may arise due to the progressive inability to clear lung secretions. This symptom is often exuberant and may scare caregivers but cause no discomfort for the patient.

Circulation is expected to progressively slow down and fail. In such process, it is common that extremities of the body, such as hands and feet, become cooler and bluish, indicating poor oxygen intake. Again, this is not uncomfortable for the patient and nothing needs to be done.

The psychological stages through which a person with an incurable disease often passes include denial, anger, bargaining, depression, and finally acceptance. It has been demonstrated that both terminally ill patients and their family caregivers may pass through these phases, but this order, however, is only the most common: they may happen in any order and not all of them will necessarily happen to a person. It is important to notice that denial and anger may be natural, healthy initial stages of a future acceptance and not a sign of permanent distress.

Psychological support for both patient, caregivers, and family may help them to accept a reality that they cannot change, decrease the despair and suffering that commonly follow a diagnosis of a fatal disease and allow people to pass through this difficult period as peacefully as possible. It may also facilitate the use of the remaining time prior to death to something enjoyable. Examples may include travels or other activities early in the course of disease or visiting a distant relative.

Psychological support also helps people to say farewell to their loved ones and give a sense of closure to their lives. This sense appears to be important in most cultures both to the remaining ones and to the patients, who often decrease their sense of psychological discomfort by having the chance of closing their own lives.

PALLIATIVE CARE AND ETHICAL QUESTIONS

Palliative care is the field of medicine that studies interventions aimed at relieving suffering and increasing quality of life as opposed to traditional medicine, which has mostly pursued prevention and cure. Palliative care is not exclusive of the period of dying: on the contrary, it is indicated whenever a medical situation cannot be cured but relieved. During a terminal disease, it is possible that every medical intervention be directed to caring instead of curing and frequently, there are several options to relieve or decrease suffering up to the last moments of life.

The knowledge on palliative care has given rise to a number of ethical questions regarding what treatment to offer a patient, because a problem will always be obviously incurable. Moreover, there are established therapeutic regimens that may be challenged to the benefit of the patient. One may take the example of cancer, which has been extensively studied and therapeutic protocols of treatment exist for most types of disease. Nonetheless, the predicted treatment may not be applicable to a frail elder patient with multiple diseases who may not support the burden of full chemotherapy that may enhance suffering without achieving cure.

Informed consent is required for any kind of medical intervention unless in emergency situations and, thus, this concept changed how doctors deal with death and dying. Even in emergencies, advance patient directives can prevent the physician from starting cardiopulmonary resuscitation or using mechanical breathing support. The same is valid in many countries for the use of life supporting devices in people with no prognosis of cure or simply not desiring their use.

EUTHANASIA, ORTHOTHANASIA, AND DYSTHANASIA

Euthanasia (from Greek for *good death*) is the practice of terminating one's life when it is perceived as intolerable, generally due to suffering associated with a terminal disease. Euthanasia is to be practiced in a painless or minimally painful way, usually with a lethal injection, a drug overdose, or disconnection of life supporting devices. Euthanasia is a controversial practice because of conflicting religious, legal, and humanist views all over the world.

Voluntary euthanasia occurs with the consent or request of either decisionally competent patients or their proxies. Nonvoluntary euthanasia occurs without the request or consent of either a competent patient or his or her proxy; in this case, the patient and proxies may not even be told of euthanasia and this is not considered a good practice even in countries where euthanasia is allowed. Involuntary euthanasia occurs with the objection of patient or surrogates; it occurs when practiced despite a specific refusal. Even in countries where euthanasia is accepted, involuntary euthanasia is considered murder. When a medical doctor does not practice euthanasia, it is often called mercy killing.

It is important to notice that palliative care that may not intentionally contribute to death is not considered euthanasia (e.g., the use of strong opioid analgesics to relieve pain, contributing to respiratory failure). The same applies to not initiating supportive treatments that be either irrelevant for patient survival or refused by patient or proxy: opposed to the withholding of an initiated treatment this is not considered euthanasia. The set of medical and multidisciplinary practices that aim at promoting a peaceful death and relieving suffering is known in palliative care as orthothanasia (from Greek for *correct death*).

Palliative care strongly opposes the use of every life-sustaining technique for keeping a terminally ill patient alive, which can actually prolong suffering. The same applies to not using analgesic or other distress-relieving drugs for fear of contributing to death. The set of measures exclusively aimed at prolonging life in spite of suffering—sometimes actually causing it—is considered a fault and has been termed *dysthanasia*, or *bad death*.

CURRENT PERSPECTIVES

With the reality of population aging virtually everywhere, which will continue in the next decades, health issues related to elderly people became as important as never before. Death and dying is obviously not a topic exclusive to the elderly, but dying in old age may be a part of a successful and healthy life, while dying young is not, for most deaths in young age became preventable with the advances of sanitation and medicine. Moreover, the same progresses mean that most deaths throughout the world occur in the elderly and, therefore, the questions raised in death and dying are fundamental for geriatric care.

Parallel to a better understanding of the process of dying, there have been efforts for the recognition of unavoidable and incoming death and responsible and adequate use of medical resources. Nowadays, it is widely recognized within the scientific community that using advanced and invasive medical resources in terminally ill patients may be a therapeutic futility if not directed toward suffering relieving, the utmost aim in caring for those who are dying.

SEE ALSO: Geriatrics; Kübler-Ross, Elisabeth; Pain.

BIBLIOGRAPHY. N. M. Goolam, "Euthanasia: Reconciling Culture and Human Rights," *Medicine and Law* (v.15/3, 1996); E. Kübler-Ross, *On Grief and Grieving: Finding the Meaning of Grief through the Five Stages of Loss* (Simon & Schuster, 2005); J. Ladbrook, "Caring for the Dying," *Nursing New Zealand* (v.4/10, 1998); M. C. Long, "Death and Dying and Recognizing Approaching Death," *Clinics in Geriatric Medicine* (v.12/2, 1996); M. M. Ross, "Palliative Care. An Integral Part of Life's End," *Canadian Nurse* (v.94/8, 1998); John Shinmers, ed., "The Art of Dying Well," *Medieval Popular Religion, 1000–1500, a Reader* (Broadview Press, 1997)

THIAGO MONACO, M.D., PH.D.
UNIVERSITY OF SÃO PAULO MEDICAL SCHOOL, BRAZIL

Death Rate

The death rate is a statistic that allows us to analyze either the total number of deaths or the number of deaths due to a specific cause in a defined population over a particular period of time. Death rates are usually expressed in terms of 1,000 or 100,000 population.

The most basic concept of a death rate is the crude death rate, the total number of deaths per 1,000 people in a population over a period of time. So, for instance, if there are 600 deaths per year in a population of 100,000, the crude death rate will be 600/100,000, or 6/1,000. While the crude death rate gives some indication of the mortality profile of a country, it can be misleading. For instance, the crude death rate of Sweden might be higher than that of Haiti, despite longer life expectancy for each individual than in Haiti, because Sweden's population is older, on average, and thus each individual is more likely to die in any given year. In order to gain a true sense of the overall mor-

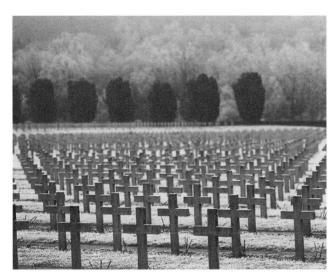

The death rate analyzes either the total number of deaths or the number of deaths due to a specific cause over a period of time.

tality picture, one must instead use an age-adjusted death rate, which compares two rates as if they were based on the same population, or a life table which tabulates life expectancies at every age.

In addition to the age profile of a nation, other factors that strongly influence the death rate are the rates of infant mortality (the number of deaths of children less than 1 year old/1,000 live births), child mortality, maternal mortality (the number of deaths due to childbearing/100,000 live births), overall nutritional standards, hygiene levels, access to medical care, access to safe drinking water, and overall levels of infectious disease.

SEE ALSO: Death and Dying.

BIBLIOGRAPHY. Economic and Social Commission for Western Asia, *Demographic and Related Socio-Economic Data Sheets for Member Countries of the Economic and Social Commission for Western Asia as Assessed in 2000* (United Nations Publications, 2002); Mary A. Freedman and James A. Weed, eds., *Vital Statistics of the United States: Mortality* (DIANE Publishing, 1999); Russell O. Wright, *Life and Death in the United States: Statistics on Life Expectancies, Diseases and Death Rates for the Twentieth Century* (McFarland, 1997).

ANNIE DUDE
UNIVERSITY OF CHICAGO

Degenerative Nerve Disease

Neurons are populations of cells which transmit information as electrical-chemical currents. Together, they form a network termed the nervous system which serves to coordinate activities such as movement with sensation and motivation. Neurons themselves are post-mitotic which means that they have lost their ability to divide and produce more neurons. In other words, once a neuron is damaged, surrounding neurons are unable to replace the lost neuron. This characteristic, in conjunction with the lack of a rigorous stem cell population within which to replace damaged neurons, makes the nervous system highly sensitive to environmental assaults.

Degenerative nerve disease is a pathological condition characterized by selective degeneration of groups of nerves. The general dogma that describes the progression of nerve degeneration begins with the accumulation of protein aggregates that are resistant to normal mechanisms of protein degradation. These proteins often have important functions in the non-diseased state. At high concentrations, however, they form insoluble sheets or aggregates which are toxic to the neuron within which they reside. In an unknown mechanism, these aggregates lead to the death of their host neuron. The disease state begins when gross neuronal death is detectable through functional deficit.

A major characteristic of degenerative nerve diseases is that they affect select groups of neurons, leading to selective loss of function. Thus, for convenience, degenerative nerve diseases will be grouped according to area or type of neuron afflicted.

DEGENERATIVE DISEASE OF THE CORTEX

Alzheimer's disease (AD) is a degenerative disease afflicting neurons of the cerebral cortex. Loss of cortical neurons initially manifests as impairment of higher cerebral function which progresses to severe memory loss with disorientation. The final outcome of AD involves the complete loss of higher cerebral function which at autopsy presents as massive cerebral atrophy. These symptoms do not usually manifest in patients before they reach the age of 50. With the aging population, AD has turned into the most common cause of dementia in the elderly.

AD is thought to be sporadic in causality although familial cases do exist. Currently, the accumulation of two major proteins has been implicated in leading to the development of AD: Aβ amyloid and tau protein. Aβ amyloid is an integral membrane protein which can be cleaved into two species, one of 40 amino acids in length, the other of 42. Although the method by which Aβ amyloid induces neuronal death is unknown, Aβ amyloid 40 is thought to be protective against AD induced by Aβ amyloid 42. Presenilin is a proteolytic enzyme responsible for cleaving and clearing Aβ amyloid protein. Thus, mutations in presenilin are often responsible for a patient's AD. Tau, on the other hand, is a protein normally associated with microtubules in axons of neurons, that serve to facilitate vesicular transport. In the disease state, tau is hyperphosphorylated, its accumulation leads to the formation cytoplasmic neurofibrillary tangles. Aggregates of these proteins in the cortex (frontal, parietal, and temporal lobes) leads to the development of neuritic plaques of twisted neural axons visible upon biopsy.

Because Aβ amyloid is coded for on chromosome 21, genetic predisposition to AD is associated with patients who suffer from Down Syndrome. Almost all patients with trisomy 21 and live into their 40s develop AD. Not only are they almost guaranteed to suffer from AD, because of increased production of Aβ amyloid, but symptoms of dementia also manifest earlier than patients with only two copies of the allele.

Allele E4 of ApoE has also been established to predispose individuals to AD. Located on chromosome 19, this gene codes for a product with high affinity for Aβ amyloid. Patients with ApoE-induced AD manifest symptoms later in life.

DEGENERATIVE DISEASE OF THE BASAL GANGLIA

Parkinsonian diseases (PD) are a collective group of chronic progressive diseases affecting dopaminergic pathways in the striatum. The striatum, which consists of the substantia nigra, caudate, putamen, globus pallidus, subthalamus, and thalamus, regulates voluntary muscle movement. As a result, symptoms of PD include involuntary tremors followed by periods of stiffness, as well as poor coordination and difficulty balancing. Dementia, depression, and visual-spatial impairment are also associated with PD.

Idiopathic Parkinson's disease is typically sporadic in origin, manifesting equally in men and women between the ages of 45–65. Biopsies reveal neurons of the substantia nigra (dopaminergic) and locus ceruleus (norepinephrine secreting) to be degenerated, filled with cytoplasmic, eosinophilic inclusions termed *Lewy bodies.* Lewy bodies are aggregates of damaged neurofilaments. Selective loss of dopaminergic neurons has directed the development of PD therapies to revolve around dopamine replacement. However, dopamine's suspected involvement with schizophrenia explains why many of these drugs produce schizoid side effects.

Other etiologies of damage to the substantia nigra include pesticides, ischemic injury, chronic carbon monoxide poisoning, Wilson's disease and encephalitis.

Huntington's disease (HD) is another common neural degenerative disease that affects the striatum. In particular, the caudate, putamen and globus pallidus are severely atrophied in HD, leading to symptoms such as chorea (involuntary dance-like rhythmic movements), muscle rigidity, and dementia. The long search for the protein responsible for this disease has come up with the Huntington gene, located on chromosome 4. Inherited in an autosomal-dominant manor, the Huntington gene consists of a cluster of trinucleotide repeats which increase in quantity with each successive generation, termed *genetic anticipation.* Interestingly, the number of repeats tends to stay the same on the allele inherited by the mother, while it increases on the allele inherited by the father.

The Huntington allele is considered mutant if it possesses more than 40 trinucleotide repeats because it is at this point that the protein becomes toxic to the neurons within which it resides. Although symptoms typically appear between the ages of 35–45 years, the more repeats that exist in the Huntington gene, the earlier the disease manifests.

DEGENERATIVE DISEASE OF THE SPINAL CORD

Lou Gehrig's disease, also known as amyelotrophic lateral sclerosis, is a degenerative disease that involves upper and lower motor neurons. Although most cases are sporadic, genetic predisposition has been associated to mutations in the superoxide dismutase I gene (chromosome 21). Symptoms of both upper motor neuron (positive Babinski sign, spastic reflexes) and lower motor neuron (muscle weakness and atrophy) damage appear usually between 40–60 years of age.

Although the above-mentioned diseases are the most common types of degenerative nerve disease, many more afflict our nervous system. Because our nervous system is so sensitive to environmental assaults, much effort in the scientific community is dedicated toward developing therapies including either reviving endogenous stem cells to replace damaged tissue or implanting neural progenitors that have been cultured from stem cells.

SEE ALSO: Alzheimer's Disease; Downs Syndrome; Huntington's Disease; Parkinson's Disease.

BIBLIOGRAPHY. Y. Furukawa, et al., "Disulfide Cross-Linked Protein Represents a Significant Fraction of ALS-Associated Cu, Zn-superoxide Dismutase Aggregates in Spinal Cords of Model Mice," *Proceedings of the National Academy of Sciences.* (v.103/18, 2006); K. Kieburtz, et al., "Trinucleotide Repeat Length and Progression of Illness in Huntington's Disease," *Journal of Medical Genetics* (v.31, 1994); Mark Rapoport, et al., "Tau is Essential to Beta-Amyloid-Induced Neurotoxicity," *Proceedings of the National Academy of Sciences* (v.99/9, 2002); Dun-Sheng Yang, et al., "Examining the Zinc Binding Site of Amyloid-β Protein," *European Journal of Biochemistry* (v.267, 2000).

KIMBERLY GOKOFFSKI
UNIVERSITY OF CALIFORNIA, IRVINE

Dementia

Dementia is a progressive loss of cerebral function which may result in a generalized disturbance in function. It is common in the developed world and its prevalence is increasing as the age of population is increasing. It involves more than one area of cerebral function, for example, memory, language, and judgment, and may result in severe dysfunction of daily life.

The prevalence of dementia is approximately 6 percent in those over 65 years and 30 percent of people aged over 90 years. Dementia is rare before the age of 60. Symptoms of dementia include loss of memory,

personality changes, and loss of executive function such as the ability to make decisions.

There are several diseases that cause dementia. The most common cause is Alzheimer's disease (AD); it accounts for 30 to 50 percent of dementia. AD is characterized early on by neuropathological changes, primarily in the hippocampus. It is stated that AD pathology is more likely to be clinically expressed as dementia in women than in men. AD is a neurodegenerative disease with histopathological features such as loss of synapses and cells and presence of amyloid plaques and neurofibrillary tangles (NFTs). NFTs are pathological protein aggregates in neurons; they are associated with the microtubule associated protein tau in the cerebral cortex particularly in the temporal lobe. The presence of NFTs may contribute to the cognitive decline such as impairment in language (aphasia), skilled movements (apraxia), and recognition (agnosia). Other symptoms of AD include loss of memory and deterioration of musculature and mobility leading to unsteady gait. AD patients generally have reduced acetylcholine activity, high concentrations of homocysteine, and folate deficiency leading to increased risk of dementia and cognitive decline. Higher plasma vitamin B-12 may reduce the risk of homocysteine-associated dementia.

Factors known to increase risk of the AD include mutations in the amyloid precursor gene and the apolipoprotein E (apoE) genotype. The apoE gene has three alleles called ε2, ε3, and ε4. The ε4 allele (chromosome 19) accelerates the age of onset of familial AD and increases the risk of developing late-onset "sporadic" AD. Its presence has been associated with an increase in β-amyloid protein (Aβ) senile plaques and neuritic plaques. ApoE in the normal brain is involved in the transport of cholesterol, redistributing lipids among CNS cells for normal lipid homeostasis, repairing injured neurons, maintaining synapto-dendritic connections, and scavenging toxins. ε4 binds to Aβ; this interaction prevents toxic aggregation of Aβ. This property is lost in AD, thus leading to Aβ accumulation and resulting plaque formation. ε4 is also associated with small vessel arteriolosclerosis and microinfarcts of the deep nuclei perhaps as a result of the plaque accumulation. Aβ protein is produced from proteolytic cleavages (using β and γ secretases) of amyloid precursor protein (APP). Aβ accumulates in the brain cortex and hippocampus of patients with AD and self-aggregates to form toxic oligomers causing neurodegeneration

Another risk factor for AD is mutations in the presenilin gene. Presenilin mutations are the main cause of familial disease. These mutations seem to result in a gain of toxic function, and a partial loss of function in the gamma-secretase complex, which affects several downstream signaling pathways. The loss of function of presenilin causes incomplete digestion of the Aβ and might contribute to an increased vulnerability of the brain, thereby explaining the early onset of the inherited form of AD. Other risk factors of AD include head injury, Down syndrome, lower premorbid intellect, and proneness to psychological distress; chronic stress is associated with hippocampal damage and impaired memory in humans.

AD is a devastating disorder for which there is no cure or effective treatment; however, various pharmacological treatments are currently employed. AD generally has a poor prognosis with a median life expectancy after diagnosis of five to six years.

The second most common cause of dementia is vascular dementias which are a group of syndromes relating to cardiovascular risk factors such as smoking, arteriosclerosis, hypertension, and diabetes. The disease occurs as a result of large hemispheral infarcts and is also associated with widespread small ischemic or vascular lesions (microinfarcts, lacunes) throughout the central nervous system with predominant subcortical lesions in the basal ganglia and white matter or in regions such as the thalamus and hippocampus. Patients who have had a stroke are at increased risk for vascular dementia. Patients often have impaired memory and altered behaviors; other signs depend on infarction distribution.

Another cause of dementia is Lewy body disease, characterized by the presence of structures called Lewy bodies which are round deposits that contain damaged nerve cells. These Lewy body proteins are found in an area of the brain stem where they deplete the neurotransmitter dopamine, causing Parkinsonian symptoms. The brain chemical acetylcholine is also depleted, causing disruption of perception, thinking, and behavior; patients also have visual hallucinations and instability. Prognosis is fairly poor, as most patients survive for about six years after diagnosis.

Rare causes of dementia include frontotemporal dementia, alcohol related, HIV infection, syphilis, subdural hematoma, and some forms of cerebral tumors. People with multiple sclerosis, motor neuron disease, Parkinson's disease, and Huntington's disease may also be more likely to develop dementia. Dementia is associated with poor prognosis in patients; most patients eventually need continuous help with everyday activities. Dementia is an important public health problem with devastating consequences for the patient and an increased burden on families.

SEE ALSO: Alzheimer's Disease; Parkinson's Disease.

BIBLIOGRAPHY. E. Ifeachor, et al., "Biopattern Analysis and Subject-Specific Diagnosis and Care of Dementia," *Proceedings of the 27th Annual International Conference of the IEEE EMBS*, Shanghai, China, September 1–4, 1005.

FARHANA AKTER
KING'S COLLEGE LONDON

Demographic Transition

Demographic transition is a term coined by F. W. Notestien in 1945 to describe the changes that occur in a population as it moves from a premodern to a modern society, or from a developing to an industrialized economy. Developing countries are characterized by a population in which there are high birth rates and high death rates. The age structure of the population is pyramidal and there are far more children than elderly. In the first stage of the demographic transition, as per capita income rises, death rates fall due to factors that may include improved hygiene, nutrition, and healthcare. Birth rates (fertility rates) remain high and there is rapid population growth. After some time, birth rates begin to decline as families decrease the number of children they wish to have. They invest more resources into fewer children and realize that most children will survive to adulthood. A new stable population state is eventually reached in which both birth and death rates are relatively low, and the age structure of the population is rectangular.

The epidemiologic transition that generally accompanies and contributes to the demographic transition involves a change in the patterns of health and disease in a population. Developing countries generally have high infant, child, and maternal mortality rates. In these countries, acute and infectious diseases such as pneumonia, tuberculosis, and meningitis are common causes of death. In industrial countries, infant, child, and maternal mortality tend to be relatively low, and cancer, heart disease, and stroke are the most common causes of death. These insidious and chronic diseases are often related to risk factors such as diet, smoking, and sedentary lifestyle. Cancers are a common cause of death in pre- and posttransition populations; however, the types of cancer vary. In developing countries, cancers are primarily those caused by microorganisms—liver, cervical, stomach, and nasopharyngeal neoplasms. However, cancers of the developed world—lung, colon, and breast—may be related to the risk factors previously mentioned. Deaths from motor vehicle accidents generally increase during the early transition period as there are more motorized vehicles in operation, and decrease in the posttransition period as laws and technology improve the safety of vehicle operation.

There is a great deal of variability in how each country and/or population experiences the demographic and epidemiologic transitions based on political and social structure, and resources. There is also great debate as to whether economic growth or other social or external factors are primarily responsible for these changes. Emerging diseases, social upheaval, and other dramatic events can interrupt or reverse the transition processes. For example, the HIV epidemic and wars have stalled reductions in mortality in sub-Saharan Africa. Similarly, massive social and healthcare system disruption have moved countries of the former Soviet Union back into a state in which vaccine-preventable and infectious diseases are a significant cause of morbidity and mortality. The concepts of demographic and epidemiologic transition are critical to understanding the health needs and the determinants of health of a population. They are also useful in designing health interventions and for health infrastructure, human resource, and social infrastructure planning.

SEE ALSO: Third World.

BIBLIOGRAPHY. P. F. Basch, *Textbook of International Health*, 2nd ed. (Oxford University Press, 1999); T. Kue Young, *Population Health* (Oxford University Press, 2005).

BARRY PAKES, M.D., M.P.H.
UNIVERSITY OF TORONTO

Dengue

Dengue is a mosquito-borne viral infection of mostly tropical and subtropical urban and semiurban areas that causes fever. In the last half of the 20th century, incidence increased 50-fold. Dengue is endemic in over 100 countries although southeast Asia and the west Pacific are most severely affected. Two-fifths of the world's population, including over 1 billion children, are exposed to the female *Aedes* mosquitoes that transmit the virus. There are approximately 50 million infections a year with 1 percent of infections developing into the potentially lethal dengue hemorrhagic fever (DHF). DHF has a global mortality rate of 5 percent. There is no treatment or vaccine for dengue, although with appropriate supportive therapy, mortality can be reduced to less than 1 percent. Although clearing an infection results in immunity against a particular serotype, there is only partial, transient cross-protection and an individual can be infected with another serotype. Sequential infection increases the probability of developing DHF.

HISTORY

The first reported cases and epidemics of dengue occurred in the 1600s. Dengue was initially considered a mild, nonfatal travelers' disease. By 1845, global pandemics arose and continue today. During the 20th century, distribution and density of *Aedes* mosquitoes expanded because of human travel and trade. Rapid rise in urban population and unplanned urbanization led to inadequate solid waste disposal and unhygienic water storage, creating mosquito-breeding grounds. While eradication efforts began in the mid-1900s, they were discontinued, and reinfestation of *Aedes* mosquitoes occurred in larger distribution and density than previously. By 2005, dengue had a global distribution comparable to malaria.

TRANSMISSION AND VIROLOGY

The most common vector is the *Aedes aegypti* mosquito, which has global distribution, though *Aedes albopictus*, found in Africa, the Americas, and Europe, is also a vector. *Aegypti* is a daytime feeder that prefers humans and lays eggs preferentially in artificial containers such as used tires and water storage drums. Female *Aedes* mosquitoes acquire the virus by feeding on an infected human and shed the virus during subsequent feeding.

The dengue virus, a flavivirus, is the most widespread arthropod-borne virus, or arbovirus. Other mosquito-borne flavivirus infections include yellow fever and West Nile disease. All four dengue serotypes have a global distribution. There is a weeklong incubation period in mosquitoes prior to infectivity. For a week after a human is infected, the virus silently replicates in organs such as the thymus and then infects white blood cells. Viremia is detectable for approximately five days. Mosquitoes acquire the virus during this time. Illness will develop about two days after onset of viremia and continue for about a week. Dengue infection during pregnancy does not cause any congenital malformations. Dengue virus cannot be transmitted between humans. Dengue infections peak in winter.

SYMPTOMS, DIAGNOSIS, AND TREATMENT

Presentation is age dependent, with children experiencing a milder infection. The three categories of dengue fever, in increasing severity, are fever, dengue fever, and DHF. Fever is the most common presentation. Dengue fever also presents with headache, muscle and joint pain, nausea, vomiting, and rash. Weakness, malaise, and anorexia may persist for several weeks. Rarely, patients experience hemorrhagic manifestations including ruptured capillaries, bruising, and bleeding of gums and nose. DHF affects mostly children and is characterized by fever, hemorrhagic manifestations, low platelet count, and objective evidence of "leaky capillaries," such as an elevated hematocrit or effusions. Without treatment, more than one in five patients dies. Fever in DHF patients can be as high as 41 degrees C (106 degrees F). The most severe form of DHF is dengue shock syndrome. After three to six days of fever, there is an abrupt temperature change, signs of circulatory failure, hypotensive shock and death within 12 to 24 hours.

Blood and urine tests showing elevated hematocrit, low albumin, or microscopic blood in urine are signs of dengue. Travel history can be important in diagnosis. Intensive supportive therapy focuses on maintaining circulating fluid volume. Treatment also includes rest, mosquito barriers, and fever and pain relief. Hospitalization is required when severe hemorrhagic manifestations or shock are present.

PREVENTION AND CONTROL

Because eradication is believed unattainable, efforts concentrate on controlling mosquito populations. Environmental management includes adequate solid waste disposal and improved water storage. Chemical management focuses on applying insecticides to larval habitats periodically. Insecticide spraying to kill adult mosquitoes has transient and variable effect because insecticide may not penetrate indoor habitats. *Aedes* mosquitoes are resistant to organochloride sprays and ultralow-volume fumigation is ineffective. Active surveillance of mosquito populations, habitats, and susceptibility is essential to prevention of dengue.

SEE ALSO: Hemorrhagic Fever; Infectious Diseases (General); Medical Entomology; Mosquito Bites; Viral Infections; Virology.

BIBLIOGRAPHY. Centers for Disease Control Division of Vector-Borne Infectious Diseases (CDC-DVBID), "Dengue Fever Publications," http://www.cdc.gov/ncidod/dvbid/pubs/dengue-pubs.htm (cited January 2007); World Health Organization (WHO), "WHO: Dengue," http://www.who.int/topics/dengue (cited January 2007).

RISHI RATTAN
UNIVERSITY OF ILLINOIS–CHICAGO

Denmark

With a per capita income of $34,800, Denmark is the 13th richest country in the world with a high standard of living and a strong safety net for the population. Danes are financially protected against illness, unemployment, and aging. Benefits in Denmark are not totally dependent on earlier employment, and programs are financed by taxes and duties. The government subsidizes housing and child-related expenses. Specific services involve health services, day care, and home help. The United Nations Development Programme (UNDP) Human Development Reports rank Denmark 15th among nations of the world in overall quality of life issues. Unemployment stands at 5.7 percent. There is virtually no poverty in Denmark, but 12 percent of females and 11 percent of males earn less than 60 percent of the median income. Primary and secondary schooling are available to all students, and enrollment is over 100 percent.

In the post–World War II era, the Danish government updated existing programs and created new ones as Denmark became a social welfare state. For instance, the National Pensions and Disablement Plan of 1957 guaranteed pensions to all citizens. Amendments in 1964 required workers to pay into the Supplementary Pension Fund. Compulsory health insurance was introduced in 1973, guaranteeing cash subsidies for Danish workers who become ill. Three years later, the Social Assistance Act was passed, enacting fixed rates for recipients.

The government is concerned with the well-being of the population, and families receive a good deal of protection in Denmark. All females are eligible for maternity leave for four weeks before and 14 weeks after birth. Fathers may take up to two weeks leave during the 14-week period, and 10 weeks leave may be shared between both parents. The new parents receive a per diem allotment, which may amount to full salary. Family allowances are given to all families with children under the age of 18, and payments are increased for single-parent families.

In 2002, the "Healthy throughout Life" plan announced that 11 ministries were working together to increase life expectancy, minimize inequalities in health, and improve the overall quality of health among the population. Target areas included smoking and obesity, and the government expressed continued commitment to reducing incidences of cancer, osteoporosis, and chronic obstructive pulmonary disease.

The Danish government spends one percent of the total budget on healthcare. Nine percent of the Gross Domestic Product (GDP) is spent on healthcare at a rate of $2,762 (international dollars) per capita. Some 83 percent of total health expenditures are provided by government funding. Private sector expenses account for 17 percent of total spending, and 92.50 percent of that amount involves out-of-pocket expenses. There are 2.93 physicians, 10.36 nurses, 0.22 midwives, 0.83 dentists, and 0.49 pharmacists per 1,000 population in Denmark.

The population of 5,450,000 experiences a life expectancy of 77.79 years, and women outlive men an average of five years. Only one percent of the population over the age of 15 is unable to read and write. The entire population has access to safe drinking water and improved sanitation. Birth control is practiced by 78 percent of female Danes, and women give birth to an average of 1.74 children each. All births are attended by skilled attendants. The adjusted maternal mortality rate of five deaths per 100,000 live births is one of the lowest in the world.

Denmark has the 17th lowest infant mortality rate in the world at 4.51 deaths per 1,000 live births. Between 1990 and 2004, infant mortality was cut in half, dropping from eight to four deaths per 1,000 live births. During that same period, under-five mortality decreased from nine to five deaths per 1,000 live births. Five percent of all infants are underweight at birth. Immunization rates are predictably high, and 96 percent of infants are vaccinated against measles. Immunization rates for diphtheria, pertussis, and tetanus (DPT1 and DPT3), polio, and *Haemophilus influenzae* type B are reported at 95 percent.

Denmark is highly industrialized, and air pollution from vehicle and power plants poses a major health threat. The North Sea has been polluted with nitrogen and phosphorus, and drinking and surface water sources are threatened by animal wastes and pesticides. The adult prevalence rate of HIV/AIDS is 0.2 percent in Denmark. While 5,000 people are living with the disease, less than 100 have died from HIV/AIDS or its complications. Meningococcal disease surfaced in Denmark in 2001, and influenza outbreaks occurred in 2003 and 2004.

SEE ALSO: Cancer (General); Chronic Obstructive Pulmonary Disease (COPD); Osteoporosis.

BIBLIOGRAPHY. Spencer Di Scala, *Twentieth Century Europe: Politics, Society, Culture* (Boston: McGraw-Hill, 2004); Sandra Halperin, *War and Social Change in Modern Europe: The Great Transformation Revisited* (New York: Cambridge University Press, 2004); Martin A. Levin and Martin Shapiro, editors, *Transatlantic Policymaking in an Age of Austerity: Diversity and Drift* (Washington, D.C.: Georgetown University Press, 2004).

ELIZABETH R. PURDY, PH.D.
INDEPENDENT SCHOLAR

Dental Health

Dental health emcompasses care of the teeth, jaws, soft structures of tongue, lips and oral mucosa (the soft pink covering inside the mouth). Teeth are made up of four types of tissue—enamel, dentin, pulp and cementum. Enamel covers the visible part of the tooth; it is the hardest body substance and does not regrow or repair itself when damages. The dentin is the calcified tooth core surrounding the pulp, made up of connective tissue, blood supply and nerves. Dentin continues to grow in healthy teeth. Cementum covers the root of the tooth and is made up of connective tissue to assist in anchoring the tooth to the jaw and cushion the impact of chewing.

For optimal dental health, individuals should brush not only their teeth, but all soft surfaces of the mouth and tongue. Flossing between the teeth, wearing a mouthguard for sports, maintaining good nutrition are also instrumental in dental health. In addition to home care, the dental health team will keep teeth healthy and treat pain or injuries. The professional team may include a dental hygienist, a general dentist and a variety of specialists as needed.

DENTAL PROBLEMS

Tooth decay. Dental cavities consist of decay caused by infectious bacteria—the most common being *Streptococcus mutans*. The bacteria feeds on sugars in foods and produces acids that can dissolve the enamel. The bacteria can also form plaque that sticks to teeth and dental work. Cavities are holes resulting from the disease from destruction of enamel and penetration into the dentin. Prevention includes removal of food particles by brushing and flossing, and routine dental visits for cleaning and removal of plaque and tartar. Treatment for lesions that haven't formed cavities include using fluorides and sealants to help maintain the enamel. If a cavity has formed, restoration includes fillings or crowns. When the decay has reached the pulp a root canal will be performed

Malocclusion. Biting (occlusion) is how teeth come together. Bite problems include teeth spacing, position of teeth, and protruding or recessing teeth. To repair these issues, an orthodontist will create braces or brackets to apply pressure to teeth (one tooth or a group) to move the teeth into alignment by reshaping the bone growth to hold the root. The process takes less time in children. In more severe cases of malocclusion, oral surgery may be necessary.

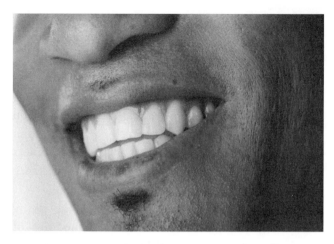

Enamel covers the visible part of teeth; it is the hardest substance in the human body and does not regrow or repair damage.

Periodontal disease. A group of diseases of the hard and soft tissue supporting structures. Bacteria found in the crevices of the gum causes infections related to the disease. Gingivitis is the first stage, and causes gums to become red, swollen, and bleed easily. In its early stages, gingivitis can be eliminated by brushing and flossing daily to remove plaque. Left untreated, gingivitis can progress to periodontitis, when bacteria attack the bone and tissue supporting the teeth. Inflammation of the bone and hard tissue is called periodontitis; if the bone dissolves, the teeth could loosen or fall out. Treatment includes cleansing (with scaling or root planing) to remove plaque and tarter on the tooth and below the gumline, and surgery to clean the roots or for restoration (reducing pocket depth, gum grafts, bone grafts).

Tooth grinding (bruxism) is the grinding and clenching of the teeth. Symptoms might include abnormal tooth wear or damage, gum inflammation, pain while chewing, infection and temperomandibular disorders (TMJ with limited jaw opening and muscle tenderness in the jaw area). Treatment depends on underlying cause and might include stress reduction, medication, or oral devices to prevent grinding, and in the case of severe damage, surgery might be required.

Wisdom teeth are the third molars. In some they occur in the mouth properly with ample room. In others, the third molar may not come through the surface of the gum, cause cysts or crowd other teeth, and surgical removal may be necessary.

In the event of tooth loss from an accident or progression of periodontal disease, false teeth (dentures or implants) must be fabricated to enable chewing.

Prosthodontists specialize in creating and inserting prosthodontics (dentures, tooth implants, and other types of artificial dental structures such as crowns or bridges).

Cosmetic Dentistry seeks to improve the appearance of the teeth and includes stain removal using bleaching, laser or light therapy, reshaping the teeth and gums, bonding (applying resin to a tooth to increase the length of the tooth, or to fill a gap) and applying veneers to the surface of the tooth.

SEE ALSO: Mouth disorders; Oral Surgeon.

BIBLIOGRAPHY. Robert K. Jackler, MD and Michael J. Kaplan MD, "Ear, Nose & Throat" *Current Medical Diagnosis and Treatment* (Lange Medical Books, 2004); Sadie S. Mestman, D.M.D. and Ariella D. Herman Ph.D. *What to do for Healthy Teeth* (Institute for Healthcare Advancement, 2004); Rebecca W. Smith and Faculty of the Columbia University School of Dental and Oral Surgery, *Columbia University School of Dental and Oral Surgery Guide to Family Dental Care* (W.W. Norton & Co, 1997);

LYN MICHAUD
INDEPENDENT SCHOLAR

Department of Energy (DOE)

The origins of the Department of Energy (DOE) can be traced to the Manhattan Project and the race to develop the atomic bomb during World War II. In 1942, the U.S. Army Corps of Engineers established the Manhattan Engineer District to manage the project. Following the war, the Atomic Energy Act of 1946 created the Atomic Energy Commission, which took over the Manhattan Engineer District's sprawling scientific and industrial complex. In response to changing needs in the mid-1970s, the Atomic Energy Commission was abolished and the Energy Reorganization Act of 1974 created two new agencies: the Nuclear Regulatory Commission to regulate the nuclear power industry and the Energy Research and Development Administration to manage the nuclear weapon, naval reactor, and energy development programs. However, the extended energy crisis of the 1970s soon demonstrated the need for unified energy organization and planning. The Department of Energy Organization Act brought the federal government's agencies and programs into a single agency. The DOE, activated on October 1, 1977, assumed the responsibilities of the Federal Energy Administration, the Energy Research and Development Administration, the Federal Power Commission, and parts and programs of several other agencies. The Department provided the framework for a comprehensive and balanced national energy plan by coordinating and administering the energy functions of the federal government. The Department undertook responsibility for long-term, high-risk research and development of energy technology, federal power marketing, energy conservation, the nuclear weapons program, energy regulatory programs, and a central energy data collection and analysis program.

Over its two-decade history, the Department has shifted its emphasis and focus as the needs of the nation have changed. During the late 1970s, the Department emphasized energy development and regulation. In the 1980s, nuclear weapons research, development, and production took a priority. Since the end of the Cold War, the Department has focused on environmental cleanup of the nuclear weapons complex, nonproliferation and stewardship of the nuclear stockpile, energy efficiency and conservation, and technology transfer and industrial competitiveness. In the 21st century, the DOE contributes to the future of the nation by ensuring energy security, maintaining the safety and reliability of nuclear stockpile, cleaning up the environment from the legacy of the Cold War, and developing innovations in science and technology.

Included under the DOE are a number of organizations dedicated to health and safety issues as they relate to energy sources and patterns of consumption. In 1989, the DOE created the Office of Environmental Management (EM) to mitigate the risks and hazards posed by the legacy of nuclear weapons production and research. Although the nation continues to maintain an arsenal of nuclear weapons, as well as some production capability, the United States has embarked on new missions. The most ambitious and far ranging of these missions is dealing with the environmental legacy of the Cold War. Like most industrial and manufacturing operations, the nuclear complex has generated waste, pollution, and contamination. However, many problems posed by its operations are unique. They include unprecedented amounts of contaminated waste, water, and soil, and a vast number of contaminated structures that will remain radioactive for thousands of years. Similarly, the Office of Civilian Radioactive Waste Management (OCRWM) is a program of the DOE assigned to develop and manage a federal system for disposing of spent nuclear fuel from commercial reactors and high-level radioactive waste from activities related to national defense.

The Office of Health and Safety and Security (HSS) focuses on maintaining and improving worker health and safety policies and assisting line management in interpreting policies and implementing worker health and safety programs. This office addresses Department-wide safety issues that impact multiple DOE sites and that would benefit from a Department-wide approach to resolution. The HSS has four subordinate offices. One office focuses on worker safety and health policy development, maintenance, and interpretation. A second office focuses on technical assistance and issues management, and will be the focal point for interface with the line management program offices, field elements, and stakeholders. The third office manages studies that evaluate domestic health effects to include health surveillance, screening, and studies. Domestic health studies, surveillance, and screening examine current and former worker health and health effects and ensure this information is used to protect workers and the public and to continuously improve worker health and safety policies. This office also supports the Department of Labor in the implementation of the Energy Employees Occupational Illness Compensation Program Act (EEOICPA). The fourth office examines the effects on populations from U.S. nuclear weapons testing or accidents and operations involving radiological materials and other international health studies. These offices work together with a major focus on helping the program offices and field elements solve problems and improve safety programs and performance. The combination of these functions into a single office with a primary mission of worker health and safety policy and technical assistance enables the HSS to focus on helping the program offices and field elements to solve the highest priority health and safety issues and to direct DOE support

resources to where they are most needed. The HSS maintains a program designed to assess the health impacts of Energy operations on employees exposed to airborne concentrations of beryllium. Energy facilitates the initiation of an integrated interagency CBD research agenda leading to improved diagnosis, prognosis, and treatment of this disease. Energy departmental elements responsible for protection and control measures for current workers, compensation for individuals who have developed CBD, and CBD research, work closely with other agencies conducting related activities.

The DOE is committed to safe operation of its nuclear facilities and activities. The Department's Office of Nuclear and Facility Safety Policy establishes nuclear safety requirements and associated guidance for nuclear facilities and activities through a combination of public rules and DOE directives. The DOE also works with nongovernmental organizations to develop standards that can be used to maintain and enhance the safety of America's facilities and activities. The Department's overall goal in relation to its nuclear safety enforcement is to improve nuclear safety performance throughout the Department's programs, sites, and contractors. Additional statutory responsibilities include enforcement of the Worker Safety and Health Program in the same manner that the nuclear safety rules are enforced.

One of the desired outcomes of this program is to promote proactive behavior on the part of contractors with the overall goal, remaining the improvement of nuclear safety performance.

SEE ALSO: Environmental Protection Agency (EPA).

BIBLIOGRAPHY. United States Department of Energy, www.energy.gov (cited October, 2006); United States Department of Energy, *Department of Energy 1977–1994: A Summary History* (Office of Human Resources and Administration, Executive Secretariat, 1994); United States Department of Energy, *Report No. 11—Department of Energy Environment, Safety, and Health Initiatives Related to Nuclear Safety* (U.S. Department of Energy Internal Working Group, Office of Environment, Safety, & Health, 1995); United States Environmental Protection Agency, *Setting Priorities, Getting Results: A New Direction for the Environmental Protection Agency.* Report to Congress (National Academy of Public Administration, 1995); United States

Office of Technology Assessment, *Hazards Ahead: Managing Cleanup Worker Safety and Health at the Nuclear Weapons Complex* (U.S. Office of Technology, 1993).

BEN WYNNE, PH.D
GAINESVILLE STATE COLLEGE

Department of Health and Human Services (HHS)

The United States Department of Health and Human Services (DHHS) is the umbrella organization for a number of government agencies that deliver social services to Americans, especially to the most vulnerable segments of the population. The roots of HHS can be traced to the creation of the Cabinet-level Department of Health, Education, and Welfare (HEW) in 1953 under President Dwight D. Eisenhower. In 1979, under President Jimmy Carter, the Department of Education assumed Cabinet status, and the Department of HEW was transformed into the Department of Health and Human Services. The Secretary of Health and Human Services is responsible for overseeing implementation of more than 300 programs that deal with issues such as health and social science research, disease prevention, food and drug safety, health coverage for and financial assistance to the elderly, disabled, and economically disadvantaged, infant health, preschool education and services, faith-based community initiatives, child abuse, domestic violence, home care and nursing home care, health services for Native Americans and Native Alaskans, and medical and emergency preparedness.

Operating under a budget of $698 billion (fiscal year 2007), HHS receives 25 percent of national government outlays; and through the Medicare and Medicaid programs alone, HHS affects the lives of a fourth of the population. Data collected through HHS are a major determinant in policy and budget decisions at all levels of government. In addition to functions carried out by eight public health service agencies, three human service agencies, and 11 operating divisions, HHS funds services administered by state, local, and county governments and by private sector grantees. HHS public health services agencies include the National Institutes of Health, which is the nation's chief medical research organization; the Food and Drug Administration, which oversees the safety and reliability of foods, drugs, and cosmetics; the Centers for Disease Control and Prevention, which protects public health through prevention and control of diseases, injuries, and disabilities and oversees the Agency for Toxic Substances and Disease Registry; the Indian Health Service, which provides services to America's Native Indian and Alaskan populations; Health Resources and Services Administration, which extends healthcare services to low-income, uninsured, or geographically isolated populations; Substance Abuse and Mental Health Services Administration, which works with states to provide treatment and counseling for the target population; and the Agency for Healthcare Research and Quality, which conducts research on U.S. healthcare systems, the quality and costs of healthcare, access to healthcare, and the effectiveness of medical treatments.

Other programs that come under the HHS umbrella include the Centers for Medicare and Medicaid Services, which also bears responsibility for the State Children's Health Insurance Program (SCHIP); the Administration for Children and Families, which administers the welfare and Temporary Assistance for Needy Families programs; the Administration on Aging, which provides essential senior services such as home-delivered meals and transportation; and the U.S. Public Health Service Commissioned Corps, which consists of some 6,000 health professionals under the leadership of the Surgeon General. HHS departments include the Office of Public Health and Science, the Office of the HHS Inspector General, and the HHS Office for Civil Rights.

HHS national headquarters is located in the Hubert H. Humphrey Building at 200 Independence Avenue, SW, Washington, D.C. 20201. A number of other HHS agencies are headquartered at various locations around the capital. In addition to the Washington offices, HHS maintains facilities for the National Institutes of Health in Bethesda, Maryland, and several thousand employees are employed by various HHS agencies located in the Parklawn Building in Rockville, Maryland. The Centers for Disease Control and Prevention and the Agency for Toxic Substances and Disease Registry are housed in Atlanta, Georgia.

HHS has established a number of major goals. These priorities include providing consumers with

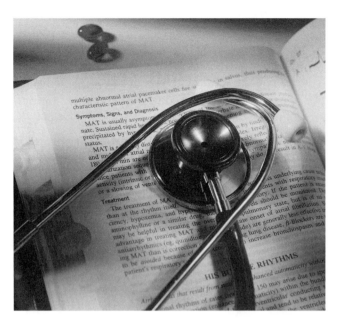

The United States Department of Health and Human Services is the umbrella organization for agencies that deliver social services.

BIBLIOGRAPHY. Russell L. Ackoff and Sheldon Rovin, *Redesigning Society* (Stanford University Press, 2003); Pascale Carayon, *Handbook of Human Factors and Ergonomics in Health Care and Patient Safety* (Lawrence Erlbaum, 2007); Department of Health and Human Services, http://www.hhs.gov/; Jerry V. Diller, *Cultural Diversity: A Primer for the Human Services* (Thomson Brooks/Cole, 2007); "Editorial: Family Planning Farce," *New York Times Online* (November 24, 2006); Sar A. Levitan, et al., *Programs in Aid of the Poor* (Johns Hopkins University Press, 2003); Kenneth J. Meier and Laurence J. O'Toole Jr., *Bureaucracy in a Democratic State: A Government Perspective* (Johns Hopkins University Press, 2006); Dennis D. Riley, et al., *Bureaucracy and the Policy Process: Keeping the Promises* (Rowman & Littlefield, 2006); Gregory L. Weiss, *Grassroots Medicine: The Story of America's Free Clinics* (Rowman & Littlefield, 2006).

ELIZABETH R. PURDY, PH.D.
INDEPENDENT SCHOLAR

the tools that allow them to make informed healthcare decisions; protecting healthcare records while providing patients and medical personnel with easy access to accurate healthcare information; facilitating prescription drug coverage for elderly Americans; providing assistance in revitalizing the New Orleans health system in the aftermath of Hurricane Katrina; personalizing healthcare in the United States; establishing prevention as a major factor in promoting public health; enhancing pandemic preparedness; and instituting emergency response and commissioned corps renewal.

Despite the HHS pledge to deliver quality health and human services to *all* Americans, critics of the George W. Bush administration have expressed grave concern over HHS's ability to serve the interests of women since the recent appointment of antiabortionist Dr. Eric Keroack to head family planning programs at HHS. Keroack is opposed to birth control, and his views on reproductive health are far from mainstream. This controversial appointment gave Keroack responsibility for financial decisions concerning the provision of healthcare to poor women in the areas of birth control, pregnancy tests, and breast care screening.

SEE ALSO: Centers for Disease Control and Prevention (CDC); National Institute of Health (NIH).

Depression

Depression is the general name for a set of diseases within the group of the mood disorders with different levels of impact. They include major depression disorder or episode, dysthymia, drug-induced depression, depression induced by a general medical condition, and depressive disorder not otherwise specified. Depressive disorders affect millions of people worldwide and major depression, the most serious of them, can be extremely incapacitating for daily activities or even lead to suicide. Depression is currently the first cause of disability in North America and it may become the second leading cause of disability worldwide by 2020. Depressive disorders affect people in all age groups.

Depressive disorders are characterized by sadness or anhedonia, a severe loss of interest or pleasures in usual activities, as well as the presence of other symptoms. Diagnosis is made based on medical history, because there are no specific tests for these disorders. While prognosis and treatment vary from disorder to disorder, options may include drug therapy, psychotherapy, and electroconvulsive therapy for some cases. Combinations of these are often used.

It is important to clarify that depression as used in common language to describe low mood or sadness that arises from disappointments or losses do not fit a medical diagnosis and better terms to describe such feelings are either sadness or demoralization. Bereavement may cause all symptoms of a major depressive disorder, but this is considered a normal, self-limited situation unless it is sustained for more than two months after the loss.

HISTORY

Depressive disorders have called attention of people since ancient times. The papyrus of Ebers contains perhaps one of the earliest descriptions of clinical depression and the symptoms leading to the suicide of the Greek hero Ajax, described in Homer's *Iliad*, is such a good depiction of a depressive disorder that it must have been based on real observations. Depression may also trace its roots to melancholia, a term used in ancient medicine to describe a predominance of black bile, one of the "four humors" postulated by Galen. The theory of the four humors postulated that there was need for equilibrium between those humors in the human body, and the excess of one of them would cause disease. When the black bile (*melancholia* in Greek) predominated, symptoms compatible with modern depression disorders arose. It is interesting to note that the modern theory of depressive disorders somehow resembles the idea of unbalanced humors: depression started to be explained by observations in the 1950s that drug-induced changes on neurotransmitter levels affected depressive symptoms, prompting the conclusion that depression was caused by an imbalance in the levels of neurotransmitters, still considered the pathophysiological basis of depressive disorders.

PREVALENCE

About 16 percent of the world population is affected by a form of depression on at least one occasion in their lives and the mean age of onset is in the late 20s. Some countries report a considerably higher incidence of depression, such as Australia, where the incidence of depression in women can reach 25 percent.

Women appear to be at a higher risk for depression, but this is decreasing and there seems to be no gender difference in the elderly. One important point is that there may be an underestimation of the incidence of depression in men; due to cultural factors, men are less likely to complain of depressive symptoms and even less likely to seek and accept treatment for depression.

ETIOLOGY

Apart from depression induced by drugs or a general medical condition, the etiology of depression is unknown. Depression is more common in first-degree relatives of depressed patients than in the general population, and concordance between twins is high, which suggests a role of genetics. A genetic tendency for depressive disorders may be triggered, though, by deep or prolonged stress. Major life-stressing episodes, such as separations and losses, may cause depressive disorders but long-lasting, multi-episode depression seem to arise only in predisposed subjects.

Neurotransmitters, which are substances produced by the neurons and used to transmit information between them, are also implicated in the etiology of depression. The production of different neurotransmitters has been found to be either diminished or abnormally regulated during depressive disorders. These include acetylcholine (involved in many cognitive functions such as learning and memory), norepinephrine and dopamine (involved mainly in motivation), and serotonin (related to the feelings of pleasure and satisfaction). Different neurotransmitters may have different levels of compromise, which may explain the diversity in the clinical manifestations of depressive disorders.

SYMPTOMS

Symptoms of depression are classified by the *Diagnostic and Statistical Manual of Mental Disorders*, 4th edition (DSM-IV) in major and minor symptoms according to their specificity for depressive disorders. The major symptoms of depression are depressive mood or sadness and anhedonia, and a loss of interest or pleasure in usual activities. The minor symptoms can be divided in psychological or physical. Psychological minor symptoms are feelings of worthlessness or inappropriate guilt, reduced ability to concentrate or make decisions, recurrent thoughts of death or suicide (thinking, planning, or attempting). The physical minor symptoms are sleep disorders (insomnia or hypersomnia), changes in weight or appetite, loss of energy, fatigue and psychomotor agitation, or retardation. Anxiety is also commonly observed but it is not considered as a depressive symptom for diagnostic purposes.

The severity of depression varies between patients and may be estimated by the number of presenting symptoms, their intensity as perceived by the patient or the physician, and the presence or absence of suicidal symptoms. Since depressive disorders can present with varied symptoms ranging from severe to mild, the diagnosis is sometimes difficult.

A depressed patient may also present to the health professional with a great variation in his or her aspect, varying from apparently normal subjects to persons with a miserable aspect, with tearful eyes and poor facial expression, low voice and poor interaction with the interviewer, wearing carelessly, and assuming a curved posture.

Psychotic symptoms may arise in some cases of depression, a situation which is more common late in life than in younger patients; nevertheless, psychotic symptoms are similar among elderly and young patients. Psychotic symptoms may include guilt about past actions and thoughts, delusions of illness, or even auditive hallucinations.

TYPES OF DEPRESSION AND DIAGNOSIS

All depressive disorders are diagnosed based on history and symptoms. Major depression is the most severe form of depression and the one which may present great risk of suicide. It is characterized by the recurrence of major depressive episodes. A major depressive episode is characterized by at least one of the major symptoms and a total of at least five symptoms, for at least two weeks and in the absence of a general medical condition or drug that may explain the symptoms or a maniac episode. This last condition would prompt a diagnosis of a bipolar disorder, which is considered a separate clinical entity. The symptoms also cannot be explained by bereavement, in which case they have to be prolonged for more than two months to be considered a major depressive episode.

Dysthymic disorder is characterized by chronic depression but less severe than a major depression. A patient has dysthymia when reporting depressed mood or appearing depressed to others for most of the day on the majority of days for two years or more. Sleep or appetite alterations, low self-esteem, and low energy are other common symptoms. Being a less severe form of depression, dysthymia may be undiagnosed for quite a long time, causing loss of life quality without impairing functioning with intensity enough for an obvious suspicion.

A minor depressive episode does not fit the five symptoms of the major depressive episode nor does it fit the duration of at least two years to be characterized as dysthymia. Thus, a patient is said to have a minor depressive episode if conditions for a major depressive disorder are present but the symptoms number from two to four symptoms including one major symptom. Currently the official diagnostic criteria of DSM-IV do not include minor depression and this set of symptoms would be characterized as a depression not otherwise specified.

TREATMENT

There are three main types of therapy for depressive disorders: antidepressant drugs, psychotherapy, and electroconvulsive therapy.

DRUG TREATMENT

Antidepressant drugs act by enhancing the levels of one or more neurotransmitters and the choice of the correct antidepressant involves the recognition of the different profiles depression can assume as well as the patient profile: Elderly people may not tolerate older antidepressants' collateral effects and many drugs used to treat chronic conditions may not be used together with a given antidepressant.

Several antidepressant drugs are currently available and they are divided into different classes according with the mechanism of action. Because these variations in the action of the antidepressants often reflect on potency, different neurotransmitter activation, and side effects, the choice of an antidepressant drug may be critical to the treatment of a depressive patient. The main classes of antidepressants are monoamine oxidase inhibitors, tricyclic antidepressants, selective serotonin reuptake inhibitors, dopamine reuptake inhibitors, norepinephrine reuptake inhibitors, tetracyclic antidepressants, and novel, atypic antidepressants.

PSYCHOTHERAPY

Psychotherapy, conducted by trained mental health professionals (psychiatrists, psychologists, or psychiatric nurses), emphasizes the need for understanding and correcting situations, habits, or problems contributing to depression. Psychotherapy offers individuals or group approaches and, by resolving factors contributing to the depressive disorder, it may achieve either the effective treatment of depression or enhance the effectiveness of other treatment strategy. Psychotherapy and drug therapy are usually coadjuvant and the simultaneous use of both is a common treatment strategy.

Successful psychotherapy may lead to a different pattern of habitual thinking, which may result in a lower relapse rate than is achievable with drug-exclusive therapy; this, however, may produce quicker results. In a crisis situation, drug therapy is usually the choice.

From the many different psychotherapeutical approaches, cognitive behavior therapy has been demonstrated to be one of the most efficient in the treatment of depressive disorders. The base of this strategy is to work on how patients think about themselves and how they behave in their relationships. The main focus is to help depressed patients to identify and substitute negative thoughts with more realistic ones and develop stronger coping strategies. It can also be used to help patients with interpersonal skills, which may allow the experience of interpersonal communication and relationship with the least possible stress.

ELECTROCONVULSIVE THERAPY

Electroconvulsive therapy (ECT), also known as electroshock therapy or, simply, electroshock, uses short bursts of an electrical current in the brain in order to elicit a brief seizure while the patient is under general anesthesia.

Most countries nowadays only allow electroconvulsive therapy to be conducted under anesthesia, in contrast to the direct electroconvulsive therapy of the past. Usually, the patient receives frequent treatment sessions per week for about one month and then the need for repeated sessions is evaluated. ECT may elicit side effects such as disorientation, headache, and short-term memory loss.

ECT offers a very fast response when compared to psychotherapy and drug therapy, but this response decays if there is no maintenance treatment with either electroconvulsive therapy or with a drug. Due to its fast action, electroconvulsive therapy is considered to be the treatment of choice in emergency situations (e.g., suicidal behavior or in catatonic depression with cessation of oral intake). Antidepressant drugs may be associated from the beginning of ECT so as to allow early discontinuation of it after drug therapy achieves control of the symptoms.

ECT has assumed a bad reputation in popular culture worldwide, but it is still considered a good treatment option if well indicated, that is, where other treatment options have failed, in severely depressed patients (especially those who have a story of previous response to ECT), in patients with significant psychotic symptoms or where antidepressants cannot be used for any reason. It is, therefore, considered to be a therapy of exception.

SUICIDAL BEHAVIOR

Suicide is the most severe consequence of depression and overwhelming suicidal thoughts are considered a medical emergency. Medical professionals advise that people who express plans of suicide seek medical attention immediately. This is especially true when the means to undertake the plans were already made available (e.g., drugs, weapons, or other means). Having a suicide plan detailed is also a great risk for suicide.

Treatments for a suicidal depressed patient may include reclusion, surveillance, or sedation with drugs until the effects of antidepressants are evident and suicidal thought vanishes. It is important to notice that most suicidal patients may inform the health professional once asked about suicidal intentions, although they will probably not inform that spontaneously. Therefore, it is important that health professionals actively search for risk of suicide in every depressed patient.

DEPRESSION IN THE ELDERLY

There are some special characteristics that make depression in the elderly a specific subject of study. As in other diseases in the elderly, differences in the aged organism may make depressive disorders difficult to diagnose. There is a smaller chance of finding depressed mood (sadness) in an elderly depressed subject as compared to anhedonia, leading to difficulty in suspecting the diagnosis. Within the minor symptoms, physical symptoms tend to be more common than psychological symptoms.

Loss of functional status is often observed, especially in the frailest elders. Cognition, especially memory, can be so severely impaired that sometimes it mimics the clinical patterns of dementia; because in these cases the cause of cognitive loss is depression and that effect is potentially reversible, such condition is called pseudodementia.

Another important feature of depression in the elderly relates to decompensation of previously compensated comorbidities: the loss of functional status may be so important that the person may lose ability or will to keep treatment for chronic conditions and it is not uncommon for the sudden worsening of a chronic condition to prompt the diagnosis of depression during emergency care. Suicidal behavior in major depression may be less frequent than in younger patients; nevertheless, studies have suggested that elderly people commit less theatrical attempts than younger patients and frailty may make elderly people more prone to die from an attempt that would not kill a younger person. These features make suspicion of suicide very important when dealing with older depressed patients.

DEPRESSION IN CHILDREN

Depression in children can be very challenging, because the clinical presentation may be blunted by different, nonspecific symptoms. A depressed child might present with learning or memory problems not previously existing, sleep problems and nightmares, irritability, loss of appetite, and important behavioral changes. Rarely do these symptoms prompt parents to seek medical help; therefore, health professionals should suspect depression when evaluating children with such symptoms.

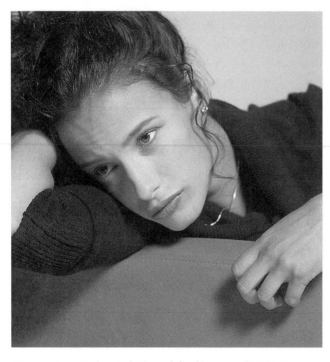

Women appear to be at a higher risk for depression, but this is decreasing and there seems to be no gender difference in the elderly.

THE ROLE OF ANXIETY IN DEPRESSION

Although anxiety and depression may occur at the same time (independently occurring together), both can occur together, with mood congruence and overlapping symptoms, a presentation that makes it difficult to separate the depression and the anxiety. This is especially true for elderly depressive patients, and "anxious depression" is a colloquial term well understood among clinicians.

SEASONAL AFFECTIVE DISORDER

Seasonal affective disorder is a kind of depressive disorder that occurs in wintertime during short daylight periods. The production of melatonin, which occurs mainly in the dark, may be abnormally stimulated by the changes in the length of daylight period and this may be in the center of seasonal affective disorder's pathophysiology. That is believed to be the reason why many patients with this condition benefit from phototherapy, the controlled exposure of the patient to bright, artificial light.

CONCLUSION

Depressive disorders are a relatively common set of diseases and the most severe form, major depression, can be very disabling. Occurring in all age groups, depression imposes a great burden on children, who often lack the diagnosis for a long time, and on elderly people, for whom the diagnosis may be difficult and the consequences of the disease may be severely incapacitating, notably in the frail elderly with different comorbidities. The most dreaded consequence of depression, which is suicide, on the other hand, can occur in all age groups. Early recognition and appropriate treatment of depressed people can be pivotal in these people's lives.

SEE ALSO: Geriatrics; Mental Health; Psychology.

BIBLIOGRAPHY. American Psychiatric Association, *Diagnostic and Statistical Manual of Mental Disorders*, 4th ed. (text revision) (American Psychiatric Association, 2000); R. C. Bland, "Epidemiology of Affective Disorders: A Review," *Canadian Journal of Psychiatry* (v.42, 1997); Edmund H. Duthie, et al., *Practice of Geriatrics*, 3rd ed. (Saunders, 1998); John R. Geddes, et al., "Relapse Prevention with Antidepressant Drug Treatment in Depressive Disorders: A Systematic Review," *Lancet* (v.361, 2003); C. J. L. Murray and A. D. Lopez, "Alternative Projections of Mortality and Disability by Cause 1990–2020: Global Burden of Disease Study," *Lancet* (v.349, 1997); J. C. Nelson, "Managing Treatment-Resistant Major Depression," *Journal of Clinical Psychiatry* (v.64 Suppl, 2003); A. R. Tyrka, et al., "Psychotic Major Depression: A Benefit-Risk Assessment of Treatment Options," *Drug Safety* (v.29/6, 2006); C. F. Reynolds III, "Treatment of Major Depression in Later Life: A Life Cycle Perspective," *Psychiatric Quarterly* (v.68, 1997); J. J. Schildkraut, "The Catecholamine Hypothesis of Affective Disorders: A Review of Supporting Evidence," *American Journal of Psychiatry* (v.122/5, 1965).

THIAGO MONACO, M.D., PH.D.
UNIVERSITY OF SÃO PAULO MEDICAL SCHOOL, BRAZIL

Dermatitis

Dermatitis is a general term used to describe the features of several skin conditions linked by the clinical finding of inflammation in the epidermis (top layer of the skin). In general it may be thought of as the skin's response to stress or irritants in the environment, and it is not contagious. There are many different types of dermatitis, which are clinically characterized by the presence of redness, scaling, pruritus (itching), swelling, and in severe cases blistering. Each type of dermatitis has an underlying pathophysiologic mechanism, which directs the appropriate therapy. Family practitioners, internists, allergists and dermatologists (a doctor who specializes in skin diseases), commonly diagnose cases of dermatitis based on the appearance and symptoms. In the event that the dermatitis is caused by an environmental allergen, prick testing with dermal needles (by an allergist) or patch testing with epicutaneous (upon the skin) chemicals applied with stickers on the skin may be necessary to determine the causative agents.

EPIDEMIOLOGY

Dermatitis occurs in people of all ages and ethnicities. According to the National Institutes of Health, people who live in dry climates or in cities have a higher risk of developing atopic dermatitis. Approximately 20 percent of children suffer from some form of dermatitis, and some of them continue to have this condition as adults.

ATOPIC DERMATITIS

Atopic dermatitis, often referred to as eczema, has a high prevalence in children, but may occur at any age. It is caused by a combination of genetic and environmental factors, and is often linked with allergies, asthma, and stress. The clinical appearance of atopic dermatitis may vary by the individual; however, the hallmark clinical picture is acute eruptions of erythematous (red), scaled, and pruritic (itching) plaques involving the antecubital fossa (inner arm crease) and popliteal fossa (behind the knee crease). The condition waxes and wanes and may have periods where the skin appears normal. Atopic dermatitis is usually controlled by identifying and avoiding triggers and maintaining the skin barrier with emollient moisturizers. In moderate to severe cases it may be necessary to treat the affected area with topical steroids or immunomodulators, and systemic antihistamines.

CONTACT DERMATITIS

Contact dermatitis is the skin's innate inflammatory reaction to an offending external environmental chemical trigger. There are three main subcategories of contact dermatitis: urticarial, irritant, and allergic.

On the other hand, with contact urticaria, the least common, hives develop by an IgE-mediated immediate type mechanism to chemical triggers such as environmental allergens or certain foods. The classical clinical presentation is characterized by a local tingling sensation and localized redness and swelling. It is usually treated with topical anti-itch creams, oral antihistamines. In moderate to severe cases systemic steroids may be necessary. As this is an immediate type reaction it may develop rapidly. A common example of contact urticaria is the allergic reaction to latex.

In irritant contact dermatitis (ICD), the most common form, irritants penetrate the skin and in doing so may remove the protective oils and moisture from the skin's outer layer. This results in chemical injury to the superficial layers of the skin with subsequent inflammation. The dermatitis in ICD usually appears within 48 hours of exposure to a caustic chemical and is generally limited to the areas of the skin which was in contact with the irritant. There may be variation in the clinical appearance depending on the strength of the chemical trigger and the strength of the skin barrier to sustain the insult. ICD can be caused by soaps, detergents, and antiperspirant, among others.

Allergic contact dermatitis (ACD) arises when an immune response is triggered in the skin after repeated contact with allergenic substances (such as fragrances and formaldehyde). The ACD-type dermatitis may be confined to the area of the skin that contacts the allergen; however, distant sites of previous exposure may also re-react with repeated exposures.

The best form of treatment for contact dermatitis is to avoid the substance that causes the inflammatory reaction. It might be difficult to determine the exact component of the substance that is causing the reaction. In ACD, patch tests may need to be performed.

SEBORRHOEIC DERMATITIS

Seborrhoeic dermatitis mostly occurs in the hair-bearing and oily areas of the skin, such as the face, scalp, genital area, and trunk. This form of dermatitis is believed to be an inflammatory reaction to a combination of the Malassezia yeast, a normal inhabitant of the skin, and decreased keratolysis (dead cells being removed) of the skin. Seborrhoeic dermatitis usually appears as dry, pink patches with waxy scale. It can be treated with the use sulfa/sulfacetamide washes and lotions, selenium, and zinc-based lotions and shampoos, topical antifungal/yeast agents (such as the azoles), and topical steroids.

NEURODERMATITIS

Neurodermatitis is a skin condition that is characterized by tremendous pruritus and subsequent excoriation. As is seen with all chronic dermatoses, the skin may increase in thickness and become rough (lichenified) in the affected area. Physicians may use patch testing, skin biopsies, or blood tests to accurately diagnose the condition, and a neurologic cause must be ruled out. Antipruritus medications such as emollients, topical steroids, and antihistamines may be needed.

PREVENTION

For prone individuals, lifestyle changes which maintain the skin barrier and include the avoidance of known triggers are paramount to the reduction of flare-ups and alleviation of symptoms.

SEE ALSO: Skin Diseases (General).

BIBLIOGRAPHY. DermNet NZ, "Dermatitis" www.dermnetnz.org (November 2005); James C. Shaw, "Overview of Dermatitis," UpToDate (2006); National Institute of Arthritis and Musculoskeletal and Skin Diseases, "Handout on Health: Atopic Dermatitis," www.niams.nih.gov (April 2003).

Shalu S. Patel
University of Michigan
Rajiv I. Nijhawan
JoAnn Tijn Kon Kiem
Independent Scholars

Developmental Disabilities

Developmental disabilities are a global health matter, affecting individuals from childhood through adulthood, presenting various special issues for families, educational, and healthcare systems throughout the world. A developmental disability, as defined by the U.S. government in Public Law 95-602, is a chronic mental and/or physical impairment, which manifests before age 22. Developmental disabilities are characterized by significant functional limitations in three or more of the following areas of major life activities: 1) self-care, 2) receptive and expressive language, 3) learning, 4) mobility, 5) self-direction, 6) capacity for independent living, and 7) economic self-sufficiency. These problems are diagnosed by comparing a child's performance with the performance norms of the child's same-age peers. As developmental disabilities are chronic, usually affecting multiple body parts or systems, and are likely to be lifelong, they often necessitate individualized multidisciplinary care. Developmental disabilities are sometimes referred to as developmental delays or disorders.

TYPES OF DEVELOPMENTAL DISABILITIES

Developmental disabilities can be categorized into nervous system disabilities, sensory-related disabilities, metabolic disorders, and degenerative disorders.

Nervous system disabilities refer to primary impairments of the brain and/or spinal cord, thereby impacting multiple aspects of learning and intelligence. The most common result of a nervous system disability is mental retardation (or low intelligent quotient [IQ]), which is a hallmark characteristic of many developmental disabilities. The most common nervous system disabilities include Down syndrome, Fragile X syndrome, and autism spectrum disorders. Autism, for example, is characterized by impairments in social interaction, communication, and restricted repetitive patterns of behavior, interests, or activities.

Sensory-related disabilities refer primarily to impairments in visual and auditory processing. They occur, not only as a primary symptom (such as deafness), but are also common comorbid problems with other developmental disabilities.

Metabolic disorders are often caused by genetic deficiencies in an enzyme, thereby affecting a person's ability to synthesize and break down substances in the body. For example, phenylketonuria (PKU) is caused by a deficiency of a certain enzyme, creating a toxic level of one amino acid and too little of another, resulting in brain damage and severe mental retardation.

Degenerative disorders refer to disabilities that are not apparent at birth but that manifest at an older age, causing the child who was developing normally to lose previously acquired skills. Functioning may regress or be lost in physical, mental, and/or sensory modalities. An example of a degenerative disorder is Rett syndrome, where persistent and progressive degeneration throughout life occurs in five areas: head circumference, hand movements, social engagement, gait, and language development.

INCIDENCE

Approximately 17 percent of children under the age of 18 have some type of developmental disability, including more mild conditions such as speech and language disorders and learning disabilities. About 2 percent of children under the age of 18 have a more serious developmental disability including mental retardation, autism, cerebral palsy, hearing loss, and vision impairment. Of these serious developmental disabilities, mental retardation is the most common.

CAUSES

The exact cause of many developmental disabilities is unknown. Some factors that contribute to developmental disabilities include trauma or infection to the brain, prenatal nutrition problems, prenatal drug or alcohol exposure, extreme premature birth, genetic and chromosomal abnormalities, and poor nutrition and medical care. Some disabilities are believed to be caused by an interaction of these biological and environmental factors.

ASSOCIATED PROBLEMS

Children with developmental disabilities have been shown to have poorer health, including increased rate of injury and need for medical attention. They also do not perform as well in school as their peers. Children with developmental disabilities have increased social problems including poor peer relationships, and increased risks of delinquency and substance abuse. They are also at increased risk for child abuse.

ASSESSMENT

Evaluation of developmental disabilities is best accomplished by a multidisciplinary team that includes the child's pediatrician, teachers, a psychologist, a speech and language therapist, an occupational therapist, and an educational specialist. Evaluations should include standardized tests of intellectual ability (e.g., the Bayley Scales of Infant Development, the Stanford-Binet Intelligence Scale, and the Wechsler Intelligence Scales), behavioral assessments (e.g., Vineland Adaptive Behavior Scale), clinical testing of speech and language, academic testing, physical and neurological examinations, and a detailed medical and developmental history. Test results are compared to norms for same-age peers to determine relative discrepancies. The *Diagnostic and Statistical Manual of Mental Disorders*, 4th edition, text revision (DSM-IV-TR) is also used for making diagnoses.

EARLY IDENTIFICATION AND SCREENING

While a developmental disability may keep a child from developing normally and reaching cognitive, behavioral, or physical milestones, specialized intensive intervention can help improve the prognosis. The key to treatment success is early intervention. Thus, early identification is crucial. Birth to 3 years of age is a critical time in a child's development, and identification and treatment during this time can improve a child's functioning, prevent associated problems, and ease the burden for the family. Proper treatment can also improve quality of life for the child and enable him or her to lead a more independent life as an adult.

Screening tools identify children who may have a developmental disability and, thus, warrant further assessment and possible treatment services. By conducting screenings early, a child may begin to receive treatment during a time when he or she is still developing and, therefore, most responsive to intervention.

Family physicians and pediatricians are in a unique position to identify children with developmental disabilities. Unfortunately, however, many fail to identify them early enough for families to provide early intervention services. The American Academy of Pediatrics recommends that primary pediatric healthcare providers use standard screening tools to conduct developmental screening of infants and children every year during the first three years of life.

TREATMENT

While there is no cure for many of the developmental disabilities, treatments are available to address a range of symptoms. For example, for autism, a multidisciplinary approach of behavioral, occupational, and speech and language therapy can help a child to use language, decrease harmful behaviors, and aid in self-care. Educational resource specialists can provide support in the school environment to facilitate the child's functioning in the regular classroom. Many research studies have shown the importance of teaching treatment techniques to parents and teachers. Skills taught to parents and teachers include feeding techniques, eye gaze, sign language, child management skills, positioning, gross motor skills, and communication skills. Medications also play an important role in treating the symptoms associated with developmental disabilities.

EARLY INTERVENTION

Research has shown that early intervention has a positive effect for many disabilities and substantial benefits for certain disorders. For example, children who are identified as having autism early in life have been shown to have significantly better cognitive, language, and motor skills and complete a higher level of education than their peers who were identified later in life. Early intervention can also improve a child's self-esteem thereby keeping him or her from a trajectory that may include substance abuse, interpersonal problems, or delinquency.

EDUCATIONAL SERVICES

For school-age children, U.S. law mandates that an evaluation called an Individualized Education Program (IEP) be conducted which documents the child's developmental level, the types of support that he or she needs to succeed, and goals for establishing independence. Parents, teachers, and school psychologists are often present at IEP meetings to ensure that there is a comprehensive approach in meeting children's needs. For younger children, a similar evaluation called the Individualized Family Support Plan (IFSP) is conducted to establish early intervention services.

It is critical that the educational program of a child with a developmental disability is at the appropriate level for him or her. For children who attend school, a range of options are available. Some children will require a separate special education classroom for their needs to be met. This is no longer the only choice available, however, as it has been in the past. Children with disabilities may now also participate fully in the regular classroom, due to a movement called "mainstreaming." Sometimes, they may have a resource specialist with them in the classroom to provide individualized support. Experts agree that the child should be placed in the least restrictive school environment possible.

Postsecondary education and vocational training is also increasingly available for people with disabilities, and legislation in some areas mandates that accommodations be made for students with disabilities.

DAILY LIVING

For adults, the scenarios in which people live and work lie on a spectrum. There was a time when people with disabilities lived segregated from the general population in institutions. Legislation and alternative support systems have made this situation less common. Many adults with developmental disabilities live by themselves, with family, or with roommates. Such individuals may have an aide who comes to the house or apartment to help with tasks of daily living on a regular basis, or who lives with them. Other people with developmental disabilities live in group homes with individuals with similar needs, where professional assistance is provided 24 hours a day. Day programs are also available, which provide a range of services from skills training, to social activities and outings, to educational programming.

Support systems for people with developmental disabilities are often based on the premise of helping them to attain the greatest level of independence possible so that they can maintain quality of life and make positive contributions to society.

SEE ALSO: Attention Deficit Disorder; Autism; Birth Defects; Blindness; Child Development; Child Mental Health;

Deafness; Down Syndrome; Genetic Disorders; Infant and Toddler Development; Mental Retardation; Metabolic Disorders; Premature Babies; Rett Syndrome; Spina Bifida.

BIBLIOGRAPHY. M. D. Batshaw, L. Pellegrino, and N. J. Roizen, *Children with Disabilities* (Paul H. Brookes, 2007); S. I. Greenspan and S. Wieder, *The Child with Special Needs: Encouraging Intellectual and Emotional Growth* (Perseus Books, 1998); F. R. Volkmar, et al., *Handbook of Autism and Pervasive Developmental Disorders* (Wiley, 2005).

DONIEL DRAZIN, M.A.
ALBANY MEDICAL COLLEGE

Diabetes

The developed and developing worlds are witnessing an epidemic of type 2 diabetes mellitus (T2DM), associated with a concomitant rise in the rates of obesity. Diabetes mellitus (DM) is the sixth leading cause of death in the United States, and its adverse health consequences, including heart disease, blindness, limb amputation, and kidney disease, represent a tremendous burden to healthcare systems. Greater than 7 percent of Americans have diagnosed DM, but the disease and its complications account for almost 14 percent of American healthcare expenditures. Moreover, the American Diabetes Association (ADA) estimated that the direct and indirect expenditures of DM, including medical costs, lost workdays, disabilities, and deaths, totaled $132 billion in the United States in 2002.

GLUCOSE METABOLISM

DM is caused by an inability of the pancreas to produce the hormone insulin in a sufficient quantity to meet the body's demands. The pancreas is an exocrine and endocrine organ located behind the stomach in the abdomen. It secretes certain important digestive enzymes into the small intestine to break down food (exocrine function), but it also secretes hormones such as insulin, glucagon, and somatostatin into the bloodstream to regulate the body's nutrient use (endocrine function). The β-cells of the pancreas secrete insulin in response to eating. This hormone acts at receptors in the liver, muscles, and other organs to allow their uptake of glucose, the

simple sugar carbohydrate that is the body's primary energy source. The tissues of the body use the energy from glucose to perform their normal physiologic functions. If there is an excess of glucose, the liver and muscles can store it for later use as glycogen, a more complex carbohydrate consisting of chains of glucose. Insulin also allows the body to turn free fatty acids (FFA) into triglycerides, the main component of adipose (fat) tissue. Without insulin, the body cannot use the glucose in the bloodstream, despite its abundance after a meal. To compensate, tissues break down protein and fats for energy, a situation similar to starvation. DM results either when the pancreas does not produce enough insulin or when the body becomes resistant to the effects of insulin. Regardless, the common outcome is hyperglycemia (elevated blood glucose levels) and a paradoxical inability of the body's tissues to use this glucose.

DEFINITION OF DM

The term *diabetes* most commonly refers to the endocrine disorders of carbohydrate metabolism known as diabetes mellitus (DM), conditions characterized by hyperglycemia. Originating from the Greek for "one that straddles" or "a siphon," the word *diabetes* alone, however, also encompasses a number of metabolic disturbances that result in increased urine production, including DM and diabetes insipidus (DI). Unlike DM, DI is a condition of increased urine output that is not caused by increased glucose levels. It is categorized by etiology. Nephrogenic diabetes insipidus (NDI) is due to an inability of the kidney to concentrate urine and can be caused by a genetic mutation or by treatment with the mood stabilizer lithium. Central diabetes insipidus (CDI) is generally caused by an inability of the central nervous system to detect and regulate the electrolyte concentration of the body's fluids; it can be caused by head trauma and some cancers. DI represents a distinct pathophysiologic process from DM and is not associated with the numerous complications of the latter.

Two laboratory tests are used to define and diagnose DM: fasting plasma glucose (FPG) and the two-hour oral glucose tolerance test (OGTT). The FPG is obtained by measuring the glucose level in the blood after a fast of eight to 12 hours. Even in nondiabetics, plasma glucose levels are elevated after eating, but high glucose levels after fasting indicate a problem with glucose metabolism consistent with diabetes. The ADA and the World Health Organization (WHO) define DM by an FPG≥126 mg/dL (7.0 mmol/L). FPG values between 100 and 125 mg/dL (5.6–6.9 mmol/L) define impaired fasting glucose (IFG), a "prediabetic" condition associated with future risk of progression to DM. The OGTT is a different measure of glucose metabolism; during this test, the participant drinks a 75-gram glucose solution and has his blood drawn two hours later. Normal individuals will be able to metabolize this glucose and reduce their plasma glucose to below 140 mg/dL (7.8 mmol/L) within two hours. DM is diagnosed at an OGTT≥200 mg/dL (11.1 mmol/L), while an OGTT between 140 and 200 mg/dL defines impaired glucose tolerance (IGT), another "prediabetic" state that has significant overlap with IFG. DM can be diagnosed with the FPG, the OGTT, or a random (nonfasting) plasma glucose >200 mg/dL in the presence of diabetic symptoms such an increased urination, thirst, blurred vision, or weight loss. Regardless, the diagnostic test should be repeated to confirm the diagnosis. Cases of DM that cannot be categorized as type 1 or type 2 (see below) may require antibody testing to identify the autoantibodies often found in type 1 DM (T1DM). In patients with certain risk factors associated with the development of T2DM, the FPG can be used as a screening test to detect the disease.

TYPES AND EPIDEMIOLOGY OF DM

While all forms of DM are marked by hyperglycemia and result from an absolute or relative insufficiency of insulin, there are distinct types of DM that differ in their etiology. In 1997, the ADA introduced the terms type 1 and type 2 diabetes mellitus to replace the previous terms *insulin-dependent* and *non-insulin–dependent* diabetes, respectively.

Formerly known as insulin-dependent (IDDM) or juvenile onset diabetes, T1DM is an autoimmune disease in which the body's own immune system destroys pancreatic β-cells, thereby eliminating the ability of the pancreas to produce insulin. T1DM affects less than 0.5 percent of the world population. Most cases occur in childhood or early adulthood, although it can occur at any age. Certain populations, including those in Scandinavia, are at greater risk for the disease than others, such as the Chinese. There is a genetic predisposition to T1DM, as evidenced by the

30-percent risk in identical twins of type 1 diabetics compared to the 0.4 percent risk in people with no family history of the disease. Some of the predisposing genetic mutations have been identified, although they are not sufficient to cause T1DM. Researchers have proposed several environmental triggers that may lead to T1DM in genetically predisposed individuals, including perinatal viral infections and exposure to certain foods like cow's milk and cereals in infancy. Most researchers believe that some environmental exposure triggers an autoimmune response in such people, resulting in antibodies directed against molecules in the pancreas necessary for insulin release. These antibodies cause the body's own immune system to destroy the pancreatic β-cells, eliminating the ability of the pancreas to secrete insulin within a few months to years. Type 1 diabetics must take insulin injections for survival. Screening for T1DM is not currently recommended for individuals at higher risk for the disease, such as children of type 1 diabetics.

Associated with obesity, T2DM comprises the majority of the current diabetes epidemic. T2DM may account for up to 95 percent of DM cases in some populations. Initially in the disease process, T2DM is characterized by insulin resistance, not by decreased pancreatic insulin production. The body's tissues, including the liver, muscles, and adipose tissue, become resistant to the effects of insulin and therefore take up less glucose from the bloodstream. To overcome this insulin resistance, the pancreas secretes greater amounts of insulin to maintain proper glucose balance. Eventually, the pancreas cannot maintain this elevated insulin secretion, and insulin production declines, resulting in hyperglycemia similar to T1DM.

Greater than 8 percent of the U.S. population carries a diagnosis of T2DM, although the true prevalence is higher due to underdiagnosis. This percentage is increasing: The prevalence of T2DM increased 38 percent between 1976–80 and 1988–94 in U.S. adults. Formerly seen exclusively in adults, T2DM is also increasing in prevalence in children and adolescents as the obesity epidemic has begun to include these generations. Although rates of T2DM are currently higher in developed countries, its prevalence is increasing most rapidly in developing countries. Wild estimated that the global prevalence of all DM will increase 39 percent from 4.6 percent in 2000 to 6.4 percent in 2030. Indeed, India and China currently have the most diabetics.

Certain ethnic groups are at greater risk for T2DM, including African Americans, Latinos, Native Americans, Asian Americans, and Pacific Islanders. Although lifestyle and socioeconomic factors may explain some of these disparities, there is also a strong genetic component to T2DM that varies with ethnicity. Having a sibling with T2DM increases one's own risk by 20 to 30 percent, and monozygotic (identical) twins have more similar risks for T2DM than dizygotic (fraternal) twins. Although rare types of DM due to single gene mutations exist, the genetic component of T2DM is likely due to mutations in several genes, each contributing a small part to the overall insulin resistance and pancreatic β-cell dysfunction.

Despite the importance of one's genetic make-up in determining one's risk for T2DM, the recent increase in the incidence of this disease gives evidence for its environmental risk factors, including weight gain, physical activity, and diet. Thus, the current paradigm for the etiology of T2DM is that certain individuals, including members of at-risk ethnic groups, have a genetic predisposition to T2DM, making them more likely to manifest the disease if they have additional environmental risk factors like physical inactivity or increased caloric intake. Some of this increased risk is mediated by a predisposition in some people to gain weight more easily than others, resulting in the insulin resistance associated with increased adiposity. The risk of T2DM increases with increasing body mass index (BMI), even within the normal range <25 kg/m². Other risk factors for the development of T2DM include an age of 45 years or older, a history of gestational DM, hypertension, and high cholesterol or triglycerides.

Gestational diabetes exists when the physiologic stresses of pregnancy cause an underlying predisposition for DM to manifest. These women have a higher risk of developing nongestational DM later in life. Several hereditary forms of DM due to single mutations have been identified, the most common of which are the various maturity-onset diabetes of the young (MODY), which are disorders due to autosomal dominant inheritance of mutations in important genes in glucose metabolism. Only about 1 to 5 percent of cases of DM are from one of the several single-mutation types; the vast majority of cases are T2DM, whose hereditary component is likely a complex picture involving mutations in several genes.

Other genetic conditions like Down syndrome and Huntington chorea are associated with an increased risk of DM. Diabetes can also be caused by diseases that damage the pancreas, including chronic pancreatitis from alcoholism and hemochromatosis, a condition marked by excess iron deposition in organs such as the pancreas. Traumatic injury to the pancreas, including any damage the pancreas may sustain during abdominal surgery, can also result in DM. Some medications can result in diabetes-like hyperglycemia, including thiazide diuretics and corticosteroids like prednisone.

NATURAL HISTORY AND COMPLICATIONS

The classic symptoms of DM are due to hyperglycemia: increased thirst, increased consumption of liquids, and increased urination. Other symptoms include blurred vision and weight loss. Especially in the case of T1DM, some individuals are found to be diabetic when they go into diabetic ketoacidosis (DKA), a life-threatening condition in which the body's inability to use glucose for energy results in the release of too much acid in the form of free fatty acids. People in DKA have abdominal pain, nausea, and vomiting and may progress to seizures or even coma without treatment, which includes insulin. Despite these possible early symptoms, many undiagnosed diabetics remain asymptomatic and may learn they have DM only because of routine medical blood tests. By this time, many of them already have one or more of the diabetic complications described below. The complications of DM are generally categorized as microvascular or macrovascular, affecting the small and large blood vessels of the body, respectively.

The microvascular complications of DM include damage to the retinas, kidneys, and nerves, while macrovascular disease involves the vessels that oxygenate the heart, brain, and extremities, resulting in myocardial infarctions (heart attacks), cerebrovascular accidents (strokes), and limb amputations. T2DM has a more insidious onset than T1DM, and thus many type 2 diabetics already have microvascular complications like eye and kidney disease at the time their disease is diagnosed.

Diabetic disease of the retinas (retinopathy) is often present at the time of diagnosis of T2DM (up to 30 percent of patients), whereas it is present in less than 3 percent of newly diagnosed type 1 diabetics. Almost all type 1 diabetics develop some retinopathy after having

DM for 20 years, while this prevalence is 50 percent to 80 percent in type 2 diabetics. Diabetic retinopathy is the leading cause of blindness in adults 20–74 in developed countries. Its progression can be slowed with good glycemic control, as monitored with hemoglobin A1c levels, and by treating coexisting hypertension. Surgical procedures such as photocoagulation and vitrectomy may be required in more advanced cases.

A second microvascular complication of DM is diabetic kidney disease (nephropathy), the leading cause of end-stage renal disease in the world. Diabetic nephropathy begins insidiously as microalbuminuria, a small amount of the protein albumin being leaked into the urine. The amount of this proteinuria increases with the progression of the kidney disease and is an indication of the amount of kidney function lost due to the scarring that DM causes in the kidneys. Once a large amount of proteinuria is present, the median time to end-stage renal disease is two and a half years, at which time kidney transplant or hemodialysis is necessary. Glycemic control and treatment with angiotensin converting enzyme (ACE) inhibitor medications can slow the progression of diabetic nephropathy.

Diabetic microvascular disease also damages nerves (neuropathy), most commonly the sensory nerves in the lower extremities but also the autonomic nerves responsible for maintaining blood pressure when a person stands up from sitting. Diabetic peripheral neuropathy often results in decreased sensation in the feet, predisposing a patient to painless sores that can become infected. The macrovascular damage to the blood vessels in the legs (peripheral vascular disease [PVD]) decrease lower extremity circulation and slow the healing of such infections. The decreased oxygenation of the legs and the increased susceptibility to infections often necessitate leg amputations, ultimately required in 5 percent of diabetics. Again, good glycemic control, regular foot examinations, and surgeries that improve blood flow to the lower extremities can reduce the foot complications associated with DM.

In addition to PVD, diabetic macrovascular disease also increases the risk of heart attack and stroke. Some studies estimate that DM increases the risk of these events by two to three times, even after adjusting for other known risk factors. Within diabetics, poorer glycemic control increases this risk even greater. Indeed, DM is considered to be a "risk equivalent" for coronary artery disease; that is, a diabetic is as likely to have a heart attack within 10 years as someone who has already had a heart attack. The World Health Organization (WHO) estimates that coronary heart disease (CHD) was the second leading cause of mortality worldwide in adults under 60 and by far the leading cause of mortality in those over 60 in 2002, followed by strokes. Given the significant risk of CHD conferred by DM, the prevention and treatment of this disease remains important to reduce its overall public health burden.

PREVENTION AND TREATMENT

Since much of the pathogenesis of T1DM, including possible environmental triggers, remains unidentified, there are as yet no effective ways to prevent this type of DM. Given the magnitude of the public health impact of T2DM, however, its prevention is a topic of great interest. Despite the significant genetic predisposition to T2DM, some cases of the disease can be prevented through lifestyle modification. The Nurses' Health Study in the United States showed that modifiable lifestyle factors associated with a lower incidence of T2DM include a BMI<25 kg/m2, moderate physical activity of at least 30 minutes per day, no smoking, and a diet high in fiber and polyunsaturated fat and low in trans fat and glycemic index.

Randomized trials have shown that the risk of T2DM in those already at high risk for the disease can be reduced through weight loss and increased physical activity. Moderate calorie restriction such as a reduction of 250 to 500 calories per day improves insulin sensitivity and glycemic control. Increased physical activity, even independent of any reduction in body weight, also improves insulin sensitivity, while sedentary activities like television watching are associated with an increased risk of T2DM.

The target of treatment for DM is glycemic control, or maintaining a diabetic's blood glucose levels within a normal range. The importance of glycemic control in diabetics was demonstrated in the Diabetes Control and Complications Trial (DCCT), a landmark prospective randomized trial in type 1 diabetics that compared conventional insulin therapy with more intensive insulin therapy that used multiple daily injections or continuous insulin pump infusion. The more intensive therapy reduced glucose levels and delayed or slowed the progression of microvascular complications, including retinopathy and nephropathy.

The United Kingdom Prospective Diabetes Study (UKPDS) similarly demonstrated the importance of glycemic control for reducing microvascular complications in type 2 diabetics. There is less evidence to suggest that glycemic control reduces the risk of macrovascular complications like coronary artery disease, but the advantages for microvascular complications clearly make glycemic control an important therapeutic goal.

Diabetics are encouraged to check their blood glucose at different times throughout the day (fasting and nonfasting) with home finger-stick glucometers and record these values in a log. If any of these values are too high or low, the patient and his physician can adjust his medication regimen accordingly. To get an overall idea of a patient's glycemic control over the last three months, physicians will check a hemoglobin A1c (HbA1c) level, a form of hemoglobin attached to sugar. Hemoglobin is a protein in red blood cells that allows them to carry oxygen, and high glucose levels in the blood cause sugar to attach to it. Normally, HbA1c comprises less than 5 percent of an individual's hemoglobin, but this percentage increases in diabetics. Diabetics should aim to keep their HbA1c levels below 7 percent, with dietary measures, physical activity, and medications.

Lifestyle modification is an essential component of the treatment of DM. Even modest weight loss can improve a type 2 diabetic's insulin sensitivity and improve HbA1c levels. This weight loss should be accomplished by reducing the total number of calories consumed daily with a diet rich in fruits, vegetables, whole grains, lean meats, and low-fat dairy products. Dietitians are key players in diabetic management, guiding patients to better food choices. Increased physical activity is also essential for weight loss and maintenance; the current recommendations from the National Institutes of Health call for 30 to 60 minutes per day of moderate intensity activity such as brisk walking.

Maintaining adequate glycemic control with diet and exercise alone is rare in a diagnosed diabetic, and so medications are important adjuncts to lifestyle modification. Producing insufficient insulin to meet the body's needs, type 1 diabetics require insulin injections or pumps, although inhaled insulin has recently been approved by the Food and Drug Administration (FDA). Different insulin preparations vary by how quickly they begin acting and for how long they act, and endocrinologists use a patient's log of home finger-stick blood glucose levels to tailor a given patient's insulin regimen. While the goal is to avoid hyperglycemia, hypoglycemia (low blood sugar) is a risk of taking too much insulin.

The symptoms of hypoglycemia include sweating, heart palpitations, and nausea, and if a hypoglycemic patient does not soon take in glucose either in the form of food or intravenous solution, he may progress to seizure or coma. In addition to type 1 diabetics, some type 2 diabetics may require insulin if oral medications do not provide adequate glycemic control.

Generally, however, type 2 diabetics are initially begun on oral diabetic medications at the time of diagnosis. There are several classes of oral diabetic medications, including the sulfonylureas, the biguanides such as metformin, the thiazolidinediones, the α-glucosidase inhibitors, and the meglitinides. Each of these classes of medications acts at a different part of the glucose metabolism pathway, including insulin sensitivity and insulin secretion, but in general they can have approximately equal efficacy in glycemic control. Each also has its own different adverse effects, which may guide physicians to choose one medication over another for a given patient. Metformin is often the first-line agent for obese patients with T2DM, since it can cause a modest degree of weight loss.

SEE ALSO: Diabetes and Pregnancy; Diabetes Type I (Juvenile Diabetes); Diabetes Type II.

BIBLIOGRAPHY. K.M. Gillespie, "Type 1 Diabetes: Pathogenesis and Prevention," *Canadian Medical Association Journal*, (v.175/2, 2006); C. Mantzoros, ed., *Obesity and Diabetes* (Humana Press, 2006); S.M. Marshall and A. Flyvbjerg, "Prevention and Early Detection of Vascular Complications of Diabetes," *British Medical Journal* (v.333/7566, 2006); S .Wild, et al., "Global Prevalence of Diabetes: Estimates for the Year 2000 and Projections for 2030," *Diabetes Care* (v.27, 2004).

JASON VASSY
WASHINGTON UNIVERSITY IN ST. LOUIS

Diabetes and Pregnancy

There are two types of diabetes mellitus (DM) in pregnancy. First, women with types 1 and 2 DM before pregnancy (pregestational diabetes [PGDM]) are at increased risk for adverse obstetric outcomes such as miscarriage and congenital malformations. Second, women who are not diabetic before pregnancy may developed impaired glucose metabolism as a result of pregnancy (gestational diabetes [GDM]). GDM also carries an increased risk of adverse events, and although it resolves after delivery, it places the mother at an increased risk for future development of nonpregnant DM.

About 4 percent of American pregnancies are complicated by DM, of which 88 percent are cases of GDM and 12 percent are in women with preexisting type 1 or 2 DM. The proportion of pregnancies with type 2 DM (T2DM) and thus PGDM is expected to rise as women delay pregnancy until later ages and as the incidence of T2DM increases with the increasing rates of obesity. Diabetic women who wish to conceive should first receive thorough physical examination, laboratory analyses, and counseling on the diabetic complications of pregnancy. Pregnancy should be avoided in women with significant coronary artery disease.

PGDM causes obstetric complications for both the mother and the fetus. Reduced kidney function and high blood pressure increase the risk of preeclampsia, a life-threatening elevation of blood pressure. During the first trimester, pregnancies in women with PGDM are at higher risk of miscarriage and congenital malformations of the fetal nervous and cardiovascular nervous systems. Preeclampsia, miscarriage, and preterm birth (delivery before 37 weeks gestational age) are risks during the second and third trimesters. Many miscarriages may be due to low fetal oxygen levels (hypoxemia) resulting from the increased metabolic rate caused by the high insulin levels found in T2DM.

Although worldwide reductions in perinatal mortality have been achieved in recent decades, diabetic pregnancies remain at a higher risk of perinatal mortality than other pregnancies. Because high maternal blood glucose levels are passed through the placenta to the fetus, PGDM is also associated with macrosomia, defined by a fetal weight greater than 4,000 grams (8.8 pounds). Pregnancies with macrosomia are more likely to be complicated by prolonged labor and shoulder dystocia of the infant at delivery, which may result in nerve damage to the shoulder and arm during difficult passage through the birth canal, especially with forceps- and vacuum-assisted deliveries. PGDM can also hinder the growth of fetuses, causing intrauterine growth restriction (IUGR), if long-standing diabetic vascular disease results in decreased maternal blood flow to the placenta and fetus.

After delivery, neonates of a PGDM pregnancy are susceptible to hypoglycemia, because they maintain an elevated metabolic state but no longer have access to the high glucose levels from their mothers. The best way to avoid the complications of PGDM is tight glucose control. For type 2 diabetics, this may necessitate switching from oral diabetic medication to insulin.

Normal pregnancy is a time of increased metabolism, and this increased demand may unmask a woman's previously hidden predisposition to glucose intolerance. Risk factors for GDM include obesity, a family history of DM, age greater than 25 years, and ethnicity including Hispanic and African. Different criteria are used to diagnose GDM. The American Diabetes Association (ADA) recommends a three-hour oral glucose tolerance test (OGTT) for diagnosis, although this may be less cost-effective than the World Health Organization (WHO) method, which uses a two-hour OGTT.

Screening guidelines also differ. While some feel that all pregnant women should be screened for GDM, the ADA recommends that all pregnant women with at least one risk factor for GDM be screened between 24 and 28 weeks' gestation or earlier if risk is greater. Pregnancies complicated by GDM are susceptible to many of the same adverse obstetric outcomes as PGDM, although these mothers do not already have some of the long-standing conditions associated with preexisting DM.

Up to 50 percent of women with GDM go on to develop DM within 10 years of pregnancy. As with PGDM, the best treatment for GDM is glucose control, through diet and insulin therapy if necessary.

SEE ALSO: American Diabetes Association (ADA); Diabetes; Diabetes Type I (Juvenile Diabetes); Diabetes Type II; Diabetic Kidney Problems.

BIBLIOGRAPHY. G. Forsbach-Sanchez, H. E. Tamez-Perez, and J. Vazquez-Lara, "Diabetes and Pregnancy," *Archives of Medical Research* (v.36/3, 2005); F. Galerneau and S. E. Inzucchi, "Diabetes Mellitus in Pregnancy," *Obstetrics and Gynecology Clinics of North America* (v.31/4, 2004).

JASON VASSY
WASHINGTON UNIVERSITY IN ST. LOUIS

Diabetes Type I (Juvenile)

The current obesity-associated diabetes epidemic has appropriately captured the attention of health professionals and the public. This epidemic is in type 2 diabetes mellitus (T2DM), a disease associated with insulin resistance followed by reduced insulin secretion. Five to 10 percent of cases of diabetes, however, are due to type 1 diabetes mellitus (T1DM), an autoimmune disease characterized by destruction of the cells in the pancreas that secrete insulin. The lifetime risk of T1DM is less than 0.5 percent, but the incidence varies with geographic region, from higher in Scandinavia to lower in Japan and China. Most cases of T1DM occur in childhood or early adulthood before age 30. In 1997, the American Diabetes Association introduced the terms *type 1 diabetes mellitus* to replace the previous terms *insulin-dependent* , or *juvenile diabetes.*

The human body's primary source of energy is the simple sugar glucose, one of the primary products of the digestion of a meal. Because of its importance for the function of the brain and other vital organs, glucose levels in the blood are normally tightly regulated by the pancreatic hormones insulin and glucagon, among others. The β-cells of a normal pancreas secrete insulin after a meal, which acts at receptors in the liver, muscles, and other organs to allow their uptake of glucose. Insulin also allows the body to turn free fatty acids (FFA) into triglycerides, the main component of adipose (fat) tissue. T1DM is an autoimmune disease in which the body's own immune system destroys pancreatic β-cells, thereby eliminating insulin secretion. Without insulin, the body cannot use the glucose in the bloodstream, despite its abundance after a meal. The result is hyperglycemia (elevated blood glucose levels) and a paradoxical inability of the body's tissues to use this glucose. To compensate for the lack of glucose utilization by the body, tissues break down protein and fats for energy, a situation similar to starvation. Once 80 percent of the β-cells in the pancreas are destroyed, the symptoms of diabetes manifest.

SYMPTOMS AND CAUSES

The classic symptoms of T1DM are due to hyperglycemia: increased thirst, increased consumption of liquids, and increased urination. The inability of the body to use glucose for energy causes other symptoms in T1DM, including weight loss despite an increased consumption of food. Such symptoms may prompt a healthcare provider to pursue a diagnosis of T1DM. Diabetes is diagnosed when the fasting plasma glucose (FPG) is ≥126 mg/dL (7.0 mmol/L) or when a random (nonfasting) plasma glucose is ≥200 mg/dL (11.1 mmol/L) in the presence of diabetic symptoms such an increased urination, thirst, blurred vision, or weight loss. Laboratory assays can also detect auto-antibodies, including anti-GAD antibodies, that cause the destruction of pancreatic β-cells. Some individuals are found to be diabetic when they have diabetic ketoacidosis (DKA), a life-threatening condition in which the body's inability to use glucose for energy results in the release of too much acid in the form of free fatty acids. People in DKA have abdominal pain, nausea, and vomiting and may progress to seizures or even coma without treatment, which includes insulin.

There is a genetic predisposition to T1DM, as evidenced by the 30 percent risk in identical twins of type 1 diabetics compared to the 0.4 percent risk in people with no family history of the disease. Some of the predisposing genetic mutations have been identified, although they are not sufficient to cause T1DM. The distribution of these mutations in the human population varies with geographic location, explaining some of the ethnic differences in the prevalence of T1DM. The most important of these are genetic mutations in the HLA (human leukocyte antigen) region of chromosome 6, which account for 40 percent to 50 percent of the genetic risk for developing T1DM. Forty percent of children with T1DM have mutations in this region compared to 2 percent of children without the disease.

Researchers have identified mutations in other chromosomes that are also associated with T1DM, albeit to a lesser degree. Genetic predisposition, however, is not sufficient to cause T1DM, since the majority of people with the higher-risk HLA mutations do not develop T1DM. Researchers have proposed several environmental triggers that may lead to T1DM in genetically predisposed individuals, including perinatal viral infections and exposure to certain foods like cow's milk and cereals in infancy. None have been definitively associated with the etiology of T1DM, however.

Most researchers believe that some environmental exposure triggers an autoimmune response in genetically predisposed individuals, resulting in antibodies directed against molecules in the pancreas necessary for insulin release, including glutamic acid decarboxylase (GAD). These antibodies cause the body's own immune system to destroy the pancreatic β-cells, eliminating the ability of the pancreas to secrete insulin within a few months to years. The resulting lack of insulin causes hyperglycemia and wasting. Since much of the pathogenesis of T1DM, including possible environmental triggers, remains unidentified, there are as yet no effective ways to prevent this type of diabetes.

Diabetes can result in many long-term medical complications during the life of a diabetic. The complications of diabetes are categorized as microvascular or macrovascular, according to the size of the blood vessels affected. Elevated glucose in the blood damages blood vessels and the organs to which they supply blood.

The microvascular complications of diabetes include eye disease (retinopathy), kidney disease (nephropathy), and nerve disease (neuropathy). Diabetes is the top cause of blindness in adults in developed countries and of end-stage renal disease worldwide. The macrovascular complications of the disease include coronary artery disease and strokes, leading causes of mortality worldwide. Diabetes is considered to be a "risk equivalent" for coronary artery disease; that is, a diabetic is as likely to have a heart attack within 10 years as someone who has already had a heart attack. The nerve and vascular damage of diabetes also make it the leading cause of leg amputations in the United States. These potential complications make routine eye, kidney, heart, and foot care an important part of a diabetic's healthcare.

TREATMENTS

Endocrinologists, physicians who treat hormone and metabolic diseases, care for type 1 diabetics. This care includes treatment with insulin, without which type 1 diabetics would not survive. In addition to survival, however, insulin helps prevent the above complications of T1DM by improving glycemic control, or maintenance of blood glucose levels within a normal range. The importance of glycemic control in type 1 diabetics was demonstrated in the Diabetes Control and Complications Trial (DCCT), a landmark prospective randomized trial that compared conventional insulin therapy with more intensive insulin therapy that used multiple daily injections or continuous insulin pump infusion. The more intensive therapy reduced glucose levels and delayed or slowed the progression of microvascular complications. There is less evidence to suggest that glycemic control reduces the risk of macrovascular complications like coronary artery disease, but the advantages for microvascular complications clearly make glycemic control an important therapeutic goal.

Diabetics are encouraged to check their blood glucose at different times throughout the day (fasting and nonfasting) with home finger-stick glucometers and record these values in a log. If any of these values are too high or low, the patient and his physician can adjust his insulin regimen accordingly. Plasma glucose levels before a meal should be 90–130 mg/dL (5.0–7.2 mmol/L), while the peak glucose level after a meal should be <180 mg/dL (<10.0 mmol/L). To get an overall idea of a patient's glycemic control over the last three months, physicians will check a hemoglobin A1c (HbA1c) level, which should remain below 7 percent.

Many different preparations of insulin exist that vary by how quickly they begin acting and for how long they act. Based on patients' glucose logs, endocrinologists often prescribe combinations of short- and long-acting insulins for injection a couple of times per day. Some diabetics choose to use insulin pumps for continually delivery of a basal amount of insulin, to which they add greater amounts of insulin in response to elevated glucose readings or in anticipation of a meal. Moreover, the U.S. Food and Drug Administration (FDA) has approved inhaled insulin. The most serious side effect of insulin therapy is hypoglycemia, or having too little glucose in the blood. The symptoms of hypoglycemia include sweating, heart palpitations, and nausea, and if a hypoglycemic patient does not soon take in glucose either in the form of food or intravenous solution, he may progress to seizure or coma.

SEE ALSO: Diabetes; Diabetic Eye Problems; Diabetic Kidney Problems; Diabetic Nerve Problems.

BIBLIOGRAPHY. K.M. Gillespie, "Type 1 Diabetes: Pathogenesis and Prevention," *Canadian Medical Association Journal* (v.175/2, 2006); A. Powers, "Diabetes Mellitus" in *Harrison's Principles of Internal Medicine*, 16th edition. (McGraw-Hill, 2005).

JASON VASSY
WASHINGTON UNIVERSITY IN ST. LOUIS

Diabetes Type II

Diabetes mellitus is being called an epidemic by the World Health Organization (WHO), and 90 percent of the more than 170 million cases of diabetes worldwide are type 2 diabetes mellitus (T2DM), formerly called non-insulin–dependent or adult-onset diabetes. In contrast to type 1 diabetes, the T2DM epidemic has occurred concomitantly with the obesity epidemic, more prevalent in, but not limited to, the developed world. Although the number of diabetics in the United States more than doubled from 5.8 to 14.7 million people from 1980 to 2004, India and China currently have the most diabetics of any country. Wild and colleagues estimated that the global prevalence of diabetes will increase 39 percent from 4.6 percent in 2000 to 6.4 percent in 2030.

Although type 1 diabetes is classically considered to be the diabetes of childhood, the prevalence of T2DM in children and adolescents has recently been increasing as these age groups are attaining a higher body mass index (BMI). Diabetes is the sixth leading cause of death in the United States, and WHO estimates that nine percent of deaths worldwide are attributable to the disease. Its adverse health consequences, including heart disease, blindness, limb amputation, and kidney disease, represent a tremendous burden to healthcare systems. Having diabetes increases an individual's healthcare costs two to three times, much of which is due to increased hospitalizations. More than seven percent of Americans have diagnosed diabetes, but the disease and its complications account for almost 14 percent of American healthcare expenditures. Moreover, the American Diabetic Association (ADA) estimated that the direct and indirect expenditures of diabetes, including medical costs, lost workdays, disabilities, and deaths, totaled $132 billion in the United States in 2002.

CHARACTERISTICS

Unlike type 1 diabetes, T2DM is initially characterized by insulin resistance, not by decreased insulin production in the pancreas. Early in the disease process, the body's tissues, including the liver, muscles, and adipose tissue, become resistant to the effects of insulin and therefore take up less glucose (sugar) from the bloodstream. This insulin resistance has been linked to obesity and specifically fat deposit in the central abdomen, although the pathway by which increased adiposity is associated with insulin resistance is not fully understood. To overcome insulin resistance, the pancreas secretes greater amounts of insulin to maintain proper glucose balance. Eventually, the pancreas cannot maintain this elevated insulin secretion, and insulin production declines, resulting in hyperglycemia and T2DM.

The etiology of T2DM is still being elucidated, but the current paradigm is that certain individuals, including members of at-risk ethnic groups, have a genetic predisposition to T2DM, making them more likely to manifest the disease if they have additional environmental risk factors like physical inactivity or increased caloric intake. The prevalence of these at-risk mutations varies with ethnicity, and certain ethnic groups are at increased risk for T2DM, including African Americans, Latinos, Native Americans, Asian Americans, and Pacific Islanders. Some of this increased risk is mediated by a predisposition in these people to gain weight more easily than others, resulting in the insulin resistance associated with increased adiposity.

Still, despite the importance of one's genetic makeup in determining one's risk for T2DM, the recent increase in the incidence of this disease gives evidence for its environmental risk factors, including weight gain, physical activity, and diet. For example, the risk for T2DM in Japanese immigrants to the United States soon matches the risk of T2DM of Americans more closely than that of native Japanese. Established environmental risk factors for T2DM include physical inactivity and increasing BMI, even within the normal range <25 kg/m^2. Other risk factors for the development of T2DM include an age of 45 years or greater and a history of gestational diabetes.

T2DM usually has a gradual onset and is asymptomatic early in the course of the disease, despite the "silent" damage that hyperglycemia causes in the body's small and large blood vessels. For this reason, many type 2 diabetics already have eye, kidney, and nerve damage at the time their disease is diagnosed. Patients with risk factors for T2DM, including ethnicity, obesity, high blood pressure, and high cholesterol, should be screened for the disease. Other symptoms may prompt a healthcare provider to test a patient for diabetes, including increased thirst or urination. Two laboratory tests are used to define and diagnose diabetes: fasting plasma glucose (FPG) and the two-hour oral glucose tolerance test (OGTT), during which a patient's glucose is measured two hours after drinking a 75-gram glucose solution. These tests can define diabetes in addition to impaired fasting glucose (IFG) and impaired glucose tolerance (IGT), "prediabetic" conditions associated with future risk of progression to T2DM. People with these conditions should institute lifestyle dietary and physical activity modification to prevent or delay the onset of T2DM.

COMPLICATIONS

The complications of T2DM are categorized as microvascular or macrovascular, according to the size of the blood vessels affected, and are the reason that diabetes is costly in terms of mortality and healthcare expenditures. Elevated glucose in the blood damages blood vessels and the organs to which they supply blood. The microvascular complications of diabetes include eye disease (retinopathy), kidney disease (nephropathy), and nerve disease (neuropathy). Diabetes is the top cause of blindness in adults in developed countries and of end-stage renal disease worldwide. The macrovascular complications of the disease include coronary artery disease and strokes, leading causes of mortality worldwide. Indeed, DM is considered to be a "risk equivalent" for coronary artery disease; that is, a diabetic is as likely to have a heart attack within 10 years as someone who has already had a heart attack. The nerve and vascular damage of diabetes also make it the leading cause of leg amputations in the United States.

The prevention of T2DM is thus an important public health initiative. Despite the significant genetic predisposition to T2DM, some cases of the disease can be prevented through lifestyle modification. The Nurses' Health Study in the United States showed that modifiable lifestyle factors associated with a lower incidence of T2DM include a BMI<25 kg/m², moderate physical activity at least 30 minutes per day, no smoking, and a diet high in fiber and polyunsaturated fat and low in *trans* fat and glycemic index. Randomized trials have shown that the risk of T2DM in those already at high risk for the disease (e.g., having impaired glucose tolerance), can be reduced with weight loss, increased physical activity and moderate calorie restriction such as a reduction of 250 to 500 calories per day.

The target of treatment for T2DM is glycemic control, or maintaining a diabetic's blood glucose levels within a normal range. The United Kingdom Prospective Diabetes Study (UKPDS) demonstrated the importance of glycemic control for reducing diabetic microvascular complications. There is less evidence to suggest that glycemic control reduces the risk of macrovascular complications like coronary artery disease, but the advantages for microvascular complications clearly make glycemic control an important therapeutic goal. Diabetics are encouraged to check their blood glucose at different times throughout the day and report these values to their healthcare provider for optimization of their medical regimen. To get an idea of a patient's overall glycemic control, physicians will check a hemoglobin A1c (HbA1c) level, a blood test correlated to the patient's glycemic control in the past three months. Normal HbA1c levels are ≤5.0 percent, but this percentage increases in diabetics. Diabetics should aim to keep their HbA1c levels below 7 percent, with dietary measures, physical activity, and medications.

Lifestyle modification is an essential component of the treatment of T2DM. Even modest weight loss can improve a type 2 diabetic's insulin sensitivity and improve HbA1c levels. This weight loss should be accomplished by reducing the total number of calories consumed daily with a diet rich in fruits, vegetables, whole grains, lean meats, and low-fat dairy products. Increased physical activity is also essential for weight loss and maintenance; the current recommendations from the National Institutes of Health call for 30 to 60 minutes per day of moderate intensity activity such as brisk walking. Maintaining adequate glycemic control with diet and exercise alone is rare in a diagnosed diabetic, and so medications are important adjuncts to lifestyle modification. There are several classes of oral diabetic medications, including the sulfonylureas, the biguanides such as metformin, the thiazolidinediones, the α-glucosidase inhibitors, and the meglitinides. Metformin is often the first-line agent for obese patients with T2DM, because it can cause a modest degree of weight loss. If one medication is insufficient for glycemic control, physicians may choose a combination regimen of two or more agents. Ultimately, some type 2 diabetics may require insulin if oral medications do not provide adequate glycemic control. Because type 2 diabetics often have other risk factors for heart disease, it is also important to aggressively treat their hypertension and high cholesterol, if present. Dietary education and routine eye and foot examination are also important components of diabetic health maintenance.

SEE ALSO: Diabetes; Diabetes Type 1.

BIBLIOGRAPHY. Christos Mantzoros, ed., *Obesity and Diabetes* (Humana Press, 2006); Sally M. Marshall and Allan Flyvbjerg, "Prevention and Early Detection of Vascular Complications of Diabetes," *British Medical Journal* (v.333/7566, 2006); Sarah Wild, et al., "Global Prevalence of Diabetes: Estimates for the Year 2000 and Projections for 2030," *Diabetes Care* (v.27, 2004).

JASON VASSY
WASHINGTON UNIVERSITY IN ST. LOUIS

Diabetic Eye Problems

One of the complications of diabetes mellitus (DM) is diabetic retinopathy, a disease of the retina or light-sensitive part of the eye. It is the most common cause of blindness in adults 20–74 years old in developed countries such as the United States. It is estimated that almost all type 1 diabetics and greater than 60 percent of type 2 diabetics have some degree of diabetic retinopathy after having DM for 20 years. About 20 percent of newly diagnosed type 2 diabetics have evidence of this condition at the time of diagnosis.

CLINICAL COURSE

The retinal changes of DM are readily seen through an ophthalmoscope. As in other locations such as the kidneys and legs, the hyperglycemia of diabetes damages small blood vessels in the retina. The first evidence of this damage is called nonproliferative retinopathy, seen as small red bulges in the vessels called microaneurysms. With time, less oxygen is delivered to the retina as a result of this vascular damage, and some areas of the retina may infarct. Patients may notice no change in vision during this early stage, although some visual acuity may be lost if the damage involves the macula, the area of the retina responsible

for the sharpest vision. New vessels grow in the retina to compensate for insufficient oxygen levels. This proliferative retinopathy can be seen on ophthalmologic examination as an overabundant number of small vessels. These new vessels can result in irreversible vision loss in two ways. They are fragile and prone to rupture, causing hemorrhage and scarring. These vessels can also contract and cause retinal detachment. In addition to retinopathy, diabetics are also more likely to get cataracts and glaucoma than the general population.

SCREENING, PREVENTION, TREATMENT

Because the damage is often irreversible by the time a person notices visual impairment, screening for diabetic retinopathy is important in the care of any diabetic patient. The American Diabetes Association (ADA) recommends that newly diagnosed type 2 diabetics receive a comprehensive dilated eye examination by an ophthalmologist at the time of diagnosis and then yearly thereafter. Type 1 diabetics should receive yearly eye examinations beginning three to five years after diagnosis and not usually before age 10. More frequent examinations are necessary if retinal damage is discovered.

Good glycemic control, as measured by blood glucose and hemoglobin A1c levels, is important in preventing the progression of diabetic retinopathy and preserving vision. Treating high blood pressure in diabetics, with drugs such as β-blockers or angiotensin-converting enzyme (ACE) inhibitors, has also been shown to slow the progression of retinopathy. Once retinopathy is seen on ophthalmologic examination, early treatment is necessary to prevent further loss of visual acuity. Standard treatment is laser photocoagulation, in which a laser is used to close or destroy the abnormal retinal vessels that are prone to rupture. While this procedure will not restore any vision that has already been lost, it has been shown to slow further vision loss. In the case of extensive damage or retinal detachment, a vitrectomy is performed, a surgical procedure in which the scar tissue and cloudy bloody fluid in the eye are removed. In the case of detachment, retinal reattachment can also be performed during a vitrectomy, although this is successful in only about half of cases.

SEE ALSO: Diabetes; Eye Diseases; Ophthalmology.

BIBLIOGRAPHY. American Diabetes Association, "Eye Complications," http://www.diabetes.org /type-2-diabetes/ eye-complications.jsp (cited June 2007); Donald S. Fong, et al., "Diabetic Retinopathy," *Diabetes Care* (v.26/1, 2003).

JASON VASSY
WASHINGTON UNIVERSITY IN ST. LOUIS

Diabetic Foot Problems

Foot disease is a prevalent complication of diabetes mellitus (DM) and is the most common cause of limb amputation in the United States. The lifetime risk of foot ulcers in DM is 15 to 25 percent and 5 percent of diabetics ultimately require amputation. Foot infections are now the leading cause of diabetes-related hospitalized days. Diabetic foot disease represents a significant cost for healthcare systems, much of which could be reduced through preventive measures.

The symptoms of diabetic foot disease include numbness and tingling in the feet that is worse at night. Foot infections manifest as redness, warmth, pain, and possibly pus around a foot ulcer. Diabetic foot disease develops for a number of reasons. Diabetic nerve dis-ease decreases the sensation in the feet and allows undetected injuries and improper foot placement during walking, which can lead to deformed foot joints and calluses. Diabetic nerve disease also decreases sweating in the feet, and the lack of moisture can predispose to cracking, which can introduce infection. Decreased blood flow to the foot also reduces oxygen delivery to the tissue of the foot, resulting in ulcers with slower healing. Certain bacteria and fungi thrive in the hyperglycemia of diabetes, and the immune response to these infections is impaired in diabetics. Fungal infections like athlete's foot can cause cracks in the feet, upon which bacterial infections can superimpose. Often beginning around the nails, infections can range in severity from local skin infection (cellulitis) to infection of the deep tissue and even bone (osteomyelitis) to irreversible death of tissue (gangrene).

Prevention with foot care is the most important intervention against diabetic foot disease. Diabetics should avoid tight-fitting shoes and may need insoles and special fitted shoes with extra depth and width. They should also wear loose-fitting cotton socks and avoid walking barefooted. The feet should be inspected daily, with a mirror if necessary, and care should be taken to avoid breaks in the skin during nail trimming, for example. The feet should be cleaned with lukewarm water and mild soap and patted dry. Diabetics should undergo yearly foot examinations by foot care specialists, including assessment of blood flow and neurologic function and inspection for ulcers and infection. Smoking cessation and tight glycemic control will slow the progression of foot disease.

Treatment of diabetic foot depends on its severity. Superficial ulcers may only require debridement (removal) of dead tissue, and superficial infections may respond to oral antibiotics. Detected by X-ray, magnetic resonance imaging (MRI), and/or bone biopsy, infection of deeper tissue or bone may require hospitalization for intravenous antibiotics, along with removal of the infected tissue and bone. Severe infections may spread to the bloodstream and cause major systemic illness. After the elimination of diabetic foot infections, relapses are common. Amputation of the leg either above or below the knee may be required for gangrene, from which the tissue will not recover. In other cases where diminished blood flow is the primary problem, vascular surgery may be able to restore blood flow to the leg.

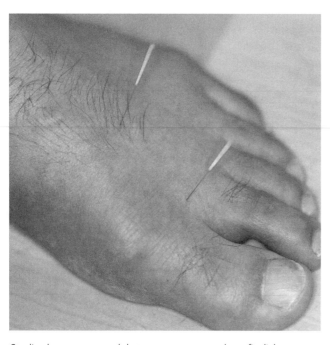

Studies have suggested that acupuncture may benefit diabetes patients with no adverse side effects.

SEE ALSO: Diabetes; Diabetes Type I (Juvenile); Diabetes Type II.

BIBLIOGRAPHY. Andrew Bolton, et al., "The Global Burden of Diabetic Foot Disease," *The Lancet* (v.366/9498, 2005); Benjamin Lipsky, "A Report from the International Consensus on Diagnosing and Treating the Infected Diabetic Foot," *Diabetes Metab Res Rev* (v.20/Suppl, 2004).

JASON VASSY
WASHINGTON UNIVERSITY IN ST. LOUIS

Diabetic Kidney Problems

Diabetes mellitus is the leading cause of kidney failure in the United States. Although the early stages of diabetic kidney disease, or diabetic nephropathy, are subtle and often go unnoticed, the disease can eventually result in end-stage renal disease (ESRD) requiring kidney transplantation or dialysis therapy. This potentially deadly complication of diabetes mellitus has grown to great public health significance, given the high cost of dialysis and the shortage of organ donations.

The U.S. Centers for Disease Control and Prevention (CDC) reported that 300,000 new cases of diabetic ESRD occurred in the United States in 2002. This absolute number continues to grow, although the proportion of diabetics who get ESRD seems to be declining. Still, ESRD treatment cost the United States Medicare system $25.2 billion in 2002. Diabetic nephropathy can occur with both type 1 and 2 diabetes mellitus, although it may occur earlier in life in type 1 diabetics, because their disease generally begins in childhood. Certain ethnic and racial groups are at greater risk for diabetic kidney disease, including African Americans and Mexican Americans. Differences in risk may be due to socioeconomic or genetic factors.

Diabetic nephropathy is considered one of the microvascular complications of diabetes mellitus, resulting from damage to small blood vessels including those in the kidneys. The high glucose levels of diabetes damage the blood vessels and kidney tissue itself, causing a gradual decline in kidney function. This microscopic damage can be seen by taking a biopsy of the kidney, although this invasive procedure is often not necessary for the diagnosis of diabetic nephropathy. The natural history of diabetic nephropathy is a gradual process that begins with albuminuria, a condition in which the kidneys leak more protein into the urine than normal, particularly the protein albumin. Normal urinary albumin excretion is less than 30 mg/day; albuminuria between 30 and 300 mg/day and greater than 300 mg/day is called microalbuminuria and macroalbuminuria (proteinuria), respectively. Microalbuminuria causes no symptoms and may already be present at the time that diabetes mellitus is diagnosed. Urinary albumin levels can be measured by using dipsticks tests on a single urine sample, by analyzing a patient's urine after a 24-hour collection period, or by testing the urinary ratio of albumin to creatinine, a waste product eliminated in the urine. With the worsening of kidney disease, microalbuminuria may progress to macroalbuminuria, which may in turn progress to an elevated creatinine level in the blood, representing the kidneys' inability to adequately remove this waste.

To track the progression of diabetic nephropathy, nephrologists, physicians who specialize in the kidney, follow a patient's blood creatinine levels and glomerular filtration rate (GFR), a measure of the kidneys' function. Kidney function may decline such that survival is not possible without kidney replacement therapy: dialysis or kidney transplant. About 2 percent of diabetics per year progress from macroalbuminuria to increased creatinine levels or ESRD. Once a person has macroalbuminuria, the median time to renal replacement therapy is 2.5 years.

The most effective way to prevent and treat diabetic nephropathy is through intensive glycemic control, measured by a patient's blood glucose levels and hemoglobin A1c (HbA1c) concentration. Treating high blood pressure in diabetics has also proven important to slow the progression of diabetic nephropathy, and the angiotensin-converting enzyme (ACE) inhibitors and angiotensin receptor blockers (ARB) are particularly effective drugs in decreasing diabetic albuminuria. Dietary protein restriction may also slow the progression of kidney disease. A patient who progresses to ESRD requires kidney transplantation or dialysis, a therapy whereby the patient's blood is cycled through a machine to remove the wastes normally filtered by the kidneys. Neither treatment is without its complications: kidney transplantation requires immunosuppressant drugs to prevent rejection of the new organ and dialysis is an invasive procedure often performed three times a week.

SEE ALSO: Dialysis; Kidney Failure and Dialysis.

BIBLIOGRAPHY. A. I. Adler, et al., "Development and Progression of Nephropathy in Type 2 Diabetes: The United Kingdom Prospective Diabetes Study (UKPDS 64)," *Kidney International* (v.63, 2003); U.S. Renal Data System, "USRDS 2004 Annual Data Report: Atlas of End-Stage Renal Disease in the United States, National Institutes of Health, National Institute of Diabetes and Digestive and Kidney Diseases, Bethesda, MD, 2004," *American Journal of Kidney Diseases* (v.45/Suppl 1, 2005).

Jason Vassy
Washington University in St. Louis

Diabetic Nerve Problems

The disease processes of diabetes mellitus cause injury to the nerves of the body. A common complication of long-standing diabetes mellitus is therefore diabetic neuropathy, a dysfunction of several of these nerves. Diabetes can affect nerves of a variety of functions and locations in the body. The most common example of diabetic neuropathy, however, is peripheral diabetic neuropathy, in which a loss of sensation first occurs in the most distal parts of the extremities, starting with the soles of the feet. Diabetics lose pain sensation in their feet and are thus unaware of small injuries to their feet, including minor sores from walking without shoes or from gravel in their shoes.

With time, these unnoticed ulcers can become infected, a process aided by the poor circulation and depressed immune function that diabetes brings. Without treatment, these infections may require limb amputation.

TYPES OF DIABETIC NEUROPATHY

Distal symmetric polyneuropathy, also known as peripheral neuropathy, is classically described as having a "stocking-glove" distribution. That is, the loss of sensation begins in the feet and, over time, progresses up to the knees before including the fingers. The loss of sensation is symmetric and includes the inability to detect pain, vibration, pressure, and joint position. In addition to the infected ulcers described above, peripheral neuropathy can also eventually result in deformed Charcot joints of the foot, because the feet do not appropriately sense and respond to the contour of the surface on which they walk. More rare, diabetics can experience painful diabetic neuropathy, characterized by burning, shooting, lightning-like pain in the legs.

A third type of diabetic nerve problem is diabetic autonomic neuropathy. The autonomic nervous system controls numerous bodily functions, such as circulation, respiration, digestion, and reproduction. Diabetic autonomic neuropathy, therefore, can manifest in many ways, including gastrointestinal and genitourinary dysfunction, rapid heartbeat, and lightheadedness on standing due to a drop in blood pressure. In addition to sensory and autonomic nerves, diabetes mellitus can also damage motor nerves, nerves that control muscle contraction. Diabetic motor neuropathy can be asymmetrical and may occur in locations such as the limbs and the muscles that control eye movements.

CLINICAL ASPECTS OF DIABETIC NEUROPATHY

Diabetic neuropathy may affect as many as 10 percent of diabetics, and its risk increases with poorer glucose control. The precise cause of diabetic nerve damage is not clear, although the high blood glucose levels and poor blood flow that are characteristics of diabetes mellitus are most likely involved. There are many other nondiabetic causes of neuropathies, and a physician must rule these out before diagnosing diabetic neuropathy. Nevertheless, the diagnosis must always be considered in a known diabetic patient, and all diabetics should receive routine neurological examinations.

Noninvasive diagnostic tests for diabetic neuropathy include the basic neurological examination that tests the motor function and sensation to pinprick, vibration, and temperature. Evidence of autonomic neuropathy is detected by monitoring changes in blood pressure and heart rate difference between sitting and standing. Definitive diagnosis requires further testing such as nerve conduction studies and nerve and skin biopsies. As with most other complications of diabetes, the best treatment for diabetic neuropathy is glycemic control, keeping the blood glucose level low through diet and/or treatment with oral diabetes medications or insulin. Reducing hyperglycemia decreases an individual's chance of getting diabetic neuropathy. Painful diabetic neuropathy can be treated symptomatically with tricyclic antidepressants and antiseizure medications such as phenytoin, gabapentin, and carbamazepine.

SEE ALSO: Diabetes;Diabetic Foot; Neurology.

BIBLIOGRAPHY. V. Bansal, J. Kalita, and U. K. Misra, "Diabetic Neuropathy," *Postgraduate Medical Journal* (v.82, 2006).

JASON VASSY
WASHINGTON UNIVERSITY IN ST. LOUIS

Diabetic Teeth and Gum Problems

Both type 1 and type 2 diabetes mellitus (DM) are associated with a higher prevalence of periodontitis, an infection of the gums and the tooth-supporting bones and ligaments of the mouth. Its symptoms include redness, swelling, and pain around the teeth, in addition to loose teeth. The disease progression includes the development of plaques between the teeth and gums, infection of the gums (gingivitis) when bacteria multiply in the plaque, and finally destruction of the tissue supporting the teeth, eventually resulting in tooth loss. About 50 percent of the U.S. adult population may have gingivitis, manifested as bleeding gums, while at least 14 percent have moderate to severe periodontitis. Although infection with oral bacteria is necessary for periodontitis, other risk factors must be present for the disease to progress. Smoking and poorly controlled DM are its major modifiable risk factors. The National Health and Nutrition Examination Survey (NHANES) III found the prevalence of periodontitis to be 17.3 percent in adult diabetics compared to 9 percent in nondiabetics. Moreover, diabetics experience earlier and more severe periodontitis than nondiabetics, and diabetics with poorer glycemic control have worse periodontal disease than well-controlled diabetics. Studies have shown no difference between diabetics and nondiabetics, however, in their response rates to the treatment of periodontitis, which consists at first of mechanical scraping and antibiotic therapy such as tetracycline or doxycycline.

DM may increase the likelihood of periodontal infections for a number of reasons. The diabetic damage to blood vessels impairs oxygen delivery to tissues, which creates a favorable environment for the growth of certain bacteria. This vascular damage also impedes the delivery of immune cells, which already have decreased function due to DM, to sites of infections. Diabetics have impaired production of collagen, a necessary protein for proper tooth attachment. DM is also associated with a higher rate of xerostomia, or dry mouth due to decreased saliva production, which may promote the progression of infection in plaques.

An alternative or complementary explanation is that some individuals may have genetic predispositions to both DM and periodontitis. An interesting idea is that periodontal disease itself may worsen diabetes. Inflammatory molecules (cytokines) released from periodontal pockets of infection may interfere with insulin and glucose metabolism. There is evidence to suggest that periodontitis may worsen glycemic control in diabetics. Additionally, temporary improvement in glycemic control has been reported after treatment of periodontitis with antibiotics.

Good oral hygiene, including brushing, flossing, and routine dental care with the removal of plaque, is important for the prevention of periodontitis in diabetics and nondiabetics alike. Gingivitis usually responds to these measures also, but more advanced periodontitis may require the surgical removal of infected tissue. Systemic antibiotics like tetracycline or doxycycline may also be administered. As with most complications of DM, good glycemic control is important and may reduce the severity of periodontitis in diabetics.

SEE ALSO: Diabetes; Diabetes Type I (Juvenile); Diabetes Type II.

BIBLIOGRAPHY. I.B Bender, A.B Bender, "Diabetes Mellitus and the Dental Pulp," *Journal of Endodontics* (v.29/6, 2003); W.A. Soskolne, A. Klinger, "The Relationship between Periodontal Diseases and Diabetes: An Overview." *Annals of Periodontology.* (v.6/1, 2001).

Jason Vassy
Independent Scholar

Diagnostic Imaging

Diagnostic imaging is the use of X-ray, ultrasound, radioactive isotopes, or magnetic resonance to generate graphical images of the inside of the human body for diagnostic purposes. More than 90 percent of all imaging can be performed using basic X-ray equipment and/or simple ultrasound machines.

Diagnostic imaging is a prerequisite for the appropriate and successful treatment of at least a quarter of all patients worldwide. The use of diagnostic imaging is justified when needed to exclude disease, to prove the existence of a pathological process needing treatment, to assist in planning of treatment, or to follow the course of a disease already diagnosed and/or treated. Diagnostic imaging makes proper treatment possible. Without such examinations, it can be more difficult for clinicians to determine appropriate treatment. For example, reports from some countries indicate that a significant portion of all abdominal surgical interventions (explorative laparotomy) may have been avoided if simple diagnostic imaging services such as ultrasound had been available. Because effective diagnostic imaging can reduce unnecessary procedures, diagnostic imaging services should be developed as an integral part of national healthcare systems. It should be planned according to country, region, or area needs, and the local social and economic structure.

X-RAYS

X-rays (radiographs) are the most common and widely available diagnostic imaging technique. Even if more sophisticated tests are needed, an X-ray is often first approached. The part of the body being pictured is positioned between the X-ray machine and photographic film, while electromagnetic waves (radiation) travel through the patient's body. Sometimes, to make certain organs stand out the patient is asked to drink or be injected with barium sulfate or a dye.

COMPUTED TOMOGRAPHY (CT) SCANS

A CT scan is a modern imaging tool that combines X-rays with computer technology to produce a more detailed, cross-sectional image of the body. A CT scan allows a doctor see the size, shape, and position of structures that are deep inside the body, such as organs, tissues, or tumors. An X-ray tube slowly rotates around the patient, taking many pictures from all directions. A computer combines the images to produce a clear, two-dimensional view on a television screen. CT scans are used when there are problems with a small, bony structure or if there is severe trauma to the brain, spinal cord, chest, abdomen, or pelvis. As with a regular X-ray, sometimes barium sulfate or a dye is used to make certain parts of the body show up better. A CT scan costs more and takes more time than a regular X-ray, and it is not always available in small hospitals and rural areas.

MAGNETIC RESONANCE IMAGING (MRI)

MRI is another modern diagnostic imaging technique that produces cross-sectional images of the body. Unlike CT scans, MRI works without radiation. The MRI tool uses magnetic fields and a sophisticated computer to take high-resolution pictures of bones and soft tissues. The MRI creates a magnetic field around the patient and then pulses radio waves to the area of the patient's body to be pictured. The radio waves cause tissues to resonate. A computer records the rate at which body's various parts (tendons, ligaments, nerves, etc.) give off these vibrations, and translates the data into a detailed, two-dimensional picture. An MRI may help doctors to diagnose torn knee ligaments and cartilage, torn rotator cuffs, herniated disks, hip and pelvic problems, and other problems. An MRI may take 30 to 90 minutes, and is not available at all hospitals.

ULTRASOUND

Medical ultrasonography uses high-frequency sound waves of between 2.0 to 10.0 MHz that are reflected by tissue to varying degrees to produce a two-dimensional image, traditionally on a television monitor. This is often used to visualize the fetus in pregnant women. Other important uses include imaging the abdominal organs, heart, male genitalia, and the veins of the leg. While it may provide less anatomical information than techniques such as CT or MRI, it has several advantages that make it ideal as a first-line test in numerous situations, in particular that it studies the function of moving structures in real time. It is also very safe to use, as the patient is not exposed to radiation and is also relatively cheap and quick to perform. Ultrasound scanners can be taken to critically ill patients in intensive care units, avoiding the danger caused while moving the patient to the radiology department. The real-time moving image obtained can be used to guide drainage and biopsy procedures. Doppler capabilities on modern scanners allow the blood flow in arteries and veins to be assessed.

ELECTRON MICROSCOPY

The electron microscope is a microscope that can magnify very small details with high resolving power because of the use of electrons as the source of illumination. Its usefulness has been greatly reduced by immunohistochemistry, but it is still irreplaceable for the diagnosis of kidney disease, identification of immotile cilia syndrome, and many other tasks.

CHALLENGES IN DEVELOPING COUNTRIES

There are many challenges in diagnostic imaging in developing countries. Mainly, there is a severe lack of safe and appropriate diagnostic imaging services (i.e., basic X-ray and ultrasound) in large parts of the world. Imaging facilities are simply not available or not functioning. The lack of equipment could be due to lack of resources or poor maintenance of existing equipment (also linked to lack of available parts). Additionally, in many countries a large number of images are of poor quality and are of no diagnostic use. However, even if proper equipment is available, there is a lack of adequately trained medical specialists including radiographers/technologists. Inadequate training means a lack of qualified personnel, and improper use of equipment as well as incorrect interpretation of images. Finally, regardless of the type of equipment and procedures used, diagnostic imaging requires a rigid infrastructure that often does not exist in developing countries. This infrastructure includes trained medical, technical, and engineering staff; radiation protection measurements; regulations; reliable supplies of clean water, electric power, spare parts and consumables; and adequate air-quality control.

The goal of the World Health Organization (WHO) working area for diagnostic imaging is to make safe and reliable diagnostic imaging services available to as many as possible, advise and support those working in the field developing and maintaining diagnostic imaging services, and promote the importance of safe and appropriate diagnostic imaging services. WHO suggests that diagnostic imaging services should be developed as an integral part of national healthcare systems, according to the needs and social and economic structure of the country, region, and area. It also suggests that the services be regulated by governments in accordance with international standards appropriate to the level of the healthcare system at which they are provided and appropriate to the therapeutic capabilities that are available.

In addition to close collaboration with various United Nations agencies, and especially with the International Atomic Energy Agency (IAEA) in Vienna, various WHO collaborating centers, and nongovernmental organizations, the most important global collaboration takes place in the Global Steering Group for Education and Training in Diagnostic Imaging. This group was officially established after a WHO meeting on Training and Education in Diagnostic Imaging held in Geneva, Switzerland, May 31–June 3, 1999, and the overall objective of this group is to try to coordinate various training activities organized by international and regional societies, and join forces to improve quality, quantity, and equity of diagnostic imaging services worldwide, but with strong emphasis on countries in most need.

SEE ALSO: Back Injuries; Fractures; Kidney Diseases (General); Pregnancy; World Health Organization (WHO).

BIBLIOGRAPHY. R. M. Califf, "Evaluation of Diagnostic Imaging Technologies and Therapeutics Devices: Better Information for Better Decisions: Proceedings of a Multidisciplinary Workshop," *American Heart Journal* (v.152/1, 2006); S. Demeter, "Socioeconomic Status and the Utilization of Diagnostic Imaging in an Urban Setting," *Canadian Medical Association Journal* (v.173/10, 2005); "Diagnostic Imaging Still Threatened by Shortages," *Lancet Oncology* (v.5/6, 2004); Lee Goldman, ed., *Cecil Textbook of Medicine*, 22nd ed. (Saunders, 1999); John Noble, *Textbook of Primary Care Medicine*, 3rd ed. (Mosby, 2000).

Barkha Gurbani
UCLA School of Medicine

Diagnostic Tests

Diagnostic tests are used by healthcare workers to help determine the presence or absence of a disease or other health condition. Diagnostic tests can be grouped into two basic categories: medical or psychological. Within these two categories, there are many subsets of tests, used for a variety of purposes. The effectiveness and reliability of a diagnostic test is an important factor that must be taken into consideration when interpreting results. An accurate test is the best means to a proper diagnosis.

The term *diagnostic test* can be misleading, because there are many reasons for using them beyond making an initial diagnosis. For example, diagnostic tests may also further define the illness, such as a cancer subtype.

A more specific diagnosis may help guide the most effective treatment protocol and can also monitor treatment effectiveness. Psychological diagnostic tests may also be used to assist in prognosis by referring to longitudinal data of outcomes of patient with similar diagnoses.

QUALITY AND EFFECTIVENESS

The quality and effectiveness of a diagnostic test is often measured by its accuracy. The accuracy of a test can be evaluated through four basic factors: sensitivity, specificity, positive, and negative predictive values. The sensitivity of a test is the probability that the test results reveal accurate diagnosis of an existing disease. The sensitivity is the proportion of accurate diagnoses correctly identified by the test. The specificity of a test is the probability that the test results will accurately identify individuals without the targeted disease. The positive predictive value of a test measures the percentage of individuals with a positive test result who actually have the disease. The negative predictive value measures the percentage of individuals with a negative test that do not have the disease.

TYPES OF MEDICAL TESTS

Analysis of body fluids commonly includes of tests of the blood, urine, as well as the fluid surrounding the spinal cord and brain (cerebrospinal fluid). Less commonly, fluids such as sweat, saliva, or fluid from the digestive tract are assessed. Body fluid analysis can be used for many different purposes, including determining whether a person has an infection to determining whether a person has cystic fibrosis. Imaging provides a picture of the inside of the body. The most common test in this category is the X-ray. Some other commonly used examples are ultrasound, radioisotope (nuclear) scans, computed tomography (CT) scans, magnetic resonance imaging (MRI), and positron emission tomography (PET) scans. The test is selected based on what the examiner is wishing to determine, and the cost of each exam varies considerably.

Endoscopy is a test that looks inside the body. An endoscope is a long flexible tube that has a camera and light inside it, permitting a physician to view images on a monitor during the procedure. An endoscope may be passed through the mouth to look at the esophagus or stomach (esophagogastroduodenoscopy), or can be passed through the rectum to look in the large intestine (colonoscopy). A newer endoscopic test consists of swallowing an extremely small capsule that contains a camera, and that takes pictures, permitting observation of areas without use of anesthesia.

Measurement of body functions involves documenting and analyzing the different activity levels of different organs. For example, an electrocardiogram (ECG) records the electrical impulses of the heart at rest and an electroencephalogram (EEG) records the electrical changes of the brain during mental activity or rest. Biopsy involves removing a sample of tissue for examination. Only small samples are required because the examination is commonly done with a microscope. Common biopsy areas include skin, breast, lung, liver, kidney, intestine, and bone.

Analysis of genetic material includes testing skin, blood, or bone marrow cells, and focuses on abnormalities of chromosomes and/or genes. DNA analysis is a component of gene analysis. Genetic testing is used with both children and adults to determine whether a disease is present, or if there is an increased risk of a disease. Genetic testing can also be done with individuals to determine the likelihood that a particular disease will be passed to their offspring.

PSYCHOLOGICAL TESTING

Psychological testing can be measured through several formats. Norm-referenced tests (NRTs) compare a person's score against the scores of people who have already taken the same exam, called the norming group. Groups can be normed by age, ethnicity,

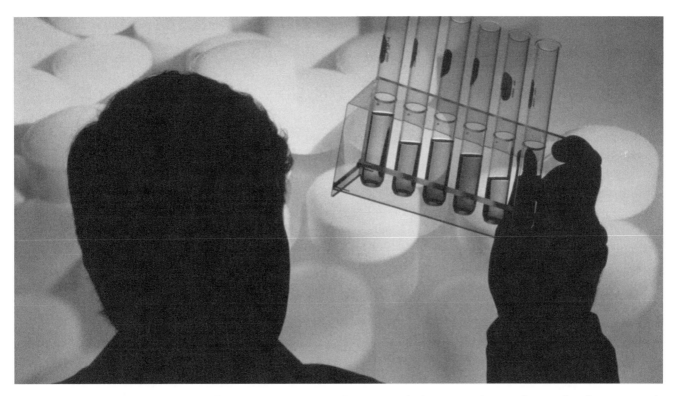

Body fluid analysis can be used for many different purposes, including determining whether a person has an infection. The effectiveness and reliability of a diagnostic test must be taken into consideration when interpreting results.

or disability. Criterion referenced tests compare an individual's performance to a level of mastery. When reviewing test results, it is important to understand that most tests are standardized, meaning there are detailed instructions for administering the test, which requires specialized training in administration and scoring. This ensures the test is administered the same way to every individual, permitting comparison of results. Standardization is important because it affects the reliability and predictability of the test. The reliability of a test refers to how accurately the test measures some trait.

In other words, if an individual is given a particular test at two different times several days apart, if environmental factors are similar, the individual should obtain similar scores. If the scores differ significantly from one session to the next, the test is not reliable. The validity of a test refers to the ability of the test to measure what it claims to measure. For example, the validity of an IQ test is based on how accurately it measures components of intelligence.

Psychological and psycho-educational tests are another category of diagnostic tests. They provide an avenue to identify and measure characteristics of an individual to norms based on age or behavior.

Intelligence Tests. Intelligence tests are designed to measure a variety of mental functions including reasoning, comprehension, and judgment. They are used to obtain an idea of a person's intellectual potential, and also to assess areas of brain dysfunction, such as in attention, memory, or visual perception. Intelligence tests are comprised of multiple subtests, which include verbal and nonverbal components. Intelligence tests are viewed as excellent predictors of academic achievement and provide a clearer picture of mental strengths and weaknesses.

Intelligence tests can be categorized into two groups. Group intelligence tests are frequently used as screening assessment of "giftedness." Commonly used tests in this category are the Otis-Lennon School Ability Test (OLSAT) and the Iowa Cognitive Abilities Test (COGAT). Individual tests of intelligence differ from group tests because they have more subtests and allow the administrator to vary the level of difficulty based on the individual's initial performance. They also allow prompting if the individual's answer is unclear. The most widely used intelligence tests are the Stanford-Binet, the Wechsler Intelligence Scale for Children (WISC), the Wechsler Adult Intelligence Scale (WAIS), and the Kaufman Assessment Battery for Children (Kaufman-ABC). The standardization and norming of these tests provide a uniform method to compare individual performance with a peer group. Intelligence testing is one of the primary tools for diagnosing children with mental retardation and learning disabilities.

Academic Tests. Academic tests are used to measure skills such as reading, spelling, vocabulary, arithmetic, and writing, and can be administered in group or individual format. Group testing is commonly done in the school system, where students are tested at a particular grade level. Scores are standardized, and can be used to compare academic achievement within the same grade locally as well as nationally. These include the Comprehensive Tests of Basic Skills (CTBS) or the Iowa Tests of Basic Skills. Individually administered achievement tests are used more frequently to help identify concerns in specific academic areas. Individual achievement tests differ from group tests because they provide flexibility to adjust degree of testing difficulty to individual level of achievement, and may also allow for prompting. Both types of tests can be used to help identify intellectual giftedness or learning disabilities, by looking for discrepancies between IQ score and components of the achievement scores.

Assessment of Personality. Personality tests can be separated into two categories and are designed to evaluate an individual's thoughts, emotions, attitudes, and behavioral traits. The first category is objective testing, which includes testing via inventories questionnaires, self-report measures, and rating scales. Some frequently used instruments in this category are the Minnesota Multiphasic Personality Inventory-Adolescent (MMPI-A), the Behavior Assessment Scale for Children (BASC), and the Beck Depression Inventory (BDI). The second category of personality assessment is projective testing. This category utilizes ambiguous stimuli open for individual interpretation. The focus of this type of testing is that an individual's reactions or responses to ambiguity will mirror facets of their personality. Projective drawing, storytelling, and inkblots are frequently used types of tests.

Neuropsychological Tests. Neuropsychological testing is often used to diagnose and monitor brain damage and dysfunction. A comprehensive assessment measures various aspects of cognitive functioning, including intelligence, attention and concentration, verbal and visual memory, language functioning, visual spatial functioning, motor abilities, sensory-perceptual processing, abstract reasoning, executive functioning (e.g., planning, self-monitoring, inhibition of impulses, and mental flexibility), and academic functioning.

Some widely used neuropsychological tests are the Luria-Nebraska, and the Halstead-Reitan. Measures such as these enable neuropsychologists to isolate and diagnose organic brain impairment. It can also assist in the development of rehabilitation programs for cognitively impaired patients.

Diagnostic tests address a broad spectrum in areas of medical and mental health. Validity and reliability are essential components of assessing diagnostic tests results. In other words, diagnostic tests should be able to identify between patients who have a particular health condition from those who do not have the health condition. In addition, diagnostics tests are helpful because they can be used to measure various stages of a disease and monitor the efficacy of different treatments.

SEE ALSO: Attention Deficit Disorders; Bladder Diseases; Bleeding Disorders; Biomarkers; Bipolar Disorder; Cancer; Child Development; Genetic Testing/Counseling.

BIBLIOGRAPHY. *A Lawyer's Guide to Psychological Assessment of Adolescents* (National Juvenile Defenders Center, U.S. Department of Justice, 2003): L. Aiken, *Psychological Testing & Assessment* (Allyn & Bacon, 2005); H. S. Levin, "A Guide to Clinical Neuropsychological Testing," *Archives of Neurology* (v.51/9, 1994); E. Benson, "Psychologists Are Broadening the Concept of Intelligence and How to Test It," *Monitor on Psychology* (v.34/2, 2003); Jerome M. Sattler, *Assessment of Children: Behavioral and Clinical Applications*, 4th ed. (Jerome M. Sattler, 2002).

GAUTAM J. DESAI, D.O.
ELIZABETH K. MCCLAIN, ED.S.
KANSAS CITY UNIVERSITY OF MEDICINE AND
BIOSCIENCES COLLEGE OF OSTEOPATHIC MEDICINE

Dialysis

Dialysis is a means of preserving one's life. It is the act of an external machine performing the function of an internal organ. When the kidneys are no longer able to filter waste products from the body, concentrate urine, or preserve electrolytes (minerals in one's blood and body fluid that affect many important aspects of normal balance in the body), then an individual is said to be in kidney failure, or renal failure. Dialysis is a cure for renal failure for many individuals. There are two types of dialysis techniques: peritoneal dialysis and hemodialysis. Peritoneal dialysis works by circulating a solution through the fluids of the abdomen. Hemodialysis works by circulating one's blood through a special machine that contains special filters to remove waste products.

Renal failure occurs when the kidneys fail to excrete harmful waste products. This may occur suddenly, acutely, or over a period of time, chronically, which may eventually lead to or end-stage renal disease (ESRD), which is a complete dysfunction of the kidneys. The etiologies of the two disease process are vast ranging from hereditary disorders to lifestyle choices. Dialysis is a treatment modality typically used to treat chronic renal failure. Diabetes and hypertension are the two most common causes of chronic renal failure and ESRD.

Peritoneal dialysis involves the use of a catheter, a soft tube. The tube is used to fill the abdomen with a dialysis solution which contains dextrose, a sugar that will pull wastes and extra fluid from the blood into the abdominal cavity, where the solution is present. The dialysis solution and the waste products from the blood are then drained out of the body via the catheter. This process of filling the abdomen and then draining it is called an exchange and takes approximately 30 to 40 minutes. The process of allowing the solution to remain the abdomen is called the dwell time, which takes approximately four to six hours. A typical regimen consists of four exchanges a day each with a dwell time four to six hours.

Hemodialysis utilizes a dialysis machine. The patient's blood is sent to the machine through what is known as a vascular access. A vascular access is a means for blood to travel from the patient, to the machine, and back to the patient. An access is surgically constructed and consists of three different subtypes: primary AV fistula, synthetic AV graft (bridge graft), and a central venous catheter. A primary AV fistula is the preferred type of vascular access. A connection (fistula) is created between an artery (A) and a vein (V) usually in the lower arm under the skin. This allows the insertion of small needles into the fistula and the flow of blood to and from the machine. The second type of access is the synthetic AV graft, or bridge graft. This method is used when a patient's arteries or veins are not able to create a fistula. In this situation, a plastic tube, graft, is used to construct a connection between the artery and vein. This tube is placed under the skin and is used similarly to an AV fistula. The third type of access is a central venous catheter. This route is performed in a more acute setting, when dialysis must be done immediately and the patient is devoid of a fistula, a graft or if a patient presents with nonfunctioning AV fistulas or grafts. Access is accomplished through placing a tube into a large vein in the neck. After the blood is collected from the body, it undergoes transformations by the dialysis machine. The machine allows contact between the patient's blood and a solution called dialysate through a membrane, which is a special filter. On one side of the membrane is the dialysate and on the other is the patient's blood. The toxic substances present in the blood shift from the blood, where it is in high concentration, to the dialysate, where it is in lower concentration or not present. This equalizes the concentration of the various substances. This method is more efficient than the natural kidneys and thus treatment is only needed intermittently. A typical regimen would include three to four hour sessions, three times a week.

SEE ALSO: Kidney Failure and Dialysis; Kidney Diseases (General).

BIBLIOGRAPHY. Thomas Golper, "Continuous Renal Replacement Therapies: An Overview," UpToDate, utdol.org (Cited September 2006); M. Manns, et al., "Continuous Renal Replacement Therapies: An Update," *American Journal of Kidney Disease* (v.32/185, 1998); R.L. Mehta, "Continuous Renal Replacement Therapy in the Critically Ill Patient," *Kidney International* (v.67:781, 2005,); P.M. Palevsky, "Dialysis Modality and Dosing Strategy in Acute Renal Failure," *Semin Dial.* (v.19/165, 2006).

Angela J. Garner, M.D.
University of Missouri–Kansas City
School of Medicine

Diarrhea

This year, over one billion people around the world will suffer from diarrhea. The disease is particularly prevalent in the developing world, where a combination of poor sanitation practices and limited access to clean drinking water act together to spread many causative organisms. Diarrhea is often ignored as a routine irritation of the gastrointestinal system, but it can rapidly progress to cause profound and life-threatening dehydration, especially in children.

According to the World Health Organization (WHO), 500 million children worldwide have at least one episode of diarrhea every year. Two million of these children die, making it the second most common cause of childhood death after respiratory infections. In fact, 20 percent of all childhood deaths (under 5 years old) are caused by diarrhea-induced dehydration, making it a leading concern for global healthcare practitioners.

CAUSES

Diarrhea, defined as excessively liquid or frequent evacuation of feces, can be caused by numerous conditions. Infectious diseases make up the vast majority of causative factors, although diarrhea can also be caused by contaminated food, as a medication side effect (particularly antibiotics), as a symptom of colorectal cancer, and as a sign of hormonal abnormalities.

Infectious organisms causing diarrhea include viruses (*rotavirus* being the most common), bacteria (e.g., *E. coli*), and parasites (e.g., *Giardia*). The gastrointestinal system, particularly the small and large intestines, are naturally populated by hundreds of different strains of nonharmful bacteria, many of which help with digestion. Infectious diarrhea can be caused either when a harmful, nonnative, biological agent colonizes the intestines or when one particular strain of native bacteria is favored over the others and takes over. This second pathway is exemplified by cases of bacterial overgrowth following the administration of antibiotics. The ingested antibiotics kill off most of the natural bacterial "flora" of the gut allowing a single disease causing variety to take over and proliferate.

The principle pathway of infectious diarrhea however, occurs through the spread of dangerous organisms through the environment. Infected individuals without access to latrines or a safe sanitation system inadvertently contaminate their own supply of water, spreading the disease to other members of their communities and creating a cycle of illness. Even with access to a clean water supply, organisms in improperly disposed of human waste can be spread to food by "vectors" like mosquitoes and other insects.

SYMPTOMS

Diarrhea by itself is often ignored by patients and considered by many to be a temporary nuisance. However, it is important to distinguish associated symptoms that indicate a more serious condition. Fever, abdominal pain, blood or mucous in the stool, nausea, and vomiting are all reasons to seek urgent medical attention. If the nausea and vomiting are severe, the patient's ability to maintain wellhydrated is at risk.

Dehydration is the biggest danger to deal with during severe episodes of diarrhea. Signs and symptoms of dehydration include lethargy, weakness, sunken eyes, an increased heart rate (greater than 110 beats per minute for a 5-year-old), and decreased urine output.

Chronic low-level diarrhea may also lead to malnutrition in children, who are unable to absorb the nutrients they need for normal growth and development.

TREATMENT AND PREVENTION

The main treatment of diarrhea is rehydration therapy, either oral or intravenous. Oral fluids should be provided to the patient in a slow and steady manner, 15 ml per 15 minutes. In the 1960s, scientists invented oral rehydration salts (ORS), comprised of sugar, sodium, and other electrolytes, which are added to water to increase the intestinal absorption of the fluid. ORS saw their first widespread use in Bangladesh after the refugee crisis resulting from the 1971 India-Pakistan war. Since then, they have become widely available throughout the developing world and the therapy is thought to have saved millions of children's lives. ORS is available for purchase in sachets manufactured under the supervision of the WHO and the United Nations Children's Fund (UNICEF). Caregivers can also be taught the following simple home recipe to make a similar solution at home: one liter of water, one fist of sugar, and one pinch of salt. Oral rehydration should continue until the diarrhea runs its natural course. Children who cannot tolerate oral intake due to nausea and vomiting should be hospitalized for intravenous fluid therapy.

Mothers should continue feeding their children during diarrhea episodes. The diet should include breast milk for breastfeeding infants, or bananas, rice, and lentils for children used to solid food. The diet should be advanced slowly, and fluid hydration should be prioritized over solid foods.

In rare cases, antibiotics may be required to treat certain strains of bacterial diarrhea. The decision to use antibiotics and the choice of agent should be left to a health practitioner, whose decision can be guided by an in-depth history of the illness and laboratory analysis (stool culture, stool analysis for ova and parasites, etc.).

The majority of diarrhea episodes can be prevented via personal and public sanitation practices. Individuals should wash their hands after using the bathroom and before cooking and eating. Where municipal water is unavailable, water should be boiled or filtered. Municipal governments can prevent diarrhea by providing a clean supply of water and by building public latrines.

Despite the consensus regarding diarrhea prevention and the ready availability of ORS, diarrhea remains a leading cause of child mortality in the developing world. Unhygienic bathroom practices and a limited access to clean water account for the continued prevalence. ORS is still used by caregivers only about 50 percent of the time to treat diarrhea.

Diarrhea prevention should include increasing access to safe water, improved hygiene, and ORS promotion. The idea must be made clear to target populations that ORS is a treatment for dehydration, not diarrhea, and that it should be used as long as the diarrhea persists.

In recent years, research has focused on developing a vaccine for rotavirus (two vaccines, rotateq and rotarix, are currently in clinical trials), which could prevent 500,000 child deaths and 2 million hospitalizations a year.

SEE ALSO: Constipation; Digestive Diseases; Drinking Water; E. Coli Infections; Giardia Infections; Infectious Diseases; Nausea and Vomiting; Travel Medicine; Traveler's Health.

BIBLIOGRAPHY. David A. Ahlquist and Michael Camilleri, "Diarrhea and Constipation," in *Harrison's Principles of Internal Medicine*, 15th ed. (McGraw-Hill Professional, 2001); Centers for Disease Control and Prevention, Richard E. Frye "Diarrhea," eMedicine, www.emedicine.com, (Cited February 2006). The Rehydration Project; www.reydrate.org; World Health Organization; www.who.int/topics/diarrhoea/en.

AMIT CHANDRA, MD, M.SC.
NEW YORK HOSPITAL QUEENS

Diesel Exhaust

At no point in human history have more humans been more exposed to air pollution than today. Rapid industrialization and urbanization are spreading this phenomenon across the globe affecting billions of people. The combustion of fossil fuels in many types of industrial and vehicular sources is responsible for the release of carbon monoxide, sulfur dioxide, nitrogen oxides, benzene, and particulate matter, among other emissions, into the environment. Most of these compounds have been shown to adversely affect human health. However, diesel vehicles and the diesel exhaust particles (DEP) they produce have been recognized as the most significant single contributors to the initiation and exacerbation of allergic airway disease and play a role in the progression of many other respiratory conditions as well.

Diesel engines are preferred because of their energy efficiency and endurance, and with rising fuel prices, they constitute an ever-increasing proportion of vehicular systems, particularly trucks and buses. Unfortunately, even new, cleaner burning diesel engines emit more gaseous fumes and up to 100 times more particular matter than nondiesel engines. As a result, diesel vehicles are the largest single source of airborne particulates worldwide.

Epidemiologic, human challenge, animal, and molecular studies have all shown a significant relationship between various types of air pollution and a myriad of respiratory and cardiovascular conditions. Gaseous (ozone and nitrogen dioxide) as well as particulate pollutants (DEP) have been shown to exacerbate asthma and chronic obstructive pulmonary disease, cause bronchitis, and lead to the slowing of children's lung development. They are also associated with higher rates of heart attacks and hospitalizations for heart problems. In addition, dramatic increases in allergic rhinitis and asthma that affect tens of million of people have been linked with DEP produced by diesel vehicles.

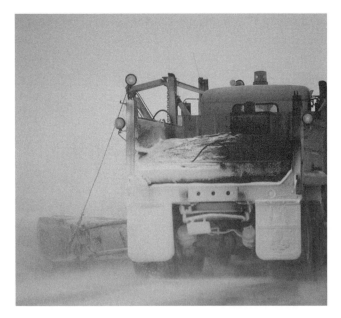

Diesel engines constitute an ever-increasing proportion of vehicular systems, particularly in trucks and buses.

Diesel exhaust particles created by the combustion of diesel fuels consist of tiny grains of carbon dust covered in many different types of toxic chemicals and metals. The sizes of the particles vary and determine where they become trapped in the lungs. Depending on where they land, the particles then cause inflammation of both the upper and lower airways. The mechanism of this inflammation is thought to be by a combination of induction of oxidative stress and irritation causing the aggregation and activation of inflammatory cells and release of cytokines (mediators of inflammation). In patients suffering from allergic disease, the particles lead to increased allergic antibody production and the augmentation of allergic sensitization.

Studies have found that children who live or play near freeways are more likely to have wheezing or severe asthma and are more likely to be hospitalized for asthma than children who do not. They are also more likely to suffer from atopy—the constellation of asthma, allergic dermatitis (eczema), and allergic rhinitis (hay fever). These effects have been confirmed in animal studies and other groups of people who are exposed to diesel pollutants as part of their jobs. It has been found that some of the symptoms of these conditions improve when the exposure to DEP pollutants is terminated. Other chronic effects of the pollution are

permanent. Some individuals are more susceptible to the effects of air pollution and diesel exhaust, but in all people, the effects are exacerbated and amplified by activities such as cigarette or cigar smoking.

Due to the constant increase in the production of and exposure to DEP, the population health effects of diesel exhaust will only become more pronounced with time. Policy and legislation are needed to regulate DEP and prevent exposure. Further research is also needed to better define which type of DEP are most dangerous, who are most vulnerable to the effects, and how the consequences of DEP can best be treated.

SEE ALSO: Pollution.

BIBLIOGRAPHY. D. Diaz-Sanchez and M. Riedl, "Diesel Effects on Human Health: A Question of Stress?" *American Journal of Physiology. Lung Cellular and Molecular Physiology* (v.289, 2005); D. Diaz-Sanchez and M. Riedl, "Biology of Diesel Exhaust Effects on Respiratory Function," *Journal of Allergy and Clinical Immunology* (v.115/2, 2005).

BARRY PAKES, M.D., M.P.H.
UNIVERSITY OF TORONTO

Dieting

Diet is what people eat. The consumption of food is necessary to maintain life. A balanced diet is one that includes sufficient quantities foods with carbohydrates for energy, meats for proteins, calcium such as milk for bones, vegetables and fruits for minerals and vitamins. A balanced diet is one that supplies healthy foods in appropriate quantities.

A casual, unplanned eating of whatever someone wants without regard to portions or to calorie expenditures is a diet that likely includes too much food or that is unbalanced can have negative consequences. One of these is that overeating can cause weight gains. While full weight is a sign of good health, it is possible for a person with an unbalanced diet to be at their full weight and still be less than the best of health. This can happened because an unbalanced diet can cause weight and poor health at the same time. An unbalanced diet can even allow the eater to be anemic or to suffer from of kinds of conditions. One of these is weight gains and obesity that require the restoration of a diet that will eliminate the excess weight. This type of diet, a nutrition plan, to achieve goal such as a weight gain or weight loss are called dieting.

Dieting is the ingesting of food in a regular planned manner to reach a particular weight goal. Most of the time the goal of dieting is weight loss; however, weight gain in the form of muscle is the usual goal of athletes. Weight lifters seeking to increase their muscle mass can be vigorous and still be overweight.

Excess weight is a ration between body weight and body height. It is a relatively small range because some people are more muscular than are others. However, in the case of a body builder, the excess weight is muscle and not fat as in the case of those who are obese.

Others who may seek to engage in a diet for gaining weight could include actors. In the case of actors playing a particular role, it may be necessary to gain a number of additional pounds in order to portray their character correctly.

Weight gain diets are important to people who have become malnourished because they were stranded without food somewhere, were ill, or for some other reason. Diets to bulk up the body's muscle mass are frequently used by athletes and soldiers.

Most dieting is done to lose weight. People who have become overweight or obese can benefit by careful development of a weight loss program. Strictly speaking, people on a diet should see to replace fat with muscle. The conversion gives strength to the body as well as reserves of energy. It also reduces the strain on the heart and other systems such as the digestive system and its endocrine parts including the pancreas.

There are a variety of eating disorders that are a very serious problem. Growing numbers of people have them. Most are cases of eating disorders, are a combination of emotional, physical, spiritual and cultural factors. Most of the people who have eating disorders are women, although men are afflicted as well. The most common eating disorders are anorexia nervosa, bulimia, and binge eating.

Anorexia nervosa is an eating disorder in which the victim seeks to reduce his or her weight to much less than his or her ideal weight. The victim has an intense phobia that she or he will become fat.

Bulimia victims experience recurring bouts of binge eating followed by purging. Depression is a common psychological condition of bulimia victims. Their weight may be nearly normal, but the problem exists.

Binge eaters eat large amounts of food off and on again. They often suffer from social emotions that make them feel out of control. Obesity and diabetes are common problems among binge eaters.

Other ailments that present eating problems are diabetes, gluten intolerance, allergies to specific foods such as peanuts, and diets for specific acute illnesses such as cancer. In the case of diabetes the pancreas no longer makes enough insulin to process the sugars digestion has placed into the blood stream. Diabetes can be managed with a combination of diet, exercise, and medication. The reduction of sugar, saturated fats and alcohol, in the diet of diabetics is a desirable dietary goal. While diabetics can eat sugar, saturated fats, and drink alcohol if these are exchanged (using the American Diabetic Association's food exchange plan), these are undesirable because they do not provide any nutrition other than sugar or fat which are either burned as calories or converted to fat. What is true for diabetics here is also true for all dieters who are seeking weight reduction.

Diets for food allergies require the careful avoidance of foods that the body cannot tolerate or which may cause allergic reactions. An advance in the public education about these problems and in packaging labels on processed foods has reduced these threats somewhat.

There are a multitude of diet plans. Many advertise themselves as the ideal or perfect diet plan. Other diet plans claim to be able to melt the fat away with the diets that is being sold to a potential dieter. However, given the great variety of people who are different ages with different body weights, body sizes, physical activities, and health problem, there is no one diet that fits all dieters. Adopting a diet plan is a matter of caveat emptor ("let the buyer beware").

A place to begin with dieting is with the Food Pyramid Guide. Whether viewed as six food groups, the pyramid rests upon carbohydrates. The carbohydrates that compose this group are breads, cereal grains such as wheat, corn, rice, millet, and other similar grains. The carbohydrate group can supply some roughage and a lot of calories. Much of its food value is converted into sugars to be used for energy. Excess amounts are converted into body fat unless combined with proteins to make muscle. These two groups include large quantities of proteins and fats. These are the building blocks for the body's nutritional chemistry.

The highest group in the Food Pyramid is the fats group. It is composed of fats from animal, some vegetables, and oils from nuts or other sources. This group is the smallest in size because it is meant to be consumed the least. The two blocks above the carbohydrate block are the vegetable group and the fruit group. These two groups are sometimes combined in other systems for grouping foods, but they supply different nutritional values. The vegetables supply carotene, a variety of vitamins and other nutritional units. The fruits supply vitamin C and other vitamins as well as other nutritional values. For the dieter, these two groups can be consumed in increased portions if the amount of carbohydrates is reduced because (especially the fruits) they supply sugars in limited quantities. The "trick" for the dieter is to not add sugar, creams, or other sauces that will turn the fresh or canned fruit into a calorie-rich desert.

Above the vegetable and fruit group in the Food Pyramid are the smaller groups of the milk group (milk, cheese, and yogurt) and the meat group. Included in the meat group are animal meats, fish, poultry, eggs, nuts, and dried beans.

There are a variety of fats found in foods. Those in meats such as choice cuts of beef or duck are rich in saturated fats. The fats are desirable from a culinary point of view because they flavor the meat. However, they are a health threat if consumed frequently over a long time because they contain saturated fats. These types of fats contain numerous hydrogen molecules in their formula. They are likely to contribute to artery blockage through artery plaque formation. They have also been linked to cancer. In small amounts, they are likely to be enjoyable, but they need to be restricted from the diet of most people unless they are engaged is hard physical activity such as hunting in the Artic or the activities of a young soldier in the field.

Fats are needed by the body for important nutritional work. They should not be completely eliminated from most diets. Vitamins E and other vitamins are absorbed by the body's fats for its metabolic use. The healthier fats to consume are the unsaturated fats. These can be found in olive oil and in other fats. They can also be used in salads, or in most cooking. The unsaturated fats do not have an abundance of hydrogen ions that can contribute to health problems.

The diets of a great many people are not balanced. Instead of diets that are in appropriate portions recommended by the Food Pyramid, their diet is quite distorted. The fat group is much larger than it should be. For many people fruit is occasional and vegetables are something rarely consumed. For many people, the only vegetables they consume are those found on pizzas that include peppers and onions.

The unbalanced diet is likely to be very fattening and lacking nutrition. Excessive amounts of carbohydrates made from refined flour, fatty meats, and over consumption of beer is a formula for unwholesome weight gains. Many people rarely drink milk. The addition of calcium and vitamins to aid the body's use of it is needed in most women and some men after menopause in order to prevent osteoporosis.

Although it is not a food and is therefore not in the Food Pyramid, table salt is needed to keep the body's use of water in balance. An insufficient supply of salt can contribute to dehydration. An excessive supply, however, can contribute to high blood pressure and to heart trouble. Most Americans get too much salt in their processed foods. Excessive amounts of salt cause retention of water and increases blood pressure. Good dieting will target the right amount of salt to consume along with other essential vitamins and minerals.

The easiest diet to follow is to eat a balanced diet of the Food Pyramid Guide while exercising portion control. The portion sizes can be slowly reduced over a period of several weeks or months. The reduction will soon add up to the loss of pounds of fat. A pound of fat is equivalent is 3,500 calories. The reduction of calorie intake of just 350 calories per day will mean the loss of a pound in 10 days or in 20 days if the reduction in calories is cut in half. In addition to calorie reduction the development of systematic exercise is very valuable for aiding weight loss on a permanent basis. The practice of exercise converts fat calories to muscle.

Exercise has a number of positive benefits and should accompany a diet plan. The burning of calories through exercise increases the strength of the body, the cardiovascular system, and the general psychology of the dieter. Few diet plans combine exercise with their numerous recipes. There are some organizations that have weight loss programs that do include an exercise plan. However, most diet plans, especially the fad diets, manipulate the balanced diet by adding more of some part of it or by eliminating some part of it. Some diets increase the amount of protein, or the amount of carbohydrates, or the amount of vegetables or fruits. Generally, diets increase some food and reduce or eliminate

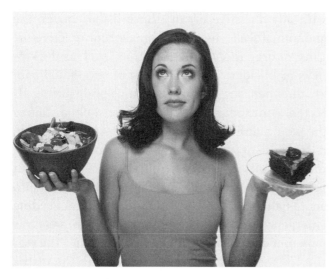

Many diet plans manipulate the balanced diet by increasing some food types and reducing or eliminating other food types.

others. The food that is increased may be fruit so that the dieter eats more grape fruit and no carbohydrates. Or the diet may eliminate carbohydrates and increase the amount of meat and vegetables.

Other diets completely eliminate food and put the dieter on a strict water-alone diet. This can result in the loss of several pounds in a few days as the body eliminates feces and some fat. However, this type of diet carries the risk of health damage. It also is likely to result in frustration after the weight loss plateaus. Some diets increase or reduce the supplements of vitamins. Others recommend more salt or more calcium or something else. These diets can accomplish some weight loss. However, they can also be damaging to health.

Another key element for any diet besides exercise is discipline. It takes systematic action to keep on a diet. Probably any diet plan will result in some weight loss; however, to reach the target weight requires discipline. The discipline needed to stay with a diet plan can be psychologically taxing or just plain boring. Many people fail to keep their diet plan with discouraging psychological results. The feeling of being a failure and that it does not matter what is attempted the weight will not come off is a common experience.

A useful tactic for staying with a diet plan is to set small target goals. It, however, is important to set rewards that are something other than food. It does little good to lose a pound and then to indulge in a triple banana split. A better tactic is to include small treats in the diet plan. This frees the dieter from the risk of identifying the desert with a reward and makes it just a part of the diet.

In the world today, a part of the world is dieting to lose weight gained from lack of exercise and usually excessively large portions of food. People in the urban settings of the Northern Hemisphere are living in a built environment that does not favor exercise. Their environment also does not favor wise eating because of the number of high calories fast foods that are easily available. The combination of cheap carbohydrates and fats in "supersized" portions combined with a lack of exercise is contributing to obesity which has become a major health hazard for millions. Sensible diets combined with sensible exercise are vital to weight loss on a permanent basis.

SEE ALSO: Anorexia Nervosa; Bulimia; Diabetes; Nutrition; Obesity.

BIBLIOGRAPHY. Elliot D. Abravanel and Elizabeth King Morrison, *Dr. Abravanel's Body Type Diet and Lifetime Nutrition Plan* (Bantam Books, 1999); T. Colin Campbell and Thomas M. Campbell, *The China Study: The Most Comprehensive Study of Nutrition Ever Conducted and the Startling Implications for Diet, Weight Loss and Long-Term Health* (BenBella Books, 2005); S. Mikielle Chatman, *Long Term Weight Reduction Management: The Advance Plan* (Fat Chance Publications. 1992); Greg Guest, *Globalization, Health, and the Environment: An Integrated Perspective* (AltaMira Press, 2005); Jean A. T. Pennington and Judith S. Douglass, *Bowes and Church's Food Values of Portions Commonly Used* (Lippincott Williams & Wilkins, 2004); James M. Rippe, *Weight Watchers Weight Loss That Lasts: Break Through the 10 Big Diet Myths* (Wiley, 2005); John Robbins and Dean Ornish, *Food Revolution: How Your Diet Can Help Save Your Life and Our World* (Red Wheel/Weiser, 2001); Shmayre Primack, *Sure-Fire Weight Reduction and Longevity Program: Solutions for Life* (Judlinsa Nutrition, LLC, 2007); Sue Rodwell Williams, *Essentials of Nutrition and Diet Therapy* (Times Mirror/Mosby College Publishing, 2000); Robert O. Young and Shelley Redford, *The pH Miracle for Weight Loss: Balance Your Body Chemistry, Achieve Your Ideal Weight* (Grand Central Publishing, 2006).

ANDREW J. WASKEY
DALTON STATE COLLEGE

Digestive Diseases (General)

The topic of digestive disease encompasses a large range of disorders and processes. It includes all disorders that can produce dysfunction of digestion. Multiple organs may be effected and the disease can be life threatening, as in certain types of cancers, or fairly benign, such as in viral infections. Today, over 60 million people in the United States have a digestive disease at some point annually. Digestive disease accounted for over 230,000 deaths in 2002 and was responsible for 9 percent of all hospitalizations in that year. To grasp a general understanding of digestive disease processes, while not going into extreme depth about individual illnesses, it is easiest to cover the function of the digestive tract, some of the more common symptoms, and the causes of these symptoms.

FUNCTION OF THE DIGESTIVE TRACT

The digestive tract serves two major functions: the absorption of nutrients and the elimination of waste. Each anatomical section of the tract is designed to process the food we eat and prepare it for either energy the body can use or disposal. Recapping the movement of food through the digestive tract is essential in understanding dysfunction of this organ system. First, the mouth houses certain enzymes in saliva that begin to break down food and then the food is pushed through the esophagus and into the stomach. It is in the stomach where food is further broken down by the highly acidic stomach contents. Next, digestion continues in the small intestine where the majority of nutrients are absorbed for the body's use. It is also in the small intestine where substances from the gallbladder, such as bile, and substances from the pancreas are added. Bile helps the absorption of digested fats. Finally, once what is left of the food is in the large intestine, water is pulled out of the stool, and thus the stool becomes more concentrated. Bacteria are also present in the large intestine and help to further ferment and break down the left over food particles. Stool is then expelled through the colon. The motility of digestion is largely caused by involuntary stimulation from our nervous systems.

ABDOMINAL PAIN

Abdominal pain is any pain that is felt between the chest and the groin. The causes of this pain are nearly endless and encompass problems associated with any digestive organ (those listed above), the abdominal wall, the spine, female reproductive organs, or organs of the urinary tract, such as the kidneys or bladder. Different types of abdominal pain result depending on what organ or body part is affected. For example, when an internal organ causes the pain, a dull vague pain usually results. However, if the cause of the pain is more externalized, it commonly results in a sharper, more precise or clear-cut pain. Abdominal pain can also be broken down into acute pain, usually occurring suddenly and needing emergent intervention, and chronic pain, which is pain that occurs over a long period of time. The reason for these differences has to do with the distribution of different branches of our nervous system. Due to the numerous causes of abdominal pain, just a few of the causes will be mentioned. These different causes will be broken down into serious illnesses causing abdominal pain and then followed by other common diseases.

The more serious causes of abdominal pain involve problems such as appendicitis, bowel perforation, and dissecting aorta aneurysm. The appendix is a blind-ended tube connected to the beginning of the large intestine. The appendix can become inflamed due to a process that is not entirely known. When this occurs, extreme pain is felt at the right lower side of the abdomen. This pain becomes worse when pressing on the skin over this area. If the appendix ruptures due to this inflammation, peritonitis (inflammation of the cavity surrounding the abdominal organs) can ensue. Bowel perforation can also result in a life-threatening peritonitis. A dissecting aortic aneurysm presents as tearing pain either felt in the abdomen or chest. This event involves the separation of layers of the aortic wall (the largest artery in the body) and can lead to rupture causing a massive amount of internal bleeding. These just account for a few of the more serious causes of abdominal pain. Others include gallstone disease, pancreatitis, peptic ulcer disease, diverticulitis, inflammatory bowel disease, and so forth.

Other common causes of abdominal pain include problems such as kidney stones and disorders associated with the female reproductive tract. Kidney stones occur more commonly in men than in women and present with severe, spasm-like pain typically. Kidney stones usually result after a long period of time where the urine has been concentrated leaving crystals or some other process. The causes of kidney stones depend largely on what substance forms the stone. Overall, drinking plenty of fluids will help prevent kidney stones from forming. Women often experience abdominal pain during menstruation or other processes involving the reproductive tract, such as a ruptured cyst of the ovary. The pain felt from a ruptured cyst is sharp, intense, and usually doesn't last long. The abdominal pain felt during menstruation is often described as cramping and is caused by the release of hormones resulting in contraction of the uterus.

NAUSEA AND VOMITING

Nausea and vomiting account for two symptoms that commonly occur in patients of all age groups. Although, these are actually two separate symptoms, they often occur together, with nausea preceding vomiting. Nausea is the urge in the need to vomit, but not necessarily regurgitating any stomach contents. Vomiting, on the other hand, is the actual process of pushing stomach contents up through the esophagus and out the mouth. Causes of these two symptoms in all age groups include medication, gastrointestinal obstruction, infections of the digestive tract, pregnancy, motion sickness, central nervous system diseases, alcoholism, and so forth. Some causes of nausea and vomiting in infants include pyloric stenosis (obstruction in the outlet of the stomach), milk allergy, gastrointestinal obstruction, and reflux (commonly known as "spitting up").

While acute or brief episodes of nausea and vomiting may just be a discomfort, prolonged vomiting can lead to severe dehydration or growth restriction in an infant. Also, prolonged or excessive vomiting in the adult can lead to aggravation of the esophagus, gastroesophageal reflux disease (GERD), and eventually may progress to esophageal cancer. Persistent vomiting is commonly associated with alcohol abuse. Dehydration caused from vomiting, when severe, is a life-threatening emergency and requires immediate medical attention to re-hydrate that individual. Hematemesis, the vomiting up of blood, is another serious condition that can occur and raises immediate concern. Causes of hematemesis are wide ranging, including ingestion of toxic substances and peptic ulcer disease. Like abdominal pain, nausea and vomiting combine with other symptoms of many disorders of the digestive tract.

DIARRHEA

Diarrhea is defined as frequent, watery, loose stools and is chronic when these types of stools last longer than four weeks. Diarrhea can either be described as an increase in frequency, urgency, or in fecal continence. A wide range of illnesses can cause diarrhea, like most digestive tract problems. The leading cause of diarrhea is viral gastroenteritis, a viral infection of the digestive tract. This infection usually lasts only a few days and is commonly referred to as the "stomach flu". Other common causes of diarrhea include malabsorption disorders (discussed later), inflammatory bowel disease, irritable bowel syndrome, and celiac disease. Like vomiting, dehydration is a major and usually the most severe consequence of diarrhea. Dehydration often has a faster onset in young children and is more concerning. As with vomiting, blood in diarrhea is also a reason for concern. Dysentery, bloody diarrhea usually caused by a bacterial infection, is associated with infections with certain types of E. coli, shigella, and salmonella. With excessive blood loss in stool, a patient must be continually re-evaluated for anemia, a lowered number of red blood cells. Food poisoning is also a common cause of diarrhea that usually resolves in a 24- to 48-hour period. Food poisoning results from drinking water or eating foods containing bacteria or parasites. Often, people can have short-lived diarrhea because of a change in diet or digestive tract irritation from certain foods. In diarrhea, as with vomiting, it is important to maintain adequate fluid intake to ensure proper hydration.

CONSTIPATION

Constipation can either be defined as infrequent stools, straining with defecation, passage of hard stools, or the sense of incomplete evacuation of stool. A more exact definition states that constipation is a lack of a bowel movement for greater than three days for an adult. Some infants may go seven days without having a bowel movement. Commonly, constipation is caused by a low-fiber diet, lack of physical activity, not drinking enough water, or waiting to defecate when having the urge to do so. Constipation, as with the other digestive disease symptoms mentioned previously, is serious if occurring in certain situations. For example, a recently born infant that hasn't passed a stool can have a congenital abnormality in their digestive tract that must be corrected rapidly or it may lead to permanent damage. Also, sudden loss of blood in the stool, hematochezia, in older people can be the first sign of a colon polyp or even colon cancer.

MALABSORPTION

Malabsorption is the difficulty of absorbing and digesting nutrients. As with the previously mentioned types of digestive disease symptoms, the causes of malabsorption are numerous. Malabsorption usually has to do with impairment of the absorption of specific sugars, fats, proteins, and vitamins; or, failed uptake of all substances in general. The causes of this problem can be from an infection, congenital, autoimmune, or caused by another illness. Autoimmune diseases are when the body's own immune system recognizes a normal part as being foreign and attacks that specific body part. Some other problems associated with malabsorption include diarrhea, growth restriction, bloating, cramping, distended abdomen, frequent stools, malodorous stools, and muscle wasting. Prolonged malabsorption causes malnutrition and/or vitamin deficiencies, which lead to many more medical problems and issues.

One of the most common causes of malabsorption in children is cystic fibrosis. This congenital disease primarily affects the respiratory system and causes recurrent bacterial infections and mucous buildup. The malabsorption component of this disease has to do with pancreatic insufficiency. This insufficiency leads malabsorption of fat and protein and eventually leading to difficult weight gain and malnutrition. Another common disease process that leads to impaired absorption is lactose intolerance (also known as milk intolerance). This illness is secondary to a deficiency in the enzyme lactase, which is found in the small intestine.

Lactase, when present, breaks down lactose, a sugar found in milk and dairy products. This deficiency usually occurs after the age of five and leads to a deficiency in vitamin D, calcium, and protein, requiring supplementation with these substances. If a person who is lactase deficient consumes dairy products, they can have symptoms such as abdominal bloating, diarrhea, flatulence, and nausea. Overall, lactose intolerance is not a dangerous disorder. Other diseases causing malabsorption include Whipple disease, celiac disease, abetalipoproteinemia, biliary atresia, and chronic pancreatitis.

Infections with certain parasites can also lead to malabsorption and those symptoms that occur with it. For example, the parasite Diphyllobothrium latum, the fish tapeworm, can lead to an infestation that inhibits the absorption of vitamin B12. Deficiency of vitamin B12 leads to a certain type of anemia. Also, Giardia lamblia is another parasite can be acquired by drinking contaminated spring water from streams or lakes and infects the small intestine. Giardia causes loss of appetite, vomiting, diarrhea, flatulence, and cramping, which all play a role in not absorbing the proper amount of nutrition. Whether it is from a parasite, or from other causes, specific supplements are needed to replace appropriate nutrients that are lost in malabsorption.

GASTROESOPHAGEAL REFLUX DISEASE

GERD is a common condition in which food or liquids travels from the stomach and back up through the esophagus. The acidity of the stomach contributes to the symptoms felt from this disorder. Stomach acid helps break down and digest food and if this acid is refluxed back into the esophagus it can cause the feeling of "heartburn". Often, GERD occurs without the presence of any symptoms. This likely occurs at some point during every person's life. A defect in the sphincter of the lower esophagus, the valve that helps prevent reflux from the stomach, often contributes to GERD. Some of the symptoms associated with reflux besides heartburn, include vomiting blood/food, nausea, belching, hoarseness, sore throat, cough, and a sour taste in the mouth.

Certain foods and activities can worsen GERD symptoms. For example, foods such as chocolate, caffeine, spicy foods, and peppermint can exacerbate these symptoms. Also, other contributors include being overweight, lying down shortly after a meal, taking medication without water, smoking tobacco, and drinking alcohol. It is important to avoid these foods and activities as part of the treatment of GERD. One of the worst consequences of prolonged gastroesophageal reflux is the change in the type of cell that lines the esophagus. Initially, this change in cell type has no meaningful consequences; however, if left unnoticed, a person may develop esophageal cancer that is life threatening. Overall, GERD is very easily managed on the right medications and if treated early.

Digestive diseases are common in every country and can range from very severe to just an overnight or one-time event. It is important to have severe illness of the digestive tract evaluated promptly and by the right healthcare worker. Also, it is important to try and prevent the less serious diseases or problems from progressing into something worse. These digestive issues will continue to be a large part of medical illnesses and will need to be evaluated earlier in order to put less strain on healthcare.

SEE ALSO: Appendicitis; Constipation; Cystic Fibrosis; Diarrhea; Gastroesophageal Reflux/Hiatal Hernia; Inflammatory Bowel Disease; Kidney Stones; Nausea and Vomiting; Peptic Ulcer Disease.

BIBLIOGRAPHY. Thomas E. Andreoli, et al., *Cecil Essentials of Medicine* (Saunders, 2004); Dennis L. Kasper, Eugene Braunwald, *Harrison's: Principles of Internal Medicine* (McGraw-Hill 2005); Medline Plus, "Medline Encyclopedia," http://www.nlm.nih.gov/medlineplus (cited March 2005) National Digestive Disease Information Clearinghouse, "Digestive Disease Statistics," http://digestive.niddk.nih.gov (cited December 2005).

ANGELA J. GARNER, M.D.
UNIVERSITY OF MISSOURI–KANSAS CITY
SCHOOL OF MEDICINE

Diphtheria

Diphtheria is a very contagious and potentially life-threatening bacterial disease that primarily affects the nasal passages, throat, and lungs. In some instances, the infection can spread or attack the skin, heart, and nervous system. Immunization efforts have been able to keep this bacterial infection out of most of the developed world and much of the developing world. However, there has been a global resurgence of diphtheria due to poorly managed vaccination programs, a lack of funding, and other preventative measures. Regionally, former Soviet Republics have seen a disproportionate increase of diphtheria infection. This is proposed to be from inadequate and nonexistent vaccine programs throughout the 1990s.

Diphtheria is caused by *Corynebacterium diphtheriae* bacteria and can be easily spread through mucous secretions by coughing or sneezing of infected persons. Cramped living conditions, poorly planned congested urban neighborhoods, lack of proper sanitation, lack of vaccination plans, and poor knowledge of the disease aid in its spread throughout the world. According to the Centers for Disease and Control (CDC), currently about 10,000 new cases are reported each year with a previous spike of some 60,000 cases reported annually during the mid-1990s. In a CDC report, it was noted that the overall case-fatality rate for diphtheria is five to 10 percent, with higher death rates (up to 20 percent) among persons younger than 5 and older than 40 years of age.

TYPES OF DIPHTHERIA

There are toxigenic and nontoxigenic strains of *Corynebacterium diphtheriae* that can cause disease. Strains that produce toxins cause an inflammation of the heart (myocarditis) and nerve inflammation and disease (neuritis and neuropathy). These toxins can also cause low platelet counts (thrombocytopenia) and protein in the urine (proteinuria). Where myocarditis experiences an early onset, it is often fatal. Neuritis often affects motor nerves and can resolve with possible paralysis of the soft palate, eye muscles, limbs, and diaphragm. Secondary pneumonia and respiratory failure are known to occur from paralysis of the diaphragm. Other complications are otitis media and respiratory insufficiency from airway obstruction. This is most common in infected infants. When the infection manifests in nonimmunized persons, the bacteria releases the toxin and subsequent damage occurs in the body. Toxigenic strains are more often associated with severe or fatal illness. This is mainly in the form of respiratory or other mucosal surface infections.

DIAGNOSIS AND TREATMENT

Diphtheria is best diagnosed clinically by identifying a gray membrane covering the throat and possibly inflamed tonsils and with an accompanying sore throat, fever and malaise. Any mucosal membrane can be infected (i.e., various nasopharyngeal, coetaneous, genital, and ocular). The diagnosis can also be confirmed with a throat culture if the laboratory capabilities exist. *Corynebacterium diphtheriae* is an aerobic gram-positive bacillus.

For those who are not vaccinated and contract the disease, active immunization and strong antibiotics are the best course of treatment. For those who are infected and are exposed to diphtheria, they must receive a booster of diphtheria toxoid plus active immunization and strong antibiotics. The most common vaccination program is the diphtheria toxoid mixed with tetanus and or pertussis vaccines. Vaccination provides the best preventative treatment.

EPIDEMIC IN POST–SOVIET COUNTRIES

The fall of the Soviet Union in 1991 engendered the Newly Independent States (NIS) and Baltic States with a fragmented health infrastructure and delays in implementing control measures. During the early 1990s, diphtheria was at epidemic levels in these states. This rapid increase in new cases of diphtheria was the first comprehensive epidemic in industrialized countries in over three decades.

Much research in the literature conclude that the main contributing factors to this epidemic include a large population of susceptible adults and children, decreased childhood immunization programs, loss of a vaccination and preventative programs, poor socioeconomic conditions, deteriorated health infrastructure, and high population movement and migration. A large-scale and well-coordinated international effort met these challenges in the mid-1990s with aggressive control strategies and high-yield outcomes.

The legacy of this epidemic includes a reexamination of the global diphtheria control strategy, new laboratory techniques for diphtheria diagnosis and analysis, and a model for future public health emergencies in the successful collaboration of multiple international partners. Diphtheria remains a global health threat and the most recent epidemic in post–Soviet nations is a stark reminder of diphtheria's potency.

SEE ALSO: Adolescent Health; Adult Immunization; Center for Disease and Control and Prevention (CDC); Childhood Immunization; Epidemic; Immunization/Vaccination; National Immunization Program (NIP).

BIBLIOGRAPHY. W. Atkinson, *Epidemiology and Prevention of Vaccine-Preventable Diseases.* eds. 9th ed. (Public Health Foundation, 2006); S. Dittmann, M. Wharton and C. Vitek, Successful Control of Epidemic Diphtheria in the States of the Former Union of Soviet Socialist Republics: Lessons Learned, *The Journal of Infectious Diseases* (v.181/Suppl 1, 2000); Stanly A Plotkin,*Vaccines,* 4th ed. (Saunders, 2003); World Health Organization (WHO), *Immunizations, Vaccines and Biologicals*, http://www.who.int/vaccines-surveillance (cited July 2006).

JOHN MICHAEL QUINN V, MPH
UNIVERSITY OF ILLINOIS AT CHICAGO

Disasters and Emergency Preparedness

The common understanding of a "disaster" assumes that some spectacular event has occurred in a particular time and space. Such a perspective is limiting because some disasters, such as famines and epidemics, or creeping environmental disasters (e.g., desertification, water depletion of lakes) involve diffuse processes occurring over long durations.

For this reason, it is best to think of a disaster in more general terms, as the convergence of sociopolitical and biophysical processes that results in an event in which there is severe physical damages and a disruption of the routine functioning of a community and/or ecosystem. By this definition, all disasters have human and material dimensions. It is particularly important to recognize this dual nature of disasters when considering how certain populations are more vulnerable than others to the effects of a disaster.

For example, analyses of the impacts of Hurricane Katrina on New Orleans, Louisiana, in 2005, and the heat wave on Chicago, Illinois, in 1995, reveal how certain marginalized communities were more heavily impacted than other groups because of the way the cities were physically and socially segregated by race and income. Similarly, analyses of the 1984 Union Carbide chemical leak disaster in Bhopal, India, reveal how those lowest on the economic scale experienced the highest fatality rate because the shanty town conditions in which these victims resided led to greater and more direct chemical exposures.

THE DISASTER MANAGEMENT CYCLE

The disaster management cycle describes a continuum of interlinked activities aimed at the reduction of risk before disaster onset and the pursuit of postdisaster recovery efforts. It is a cycle because what is learned during the recovery phase can be used to produce more effective risk-reduction activities for similar disasters that may occur in the future. The disaster management cycle consists of five parts. The recovery phase consists of 1.) response, 2.) rehabilitation, and 3.) reconstruction activities, while the reduction phase involves 4.) mitigation and 5.) emergency preparedness. Mitigation and emergency preparedness are complementary. The former involves those measures intended to reduce the vulnerability of places to disaster and to reduce the disaster impacts. Mitigation includes such things as the enforcement of building and land use regulations, the control of hazardous substances, and the implementation of safeguards to protect critical infrastructure elements such as power supplies and communications networks. The overall objective of emergency preparedness is to ensure that appropriate systems, procedures, and resources are in place to provide prompt and effective assistance to disaster victims. In essence, it involves those measures that enable organizations, communities, and individuals to rapidly and effectively respond to disasters. The emergency preparedness component includes the formulation of disaster plans; the special provision for emergency action (i.e., evacuation plans, temporary safety shelters, the mobilization of relief

agencies, emergency warning, and communication systems); and public education/awareness programs and training programs (i.e., practice exercises and drills). Although related to other stages of the disaster management cycle, preparedness measures tend to be more strongly oriented toward action by organizations such as police and fire departments, utility companies, hospitals, social service agencies, military, mass media, and nongovernmental agencies.

There are many disruptive elements associated with disasters, including property damage, loss of livelihood, interruption of essential services, economic losses, physical and mental health impacts. Notwithstanding their dual nature, disasters may be classified as natural or technological depending on the nature of the particular causative agent. Examples of the former include earthquakes, tornadoes, hurricanes, and floods, while the latter includes chemical spills, industrial explosions, and nuclear accidents.

TECHNOLOGICAL DISASTERS

On a macroscale, globalization has contributed to issues of vulnerability and marginalization in the context of technological disasters and has played a role in the unequal distribution of risks and hazards around the world. For instance, in the aftermath of the Bhopal tragedy, it was found that Union Carbide's sister companies in developed countries had more stringent safety measures and occupational health practices in place to protect workers and prevent industrial accidents. The significance of such differences is that the potential for industrial disasters may be higher in the developing world relative to the developed world.

Furthermore, multinational corporations may choose to locate some of their companies in impoverished areas because it is less costly (because they will not have to abide by stringent environmental and health regulations and standards). Those living in such areas are more likely to accept these risk-producing industries because they have no other options to consider in regard to economic gains. This is also true for the location of toxic waste sites and other activities that have a high disaster potential. For example, research has found that toxic waste sites in the United States are more likely to be found near poor African-American neighborhoods, thus increasing the disaster potential for this social group.

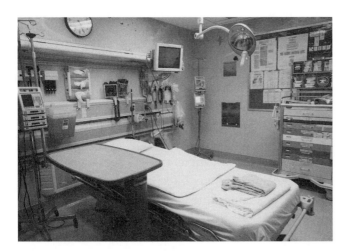

The objective of emergency preparedness is to ensure that appropriate resources are in place to provide effective assistance.

In the aftermath of a technological disaster such as a chemical contamination event, community members sometimes suffer for decades on a number of fronts (i.e., emotionally, mentally, physically, socially, financially, etc.). Further, low levels of contaminants may sometimes remain in the environment long after the disaster onset, thereby contributing to the experience of chronic, debilitating disease and illness—in effect leaving behind a toxic legacy. Such problems were experienced, for example, by survivors of the nuclear disaster in Chernobyl (1986), and those living in the contaminated Love Canal, New York, site (which brought to the fore the issue of toxic waste in 1978) as well as those residing near the many abandoned industrial sites (known as brownfields) throughout the world. Technological disasters of this type may have severe mental health impacts often described in terms of the syndrome of post-traumatic stress disorder (PTSD). Symptoms of PTSD include nightmares, emotional numbing, withdrawal, insomnia, and irritability. These may be exacerbated by the social conditions that emerge in the posttechnological disaster milieu.

Unlike natural disasters where the physical harm to the body is immediately apparent (e.g., a broken arm caused by falling off a tree), with a technological disaster such as a nuclear or chemical contamination event, the harm is much more insidious. For example, exposure to chemical contaminants may lead to feelings of dread and anxiety because of the uncertainty caused by the lag time between exposure and the development of the disease (e.g., cancer). Moreover, because a technological disaster is often attributed to a human error, victims in the disaster aftermath are often involved in stressful legal cases involving compensation, blame, and the search for those responsible. These circumstances lead to a corrosive community that is characterized by a lack of trust, suspicion, and fragmentation which also contribute to the mental health impacts of a technological disaster. On the other hand, in the face of natural disasters, a sense of community cohesiveness emerges with the common rationalization that the disaster was merely an unfortunate and nonpreventable act of nature. In these circumstances, a therapeutic community may emerge in which people band together in a spirit of goodwill to respond to the natural disaster. Both types of social responses should be considered in developing appropriate emergency preparedness plans.

NATURAL DISASTERS

Popular accounts of natural disasters tend to "naturalize" the disaster. Unlike the case of human-made disasters where failures in technology represent a *loss* of control over systems we have created, natural disasters are often viewed as the inevitable *lack* of control over natural agents. Consequently, the social and political underpinnings of the "natural" disaster are not considered as part of emergency planning. The impacts of a natural disaster, however, are the result of the interplay of human activities related to land use, living standards, and public policies in addition to the natural agent itself.

For example, in the case of the Chicago heat wave, it was found that intense heat was deadly only in combination with particular social and physical circumstances in which socially isolated members of the black community (such as elderly individuals who were poor and lived alone) were afraid, or unable to, venture out in dangerous neighborhoods to seek air conditioning, nor could they leave their doors and windows open for fear of crime. The city's emergency plan did not consider this. Similarly, Hurricane Katrina revealed the inadequacy of the emergency plans in New Orleans by emphasizing evacuation by car, neglecting those who simply could not afford this luxury and as a result were stranded in the flood conditions.

Ideally, the development of effective and efficient emergency preparedness strategies should incorporate the lessons learned from the mistakes made in response to similar disasters of the past. In a positive light, this did, in fact, occur in 1999 when Chicago experienced another severe heat wave. In this instance, issues related to vulnerable and marginalized groups were more effectively addressed.

EMERGENCY PREPAREDNESS MYTHS

Preparedness measures defined in many emergency management plans are often inadequate. These deficiencies may be partially addressed by focusing more attention on tighter coordination among organizations who work with vulnerable groups (such as social service organizations, police, and nongovernmental agencies). Furthermore, attention should focus on measures to ensure clearer communication among people who need information; and greater cooperation among individuals and organizations, particularly between the military and civilian groups.

Second, in drafting emergency preparedness measures, disaster managers should take into consideration the myths and realities of disasters. The Pan American Health Organization (2000) lists several of these. For example, it is a myth that medical volunteers with any kind of medical background are needed at times of emergencies because it is the local population who almost always covers the immediate lifesaving needs. As such, only those medical personnel with those specialized skills that are not available in the affected area may be needed. Similarly, it is a myth that any kind of international assistance is needed, and that it is needed immediately. The reality is that a hasty response that is not based on an impartial evaluation only contributes to the chaos. It is, therefore, better to wait until the genuine needs have been assessed because in actuality, most needs are met by the victims themselves and their local agencies, not by foreign intervenors. It is popularly thought that disasters bring out the worst in human behavior, such as looting and rioting, but in reality, this is not always true. Although there may be some isolated cases of antisocial behavior (that is often emphasized in media accounts, perhaps for the dramatic effect, as was the case in the Hurricane Katrina coverage), for the most part, people respond spontaneously and generously during disasters. It is also commonly thought that the affected population will be too shocked and helpless to take responsibility for their own survival. However, studies have shown that many find new strength during an emergency, as seen for example, by the thousands of volunteers who spontaneously united to sift through the rubble in search of victims in the aftermath of the 1985 earthquake in Mexico City. It is also a myth that disasters are random killers, because as we have discussed above, the fact of the matter is that the impact of disasters are felt most by vulnerable groups such as the poor, the elderly, women, and children.

Emergency preparedness may be enhanced by incorporating elements of vulnerability analysis. This includes an integrated multidisciplinary approach that seeks to understand those circumstances that put people and places at risk based on an analysis of the complex interactions between social, natural, and engineered systems. By providing information about the sectors at risk such as the physical (e.g., buildings, infrastructure, critical facilities), the social (e.g., vulnerable groups, livelihoods, local institutions, poverty),

and the economic (i.e., direct and indirect financial losses) as well as by focusing on the kind of risk (e.g., damage to public infrastructure, housing, or casualties), a more integrated approach to emergency preparedness may be developed—one that is sensitive to the totalizing nature of all disasters.

As illustrated by our discussion of technological and natural disasters, the fact that all types of disasters have a sociopolitical basis should be taken more seriously in emergency preparedness planning. This could be accomplished, for example, by taking into account grassroots input and local knowledge into emergency preparedness planning by collaborating with lay participants, community members and environmental justice activists on specifically action-oriented strategies. Lay–expert collaborations have been found to be a necessary component for more successful regulatory processes and policies in general. This would also hold true for the development of sound emergency preparedness plans and measures because the success and failure of such efforts will ultimately depend on citizen understanding and public buy-in.

SEE ALSO: Environmental Health; Pan American Health Organization (PAHO); Post-Traumatic Stress Disorder.

BIBLIOGRAPHY. W. Nick Carter, *Disaster Management: A Disaster Manager's Handbook* (Asian Development Bank, 1991); Lee Clarke, *Mission Improbable: Using Fantasy Documents to Tame Disasters* (University of Chicago Press, 1999); Eric Klinenberg, *A Social Autopsy of Disaster in Chicago: Heat Wave* (University of Chicago Press, 2003); Pan American Health Organization, *Natural Disasters: Protecting the Public's Health* (Pan American Health Organization, 2000).

S. Harris Ali, Ph.D.
Ann Novogradec, Ph.D.
York University, Toronto

Disease and Poverty

There is a direct correlation between poverty and disease. Poverty creates a cyclical relationship with disease for vulnerable groups and countries in that poverty causes people and countries to be hopeless, unaccountable, and irresponsible and these in turn create the conditions for disease to fester and spread. Thus, from a human behavior perspective, many of the diseases that are causing so much suffering in our world today could be prevented if individuals and governments would be responsible in their behavior. While this may come as a harsh indictment, an analysis of the causes and spread of some of the deadliest diseases will reveal that they could be contained if governments and individuals acted in ways that would minimize the outbreak and spread of some diseases. However, governments and people in poor countries have not acted to curb diseases because they do not have the resources with which to act in the first place. Therein lies the dilemma and hopelessness of disease control in poor countries. The deadliest diseases are found predominantly in the poorest regions of the world. The poorest people in these places are the most vulnerable, as well. Sub-Saharan Africa and southeast Asia are the two regions in the world where the human cost of disease is greatest and poverty levels are highest. Indeed, sub-Saharan Africa is the only region in the world now where poverty levels keep rising and more people are afflicted with killer diseases every year.

In a feature article in *Time* in March 2005, Jeffrey Sachs drew attention to the persistence of poverty in Africa by stating that "while the economic boom in East Asia has helped reduce the proportion of the extreme poor in that region from 58 percent in 1981 to 15 percent in 2001, and in south Asia from 52 percent to 31 percent, the situation is deeply entrenched in Africa, where almost half of the continent's population lives in extreme poverty—a proportion that has actually grown worse over the past two decades as the rest of the world has grown more prosperous."

The magnitude of poverty in Africa can be appreciated from the Live 8 Concerts that Bob Geldof, in association with other activist musicians, organized in different cities across the globe to draw the attention of G-8 leaders meeting in Scotland in July 2005 about poverty in Africa. Geldof organized a similar concert in 1985 to raise money to fight African poverty in Ethiopia. Twenty years later, the situation appears to have worsened. One of the clearest expressions of the links between disease and poverty is the HIV/AIDS pandemic.

HIV/AIDS PANDEMIC
In the 1980s, when doctors and scientists were grappling with the cause and mode of spread of AIDS, a staff writer for *Time* magazine wrote that more than 2 million Africans were infected with the HIV virus. Less than 20 years later, in 2002, the World Health Organization (WHO) estimated that there were 29.4 million Africans living with HIV. In 2005, there were an estimated 35 million people worldwide living with HIV/AIDS and the greatest number lived in sub-Saharan Africa.

Sue Sprenkle of the Southern Baptist Convention International Mission Board wrote in 2001 that "only 10 percent of the world's people live in Africa, yet it is home to 70 percent to the world's HIV-infected people." Countries in southern Africa are the worst hit. According to estimates, one in every four people in Botswana is HIV positive; it is one in three in Zimbabwe. South Africa is perhaps the worst case in the world. In 1986, HIV prevalence in adults in that country accounted for only about one percent; by the end of 2001, it had risen to about 39 percent.

Not surprisingly, of the 3.1 million people worldwide who died of AIDS in 2002, 2.4 million were living in sub-Saharan Africa. For South Africa alone, WHO has estimated that for the age group 15–34 years living with AIDS, 1.3 million would die between 2000 and 2005, and a further 1.7 million the next five years. The United Nations projects that there will be 40 million AIDS orphans in Africa by 2010. Some of these orphans would be carriers of the AIDS virus. The problem of HIV/AIDS in Africa thus reflects the deepest levels of misery and hopelessness.

When we contrast the prevalence of HIV/AIDS in the world's poorest regions with that in developed countries, an interesting scenario emerges. In first world countries, the incidence of AIDS is greatest among third world communities, that is, communities in developed countries that mimic conditions of life in third world countries.

In the United States, for example, a Centers for Disease Control and Prevention (CDC) report that appeared in June 2005 estimated that more than 1 million Americans were living with the HIV/AIDS virus, up from between 850,000 and 950,000 in 2002. The report explained that the increase is due to the fact that people suffering from AIDS are living longer because of the availability of powerful drugs. Importantly, the report indicated that African Americans make up 47 percent and gay and bisexual men represent 45 percent of HIV/AIDS cases in the United States.

The categories "black," "gay," and "bisexual" represent marginalized and underresourced groups in the United States; however, they do not give a good measure of comparability. The demographics for 2003 are rather revealing. For every 100,000 people in given populations, the rates of HIV/AIDS infection were as follows: 58 for blacks, 10 for Hispanics, 8 for American Indian/Alaska, 6 for whites, and 4 for Asian/Pacific Islanders. The rates for all other groups combined are less than half of the rate among the black population. One wonders whether this is coincidence or an accident; it is as if to suggest that black people everywhere have been especially marked for the disease.

OTHER DEADLY DISEASES

In addition to AIDS, there are other deadly diseases that afflict millions of poor people worldwide. A WHO report in April 2005 stated that outbreaks such as Ebola and Marburg in Africa and severe aute respiratory syndrome (SARS) in Asia may arouse genuine fears in people, but they are not the biggest killers. Diseases such as malaria, diarrhea, tuberculosis, measles, meningitis, tetanus, and syphilis continue to kill millions in nations in Africa and southeast Asia, although in absolute terms the rate of death is greatest in Africa than anywhere else.

According to the report, malaria kills between one and five million people around the world every year, and 90 percent of the deaths occur in Africa where a child dies of malaria every 30 seconds. A CNN news report in April 2005 stated that malaria costs Africa $12 billion a year. In southeast Asia, a similar trend can be observed. The WHO director for the region, Dr. Uton Muchtar Rafei, told a conference on tuberculosis (TB) and malaria in Dhaka, Bangladesh, in November 2000, that about 25 million people suffered from malaria and over 1.25 billion people were at risk of infection in the region. With reference to TB, Rafei said that about 40 percent of the people in southeast Asia were infected and more than 1.5 million died in 1999 alone. He said that 95 percent of TB cases worldwide occur in poor countries and that in these countries, poor people are the most vulnerable.

In addition, in southeast Asia, a joint mission of international donors visiting Afghanistan in April 2002 drew attention to the appalling state of health delivery in the war-ravaged country, especially in rural areas where the doctor–patient ratio is one to 100,000. The mission reported that only 65 percent of Afghans had access to health facilities, while only 32 percent of children were immunized against childhood diseases. The mission recommended that donors would have to invest $200 million in healthcare to enable Afghans to move beyond the cycle of disease and deprivation.

HOW DISEASE OCCURS

Given the spread of diseases in poor countries it is necessary to examine how they occur. HIV/AIDS is a good example. Some people, mostly a few evangelical Christians, have suggested that HIV/AIDS is divine punishment to curb promiscuity and homosexuality. There is even an apocalyptic ring to that suggestion and it says that in the last days incurable diseases will afflict humanity. To some Christians, then, HIV/AIDS and other deadly diseases point to the end of the world. To the extent that the medical and scientific community has not yet developed a cure for HIV/AIDS, these Christians may continue to hold their unique perspective on the disease.

Indeed, HIV/AIDS is largely a sexually transmitted disease; however, it is not solely the disease of the sexually promiscuous, although such people stand a greater risk of infection. Millions of children have been born with the disease through no fault of their own, while others have contracted the virus through blood transfusion or intravenous needle-sharing with infected persons. What is evident is that HIV/AIDS has emerged as the disease of the poor both in developed and developing nations.

One important factor regarding the spread of AIDS is that of government intervention and public responsibility. In rich countries, governments spend millions of dollars educating people and funding research to find a cure for the deadly disease. An MSNBC news report of July 5, 2005, states that the U.S. government passed a law that required all expectant mothers to undergo an HIV/AIDS test. The purpose was to protect unborn babies from contracting the virus from mothers who may be infected.

This was a great preventative measure that served as the first line of defense against the disease in children. The government could pass this act because it had the resources to carry out the tests. But it is one thing to diagnose a disease and another thing to offer a cure to the afflicted. About 39 million Americans do not have health insurance, meaning that they do not have access to quality healthcare. If any of them contracts the HIV/AIDS virus they would not know that they are carriers and would unknowingly pass it on to partners. Thus even in the richest country in the world, the danger of AIDS is a factor of poverty.

The situation is worse in poor countries where governments cannot fund research or import retroviral drugs to curb the spread of HIV/AIDS. In terms of educating the public about safe sex, governments in these countries face an uphill battle because of illiteracy, ignorance, and poverty. Radio and television advertisements have not been effective because the target group does not have access to such technology. Myths about the causes of the disease and traditional ideas about sex have inhibited efforts to curb the spread of the disease.

In a February 2001 edition of *Time*, Johanna McGreary offered insights into how myths fed the spread of the disease in Africa. Some attributed infection to witchcraft, action by angry ancestors, or, in the case of South Africa, a ploy by whites to control the black population when apartheid finally ended. These beliefs could hardly help the people to understand the enormity of the danger with which they were confronted.

And when they finally understood what they were up against, the stigma attached to the disease (because it is sexually transmitted) led infected persons to keep quiet about their condition.

In the United States and Canada, people testing positive for the virus are required by law to inform their spouses if they are married. In Africa there is a "don't tell" culture surrounding the disease. Even doctors do not indicate on death certificates that patients died of HIV/AIDS, in accordance with local practices. In the majority of cases, infected people did not know that they carried the virus and attributed its manifestation to malaria, TB, diarrhea, or any other disease that would crumble their already compromised immune system. These carriers would unknowingly spread the disease until they are too weak to engage in sex.

By then, their partners might have carried it on to others, creating a ripple effect that is difficult to arrest. Once people have contracted the virus, they wait to die. In rural areas where patients may not have access to clinics, these people are treated as outcasts, condemned, and neglected because of their particular type of disease. Those who end up in hospitals may live a little longer because of the rudimentary treatments that they receive. Governments are now struggling to increase the importation of generic drugs to prolong the lives of people carrying the HIV/AIDS virus.

When we move beyond AIDS and consider diseases such as malaria, cholera, and TB, we see how poverty couples with ignorance to make people irresponsible. Malaria is spread by mosquitoes, and mosquitoes breed in stagnant water, dead weeds, and damp and dirty surroundings. The hot and humid climate in Africa and parts of Asia is ideal for mosquitoes to thrive; incidentally, these are places where drainage systems are poor and sanitation is worse. People dispose of garbage and human waste in utter disregard of the health consequences.

Huge garbage dumps spring up in residential areas where mosquitoes breed in large numbers. The majority of people sleep without treated mosquito nets, thus becoming vulnerable to mosquito bites. Governments do not have enough resources to spray the mosquitoes or import medicines. And so like HIV/AIDS, people suffering from malaria only hope that they will be lucky. If not, they die. That is the sad reality of the impact of poverty on human health.

In rural areas in western Africa, for example, villagers dig pits as places of convenience. These open pits attract flies that may settle on food. When it rains, feces washes into streams that may also serve as sources of drinking water for other rural populations. In towns, human-waste management is left in the hands of "night soil men" (men who clear pan loads of feces every night) who dig bigger pits where they dump the waste. The problems associated with human waste in rural areas occur in towns on a larger scale.

Although city populations have potable water they still live with the stench and flies that have feasted on the feces. Even houses and facilities that have water closets are not entirely free from the problem of human waste. Cesspools are poorly constructed and easily spill over, leaving dark streams of toxic human waste that pollute the atmosphere. As the world waits for G-8 leaders to take action on world poverty, a British government official has said that people expecting total eradication of poverty would be disappointed. Some may see the comment as bad for its timing, but sadly, it is true. Even if rich nations create clean financial slates for poor African countries, they would have to find strategies to deal with disease on the continent. McGreary summed it up best when she said that "Here [Africa] the disease

[HIV/AIDS] has bred a Darwinian perversion. Society's fittest, not the frailest, are the ones who die." When the generation of working people is dying out because of disease, there is no amount of debt relief that can salvage sub-Saharan Africa from despair and demise unless disease has been brought under control.

SEE ALSO: AIDS; Nutrition; South Africa.

BIBLIOGRAPHY. Tony Barnett and Alan Whiteside, *AIDS in the Twenty-First Century: Disease and Globalization* (Palgrave Macmillan, 2003); CNN, "WHO Finds TB, Malaria Return as Killer Diseases," www.cnn.com (cited June 2005); Denise Grady, "Just How Does AIDS Spread?" *Time* (March 21, 1988); Johanna McGreary, "Death Stalks a Continent," Time (February 12, 2001); Christine McMurray and Roy Smith, *Diseases and Globalization: Socioeconomic Transitions and Health* (Earthscan/James & James, 2000); Jeffrey Sachs "The End of Poverty," *Time* (March 14, 2005).

MARTHA DONKOR, PH.D.
EDINBORO UNIVERSITY

Disease Prevention

Disease prevention is essential in preserving lives, maintaining quality of life, and mitigating the enormous financial burden associated with unhealthy populations. Around the world, the leading causes of death are largely preventable by making alterations in lifestyles and practicing basic safety measures that prevent the spread of infectious diseases and help to forestall accidents. In developed countries, the leading causes of death are ischemic heart disease, cerebrovascular disease, chronic obstructive pulmonary disease, lower respiratory infections, trachea, bronchus, and lung cancers, vehicular accidents, stomach cancer, hypertensive heart disease, tuberculosis, and suicide. While the developing world shares some of the affects of lifestyle-related diseases, they also have unique vulnerabilities to diseases that are generally under control in the developed world. The leading causes of death in developing countries are HIV/AIDS, lower respiratory infections, ischemic heart disease, diarrheal disease, cerebrovascular disease, childhood diseases, malaria, tuberculosis, chronic obstructive pulmonary disease, and measles.

At the global level, the major steps in disease prevention include combating poverty, increasing surveillance of disease outbreaks, providing assistance to countries that report health problems, restricting transport of people and goods out of infected areas, developing tests that provide early detection capabilities, and making vaccines and antiviral drugs available wherever needed. At the national level, all countries need well-established infrastructures that guarantee access to healthcare, ensure safe drinking water and improved sanitation, and monitor public health. Both national governments and international organizations need to take greater responsibility for promoting preventive care at the individual level through information dissemination and programs designed to encourage populations to practice preventive measures that include avoiding tobacco and excessive alcohol consumption, obtaining prenatal and postnatal care, maintaining healthy weight levels, eating more fruits and vegetables and less fat, salt, and sugar, being physically active, immunizing children against preventable diseases, washing food, hands, and utensils to avoid food contamination, practicing birth control and safe sex, controlling chronic diseases such as diabetes and high blood pressure, practicing home and vehicular safety, and maintaining good mental health.

In the poorest countries of the world, disease prevention and treatment require concentrated efforts by international organizations such as the United Nations, the World Health Organization (WHO), and the United Nations Children's Fund (UNICEF) as well as by national and private organizations. The United Nations Millennium Goals recognize that the key to disease prevention is fighting poverty. Specific goals include reducing child mortality by two-thirds, cutting maternal mortality by three-fourths, and reversing current trends in infectious diseases such as AIDS, tuberculosis, and malaria. The Global Fund to Fight AIDS, Tuberculosis, and Malaria awards grants for programs designed to prevent and treat these diseases while requiring accountability and success in meeting target goals. The United States government has earmarked funding for disease prevention and treatment through the Millennium Challenge Account and the President's Emergency Plan for AIDS Relief. In June 2007, at the annual summit of the Group of Eight (G-8) industrialized nations, delegates pledged $60 billion a year earmarked for prevention and treatment programs for HIV/AIDS, malaria, and tuberculosis in Africa and for strengthening health systems in the least developed countries.

Private funding is also essential in dealing with disease prevention at the global level. For instance, in June 2007, the Sabin Vaccine Institute, an organization devoted to eradicating diseases associated with poverty announced that actress and humanitarian Alyssa Milano had been named a founding ambassador of the newly created Global Network for Neglected Tropical Diseases (NTDs). The institute is dedicated to calling public attention to the 13 chronic and disabling bacterial and parasitic infections that are collectively known as "diseases of poverty." Those diseases, which include hookworm, schistosomiasis, river blindness, and elephantiasis, currently affect a billion people in developing countries. Milano's personal pledge of $250,000 and a matching grant are being used to eliminate lymphatic filariasis (LF) in the southeast Asian nation of Myanmar under the direction of the Lymphatic Filariasis Support Centre of the Liverpool School of Tropical Medicine. An earlier $8.9 million grant is being used to eliminate NTDS in Rwanda and Burundi.

PROMOTING HEALTHY LIFESTYLES

Disease prevention also involves educating the public about what is involved in leading healthy lifestyles. The elimination of tobacco products may be the single most important factor in preventing a number of diseases. While most of the emphasis on the dangers of smoking has focused on risks to smokers, newer research has documented an alarming trend in conditions and diseases linked to passive smoke, including eye irritation, headache, cough, sore throat, and dizziness. Passive smoke can also exacerbate existing health problems. In homes where anyone smokes, all members of the household have a 25 percent higher risk of developing lung cancer and heart disease; and smoking and heavy alcohol consumption have been linked to cancers of the upper and lower gastrointestinal tract. Children in homes where someone smokes are susceptible to low birth weight, respiratory illnesses, middle ear infections, and mortality. Infants are at an increased rate for sudden infant death syndrome (SIDS).

Good nutrition is one of the building blocks of disease prevention. The human body is designed to extract vitamins, minerals, and other substances from food to maintain health and energy. In developing countries, the poorest segments of the population are often undernourished. Consequently, residents suffer from poor overall health and are vulnerable to diseases. Deficiency diseases such as xerophthalmia, anemia, scurvy, and pellagra that have been virtually eradicated in the developed world continue to occur in developing nations. Populations in developing nations are also extremely vulnerable to food and waterborne and vectorborne diseases.

Throughout the world, dietary alterations are key factors in disease prevention. Dietary habits are major factors in 60 percent of male cancers and 40 percent of female cancers. Salt reduction is instrumental in reducing incidences of high blood pressure. The recognition that saturated fats are strongly linked with cardiovascular diseases has halved incidences of fatal heart attacks in the United States. The addition of folic acid to the diet of women of childbearing age has reduced the incidence of birth defects by approximately 70 percent. Adding calcium to diets helps to prevent osteoporosis. Zinc and antioxidants are believed to halt the progress of muscular degeneration, which is the leading cause of irreversible blindness. Consumption of fruits and vegetables has been associated with reducing risks of certain cancers. Fiber and possibly calcium are considered deterrents to the development of colon cancer.

INFECTIOUS DISEASES

Some 40 new diseases have been identified over the last few decades, and all have major global implications. Some of these new diseases are mad cow disease, the hanta virus (a pulmonary syndrome caused by contact with infected rats), *E. coli*, Lyme disease, sudden acute respiratory syndrome (SARS), and avian flu. Older diseases such as dengue fever, cholera, and tuberculosis have resurged. Malaria is one of the major causes of death among the children of Africa and is the seventh leading cause of death in developing countries. There has been a fivefold increase in the number of foodborne diseases over the past few decades. Globalization plays a major role in the spread of infectious diseases because travelers, immigrants, and goods may transport diseases from country to country. The most striking example of the link between globalization and disease occurred with the

SARS outbreak. The disease moved from a small village in rural China to the other side of the world with the result that Canada became a hotspot for SARS. By 2003, 8,100 cases of SARS had been reported worldwide and 800 people had died. The outbreaks exacted a heavy toll on the tourist industry at a cost of $7.6 billion and the loss of 2.8 million jobs.

In 1985, a shipment of tires from Japan arrived in the United States containing pockets of water in which Asian mosquitoes were breeding. These mosquitoes are capable of spreading a new and more virulent form of dengue fever. The disease had been eradicated in North and Latin America for decades through pesticides. However, in the early 1980s, 800,000 new cases were reported. By the end of the decade, the incidence rate had reached over a million. Outbreaks of avian flu resulted in a worldwide scare after the disease jumped from birds to humans. Marburg fever, a deadly hemorrhagic disease, was first identified in Germany in 1967. When Marburg fever reached Angola in May 2005, 90 percent (300 people) of those infected with the disease died. Peru experienced a major cholera outbreak in the 1990s when contaminated water infected fish and shellfish. Infected fish were subsequently eaten by Peruvians. After treatment systems failed to remove the disease from water supplies, infected water was unknowingly pumped into Peruvian homes where it was ingested by unsuspecting residents. Before it was checked, cholera had spread throughout South America. In spring 2004, a polio outbreak that originated in Niger spread to Indonesia. Polio continues to be a major risk in Muslim countries where populations refuse to endorse Western vaccinations. Because of the resurgence of the disease, the WHO has accepted the responsibility for tracking polio.

HIV/AIDS, which was first identified in New York and Los Angeles in 1981, is the leading cause of death in developing countries. There are approximately five million new cases of HIV/AIDS reported each year despite the fact that the disease is entirely preventable if individuals practice safe sex and refrain from sharing needles with other drug users. Strict testing of blood supplies has virtually wiped out transmission from blood transfusions in developed countries. Worldwide, about 3 million people die each year from the virus. Sixty percent of all cases are found in sub-Saharan Africa where HIV/AIDS continues to decimate populations in countries such as Swaziland (38.86 percent adult prevalence rate) and Botswana (37.30 percent adult prevalence rate.

In the United States, with a 0.60 percent adult prevalence rate, most HIV/AIDS is spread through male-to-male sex and through unprotected heterosexual sex with infected partners. Three-fourths of all infected Americans are male. Forty-nine percent are African American, and 31 percent are white. According to the Centers for Disease Control and Prevention, out of 956,666 persons diagnosed with HIV/Aids since 1981, 530,756 have died. Widespread testing to identify individuals with the virus and landmark advances in drug therapies have resulted in lower death rates from HIV/AIDS.

CHILDREN

Prenatal care is an essential element in producing healthy children, and immunizations and prompt medical attention protect children from conditions that threaten health after they are born. Each year, more than 10 million children die from preventable diseases. The most common of these are polio, diphtheria, tetanus, whooping cough, measles, mumps, rubella, Haemophilus influenza type B (Hib), Hepatitis B, chicken pox, pneumonia, sepsis, and skin and throat infections. Children under the age of five are particularly vulnerable to these diseases. Before the Haemophilus influenza type B vaccination was introduced in the United States in 1992, one of every 200 children contracted bacterial meningitis. Among infected children, one in 20 died, and from 10 to 30 percent suffered permanent brain damage.

Acute diarrhea is one of the leading causes of death among children. Because children with diarrhea are vulnerable to dehydration, rehydration therapies that restore the proper balance of fluids and electrolytes are essential. Educational efforts to teach mothers to care for children with diarrhea have been highly successful in a number of developing countries. In Bangladesh, for example, poor women were taught to concoct a rehydration formula using a little salt and sugar added to a cup of water. They then taught the method to other mothers. For a total cost of $9 million in aid, the death rate from acute diarrhea in Bangladesh was slashed from 50 percent to less than one percent.

In countries where malaria is endemic, inexpensive insecticide-treated bed netting saves lives. Seven countries in southern Africa followed the example of South American countries that had been successful in eradicating malaria and sent out teams of volunteers to educate the population about malaria prevention. A subsequent campaign was designed to ensure that all children between the ages of nine months and 14 years were vaccinated against measles. International aid bore the cost of $1.10 per child with the result that in six of the countries, incidences of measles dropped 60,000 in 1996 to 117 in 2000. In Nepal, grandmothers conducted house-to-house campaigns to inform the population about polio and encourage parents to vaccinate their children.

UNITED STATES

The United States spends more than twice as much on healthcare as any other nation in the world; yet, the population is one of the unhealthiest among industrialized nations. Much of that ill health is due to unhealthy life style choices that include diets that are high in fats and sugars, smoking, alcohol consumption, and limited physical activity. However, a deeper issue involves lack of access to healthcare that has been precipitated by rising health costs and the increasing number of uninsured Americans. While every state has its own health department and a plethora of government and private organizations are devoted to every aspect of health, there is a tendency for Americans, particularly those in the working class who do not qualify for government-assisted medical care and who may not be able to afford private insurance, to neglect preventive care, focusing on treating illness after they develop. Even among those who have Medicare and/or Medicaid, medications and treatments are not always affordable.

A major reason that Americans are unhealthier than in the recent past is due to government complaisance. Before 1970, government spending on public health continued to rise. At that time, funding was cut by half. Additional cuts by the Reagan/Bush administrations in the 1980s continued to limit the ability of the government to engage in disease prevention. In 1989, for instance, there was a rise in incidences of tuberculosis. After terrorist attacks on the United States on September 11, 2001, George W. Bush made Americans more vulnerable to ill health by shifting funding away from general health programs to antiterrorism programs.

According to a report by the World Bank, when mortality rates are age-adjusted, the United States ranks 24th in the world in mortality. Studies show that about one-fifth of Americans never fill prescriptions from their physicians, and approximately half on those who do fill them neglect to take medications consistently. In the 1950s, the United States had the sixth lowest infant mortality rate in the world. By 2007, the American had dropped to 42nd lowest (6.37 deaths per 1,000 live births) and ranked 45th in life expectancy (78 years). Because of the controversy surrounding abortion, birth control, and sex education, teen pregnancies, which present high risks to both mother and child, continue to be the highest in the Western world. A million teenage mothers give birth each year. Roughly a third abort, another third miscarry, and the final third give births.

Disease prevention and preventive care are the focus of the Healthy People 2010 initiative, which has targeted 467 issues in 28 separate areas designed to make Americans healthier. Major goals include improving quality of life, eliminating health disparities, reducing obesity, increasing fruit and vegetable consumption, and decreasing consumption of fats and sodium. Focus areas include preventing and treating diseases such as arthritis, osteoporosis, cancer, kidney disease, diabetes, respiratory diseases, and sexually transmitted diseases (STDs) and promoting oral health, family planning, food and drug safety, mental health, and occupational safety and health.

SEE ALSO: AIDS; Birth Defects; Cancer (General); Centers for Disease Control; Diabetes; Gastroenterology; Immunization/Vaccination; Infant and Toddler Health; High Blood Pressure; Medicaid, Medicare, Pregnancy, Preventive Care; Sudden Acute Respiratory Syndrome (SARS); Sexually Transmitted Diseases; Sudden Infant Death Syndrome (SIDS); Suicide; United Nations Children's Fund (UNICEF); Vitamin and Mineral Supplements; World Health Organization (WHO).

BIBLIOGRAPHY. Adrianne Bendich and Richard J. Deckelbaum, eds., *Preventive Nutrition: The Comprehensive Guide for Health Care Professionals* (Humana Press, 2005); Centers for Disease Control and Prevention, "Smoking and Tobacco Use Fact Sheet" www.cdc.gov (cited February 2007); Larry Cohen, et al, *Prevention Is Primary: Strategies for Community Well Being* (Jossey-Bass, 2007); Tom Farley and Deborah A. Cohen, *Prescription for a Healthy Nation: A New Approach to Improving Our Lives by Fixing Our Everyday World* (Beacon, 2005); William H. Foege, et al., eds., *Global Health Leadership and Management* (Jossey-Bass, 2005); George Fried and George J. Hademenos, *Schaum's Outline of Theory and Problems of Biology* (McGraw-Hill Professional, 1999); William. A. Gunn, et al, *Understanding the Global Dimensions of Health* (Springer, 2005); Kelly Lee, *Globalization and Health: An Introduction* (Palgrave Macmillan, 2003); Alan D. Lopez, *Global Burden of Disease and Risk Factors* (Oxford University Press, 2006).

Elizabeth R. Purdy, Ph.D
Independent Scholar

Diverticulosis and Diverticulitis

A diverticulum is an out pouching of the wall of the gastrointestinal tract that is sac-like in appearance. Diverticula can appear at any level of the gastrointestinal tract including the esophagus, stomach, or the small intestine; however, the most common location is the left side of the colon. Diverticulosis means that unless otherwise specified, diverticula are present within the colon. Diverticulitis is a state of inflammation within a diverticuli. While diverticulosis is rare in a patient under age 30, in Western society the prevalence approaches 50 percent in adults over age 60 and up to 25 percent of these will have complications.

Given the prevalence of diverticulosis in developed societies and the relative infrequency of the disease in nonindustrialized countries, it is thought that environmental and lifestyle factors contribute to the development of diverticula. The wall of the colon is marked by longitudinal bands of muscle that are penetrated by nerves and blood vessels. The sites of penetration of these structures create defects in the muscle wall that are points of weakness for diverticula formation. The herniation of the colonic wall through these defects in the muscle can happen if there is prolonged, exaggerated contraction of the musculature as is seen when there is reduced stool bulk. A diet high in fiber will increase stool bulk and prevent the exaggerated contractions that will cause

diverticula formation. The trend in industrialized societies to diets high in carbohydrates, protein, and saturated fats explains the higher prevalence of diverticulosis in these nations. The diagnosis of diverticulosis is often incidental, found during testing for other reasons such as a screening colonoscopy. The majority of people with diverticulosis will remain asymptomatic.

Diverticulitis, or inflammation of diverticula, occurs when there is erosion of the wall of a diverticuli as a result of decreased local blood flow. The decreased flow may be a result of increased colonic wall tension or the impaction of stool within the diverticuli. Diverticulitis can be divided into simple and complicated forms. The overwhelming majority of cases, around 75 percent, are considered simple diverticulitis, which is not associated with complications and will respond to medical management.

Surgical intervention is rarely necessary. Conversely, complicated diverticulitis will often require surgical intervention. As the wall of the intestine is eroded by inflammation, symptoms can develop which include abdominal pain or cramping, nausea and vomiting, diarrhea or constipation, and urinary symptoms. Complications of diverticulitis can include abscess formation within the diverticuli, obstruction of the colon, and perforation of the colon leading to peritonitis and sepsis. In addition, a fistula, or an abnormal connection between two structures, can develop between the bowel and the surrounding anatomy such as the bladder or the vagina.

Treatment of diverticulitis varies depending on the severity of disease. Patients with asymptomatic diverticulosis are often advised to increase fiber intake to prevent development of new diverticula. Patients with simple diverticulitis and mild symptoms can be treated on an outpatient basis with oral antibiotics and a clear liquid diet. If severe symptoms are present, the patient may be admitted to the hospital for intravenous fluids and antibiotics while being kept fasting. If there is obstruction, fistula formation or peritonitis surgery may be necessary to resect the diseased area of the colon or to close the fistula. In conclusion, diverticulosis is a mostly benign condition that can develop complications leading to hospitalization and surgical intervention.

SEE ALSO: Colonic Diseases (General); Gastroenterology.

BIBLIOGRAPHY. Vinay Kumar, Abul Abbas, and Nelson Fausto, *Pathologic Basis of Disease* (Elsevier Saunders, 2005).

KRISTEN MAMELIAN
UNIVERSITY OF MISSOURI, KANSAS CITY

Dizygotic Twin

Two siblings who come from separate ova, or eggs, that are released at the same time from an ovary and are fertilized by separate sperm. Dizygotic twins are also known as fraternal twins. The term originates from *di* or two and *zygote* or eggs. In order for this to occur, two eggs need to be present, referred to as double ovulation, as well as the presence of two separate sperm. This is very rare and the causes are still under study and research. Across the world, the occurrence of dizygotic twinning varies. Throughout the world, dizygotic twins can be seen as a family blessing or financial curse.

Dizygotic twins develop in the uterus separately. Each zygote develops with its own chorion or outer sac. This chorion is connected to the placenta which is the outermost protective membrane around the developing fetus. The placenta lines the uterine wall, partially envelopes the fetus, and is attached to the umbilical cord. The placenta exchanges nutrients, wastes, and gases between maternal and fetal blood. Each zygote also has its own inner sac that contains amniotic fluid. Dizygotic twins each have its own placenta; however, if the two zygotes implant in the uterus close together, it may appear on an ultrasound as one placenta.

Dizygotic twins may have different fathers, meaning that one egg is fertilized by one sperm and the other egg is fertilized by a different father with different sperm. These cases are rare and few have been documented. Due to their being two separate zygotes, the genetic makeup is different and dizygotic twins are not identical. On average, these twins will share half of their genes, just like any other siblings. Two-thirds of twins are fraternal and may be the same sex or be a male and female pair.

Dizygotic twins are most common for older mothers, with highest rates for mothers over the age of 35 years. With the advent of technologies and techniques to assist women in getting pregnant, the rate of fraternal twins has increased markedly. Other possible predispositions to dizygotic twins are mothers who are taller and heavier, the recent discontinuation of oral birth control, possible genetic predispositions that involve excess secretion of follicle-stimulating hormone (FSH), emotional stress, and diet. Diet may play a role as seen in African mothers from Nigeria in the Yoruba tribe that have high frequency of dizygotic twins and have a significant diet of yams.

Last, environmental stress from chemical agents in highly polluted areas may reduce sperm count, thus decreasing the frequency of fraternal twinning. The key concept here is that while certain background factors may be important, fraternal twinning is influenced by a complex mix of events that are poorly understood. In poorer countries, fraternal twins may cause financial hardship. However, in some cultures throughout the world, dizygotic twins are seen a gift to the family and society.

EPIDEMIOLOGY

Historically, about one in 100 to 125 human births results in a twin pregnancy in North America. In Japan, rates vary from one or two per 1,000 and can be as high as 14 per 1,000 in Africa. The rate of twinning varies greatly among ethnic groups. The widespread access and use of fertility medications has aided in an increase in the birth of fraternal twins. Fertility medications may cause a stimulated release of multiple eggs by the mother that cause dizygotic twins.

SEE ALSO: Birth Rate; Fraternal Twins; Monozygotic Twin.

BIBLIOGRAPHY. Nancy Segal, "Chapter 1: Identical and Fraternal Twins: Living Laboratories," in *Entwined Lives: Twins and What They Tell Us about Human Behavior* (Penguin, 1999).

JOHN M. QUINN V, M.P.H.
UNIVERSITY OF ILLINOIS AT CHICAGO

Dizziness and Vertigo

Dizziness is a common complaint for which patients seek medical advice. Dizziness is typically defined as one of four types: vertigo, lightheadedness, disequilibrium, and presyncope. Differentiation of these types is necessary in the diagnosis, management, and treatment. However, this can be challenging because symptoms associated with each of these conditions (including nausea, vomiting, and diaphoresis) may be difficult for patients to describe. Additionally, comorbid chronic conditions over time may confound the picture. It is difficult sometimes to discern if symptoms are related to an acute illness or a new symptom of a chronic disease.

The differential diagnosis of the symptom of dizziness is large and may be a side effect of many of the body's systems. Seizure disorders may present with dizziness as a symptom, as well as psychiatric disorders and motion sickness. Ear disorders including otitis media and impacted cerumen may also present with dizziness.

Vertigo specifically is the illusion of movement (typically rotational motion). Vertigo is also the most prevalent type of dizziness. It is important to differentiate whether the symptoms of vertigo are from peripheral vestibular causes, from central causes, or from other conditions such as drug side effect or chronic neurologic disease.

To determine if the patient truly has vertigo or another type of dizziness, it is common to inquire if the patient "feels lightheaded" or if "the room appears to be spinning around." Often, patients with true vertigo will respond that the room appears to be spinning.

An accurate history must be performed to help narrow the differential diagnosis. Inquiring about the timing and duration of the dizziness, exacerbating and remitting factors, associated neurologic symptoms, and any hearing loss should be performed as well as queries about medications, toxic exposures, and trauma.

Diagnosis of dizziness and vertigo further depends upon physical examination, with particular attention to examination of the head and neck, cardiovascular system, and neurologic findings. Orthostatic changes in systolic blood pressure and pulse may identify patients with underlying dehydration or autonomic dysfunction, in addition to changes in blood pressure resulting from medical treatment of hypertension. Orthostatic hypotension, defined as a drop in blood pressure of at least 20 mm Hg systolic or 10 mm Hg diastolic within three minutes of standing may be diagnostic of the problem. Additionally, a resting pulse >100 may indicate some volume depletion. Irregular-

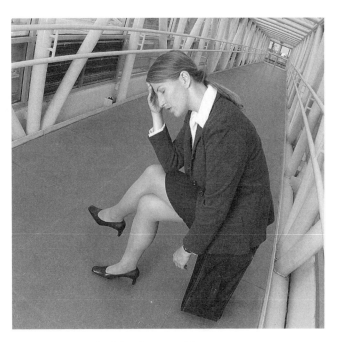

Dizziness is typically defined as one of four types: vertigo, lightheadedness, disequilibrium, and presyncope.

ity of the pulse which includes both bradycardia, or slowing of the heart, and tachycardia, or increasing the speed of the heart rate, may further contribute to underlying cardiovascular abnormalities that may lead to vertigo as a symptom of presyncope, or an actual syncopal, episode.

The Dix-Hallpike maneuver may assist in the diagnosis of benign paroxysmal positional vertigo (BPPV). Because this procedure sometimes provokes the symptoms, the patient must be aware that the symptoms may temporarily worsen while performing the procedure. Through some specific movements, the physician moves the patient's head from an upright position to a supine position, resulting in minimal hyperextension of the neck. A positive test results in horizontal nystagmus which changes direction when the patient sits upright again. Although a positive Dix-Hallpike maneuver may be helpful to differentiate the diagnosis of patients with vertigo, it is not absolutely pathognemonic for BPPV.

Peripheral causes of vertigo include factors that exacerbate the normal functions of the organs of the ear. Commonly, a viral or bacterial infection can inflame the labyrinthine organs. Additionally, the vestibular nerve itself can become inflamed, usually from a self-limited upper respiratory viral infection, while the vesicular eruption of herpes zoster may, in addition to causing skin symptoms and pain associated with this infection, also affect the ear and cause vertigo.

While BPPV causes transient episodes of vertigo symptoms because of calcium debris in the semicircular canals, the etiology of Ménière's disease appears to be caused by an increased amount of endolymph in the semicircular canals of the ear. A cholesteatoma, a benign cyst-like tumor filled with debris, can involve the middle ear and mastoid which may also cause vertigo. Over time, thickening of the tympanic membrane caused by age or chronic recurrent infections may cause otosclerosis which contributes to hearing loss and subsequent vertigo. Trauma, either a direct blow to the ear or indirectly from barotrauma of scuba diving or heavy weight bearing, for example, may cause perilymphatic fistulas to form which may result in vertigo.

Central causes of vertigo are those etiologies that involve the brain. The location of certain tumors may cause symptoms, as may cerebrovascular disease affecting arterial flow to the brain, or subsequent ischemia or infarction resulting in transient ischemic attack or stroke. Some migrainous headaches cause vertigo as part of its pattern, either as part of the aura preceding the headache or part of the migraine itself. Other chronic neurologic conditions, such as multiple sclerosis, which causes demyelinization of the white matter in the central nervous system, may also contribute to the symptoms.

Other causes of vertigo exist. Occasionally, vertigo may result from somatosensory input from head and neck movements. Adverse reactions from medications or drugs may contribute to vertigo. Additionally, psychologic stress may cause a symptom of vertigo, as it relates to hyperventilation associated with anxiety and panic attacks.

Laboratory testing should be considered in the diagnosis of vertigo, especially if there are additional symptoms or if there is a concern about medication side effect or electrolyte abnormality. Also, a formal audiometry test should be considered for those patients complaining of hearing loss. Radiologic studies should be considered in patients with additional neurologic symptoms, patients with risk factors for cerebrovascular disease, or progressive unilateral hearing loss and consideration for neuroimaging should also occur for any localizing neurologic symptom.

Treatment of dizziness and vertigo depends upon the etiology of the symptom. Several medications exist to treat the concurrent nausea and vomiting associated with the disorder. However, those medicines are usually treating the side effects of the vertigo, not the underlying cause, which is why diagnosis is so imperative.

SEE ALSO: Arrhythmia; Ear Disorders; Fainting; Multiple Sclerosis; Neurologic Diseases (General).

BIBLIOGRAPHY. Jon E. Isaacson and Neil M. Vora, "Differential Diagnosis and Treatment of Hearing Loss," *American Family Physician* (v.68/6, 2003); Ronald H. Labuguen, "Initial Evaluation of Vertigo," *American Family Physician* (v.73/2, 2006); Thomas H. Miller and Jerry E. Kruse, "Evaluation of Syncope," *American Family Physician* (v.72/8, 2005); Randy Swartz and Paxton Longwell, "Treatment of Vertigo," *American Family Physician* (v.71/6, 2005).

ANN M. KARTY, M.D.
KANSAS CITY UNIVERSITY OF MEDICINE
AND BIOSCIENCES

Djibouti

Djibouti is located on the eastern coast of Africa, a small, narrow country between Eritrea to the north, Ethiopia to the west and south, and Somalia to the southeast. Yemen is 12 miles off the coast, across the Gulf of Aden. The country has historical ties to France. Ninety-two percent of Djiboutians are Muslim, with 60 percent belonging to the Issa people, 35 percent to the Afar, and the remainder a mix of Arab, Ethiopian, and European.

The population is 486,500, growing at a rate of 2.2 percent annually. The birth rate is 39.53 per 1,000 and the death rate is 19.31 per 1,000.

With its favorable location at the end of the Red Sea, Djibouti's economy is almost entirely reliant on shipping. Most of the population, 86 percent, lives on the coastline, with just a minority of nomadic peoples subsiding in the hot, dry interior. Unemployment in Djibouti is 50 percent, and per capita income is $1,030 per annum.

Life expectancy at birth is 54 years for males and 57 years for females, with healthy life expectancy at 42.5 years for men and 43 years for women. Infant mortality is 102 deaths per 1,000 live births. The death rate for children aged 1–5 years is 126 per 1,000. Maternal mortality is high at 730 deaths per 100,000 live births. About 60 percent of births are monitored by a trained attendant.

Sanitation within the country is limited, with 80 percent of Djiboutians having access to clean water and 50 percent having sanitary facilities. Hepatitis A and E, typhoid, malaria, and dengue fever are common. Djibouti has a high rate of tuberculosis infections, with 100 cases per 100,000 people. Polio has been identified in all neighboring countries and is suspected to be present in Djibouti as well. Immunization rates for children against polio and other illnesses are about 60 percent. A single case of avian flu was detected in May 2006.

The human immunodeficiency virus (HIV)/AIDS rate is 2.9 percent, with an estimated 9,100 Djiboutians infected with the virus and 690 deaths from this disease. The highways passing through Djibouti from Ethiopia are among the busiest on the Horn of Africa, and an active sex trade exists between truckers and the poverty-stricken women who live along the way. A 2005 survey by the United Nations Children's Fund (UNICEF) found that 48 percent of Djiboutians under age 24 did not know that using condoms could help prevent the disease. UNICEF set up an education center in an old shipping container left by the side of a highway; it also hands out an average of 300 condoms a day.

Female genital mutilation (FGM) is widely practiced in Djibouti, with the U.S. State Department estimating that 90 percent to 98 percent of girls under age 10 are undergoing the procedure. Girls from the Issa and Afar tribes are usually given type II FGM, called excision—the removal of the clitoris and the labia minora. Girls from Yemeni tribes are generally given type III, also known as infibulation—the removal of the clitoris, labia minora, and labia majora, with the vagina sewn up with only a tiny hole left open for the passage of urine and menstrual blood.

Medical services are limited and are largely restricted to Djibouti City and outlying towns. Those who live in the interior have little access to healthcare. In 2004, the World Health Organization counted 129 physicians and 257 nurses working in the country.

SEE ALSO: Healthcare, Africa.

BIBLIOGRAPHY. James Morrow, *Djibouti (Modern Middle East Nations and Their Strategic Place in the World Series)* Mason Crest Publishers, 2002); Peter J. Shraeder, Erick J. Mann, *Djibouti*, (ABC-CLIO, 1991).

HEATHER K. MICHON
INDEPENDENT SCHOLAR

DNA

DNA is the abbreviation for the double helix molecule, deoxyribonucleic acid. It is a long chain polymer (polynucleotide) which is found is all living cells. Using its chemical patterns it directs the formation, growth, operations and reproduction of individual cells and thus of organs and of living organisms. The DNA molecule is very long and is like a spiral staircase or a double helix in structure. The structure of DNA was first discovered by James D. Watson and Francis H. C. Cricket in 1953. The discovered of the structure opened the way for detailed understanding of the chemistry of the DNA molecule and of genetics as well.

DNA molecules are composed of two polynucleotide strands wrapped around each other to form a double helix. They consist of two long nucleotides composed of a sugar molecule and a phosphate group bonded to a DNA base. This sequence is repeated numerous times to form genes and chromosomes. The legs of the DNA spiral staircase have major and minor groves. Other chemicals form the connecting steps. The whole molecule is composed of thousands of smaller chemical units called nucleotides which are bonded together to form polynucleotides.

Nucleotides are composed of a phosphate, a sugar (deoxyribose) and another compound which is called generally a base. The sugar is 2'-deoxyribose which has five carbon atoms. The carbon atoms in the sugar molecule are named 1' (prime), 2' and so forth. Hydrogen bonds between bases on the two DNA strands stabilize the double helix.

There are four types of bases: adenine, guanine, thymine, and cytosine. The adenine and guanine bases have two carbon-nitrogen rings and are purines. The thymine and cytosine bases have a single ring and are pyrimidine. The bases are attached to the 1' carbon of the deoxyribose. It takes a sugar plus a base to make a nucleoside. Nucleotides have one, two, or three phosphate groups. These are attached to 5'-carbon atom of the sugar molecule.

The bases vary in the nucleotides, but the sugar and the phosphate are the same in all DNA nucleotides. Nucleotides may be individual molecules or they may be polymers of DNA or ribonucleic acid (RNA). It is the varying combinations of bases that create the power of the DNA molecule to replicate itself thus to grow new living cells. The nucleotides bonded as triphosphates of the four bases that are boned into DNA polynucleotide chains.

The base adenine is a heterocyclic aromatic organic compound. It is composed of a pyrimidine ring which is fused to an imidazole ring. There are two types of nitrogenous bases—purine and pyrimidines. Purines are the essential part of both deoxyribonucleotides (DNA) and ribonucleotides (RNA). In addition to its role in DNA and RNA adenine is an important part of many organic chemical reactions and processes. The reactions include protein synthesis and cellular respiration.

In earlier chemistry adenine was often identified as vitamin B4, but understanding has been modified. Adenine combines with two of the B vitamins—niacin and riboflavin. These form into essential cofactors. Some evolutionists have argued that adenine was synthesized from hydrogen cyanide (HCH) to begin the formation of life; however, this view is not universally held.

Adenine forms nucleotides of DNA from its purine nucleobases. Its hydrogen molecules bond in DNA with thymine. In RNA adenine bonds with uracil and is a part of protein synthesis. Other reactions involving adenine include the formation of adenosine by bonding with ribose and deoxyadenosine by bonding with deoxyribose. It also bonds with phosphate groups to form denosine triphosphate (ATP). Cellular metabolism uses chemical energy from chemical reactions through adenosine triposphate.

The DNA base guanine ($C_5H_5N_5O$) is a purine with a pyrimidine-imidazole ring system with conjugated double bonds. It has a keto form and an enol form. With three hydrogen bonds it binds to cytosine which acts as an hydrogen donor. Specific locations in the guanine structure act as hydrogen acceptors. It is present in both DNA and RNA.

Thymine (5-methylluracil) is a DNA base that is a pyrimidine nucleobase. It is a derivative of methylation of uracil at the fifth carbon atom. It is a part of the DNA molecule. However, in RNA it is replaced by uracil. In DNA, thymine (T) bonds with adenine (A). The atomic structure of the nucleic acid is stabilized with two hydrogen bonds. Deoxyribose combines with thymine to form nucleoside deoxythymidine known as thymidine. It can bond with phosphates to form posphorylated molecules on the one, two, or three phosphoric acid groups. These form, respectively, TMP, TDP, or TTP.

DNA REPLICATION

In DNA replication a common mutation occurs with two thymines or a cytosine are exposed to ultraviolet (UV) light. The UV light causes thymine dimmers to form. This causes pattern disorder in the DNA molecule and blocks its normal functioning.

The DNA base cytosine was first discovered in 1894. It is a phyimidine derivative with a heterocyclic aromatic ring. Isolated from the thymus tissue of a calf it was within 10 years synthesized in laboratory experiments. Its atomic structure was understood by 1903. It is one of the nucleotide bases of DNA. It has a key role in genetic information transmission. Cytosine bonds with guanine with three hydrogen atoms.

DNA has the ability to transmit genetic information that is needed by living cells to reproduce. This ability is closely related to the structure of DNA. While DNA is a polymer it is composed of long chain monomer (nucleotides). In each nucleotide is a sugar, a nitrogen molecule in the form of a molecular ring (base) and a phosphate base. The characteristic double-helix structure is a repetition of bands in a regular pattern. The DNA helix executes a turn after set of 10 base molecules. From a top view the DNA molecule looks like a stack of plates set on top on one another. From a side view it has on the opposing strands a distance that makes it "antiparallel."

Variants of DNA forms occur when the molecule and crystalline forms of the molecule form under different conditions. The A form is more compact than the B form found in living cells. The C, D, E forms also exist. The Z form takes a left-handed double-helix shape.

Complementary base pairing between the two polynucleotide chains is fundamental to the structure and functioning of DNA. The bases of the two polynucleotides interact with one another. This is possible because the space between the two polynucleotides is at a distance that allows the two-ring purine molecules to engage the single ring pyrimidine molecules.

The bases of the two polynucleotide chains interact with each other. Adenine and react with thymine because the two ring purine molecules react with single ring pyrimidine. Guanine reacts with cytosine. The hydrogen bonds that bond between the bases are stabilizing. Two hydrogen bonds form between A and T, while three hydrogen bonds from between G and C in complementary base pairing. The sequence is predictive because they bonding must follow a pattern. It allows one strand to compliment and thus to replicate the other strand.

The bonding of A to T and G to C a sequential pattern is formed. Because of the size of the molecules A and G or C do not bond because they cannot fit into the double helix nor may hydrogen bonding occur.

The complementary bonding of the base pairs allows one strand to replicate the other strand. It is this vital mechanism that allows the expression of genetic information via messenger RNA molecules.

The structure of RNA is similar to DNA, but with some significant differences. The RNA molecule replaces 2'-deocyribose and the base thymine with uracil. It can base pair with adenine. Moreover, RNA molecules exist normally as a single polynucleotide strand and not as a double helix. However, it is possible for it to have base pairings that occur for a short period of time creating double stranded regions.

The DNA polymer encodes genetic information in the sequences of the bases in the DNA molecule. It does so in a series of genes. Genes are units of information. They correspond to specific segments of the DNA. They encode the amino acid sequence of a polypeptide. Human cells have 23 chromosomes. They genes are dispersed along the DNA molecule. In between the genes lie noncoding intergenic DNA sequences. Because of the coding sequencing can act as template strands DNA molecules have a vast range of genetic informational coding possibilities.

Some of the genes are arranged in clusters. Operons occur in bacteria and contain coregulated genes. Higher organisms have multigene families. These genes are identical or similar, but they are not regulated in a coordinated manner. The expression of the genetic information in the genes in DNA is done by the genes. The expression process has a RNA copy made of the gene. It then makes a protein which allows cells to function. Cells use many proteins to in a orchestrated manner. The success of gene expression manufactures proteins at the right place and time.

Gene expression is very restricted because while a number of genes may be present in a cell only a few are active. In addition, different types of tissue cells express different genes. The promoter which is a related segment of DNA regulates the coding sequence. A series of segments called exons are separated from the non-coding sequences (introns). The exons are responsible for most of the coding sequencing. The promoter binds RNA polymerase and associated transcription factor proteins. It also begins the process of synthesizing an RNA molecule. In replication the introns are removed from RNA transcripts of the gene's code. Between genes the number and size of introns varies. Splicing eliminates them from replication. In this process mistakes can occur. There are pseudogenes which are simply mistakes that are nonfunctional.

Physically a gene is a discrete segmane of DNA with a base sequence that encodes the amino acid sequence of a polypeptide. Gene segments of DNA vary widely in size. They may have as little as a hundred base pairs. Or they may have several million base pairs. Higher organisms including humans have gene sequences arranged in a very long sequence of DNA molecules called chromosomes. In humans there are at least 20,000 to as many as 25,000 genes arranged on 23 chromosomes.

Intergenic DNA molecules separate the genes from one another. The intergenic DNA material does not seem to have a role in replication. The biological information is carried on just one of the strands of DNA. It is

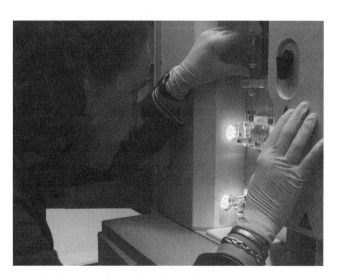

National Human Genome Research Institute researcher Elizabeth Gillanders, Ph.D., monitoring a DNA sequencing machine.

the template strand and it produces the complementary RNA molecule sequence which orders the synthesis of a polypeptide. The nontemplate strand of DNA has potential to act as a template strand. The strands of DNA are also called sense and antisense strand or coding and noncoding strands.

In general genes are spread along the chromosomes in a random fashion. However, some are clustered into groups. There are two types of clusters of genes: operons and multigene families. Operons are found in bacteria. They are genes that act in a coordinated fashion so that they can encode proteins in a closely regulated manner. For example in *E. coli*, the lac operon has three genes. These encode enzymes that break down lactose. The bacterium uses the lac operon to enzymes to break down lactose as an energy source in a coordinated manner so that they switch on and off together.

Higher organisms do not have operons. Instead clustered genes are multigene families. The genes in multigene families are very similar or identical which is different from the genes in operons. It has been speculated that during the evolutionary process that genes clustered in order to fulfill a need for multiple copies of the gene. Different chromosomes contain multigene families which may have developed during evolution when DNA rearranged.

Simple multigene families have identical genes. For example many cells need the gene product 55 ribosomal RNA. There are about 2,000 genes that produce it exiting as clustered copies.

Complex multigene families have similar, but non-identical genes. For example the globin gene family produces a series of polypeptides. These differ from each other as α, β γ, ε, χ globin molecules. These forms of globin have different amino acid groups attached to produce the difference between them. The globin polypeptides form complexes join with heme to form hemoglobin the chemical that carries oxygen to cells.

Gene expression is the process by which the biological information in the DNA molecule is used by the cell. The central dogma (a term coined by Francis Crick) stated that information is transferred fro DNA to RNA to a protein. The central dogma says that the transfer of genetic information is asymmetrical. It flows in only one direction. It cannot reserve engineer a product. The process of gene expression occurs when DNA molecules copy their genetic information to a RNA molecule which it synthesizes.

The RNA molecule is created by the process of transcription. The RNA molecule then directs the synthesis of a polypeptide that has an amino acid sequence. The specific amino acid sequence is determined by the base on the RNA in the process of translation. The amino acid sequence now has a function dictated by its protein.

The number of possible different human beings is limited by the number of possible combinations of bases into genes. The bases (A, G, T, C) can combine four ways. However, a gene may have three hundred bases. This gene could have a total of 4,300 possible arrangements. Every one of the possible permutation could then produce a different gene and a slightly different human. Given a total of 25,000 genes in all humans there are nn(25,000) possible combinations of bases. This is a very high number, but not an infinite one. Some of these base sets acting as genes might be lethal combinations so that the individual might not survive to birth or long afterward. However, perhaps more important than DNA is the development of a human being is their environmental experiences.

SEE ALSO: Chromosome; DNA Repair; Gene Array Analysis; Gene Mapping; Gene Pool; Gene Silencing; Gene Transfer; Gene and Gene Therapy; Genetic Code; Genetics.

BIBLIOGRAPHY. Terry Brown, *Gene Cloning and DNA Analysis: An Introduction* (Blackwell Publishing Professional, 2006); Hugh Fletcher, Ivor Hickey, and Paul Winter, *Bios Instant Notes: Genetics.* 3rd ed., (Taylor & Francis, 2007); Arthur Kornberg and Tania Baker, *DNA Replication* (University Science Books, 2005); Benjamin Lewin, *Genes VIII*, (Benjamin Cummings,m 2003); Arseni Markoff, *Analytical Tools for DNA, Genes and Genomes: Nuts & Bolts* (DNA Press, 2005); Ulrike Nuber, ed., *DNA Microarrays* (Taylor & Francis, 2005); Matt Ridley, *Genome: the Autobiography of a Species in 23 Chapters* (HarperCollins, 2006); James D. Watson, *Double Helix: A Personal Account of the Discovery of the Structure of DNA* (Simon & Schuster, 2001); James D. Watson, et al., *Recombinant DNA: Genes and Genomes – A Short Course* (W. H. Freeman, 2006); Michael R. R. Winfrey, Marc A. Rott, and Alan T. Wortman, *Unraveling DNA: Molecular Biology for the Laboratory* (Benjamin Cummings, 1997).

Andrew J. Waskey
Dalton State College

DNA Repair

DNA repair refers to the mechanisms by which a cell maintains the integrity of its genetic code. This integrity not only ensures the survival of a species, which requires that parental DNA be inherited as faithfully as possible by the offspring, but it also preserves the health of an individual. Mutations in the genetic code can lead to cancer and other genetic diseases.

Successful DNA replication requires that the two purine bases, adenine and guanine, pair faithfully with their pyrimidine counterparts, thymine and cytosine. There are three types of damage that can prevent correct base pairing: spontaneous mutations, replication errors, and chemical modification. Spontaneous mutations occur when DNA bases react with their environment, as when water hydrolyzes a base and changes its structure, causing it to pair with the wrong base. Replication errors are minimized when the DNA replication machinery "proofreads" its own synthesis, but sometimes the mismatched bases escape proofreading. Chemical agents modify bases and interfere with DNA replication. Nitrosamines, found in beer and pickled food products, aklylate bases and the DNA backbone. Oxidizing agents or ionizing radiation create free radicals in the cell that oxidize bases, especially guanine. Ultraviolet (UV) rays fuse adjacent pyrimidines, preventing DNA replication. Ionizing radiation or drugs such as bleomycin can also block replication, by creating double-stranded breaks in the DNA. Base analogs or intercalating agents can cause abnormal insertions and deletions in the sequence.

There are three types of repair mechanisms: direct reversal of the damage, excision repair, and recombination repair. Direct reversal repair is specific to the damage. For example, in a process called photoreactivation, pyrimidine bases fused by UV light are separated by DNA photolyase. For direct reversal of akylation events, a DNA methyltransferase detects and removes the alkyl group. Excision repair can be specific or nonspecific. In base excision repair, DNA glycolyases specifically identify and remove the mismatched base. In nucleotide excision repair, the repair machinery nonspecifically recognizes distortions in the double helix caused by mismatched bases and excises the distorted region. Recombination repair takes advantage of the fact that mammalian chromosomes come in pairs, and uses the sequence from an undamaged sister chromosome to repair the damaged one.

Often when DNA is damaged, the cell chooses to replicate over the lesion instead of waiting for repair (translesion synthesis). Although this may lead to mutations, it is preferable to a complete halt in DNA replication, which leads to death. On the other hand, the importance of proper DNA repair is highlighted when repair fails. The oxidation of guanine by free radicals leads to G-T transversion, one of the most common mutations in human cancer.

Hereditary nonpolyposis colorectal cancer results from a mutation in the MSH and MLH proteins, which repair mismatches during replication. Xeroderma pigmentosum (XP) is another condition that results from failed DNA repair. Patients with XP are highly sensitive to light, exhibit premature skin aging and are prone to malignant skin tumors, all because the XP proteins, which mediate nucleotide excision repair, can no longer function.

SEE ALSO: Cancer; Colorectal Cancer; DNA; Genetic Code; Genetics; Skin Cancer.

BIBLIOGRAPHY. J. O. Andressoo, J. H. Hoeijmakers, and J. R. Mitchell, *Nucleotide Excision Repair and the Balance between Cancer and Aging* (Cell Cycle, 2006); Donald Kufe, et al., eds., *Cancer Medicine,* 6th ed. (Hamilton, 2003); James Watson, et al., *Molecular Biology of the Gene* (Benjamin Cummings, 2003).

CINDY CHANG
COLD SPRING HARBOR LABORATORY
SUNY STONY BROOK

Dominica

Dominica is a small country located in the Windward Islands of the Caribbean, between the islands of Guadeloupe and Martinique. Its virtually unspoiled beauty has won it the nickname of "the nature island of the Caribbean." The island is 289.5 square miles (754 square kilometers) and has eight active volcanoes; 65 percent of the country is covered with rainforest. Dominica is home to the world's second largest "boiling lake," a fumarole, or opening, in the Earth's crust that allows volcanic gases to heat lake water to almost 200 degrees F. The site was declared a World Heritage Site in 1997.

Dominica's population is 68,900, with a growth rate of minus 0.08 percent annually. The migration rate is minus 9.3 per 1,000, as natives leave in search of work and opportunity. The economy is based on agriculture, particularly the cultivation of bananas. The industry has been in decline since the 1990s, leading to high rates of unemployment. The country's geographical location in the "hurricane belt" leaves it vulnerable to heavy rainfall, flash flooding, and landslides. Volcanic activity and earthquakes are common.

Life expectancy is high, at 72 years for males and 78 years for females. Child mortality is quite low, at 13 deaths per 1,000 for infants under age 1, and 15 deaths per 1,000 for children aged 1–5. Maternal mortality is reported at 67 deaths per 100,000 live births. All births in Dominica are attended by trained personnel, and 100 percent of women receive prenatal care.

Immunization rates for children are high, and all schoolchildren are tested for hearing and vision problems, as well as growth and development issues. Adolescents accounted for 53 percent of attempted suicides reported between 1996 and 1999.

Dengue fever is the most common vector borne disease present in Dominica. Malaria was eradicated in 1962, although there are some sporadic "imported" cases. Gastrointestinal diseases such as *E. coli*, giardia, and typhoid are frequently reported. There was a single case of leprosy diagnosed in 1998. Mortality is driven by accidents and violence, cardiovascular disease, and cancers. Diabetes is becoming more of a health problem for Dominicans. It is the second leading cause of hospital and clinic visits and the fourth leading cause of death in adults. In 2000, there were an estimated 3,000 cases of diabetes on the island. Dominica is almost free of HIV/AIDS, with only 69 cases confirmed in 2002. There are no known tuberculosis/HIV co-infections.

The Dominica healthcare system is small, with 38 doctors and 317 nurses reported in 1997. Per capita government expenditures on health are $151 annually, although citizens generally pay 100 percent of medical expenses out of pocket. The Ministry of Health monitors seven health districts, including general hospitals and community-based clinics. The

government has been active in developing programs for specific populations in need, particularly children and the elderly.

SEE ALSO: Dengue; Diabetes.

BIBLIOGRAPHY. Pan American Health Organization "Dominica, General Situation and Trends," http://www.paho.org/english/HIA1998/Dominica.pdf (cited July 2007); World Health Organization, "Dominica," http://www.who.int/countries/dma/en/ (cited July 2007).

HEATHER K. MICHON
INDEPENDENT SCHOLAR

Dominican Republic

Located in the Caribbean, this nation occupies the eastern end of the island of Hispaniola, and was a Spanish colony until gaining its independence on February 27, 1844. It has a population of 8,834,000 (2004) and there are 216 doctors and 30 nurses per 100,000 people. There are also 516 dentists in the country. Until relatively recently, the health services in much of the Dominican Republic were fairly rudimentary.

It is believed that Christopher Columbus, on his first voyage in 1492, may have landed on the Samaná peninsula which was then a separate island off the north coast of the Dominican Republic. On his second voyage in 1493, he built a base at what is now Santo Domingo, and it was during this visit that he and his sailors noticed the local Taino people smoking rolled leaves of tobacco. Some tobacco leaves were then brought back to Europe, with a major effect on the healthcare around the world to the present day.

The major health problems facing people in the Dominican Republic include malaria, especially in rural parts of the country; heat exhaustion and heat stroke, and schistosomiasis (bilharzia). The latter comes from parasitic worms which live in infected freshwater snails and are commonly found in rivers, lakes and especially near dams. Tourists are thus advised not to swim except in chlorinated swimming pools. There have also been cases of dengue fever, and a prevalence of human T-cell leukemia lymphona virus in some black former slave communities in the country. By 1988, there had been 701 cases of the acquired immune deficiency syndrome (AIDS), of which 65 had died. Subsequently, AIDS increased dramatically, and HIV and AIDS are now widespread.

Healthcare in the Dominican Republic is run by the Secretariat of State for Public Health and Social Welfare, with the Secretary of State having a position in the cabinet. The Asociatión Médica Dominicana (Dominican Medical Association), founded in 1941, operates from Santo Domingo, the country's capital, and publishes the *Revista Médica Dominicana*. It has 1,550 members. Founded in the same year, the Asociatión Médica de Santiago (Santiago Medical Association) operates from the city of Santiago de los Cabelleros, in the north of the country, and publishes *Boletin Médico*, and has 65 members. Mention should also be made of the Dominican Medical Congress which has been in operation since 1844.

There are a number of medical schools throughout the country, the main one being the Faculty of Medicine in the Universidad Autónoma de Santo Domingo, the university founded in 1538 making it the oldest university in the Americas. There is a Faculty of Health Sciences at the Pontificia Universidad Catolica Madre y Maestra; a Faculty of Medicine at the Universidad central del Este; a School of Public Health at the Universidad Eugenio Maria de Hostos, the Faculty of Health Sciences at the Universidad Nacional Pedro Henriquez Urena and at the Universidad Tencnológia de Santiago.

From the mid-1970s, there has been a major government attempt to improve healthcare throughout the country. As a result, by the early 1980s, there were some 5,000 rural health clinics, health subcenters and some satellite clinics. Pharmacies are now common throughout the country. Doctors were required to serve for one year in remote or poor districts, but there were complaints that some poorly trained local health workers were not sufficiently trained in how to teach about health problems and disease prevention. To alert the public to health care concerns, and raise money for charity, the postal authorities of the Dominican Republic have issued large numbers of postage stamps to raise money for medical charities.

SEE ALSO: Leukemia; Malaria.

BIBLIOGRAPHY. *Congreso Médico Dominicano del Centenario 1844–1944: Memoria* (Editorial El Diario, 1945); Frank Moya Pons, ed., *El Ejercicio de la Medicina en la República Dominicana* (Editora Amigo del Hogar, 1983).

JUSTIN CORFIELD
GEELONG GRAMMAR SCHOOL, AUSTRALIA

Double-Blinded Study

A randomized clinical trial is regarded as the most highly influential study design that provides the highest level of evidence in the assessment of therapeutic outcome in medical science because it increases the validity of the study by eliminating potential study-related biases. However, to address potential study-related biases, various criteria have been established to maintain such high level of evidence and are largely based on the quality of the trial. Thus, trial quality is an imperative component in any randomized clinical trial. If steps are taken to reduce potential bias, the appropriately size and direction of the intervention effect can be properly obtained. One method utilized to decrease the risk of potential bias that could mislead the intervention effect is double blinding.

Prior to the start of a randomized clinical trial, generation of the allocation sequence is imperative. In clinical trials, defining the manner as to how the allocation sequence is generated characterizes the type of study design as being randomized, quasi-randomized, or a controlled clinical trial. If the generation of the allocation sequence was unpredictable, the two groups being compared are associated with less confounds between them and a true measure of the treatment effect can be obtained. Compromising the allocation sequence could contribute to selection bias.

According to the latest statement by the CONSORT group regarding improving quality trials in randomized clinical trial, allocation concealment represents the method utilized to employ the random allocation sequence. Such a method clarifies whether the allocation sequence was or was not properly concealed until interventions were assigned. Proper allocation concealment prevents the participants and the investigators from knowing in advance what treatment the subjects will receive. Therefore, both the participants and the investigators or the researcher responsible for the assessment of the intervention are both blinded (double blinding) to the treatment administered. Thus, adhering to allocation concealment by double blinding prevents influencing the subjects whether or not to enroll, adhere, or respond to a treatment regime; thereby, decreasing the risk of selection bias. In fact, a meta-analysis of various trials assessing if allocation concealment was inadequate/unclear or adequate indicated that trials with inadequate/unclear concealment yielded an overestimated treatment effect by 30 percent. The overestimated effect of lack of allocation concealment was twofold in comparison to the assessment of nonblinding versus blinding. Thus, allocation concealment is an imperative component to trial quality.

The lack of double blinding can further affect the true estimate of the treatment and contribute to performance bias by the patient and detection/measurement bias by the study investigators. Knowledge of the treatment by the study investigators and subjects could affect the outcome being expressed and measured; thus, affecting the true effect of the treatment. In addition, not accounting for study withdrawals or dropout rates, also referred to as attrition bias, may contribute to unbalanced sample groups; thus, the effects of the treatment could be inappropriately estimated. Methodological quality in randomized clinical trials is largely based upon the proper execution of the generation and concealment of the allocation sequence, and the assessment of withdrawals or dropouts. However, to properly perform such methods or avoid deleteriously affecting certain study events that may influence the treatment effect, double blinding is paramount.

SEE ALSO: Clinical Trial; Crossover Study; Prospective Study; Randomized Clinical Trial.

BIBLIOGRAPHY. Centre for Evidence Based Medicine, "Levels of Evidence and Grades of Recommendations," www.cebm.net/levels_of_evidence.asp (cited October 2006); Matthias Egger, Shah Ebrahim, and George Davey Smith, "Where Now for Meta-Analysis," *International Journal of Epidemiology* (v.31, 2002); David Moher, et al., "Does Quality of Reports of Randomised Trials Affect Estimates of Intervention Efficacy Reported in Meta-Analyses?" *Lancet* (v.352, 1998); David Moher, Kenneth F. Schulz, and Douglas G. Altman, "The CONSORT Statement: Revised Recommendations for Improving the Quality of Reports of Parallel-Group Randomized Trials," *Journal of the American Medical Association* (v.285, 2001); David L. Sackett and Michael Gent, "Controversy in Counting and Attributing Events in Clinical Trials," *New England Journal of Medicine* (v.301, 1979).

DINO SAMARTZIS, D.SC., M.SC., DIP. EBHC
HARVARD UNIVERSITY AND ERASMUS UNIVERSITY

Doula

This word, coming from the Greek, refers to a woman who helps another woman, and in medical terminology has come to mean a person, often a woman, who is a nonmedical assistant in prenatal care, childbirth, and in looking after a baby soon after he or she has been born.

Initially, the term in Greek generally referred to a slave, with the medical anthropologist Dr. Dana Raphael being one of the first to use the term when she referred to experienced mothers among the Ilocanos in Luzon in the Philippines helping mothers who had just had their first babies. Although relatives such as grandmothers and aunts often helped people in village societies where there were extended family networks, there was also heavy use of nonrelated women. The more experienced women were able to help with breastfeeding and newborn babies. As a result, this was largely dealing with the postpartum period (i.e., after birth), but gradually came to be used to refer to people who helped before birth as well. Work by medical researchers Marshall H. Klaus, John H. Kennell, and Phyllis H. Klaus, in their book *Mothering the Mother* (1993) showed the importance of the doula attending birth, and as a result, the process became more common in nonvillage societies such as in cities.

Nowadays, doulas involved in labor support are trained in dealing with the emotional and physical comfort needs of women about to give birth. Some work attached to hospitals and clinics, but many, especially in third world countries, work on a semiformal or informal basis visiting expectant women, and those who have recently given birth, in their homes. Their role has often been increased to involve them with helping mothers in recovery after childbirth by doing housework, preparing meals, and buying food when the woman has no other social network on which she can call. On another level, they can also advise authorities if the mother is having any problems before or after birth.

Although doulas in the United States and Canada are not required to be certified, this is possible, and many have completed long courses and built up years of experience. They have also been involved in providing medical advice to mothers, drawing up exercise regimens during pregnancy, and giving advice on diet and other areas. They suggest positions that the woman can adopt during labor, which is particularly important when labor pains begin unexpectedly. They also advise the partner of the mother, can be present at birth, and help with immediate postnatal care.

SEE ALSO: Pregnancy; Prenatal Care.

BIBLIOGRAPHY. Marshall H. Klaus, John H. Kennell, and Phyllis H. Klaus, *Mothering the Mother: How a Doula Can Help You Have a Shorter, Easier, and Healthier Birth* (Addison Wesley, 1993); Amen Ness, Lisa Gould Rubin, and Jackie Frederick, *Birth That's Right for You: A Doctor and a Doula Help You Choose and Customize the Best Birth Option to Fit Your Needs* (McGraw-Hill, 2006); Dana Raphael and Flora Davis, *Only Mothers Know: Patterns of Infant Feeding in Traditional Cultures* (Greenwood, 1985); Karen Salt, *A Holistic Guide to Embracing Pregnancy, Childbirth and Motherhood: Wisdom and Advice from a Doula* (Da Capo, 2002).

JUSTIN CORFIELD
GEELONG GRAMMAR SCHOOL, AUSTRALIA

Down Syndrome

Down syndrome, also called Down's syndrome or trisomy 21, is a congenital disorder caused by the presence of all or part of an extra 21st chromosome. This gives people with Down syndrome 47 chromosomes, rather than 46. It acquired the name after the British doctor John Langdon Haydon Down (1828–1896) who first described it in 1866. The outward physical signs of the disorder, usually identified at birth, are a range of major and minor differences in body struc-

ture, including an impairment of cognitive ability and also physical growth.

The incidence of Down syndrome is estimated at 1 for every 800 to 1,000 births, and it was first recognized by John L.H. Down as a different form of mental retardation in 1866, and four years later he published his report "Observations" on an Ethnic Classification of Idiots which was published in the Clinical Lecture Reports from London Hospital. Down, born in Torpoint, Cornwall, was from a well-connected family—his great-great grandfather on his father's side was the Roman Catholic Bishop of Derry, and the daughters of his sister married into the Darwin and Keynes families. Apprenticed to his father, a village apothecary, Down later went to work as a surgeon in London, and then to the Royal London Hospital and the Royal College of Surgeons, and became a Fellow of the Royal College of Physicians. He then worked at the Earlswood Asylum for Idiots in Surrey, and conducted much of his work at the Normansfield Asylum, in Teddington, Middlesex. His work used many terms such as mongolism which have long since stopped being used. There were various programs in the United States and also Nazi Germany involving identifying people suffering from Down syndrome, and then embarking on forcible sterilization, even though the cause remained unknown at the time, but was believed to be genetic.

In 1961, some 19 prominent geneticists wrote an open letter to *The Lancet* in which they argued that the "mongoloid" description should be dispensed with, and the journal supported the new term *Down's Syndrome*. Four years later, the delegate to the World Health Organization from Mongolia also objected to the term, forcing it to be dropped as an official term.

The vast majority of the people who suffer from Down syndrome have a third chromosome which is associated with the chromosome 21 pair. This is why the disorder is often known as trisomy 21. There are also some 4 percent of sufferers who have an abnormal condition known as translocation. This is because in their bodies, the extra chromosome in the 21 pair has broken off and attached itself to another chromosome. In spite of much research into the cause of Down syndrome, the reason for the chromosomal abnormalities is still unknown although it has been shown that there is a higher incidence of Down syndrome in the offspring of women who give birth over the age of 35. Although statistically the number of Down syndrome births in children remains one in 800–1,000, the level of incidence in women who give birth over the age of 40 are one in 40. This has led to a range of tests which can be used to diagnose Down syndrome prenatally by checking for the presence of the abnormal chromosome in samples of the fetal cells which can be collected from the amniotic fluid.

As well as an extra chromosome, there are many common physical features associated with Down syndrome. These involve having shorter limbs and neck, poor muscle tone, and a single transverse palmar crease. Those affected with Down syndrome also usually have an enlarged protruding tongue and lips, a sloping underchin, and eyes which have an almond shape, sometimes with an inner epicanthal fold, and low-set ears. There are also several problems such as a lower-than-average cognitive ability, at its most extreme involving moderate mental retardation, with some having severe mental retardation, as well as heart and kidney malformations. Some 40 percent of people with Down syndrome also tend to suffer from congenital heart disease.

A number of notable people who suffered from Down syndrome include the German actor Bobby Brederlow, the New York actor Chris Burke, the Belgian actor Pascal Duquenne, the London actor Max Lewis, the Scottish film actress Paula Sage, the artist Judith Scott, and the Argentine singer Miguel Tomasin who sung with the avant-rock band Reynols. In addition, Stephanie Ginnsz, an actor, was the first with Down syndrome to take the lead part in a motion picture. Anne de Gaulle (1928–1948), daughter of the French politician Charles de Gaulle, suffered from Down syndrome; and there has been retrospective speculation that Charles Waring Darwin, son of the naturalist Charles Darwin, was also a sufferer from Down syndrome, evidence for this included the fact that Darwin himself conducted a correspondence with John Langdon Haydon Down.

Modern healthcare has meant that many people with Down syndrome now live into adulthood, although those with major heart defects that cannot be subjected to corrective surgery die as children. Overall in the United States and western Europe, people with Down syndrome have a life expectancy of about 55, lower than normal adults, mainly because the condition means that they age prematurely. Many have managed to be self-supporting to a large degree, being able to work in the home, or a sheltered workshop. With increasing tolerance in the wider society, and the greater awareness of Down syndrome, there is a much more general acceptance of the disorder and people with the disorder which was not the case even 30 years ago when many Western countries had asylums where sufferers would spend most of their lives. The work undertaken by the National Down Syndrome Society in the United States, which holds Down Syndrome Month each October, has been very effective in raising the profile of the disorder. The Down Syndrome Awareness Day is held on October 20 each year in South Africa.

SEE ALSO: Degenerative Nerve Diseases; Healthcare, U.S. and Canada.

BIBLIOGRAPHY. Valentine Dmitriev, *Early Education for Children with Down Syndrome: Time to Begin* (Pro-Ed, 2001); Margaret Farrell and Pat Gunn, *Literacy for Children with Down Syndrome: Early Days* (Post Pressed, 2000); Lynn Nadel and Donna Rosenthal, eds., *Down Syndrome: Living and Learning in the Community* (Wiley-Liss, 1995); Kristina Routh, *Down's Syndrome* (Heinemann Library, 2004); Carol Tinget, ed., *Down Syndrome: A Resource Handbook* (Taylor & Francis, 1988); O. C. Ward, *John Langdon Down, 1828–1896* (Royal Society of Medicine Press, 1998).

JUSTIN CORFIELD
GEELONG GRAMMAR SCHOOL, AUSTRALIA

Drinking Water

Drinking water is potable water or water that can be drunk or ingested by human beings. Water is a vital necessity for humans, without which they quickly die.

The modern world is now rapidly growing more urban than rural and has a population projected to reach as high as 12 billion people by the year 2050. Securing potable water for all people is challenging the limited supplies.

Although almost 70 percent of the surface of the Earth is covered by water in the world's oceans and seas its saline content is too high for humans to drink. In addition, enormous amounts of water are locked in ice caps in Antarctica, Greenland, and elsewhere. Other large quantities exist as water vapor in clouds or in the atmosphere. As a consequence, only about one or two percent of the water on the surface of the earth is fresh water available to people for drinking.

Virtually all of the water that people drink begins as rain water. It is gathered by nature and is available in very unevenly distributed places. As a result, drinking water comes from the surface of the Earth or from relatively shallow sources underground. The most common natural water sources for potable water are springs, lakes, streams, rivers, rain collectors, underground aquifers, or other natural sources.

The fresh water supplies needed as drinking water are competed for by agricultural, industrial, and recreational users. In addition, it is simply not possible to sustain the ecology if all of the waters of lakes and streams are diverted for human use. As a consequence, much of the water drunk by people in urban areas is purified water. This is water that may have been used previously for industry, sewage, agricultural runoff, or other polluting and toxic uses. However, the science of water purification is advanced to the level where water can be used and then purified as is moves down stream to the sea in city after city.

The use of purification systems would be required even if the water supplies were not polluted by prior human use. There are a variety of diseases that come from microbes in water such as *E. coli* or typhoid that would imperil human health without purification. Modern water purification uses chemicals to purify the water people drink. Chlorine or other chemicals are used to kill germs. The use of chlorine or chlorine compounds carries a small risk because it is an element that is a known carcinogen. However, the risk is very small that chlorine may cause cancer versus the very high likelihood that large numbers of people will sicken and die from untreated water.

Innovative ideas offered the sources for new supplies of fresh water have included melting frozen water and in Libya pumping water trapped in earlier geologic eras across the Sahara Desert to population centers. Another important possible source that has been offered is the used of desalination plants that can extract fresh potable water from sea water.

There are currently problems associated with the used of desalination processes. The problems include the high amounts of energy that are required to de-salinate water and the quality of the water itself. If it is sterile water, that is just pure evaporated water then it will taste flat and it will also be lacking in minerals that are found in natural water. Strictly speaking, all water on Earth is mineral water. As rain falls, it can collect minerals from the air. When it hits the ground, it will usually absorb some combination of minerals from rocks and soils it passes through.

The minerals in the water people drink is one source of the minerals that are dietary supplements needed by people. Iodine is just one such mineral. The recognition that minerals are important to health has historically led people to seek out mineral springs. There, especially at hot springs, people have drunk and bathed in the mineral waters. There are also mineral springs that bottle and sell their waters around the globe.

Famous bottle mineral waters include Apollinaris from Neuenahr, Germany; Badoit from Saint Galmier, France; Bru from Chevron, Belgium; Caddo Valley water and Mountain Valley water from near Hot Springs, Arkansas; Evian from Evian-les-Bains, France; Fiuggi from Italy; Gerolsteiner Srudel, from Gerolstein, Germany; Mattoni from Kysebel-Kyselka, Czech Republic; Perrier from Vergeze, France; Poland Water from Poland, Maine; San Pellegrino, from Bergamo, Italy; Vittel water from Vittel, France. Some of these bottle mineral waters are "sparkling" water, that is, they contain carbon dioxide that is found in the water at the spring from which it is drawn. Other commercial mineral waters are "still" mineral waters, that is, they do not have a significant gaseous content.

The mineral content of mineral waters varies. There are springs that contain sweet-tasting limestone minerals. Other springs contain concentrations of alkali and can be unpleasant in tastes, but desired for bathing. In some places sulfur in the water gives it a rotten egg smell, which is however often desired as a natural mineral water for drinking and bathing in a spa.

Some commercial mineral waters such as Apollinaris have a high mineral content. Others such as Poland Water from Maine have a low mineral content. Many claims have been made about the health benefits that come from drinking these mineral waters. Europeans have long made a variety of health claims about their mineral waters. In the United States, the Food and Drug Administration which supervises such claims has a very tough policy that requires rigorous scientific proof for such claims before they can be made.

There are hundreds of brands of bottled water in the United States. Some are "spring" water, that is, bottled from some spring, but not necessarily at the spring itself. All mineral waters that are sold must be bottled at the source.

Most bottled water sold in the United States is bottled tap water. For example, it is possible to purchase Miami tap water from nationwide grocery chain stores. There is nothing impure about these many brands of bottled water; however, many purchasers are misled into thinking that they are drinking spring water rather than purified water. In addition, some commercially available bottled water is sold as "sparkling" water; however, the carbon dioxide fizz has been inserted from industrially produced carbon dioxide. A test that can be used is if the water freezes without any bubbles, it is distilled water. If it has a white deposit at the center, it is hard water. It if has numerous bubbles, it is cloudy and is soft water.

Historically, people were able to drink fresh water that was untreated from springs, streams, or other sources. This can still be done in some remote locations such as Alaska, northern Canada, or Patagonia or the Andes in southern Chile. Fresh untreated water is still consumed by great numbers of people around the Earth from springs or mountain streams. In addition, fresh water that is untreated but pure

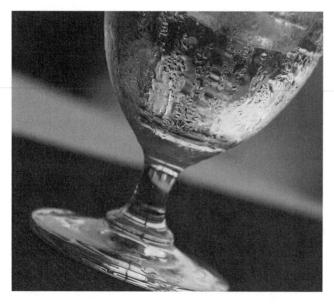

The fresh water supplies needed as drinking water are in competition with agricultural, industrial and recreational uses.

enough to drink straight out of the ground is available from water wells.

Large numbers of people in the United States or around the world get their drinking water from wells. Drilling or digging holes into the ground to get water is an ancient practice that has been able to reach ever-deeper sources of ground water through modern well drilling technology. Hand dug shallow wells are wells dug with hand tools during a dry season to the water table below. In many cultures, a man or woman called a dowser in the United Sates is believed to have special powers for locating pure water has been summoned to identify the place where the new well will be dug. Using a "divining or witching" rod, they will walk an area until the diving rod shows them the best place for water. Such practices go back for thousands of years. Claims made for the success of dowsers are not universally accepted.

For thousands of years, shallow hand-dug wells have been a major source of water for people. Wells are considered shallow if they descend to less than 50 feet in depth. Shallow wells reach either the water table (water table wells), which is the level at which the soil is saturated with water, or a well may be dug through an impermeable layer of clay or rock to an aquifer, which is a permeable layer of either soil or rock through which water flows but which is capped by at least one impermeable layer (aquifer wells).

The well is a hole that is dug to the place where water is found and then some deeper. The bottom of the well is filled with clean gravel. Stones or burnt bricks or some other solid material is used to form the sides of the well. The sides keep the soil from collapsing into the well and ruining it. In modern water wells, the casing of the sides is often cement. The water table rises in the well and reaches greater heights during wet seasons.

For millions of people in rural areas of the world, and especially in the third world shallow water wells supplying water to their village means that they do not have to share a water hole with wild beasts. The water will therefore not be polluted with their droppings or contaminants. Well water is healthier to drink from than is a water hole as long as the well is properly capped and ground water with pollutants does not sweep into it.

In many third world countries, shallow wells are still being dug and used by people as a substitute for sharing a waterhole with wild animals. These wells are dug at villages in the bush that are remote and can be reached only by a beaten track.

Wells can be drilled with machinery as well as dug with hand tools. The drilling of wells began in the mid-1800s. The well diggers of that time adopted a machine that drove or "pounded" a bit into a hole into the ground. The bit was attached to a cable and was dropped repeatedly into the drill hole. The cable tool drilling method was slow and inefficient. It was replaced by the rotary drilling method in the 1900s.

The rotary drill bit is made of tungsten steel or other tough metals. Attached to a drill pipe, it is rotated to grind up rock that it encounters in drilling the well. It is operated inside of a larger pipe which is regularly flushed with water to cool the drill bit and to wash out the cuttings, dirt, gravel, and sand. The outer pipe acts as a wall and prevents the drill hole from collapsing which would block the drill hole. As the drilling progresses, the well driller keeps an accurate log of the depths of the drilling and the levels at which water is encountered.

Millions of other rural homes on other continents are supplies with potable water from water wells. Today the vast majority of wells used in the United States are drilled wells. Probably half of the households in rural America used well water. The number around the world is enormous.

Obtaining adequate potable water supplies is a growing global problem. Diseases from a range of pathogens including parasites plague millions in third world countries. In many desert and semiarid areas the growth of populations is taxing all available water supplies. The carrying capacity of an ecological system is very much tied to the availability of water. For perhaps as many as a billion people on the globe, potable water, safe for humans to drink, is difficult to obtain. As a consequence, the threat to the health of large numbers of people is grave.

Standards for water quality are set around the world by many governmental agencies. The World Health Organization sets international drinking water standards. In the United States, the Safe Drinking Water Act of 1974 (SWDA) (42 U.S.C. 300j-9(i) requires the Environmental Protection Agency to set national standards. It also allows water treatment employees the right to report violations as protected whistle-blowers. Their reporting of water treatment standards violations would go to the Occupational Safety and Health Administration (OSHA).

Tests for water safety include tests for bacterial contamination from pathogens like *Escherichia coli* (*E. coli*). The laboratory examination of water samples will reveal the presence of sewage that can cause serious health threats. The health of an individual and of a country's population as well is an indicator of their capacity for productive work. The wealthier an individual or a country is, the greater its capacity to obtain safe drinking water.

The World Health Organization estimated that in the low- and middle-income countries of the world, as many as a billion people do not have access to safe water. In addition, proper sanitation facilities are not available for another one billion people. In a great number of countries, a lack of water is not the problem instead, it is the absence of adequate water treatment facilities that keeps drinking water supplies from being safe. Even in water, rich countries the threat to the safety of drinking water, especially from tap water, are pathogens or industrial pollutants.

The main reason for poor access to safe water is the inability to finance and to adequately maintain the necessary infrastructure. Overpopulation and scarcity of water resources are contributing factors.

SEE ALSO: E. Coli Infections; Food and Drug Administration (FDA).

BIBLIOGRAPHY. American Water Resources Association Staff, *Water Quality and Treatment Handbook* (American Water Works Association, 1999); Joshua I. Barzilay, Winkler G. Weinberg, and J. William Eley, *Water We Drink: Water Quality and Its Effects on Health* (Rutgers University Press, 1999); Michael D. Campbell and Jay H. Lehr, *Water Well Technology: Field Principles of Exploration, Drilling, and Development of Ground Water and Other Selected Minerals* (McGraw-Hill, 1973); Jerry Dennis, *The Living Great Lakes: Searching for the Heart of the Inland Sea* (St. Martin's Press, 2004); Michael Detay, *Water Wells: Implementation, Maintenance and Restoration* (Wiley, 1997); R. Allan Freeze and John A. Cherry, *Groundwater* (Prentice-Hall, 1979); Ulric P. Gibson and Rexford D. Singer, *Water Well Manual: A Practical Guide for Locating and Constructing Wells for Individual and Small Community Water Supplies* (Premier Press, 1971); P. Howsam, *Water Wells—Monitoring,*

Maintenance, Rehabilitation: Proceedings of the International Groundwater Engineering Conference Cranfield Institute of Technology (Taylor & Francis, 1990); Brian Kronvang. Jadran Faganeli and Nives Ogrinc, eds.. *Interactions Between Sediments and Water* (Springer-Verlag, 2006); Gordon A. McFeters, ed., *Drinking Water Microbiology* (Springer-Verlag, 1990); *Nutrient Management in Agricultural Watersheds: A Wetlands Solutions* (Wageningen Academic Publishers, 2005); National Academies Press, *Identifying Future Drinking Water Contaminants* (National Research Council, 2000); Kerwin L. Rakness, *Ozone in Drinking Water Treatment: Process Design, Operation, and Optimization* (American Water Works Association, 2005); Steven Schwartz, *The Book of Waters* (A&W Visual Library, 1979); Frank R. Spellman, Steve Strauss, and Joanne Drinan, *Drinking Water Handbook* (CRC Press, 1999); James M. Symons and Bradley Lee, Jr., *The Drinking Water Dictionary* (McGraw-Hill, 2001).

ANDREW J. WASKEY
DALTON STATE COLLEGE

Drug Abuse

Drug abuse refers to repetitive, nonmedical use of any substance that is detrimental to the physical, psychological, or social health of the user and negatively impacts the welfare of others. One of the most complex and widespread epidemics in the world, drug abuse cuts across economic, social, ethnic, gender, and age strata and affects people in developed and underdeveloped countries alike. Drug abuse poses significant threats to the health, social and economic stability, and functionality of families, communities, and nations.

The World Health Organization indicated in the 2002 *World Health Report* that there are 2 billion alcohol users, 1.3 billion smokers, and 185 million drug users, and drug abuse accounted for an estimated 8.9 percent of deaths worldwide. Yet, that estimate does not take into consideration deaths indirectly related to substance abuse, such as suicide, cancer, accidents, or violence, signifying that drug abuse contributes to far more global illness and death than the statistics reveal.

DRUGS

Drugs fall into one of three categories: legal or licit, prescription, and illicit. They include, but are not limited to, the following substances: alcohol, cannabinoids (e.g., marijuana, hashish), cocaine, hallucinogens (e.g., LSD, mescaline), inhalants (e.g., toluene, acetone), opioids (e.g., heroin, morphine, methadone), sedative hypnotics (e.g., barbiturates, nonbarbiturate sedatives, benzodiazepines), stimulants (e.g., amphetamines, anorectic agents, preparations of *Catha edulis*, ecstasy), and tobacco. All drugs are characterized by the ability to change the consciousness, mood, senses, or thinking patterns of the user. Legal or licit drugs, like alcohol, cigarettes, and even caffeine, do not induce harmful effects when use is limited; however, when such drugs are taken in excess, they have potentially psychoactive and addictive effects. Prescription drugs are considered helpful, not harmful, when taken under the guidance of a licensed medical practitioner; however, when abused, they are considered detrimental to individual health and well-being. Substances deemed illicit either by international standards or local legislature are generally deemed more problematic with the potential to greatly inhibit the welfare of individuals and their communities.

There is much debate about the distinction between drug use, drug abuse, addiction, and dependence. The terms are often interchangeable, although they have subtly different implications in the realms of public health, mental health, law, and the mass media. Here, drug use indicates neither the problematic nor habit-forming use of any substance. Drug abuse results from the complex physiological and psychological interactions of the substance, the individual, and social and environmental factors. It refers to a pattern of self-destructive behavior of repeated use of drugs that fall outside the realm of accepted medical or social norms, despite negative health and social consequences.

Drugs may elicit either physical or psychological dependence or both. Drug dependence is a physical phenomenon caused by the biochemical activity of repeated use of the drug in the body and is characterized by marked physical disturbances when the drug is withdrawn. The dependence potential of a substance is determined by its pharmacological properties, mode of administration, and frequency of use. Psychological dependence, labeled *addiction*, describes the overwhelming craving or compulsion a user feels to use the drug(s) to function or survive. The attainment and use of the drug often override the individual's other personal, social, and/or occupational responsibilities, leading to a pattern of self-destructive and socially destructive behavior. Drug addiction tends to evolve during periods of abuse and may or may not involve a chemical dependency. Like drug abuse, drug addiction is regarded as a chronic mental health disorder that is precipitated by a complex combination of genetic, environmental, biological, and pharmacological factors.

Most drugs of abuse generate physical dependence and all induce a psychological dependence. Interestingly, addiction may occur without dependence, but the converse is not necessarily true. For example, inhalants and LSD do not mediate a physiological addiction, yet the individual seeks the sensations experienced induced by the drug and continues use. Conversely, some drugs create a physical dependence, such as chlorpromazine, but are not abused due to the lack of development of a psychological dependence or addiction.

RISK FACTORS

Drug abuse is not a singular problem involving a specific substance, but rather a multitude of problems resulting from the abuse of a multitude of substances. The complexity of the problem renders the identification of the causal pathway complex and difficult to determine. It is not entirely understood why some people use drugs in a controllable, predictable, and nondestructive manner, while others develop addiction and dependence.

There exists a gamut of underlying physical, psychological, and environmental factors that contribute to drug abuse, yet there is no clear causal pathway from any single risk to the eventual outcome of drug abuse. Physical factors include a genetic disposition to addiction, the inability to manage stress and emotions, and the age of initiation of drug use, with those starting at a younger age more likely to develop drug abuse problems. Psychological factors relate underlying mental health conditions and personality characteristics to the propensity to abuse drugs. Environmental factors range from the influence of the family to the norms of society. Family instability, family members suffering from drug abuse, and domestic or societal violence all correlate to the potential of an individual to develop a drug abuse disorder. Poverty

and unemployment may contribute to the stress of a family or an individual to satisfy their quality of life and lead them to use and abuse drugs.

Organized crime, the increased availability of drugs, a culture of drug use, and even the surge of medical prescription correlate to an outcome of drug abuse. Again, there is not clear causal pathway from any one risk factor to the eventual outcome of drug abuse: There are individuals who possess a number of risk factors and never develop abuse, just as there are individuals with few risk factors who ultimately exhibit symptoms of abuse.

ASSOCIATED HEALTH PROBLEMS

Drug abuse relates directly and indirectly to an array of causes of morbidity and mortality. The inconsistency of epidemiological methodology and the lack of data from several countries inhibit a comprehensive review of the total global burden of disease instigated by drug abuse. The contribution of drug abuse to morbidity and mortality rates is frequently underestimated because It may be one several contributing factors to the outcome of illness. The extent of health problems resulting from drug abuse depend on the type(s) of substance(s) abused, the mode of administration, the frequency of use, the age of initiation, and the underlying genetic factors of the individual. The health problems derived from drug abuse can be categorized into three broad categories: 1.) physical problems, 2.) psychological/psychiatric problems, and 3.) social and economic problems.

PHYSICAL PROBLEMS

Drug abuse is related to a plethora of chronic and acute health sequelae. Abusing drugs holds the potential to cause morbidity in nearly every organ system in the human body. It increases a person's risk for cardiovascular hypertension, stroke, coronary artery disease, gastrointestinal and biliary ulcers, pancreatitis, cancer of the gastrointestinal tract and lungs, cirrhosis of the liver, chronic obstructive pulmonary artery disease, neuropathy, vitamin deficiencies, hematopoietic anemia, and death by overdose. Furthermore, trauma accidents in air, land, or water including car crashes, drownings, fires, electrocution, and injury from falling are common when an individual is under the influence of drugs.

The risk of contracting communicable and infectious diseases rises with drug use. Alcohol, opioids, and cannabinoids have been proven to suppress the immune system by markedly decreasing lymphocyte proliferation, antibody formation, and cytotoxic activity. As a result of decreased immune function, susceptibility to infectious diseases increases. Drug users face a greater susceptibility to bacterial, viral, and fungal etiologic agents that cause diseases such as syphilis, community-acquired pneumonia, herpes, hepatitis, and human immunodeficiency virus (HIV)/AIDS. In addition to immunosuppression, injection drug users (IDUs) put themselves at further risk for blood-borne infections such as hepatitis and HIV/AIDS when sharing needles or using contaminated paraphernalia.

Drug abuse has been a factor in the spread of HIV/AIDS and other sexually transmitted diseases as it correlates with increased sexual risk taking. Intoxication with alcohol, cannabinoids, cocaine, inhalants, opioids, or stimulants lessens the user's sense of social inhibitions and paves the way for promiscuous behaviors. In short, drug abuse increases the susceptibility of infection by immunomodulation and the exposure to infectious agents by increasing the impulse to engage in harmful health behaviors. In eastern Europe and Russia, injection drug fueled the transmission of HIV/AIDS and shaped the epidemic in the region.

Unplanned pregnancies are not uncommon with drug abusers as they have relatively more sexual partners and more pregnancies than nonusers. With the increased potential to contract an infectious disease, drug-abusing mothers bear a greater probability of transmitting infectious diseases to their babies. Mother-to-child transmission plays a significant role in the spread of diseases such as HIV/AIDS and syphilis, particularly in underdeveloped countries where HIV/AIDS education and healthcare are inadequate. Furthermore, all drug use—from tobacco and alcohol to cocaine and opioids—during pregnancy causes mild to serious fetal developmental defects and sometimes death.

PSYCHOLOGICAL/PSYCHIATRIC PROBLEMS

The American Psychiatric Association's *Diagnostic and Statistical Manual of Mental Disorders* (DSM) classifies substance abuse as a mental health disorder. Drug abusers develop a range of short- and long-term mental health disorders as well as exacerbate any previous mental health conditions. The effects of many drugs cause, as well as mimic, psychiatric disorders such as anxiety, paranoia, delusions, depression, or mood changes. Depression is the most notable symptom of drug abuse. Depression affects an individual's quality of life and physical health as well as the health and well-being of those around them. There is also a strong relationship between drug abuse and suicidal ideation, attempts, and acts, which are mediated by depression.

SOCIAL AND ECONOMIC PROBLEMS

The social and economic repercussions of drug abuse reach far beyond the individual, affecting families, communities, and nations. Family and loved ones of addicts usually support the greatest financial and emotional onus produced by drug abuse. The physical and psychological illnesses resulting from drug abuse create excess tension in the household and ultimately undermine the stability of the family. Further discord disrupts and sometimes destroys households with the combination of the economic need of the addict to maintain the drug supply and the financial demands of healthcare for subsequent illnesses. Family members who care for addicts report a decreased quality of life and an increase in mental health disorders, including depression. Drug-induced memory lapses, impulsive behaviors, and a preoccupation with acquiring and using drugs strain the social relationships of drug abusers.

The children of addicts suffer in myriad ways, as they are deprived of their physical, emotional, and educational needs due to irresponsible parenting. Subjected to a climate of drug abuse, a risk factor in initiating drug use, children of addicts are more likely to become addicts, thereby driving the vicious cycle of drug abuse from generation to generation. In countries with social welfare systems, the children of addicts frequently end up in foster homes, shelters, or correctional facilities. In countries with little social infrastructure, the children of addicts may end up living with incarcerated parents in jail, abandoned, or living on the streets. On the streets or in parentless households, children are deprived the basic human rights of food, shelter, and education. Moreover, they become more vulnerable to sexual and labor abuse and exploitation.

Communities feel the impact of drug abuse in the forms of crime, violence, and a loss of economic productivity. Drugs and alcohol are associated with crimes ranging from petty theft to rape and homicide. Some crimes, like thefts, are motivated by the addicts' need for funds to support their drug abusing habit. Other crimes are committed under the influence of drugs when moods, impulses, and perceptions are tainted by intoxication. The direct relationship between drug abuse and crime mean greater local and national expenditures on crime prevention and managing the criminal justice system. The HIV epidemic coupled with the increase of crimes and incarcerations attributed to drug abuse and trafficking continue to propel the cost of drug abuse prevention and treatment to spiral upward. In the workplace, drug abuse leads to significant declines in productivity, which, depending on the extent of the drug abuse problem, triggers public health repercussions on national and international levels. For example, unemployment and homelessness may result from poor job performance. The local communities and national economies—not the drug abusers—bear the brunt of the burden of subsequent healthcare, legal, and educational costs.

GLOBAL BURDEN OF DRUG ABUSE

Few, if any, countries are immune to the deleterious effects of drug abuse. Worldwide, the regulation and treatment of drug abuse are the cause of staggering economic and social costs, permeating all cultural and geographic boundaries. Few comprehensive international studies have been undertaken to measure the global costs of drug abuse to society. The World Health Organization is the only organization working to document and control all drugs regardless of their legal status. As previously mentioned, in its 2002 *World Health Report*, it found that 8.9 percent of deaths worldwide were directly attributable to drug abuse, In other words, tobacco and alcohol accounted for 4.1 percent and 4.0 percent, respectively, of the burden of ill health in 2000, while illicit drugs accounted for 0.8 percent.

With globalization bringing about improved transportation and communication capacities around the globe, people, capital, and goods are able to move more easily and more frequently across borders than was previously the case. While the trend in globalization has facilitated the growth and development of legitimate international businesses, it has also paved the way for drug producers and traffickers to organize themselves on a global scale. According to the United Nations Office on Drugs and Crime, the value of the global illicit drug market in 2003 was estimated

at \$13 billion at the production level, \$94 billion at the wholesale level, and at \$322 billion based on retail prices, taking seizures into account at all levels. The drastic increase in value of drugs as they move from production to market illustrates the economic extent of the business and the demand for the product.

While those involved in the upper echelons of the drug trade reap the economic benefits, society around the globe pay the price. The Office of National Drug Control Policy estimated that the costs of drug abuse incurred by government and society between the years of 1992 and 2002 were \$15.8 billion for healthcare, \$128.6 billion for lost productivity, and \$36.4 billion for law enforcement and social welfare. Additionally, countries must deal with the fact that many of the funds earned by illegal trafficking are siphoned into gangs and terrorists groups to support illegal and violent activities. In fact, much of the violence attributed to drug abuse is associated with its illegal trafficking and sales and with its biological effects on the abuser. The comorbidity of drug abuse with other social problems suggests that addressing greater social problems, like crime, poverty, or the development of health educational infrastructure, may mitigate the negative health, social, and economic impacts of drug abuse on individuals and communities.

CONTROL AND PREVENTION

The World Health Organization and individual nations strive to prevent and reduce the negative health and social consequences of drug abuse through public health programming and policy. Public health programs try to inform the public of the perils of drug abuse and provide alternative activities for youth to prevent the initiation of drug use. Taxation of legal drugs such as alcohol and tobacco has proven to be an effective means of countering the economic drain due to drug abuse as it generates enormous revenue for the government and allows for employment opportunities within the industries.

The principal manner to control drug abuse has been to make drugs illegal and enforce the control of production, distribution, and use around the globe. The drawback is that the majority of costs due to drug abuse arise from police, legal, and incarceration expenses along with lost productivity of incarcerated criminals and of victims of crimes. Furthermore, as seen with prohibition in the early 20th-century America, an illegal or black market is harder to uncover, regulate, and control. These issues have prompted some social and political groups to lobby for the legalization of drugs. Proponents for the legalization of drugs argue that eliminating the black market and creating stricter business regulation for drug handlers would minimize on the crime associated with the current black-market style of drug trafficking. Some researchers believe that the economic costs associated with drug abuse can be reduced by legalizing now-illegal drugs. Legalization would allow for taxation as with alcohol and tobacco to augment government income and help cover the costs of the damaging health and economic sequelae of drug abuse. Opponents to the legalization of drugs argue that legalizing drugs would only increase drug production, supply, and drug abuse, further intensifying the heath, social, and economic problems linked to drug abuse. They also assert that the legalization of drugs would send a message of approval of drug abuse to youth, which may stimulate a more severe epidemic in the future.

Countries with indigenous populations encounter other challenges in policy development. They struggle to reconcile the conflicting modern-day political, social, cultural, and medical viewpoints on drug abuse with the historical and cultural significance of drug use embedded in the traditions of indigenous groups.

TREATMENT AND REHABILITATION

There exists neither a quick solution nor cure for drug abuse. All treatment programs, aside from harm reduction, have a twofold purpose: 1.) helping individuals live without the use of drugs and 2.) reintegrating affected individuals into society to function as productive members. Treatment is a continuing process that employs medical or behavioral therapies or both.

Medical therapies are available for some drugs, including opioids and tobacco. They offer help in overcoming the physical symptoms of drug withdrawal during detoxification by mimicking some of the effects of drugs in the body. Medical therapies are also available to help reestablish normal brain function and prevent relapses later on in the rehabilitation process.

Behavioral programs aim to engage the recovering addict in the rehabilitation process and to motivate, condition, or teach them to change harmful attitudes and behaviors. These programs are usually religious or socially based and incorporate group and individual counseling as well as self- or mutual-help groups. Most programs require a residential stay in a clinic or in a therapeutic community, where the recovering addict has the opportunity to focus on rehabilitation without the distractions, stresses, and temptations of everyday life. Popular around the world are Alcoholics Anonymous and Narcotics Anonymous, 12-step rehabilitation programs incorporating peer support networks and individual and group counseling. Nearly all rehabilitation programs promote absolute abstinence from drugs for life. Accordingly, no treatment program asserts to cure drug abuse; rather, they enforce the fact that rehabilitation requires a constant, active effort to sustain rehabilitation and sobriety.

Comparatively, harm reduction represents a major paradigm shift in the treatment of drug abuse. Harm reduction asserts that drug abuse will persist despite all efforts to curtail it. Under this presumption, harm reduction seeks to minimize the harmful effects of drug use and abuse, rather than promoting abstinence like treatment programs. Such methods and strategies are becoming more common in public health programs striving to minimize the spread of HIV among IDUs. One example of harm reduction strategies employed to achieve this goal are needle exchanges, where needles are distributed or exchanged, free of cost, to IDUs to reduce the chances of transmission by sharing contaminated needles.

SEE ALSO: AIDS and Infections; Alcohol and Youth; Alcoholism; Drug Industry; Mental Health; Pregnancy and Substance Abuse.

BIBLIOGRAPHY. American Psychiatric Association, *Diagnostic and Statistical Manual of Mental Disorders DSM-IV-TR 4th Edition* (Text Revision) (American Psychiatric Publishing, 2000); Herman Friedman, Susan Pross, and Thomas W. Klein, "Addictive Drugs and Their Relationship with Infectious Diseases," *FEMS Immunology & Medical Microbiology* (v.47/3, 2006); Hamid Ghose, *Drugs and Addictive Behavior: A Guide to Treatment* (Cambridge University Press, 2002); Zili Sloboda, ed., *Epidemiology of Drug Abuse* (Springer, 2005); World Health Organization, *Alcohol in Developing Societies: A Public Health Approach* (World Health Organization, 2002).

Katherine Schlaefer, M.P.H.
Amino al Cambio

Drug and Medical Device Safety

For decades, drug and medical device safety has been, and continues to be, an important global health issue. Several major drug-related tragedies have demonstrated the need for effective drug and medical device safety systems. Clinical trials and postmarketing surveillance help to ensure some degree of safety among marketed medical interventions. Recent safety concerns substantiate the need for improved systems to ensure drug and device safety.

A GLOBAL HEALTH CONCERN

In 1961, the world experienced the infamous "thalidomide disaster." Thalidomide was a prescription drug marketed in several countries to alleviate morning sickness in pregnant women. Shortly after its launch, health practitioners observed a dramatic increase in phocomelia, a rare birth defect in which children are born without limbs. Epidemiological studies demonstrated that phocomelia was associated with exposure of the fetus to thalidomide.

Despite national and international efforts intended to prevent and mitigate future drug-related tragedies, such as the establishment of the World Health Organization (WHO) Programme for International Drug Monitoring, drug safety issues persist into the 21st century. In 2004, the COX-2 inhibitor rofecoxib was removed from the markets in many countries due to serious safety concerns related to potentially fatal cardiovascular complications. Two years later, in September 2006, the Institute of Medicine (IOM), a not-for-profit subsidiary of the National Academies in the United States, which exists to provide science-based advice on matters of biomedical science, medicine, and health, published a landmark report on drug safety—*The Future of Drug Safety: Promoting and Protecting the Health of the Public.*

DRUG DEVELOPMENT AND APPROVAL

The IOM report, and the publicity surrounding it, underscores the importance of drug safety to public health. Each year, more and more drugs are introduced to the world market. Bringing a new drug to market involves a complicated, time-consuming, and costly research and development process. A major component of the development and approval process is a three-phase clinical study period in which an investigational new drug is tested in human subjects to assess its safety and efficacy. Phase 1 studies involve the initial introduction of an investigational new drug into healthy human volunteers and are designed to determine the metabolic and pharmacologic actions of the drug in humans and the side effects associated with varying doses. Phase 2 includes early controlled clinical studies conducted to obtain preliminary data on the effectiveness of the drug in patients with a particular disease or condition.

These studies are typically well-controlled, closely monitored, and conducted in a relatively small number of patients and can help determine the common short-term side effects and risks associated with the drug. Phase 3 studies are basically expanded Phase 2 studies that are performed after preliminary data suggesting effectiveness of the drug are obtained, and are intended to gather additional information about effectiveness and safety that is needed to evaluate the overall benefit–risk relationship of the drug.

POSTMARKETING SURVEILLANCE

Even though one of the primary objectives of the drug development and approval process is to ensure that drugs are safe before marketing commences, conventional randomized, controlled trials used in clinical testing are often inadequate to detect and assess rare adverse events associated with a new drug. Since these studies are conducted in relatively small numbers of people, rare adverse events associated with a new drug may not be detectable until more people are exposed to it.

To identify safety issues associated with a newly marketed drug, postmarketing surveillance methods, or pharmacovigilance, have developed. Pharmacovigilance is a process of continual monitoring for deleterious effects of marketed drugs. In practice, pharmacovigilance refers almost exclusively to spontaneous reporting systems. These systems, such as the MedWatch system maintained by the Food and Drug Administration (FDA) in the United States, allow regulators and healthcare providers to report adverse drug reactions to a central agency (e.g., FDA), which can then combine reports from many sources to produce a more informative drug safety profile.

MEDICAL DEVICE SAFETY

Like drugs, medical devices are subject to safety evaluation. The term *medical device* covers a broad range of entities typically including instruments, apparatuses, machines, implants, and contrivances intended for use in diagnosing, treating, or preventing disease. Specific examples include electronic blood glucose monitors, pacemakers, contact lenses, and hearing aids. The FDA recognized three classes of medical devices based on the level of control necessary to assure the safety and effectiveness of the device: general controls, general controls with special controls, and general controls and premarket approval. The amount of information that must be obtained prior to marketing varies by class according to the potential for risk posed by the device. Once a device is marketed, sponsors must follow good manufacturing practices and monitor the safety of their products. Devices are also subject to inspections by appropriate regulatory agencies.

SEE ALSO: Clinical Trial; Food and Drug Administration (FDA); Food Safety; Pharmacoepidemiology; Randomized Clinical Trial.

BIBLIOGRAPHY. Committee on the Assessment of the US Drug Safety System, et al., *The Future of Drug Safety: Promoting and Protecting the Health of the Public* (The National Academies Press, 2006); Food and Drug Administration, "U.S. Food and Drug Administration Homepage," www.fda.gov (cited October 2006); Brian L. Strom, *Pharmacoepidemiology* (Wiley, 2005); "WHO Programme for International Drug Monitoring," www.who-umc.org (cited October 2006).

JOSHUA J. GAGNE, PHARM.D.
JEFFERSON MEDICAL COLLEGE

Drug Enforcement Administration (DEA)

In compliance with federal law, the United States Drug Enforcement Administration (DEA) is responsible for the oversight of all controlled substances. DEA has the authority to levy federal and/or civil charges against violators who grow, manufacture, or distribute illegal substances. The DEA also works with state, local, and international officials to bring individuals and organizations to justice whenever they violate drug enforcement laws in those jurisdictions. The DEA is headquartered at 2401 Jefferson Davis Highway, Alexandria, Virginia 22301. Information on the agency is available by telephone (1-202-307-1000), through the 21 regional offices, and on the internet (http://www.dea.gov/).

The DEA's major responsibilities include investigating charges against suspected violators, preparing cases for prosecution by appropriate individuals; managing the national drug intelligence program; implementing the seizure and forfeiture of assets proved to be associated with drug trafficking; enforcing the sections of the Controlled Substances Act that deal with the manufacture, distribution, and dispensing of legally produced controlled substances; working with governments at all levels to stop violators who perpetrate crimes across borders; and implementing measures to control illegal substances through such activities as crop eradication, crop substitution, and training of foreign officials engaged in drug enforcement. The DEA also works with the secretaries of state and U.S. ambassadors to coordinate international drug enforcement activities and serves as a liaison in the area of drug enforcement between the United States and the United Nations, Interpol, and other international crime-fighting agencies.

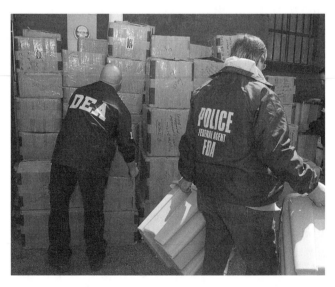

DEA and FDA agents caught e-traffickers who used websites to illegally distribute controlled substances in Operation "Cyber Chase."

In 1915, the Bureau of Internal Revenue was assigned the responsibility of drug enforcement. With the passage of the Eighteenth Amendment in 1919, Prohibition expanded the scope of the Bureau's activities as speakeasies sprang up around the country, and as moonshining activities expanded in rural areas. Organized crime was an offshoot of Prohibition, and DEA agents were engaged in fighting crime on a major scale. In 1968, President Lyndon B. Johnson introduced Reorganization Plan 1, combining the Bureau of Narcotics (FBN), which, as an agency of the Treasury Department, had been responsible for controlling marijuana and narcotic drugs, and the Bureau of Drug Abuse and Control (BDAC), which operated under the auspices of the Department of Health, Education, and Welfare to control depressants stimulants, and hallucinogens. The new agency became the Bureau of Narcotics and Dangerous Drugs (BNDD), operating under the Department of Justice to enforce all federal laws on controlled substances. In 1973, as part of the global war on illegal drugs, President Richard Nixon introduced Reorganization Plan 2, consolidating all federal drug enforcement responsibilities into the current DEA.

The decision to consolidate drug enforcement responsibilities was in large part a reaction to the emergence of the drug culture that had become a permanent element of American society. Those responsibilities took on new meaning in the latter decades of the 20th century when schools became a frequent target of drug dealers, many of whom were students themselves. DEA data indicate that the number of people using illegal drugs grew from 4 million in 1960 to 74 million in the first years of the 21st century. During that same period, international drug-trafficking syndicates, such as those from Colombia and Mexico, made the DEA's efforts to control illegal drugs even more difficult. Between 1960 and 1974, the DEA opened offices in 43 foreign countries, covering the globe from Paris to Hong Kong to Mexico to the Philippines to Canada to the Netherlands.

In 1970, Congress passed the Controlled Substances Act as Title II of the Comprehensive Drug Abuse Prevention and Control Act, consolidating 50 separate laws into a single package to control narcotic and psychotropic drugs. Substances were classified according to their potential for abuse and addiction and whether they had a legitimate medical value. In amended form, this legislation continues to provide the framework for the DEA classification of drugs. In 1971, the Diversion Control Program established measures for dealing with the practice of diverting legal drugs such as amphetamine and methamphetamine into illegal channels.

In 1973, the DEA Intelligence Program was established to provide up-to-date information that allowed the newly established DEA to track and access criminal activity for use in identifying and prosecuting violators and in establishing long-term strategies. The National Narcotics Intelligence System was also set up as the first national law enforcement automated index. The following year, the Drug Abuse Warning Network (DAWN) was founded to generate data on the scope of drug abuse in the United States. Over time, the DEA added additional capabilities in aviation, training, technologies, and laboratories. In the late 1990s, DEA agents began devoting a good deal of attention to monitoring synthetic drugs such as ecstasy, and the potential use of illegal substances by terrorists became a focus of increased activity after the attacks on the United States on September 11, 2001.

SEE ALSO: Drug Abuse; Drug and Medical Device Safety.

BIBLIOGRAPHY. Drug Enforcement Administration, www.dea.gov; *Drug Enforcement Administration: A Tradition of Excellence, 1973–2003* (Department of Justice and Drug Enforcement Administration, 2003); Kenneth J. Meier and Laurence J. O'Toole Jr., *Bureaucracy in a Democratic State: A Government Perspective* (Johns Hopkins University Press, 2006); David F. Musto and Pamela Korsmeyer, *The Quest for Drug Control: Politics and Federal Policy in a Period of Increasing Substance Abuse, 1963–1981* (Yale University Press, 2002); Dennis D. Riley, et al., *Bureaucracy and the Policy Process: Keeping the Promises* (Rowman & Littlefield, 2006); David Robbins, *Heavy Traffic: Thirty Years of Headlines and Major Ops from the Case Files of the DEA* (Chamberlain, 2005).

ELIZABETH R. PURDY, PH.D.
INDEPENDENT SCHOLAR

Dyslexia

Dyslexia, also known as a reading disorder, is the most common and best studied of the learning disabilities. A reading disorder refers to children who do not begin

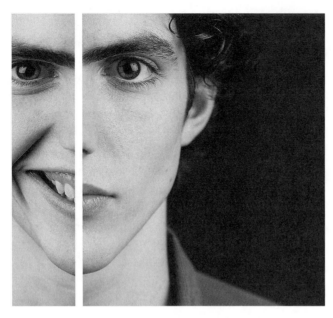

Learning disabilities can persist into adulthood and it is estimated that dyslexia affects between 4 and 15 percent of the population.

to read at the appropriate time and have no obvious reason for failure to do so. Dyslexia is diagnosed when achievement on individualized, standardized tests is substantially below what is expected. It must be differentiated from normal variations in learning, mental retardation, and from environmental causes such as lack of opportunity to learn, poor teaching, or the presence of significant cultural factors. Without recognition and treatment, having a learning disability can lead to demoralization, low self-esteem, and difficulties with social adjustment. Learning disabilities can persist into adulthood and it is estimated that dyslexia affects between 4 and 15 percent of the population. Living in an industrialized country where reading is fundamental to lifetime learning and job requirements, dyslexia can be a major disability. Early identification of affected individuals has the potential to make a significant impact on society in general.

Establishing whether a child has dyslexia is not a simple task as there are no universally accepted definitions for categorizing an individual as having a developmental disability. The U.S. Office of Education, provided as part of Public Law 94-142, lists guidelines for determining the existence of a specific learning disability. The American Psychiatric Association has published the *Diagnostic and Statistical Manual of Mental Disorders*, 4th edition (DSM-IV), which spec-

ifies criteria that must be met in order to diagnose a reading disorder. The essential diagnostic feature is that one's reading achievement is substantially below that expected given the individual's chronological age, measured intelligence, and age-appropriate education. In addition, the reading disturbance must significantly interfere with academic achievement or with activities of daily living. If the child has a vision or hearing impairment, neurological, or other medical condition, the reading difficulties must be in excess of what would be expected in those situations.

One of the major tasks for school-aged children is learning to read. Early symptoms of reading difficulty may include inability to distinguish among common letters or to associate common sounds with syllables. For the dyslexic, oral reading is characterized by distortions, substitutions, or omissions. Both oral and silent reading is characterized by slowness and errors in comprehension. Federal legislative action, noted in Public Law 99-457, has provisions that guarantee that diagnostic and interventional services will be made available to those who display significant developmental delays or have been diagnosed with physical or mental conditions that have a high probability of causing developmental delays. Although symptoms of reading difficulty may appear as early as kindergarten, a reading disorder is seldom diagnosed before the end of kindergarten or the beginning of first grade because this is when formal reading instruction usually begins in most school settings. Unfortunately, this alone does not guarantee early recognition of the disability. When a child is very bright, he or she may be able to function at or near grade level, so that the problem is not identified until fourth grade or later.

Dyslexia is a complex disorder that requires careful team evaluation to rule out other disorders that may mimic it. Deficits in visual perception, linguistic processes, attention, and/or memory may be involved. There may be underlying abnormalities in cognitive processing that precede or are associated with learning disorders. Many individuals with psychiatric disorders diagnosed in infancy and early childhood also have learning disorders. These include conduct disorder, oppositional defiant disorder, attention deficit hyperactivity disorder, and major depression.

When a child is noted to be struggling academically, he or she should be referred for evaluation. Psychologists are professionals trained to administer and interpret testing results. Reading ability is correlated with intelligence and diagnosed using discrepancy scores. There are standardized tests available to determine intelligence (IQ) and academic achievement. A variety of statistical approaches are then used to establish that a discrepancy is present. A significant difference between IQ and academic achievement scores is usually defined as more than two standard deviations or two years below what is expected for chronological age. In mental retardation, learning difficulties are consistent with their lower intelligence scores. Children from backgrounds where English is not the primary language or where teaching has been inadequate may score poorly on achievement tests and this must be taken into consideration before making a diagnosis.

It is rare for a reading disorder to be diagnosed in isolation; mathematics disorder and disorder of written expression are commonly identified in the same individual. The majority of individuals diagnosed with a reading disorder are males. However, this is thought to be due to a bias in referral as boys tend to be more problematic in the classroom. The diagnosis is found to occur at more equal rates in males and females when careful referral and stringent diagnostic criteria are used. Clustering of dyslexia in families has been noted since the early 1900s and reading disorders are more prevalent among first-degree biological relatives of individuals with learning disorders.

At this time, the causes of reading disorders are not known but appear to be multifactorial. Learning disabilities are frequently found in association with a variety of medical conditions such as lead poisoning, fetal alcohol syndrome, and Fragile X syndrome. Genetic predisposition, injury during the birthing process, and various neurological or other medical conditions may be associated. On the other hand, many individuals with no such history have a learning disability. The cause of dyslexia has been the subject of much speculation. Behavioral, social, and neurobiological factors continue to be recognized as possible important factors. Different subtypes of dyslexia, with proposed etiologies and neuropsychological rationales for treatment exist. Among the leading speculations being considered are phonological deficiencies, deficits in auditory processing, abnormal cortical asymmetry, a rapid automatic naming dysfunction, a cerebellar deficit, a deficit in temporal processing, and visual deficits.

Remarkably, little research on the treatment of developmental dyslexia has been published during the last 25 years; however, there are many studies in progress and with advancing technology, the answer may not be far off. There are hundreds of institutes all over the world that offer programs to facilitate the reading of dyslexic children. The important question is, and remains, what is the best learning environment for a particular child hampered in the ability to read? Despite the unanswered questions, it appears that with early identification and intervention, having a reading disorder has a good prognosis in a significant percentage of cases.

SEE ALSO: Child Development; Child Mental Health; Learning Disorders; Psychologist; Psychiatry.

BIBLIOGRAPHY. Dirk Bakker, "Treatment of Developmental Dyslexia: A Review," *Pediatric Rehabilitation* (v.9, 2006); *Diagnostic and Statistical Manual of Mental Disorders*, 4th ed. (American Psychiatric Association, 2000); Kimberly Noble and Bruce McCandliss, "Reading Development and Impairment: Behavioral, Social, and Neurobiological Factors," *Developmental and Behavioral Pediatrics* (October 2005); Steven Pliszka, Caryn Carlson, and James Swanson, *ADHD with Comorbid Disorders: Clinical Assessment and Management* (Guilford Press, 1999).

DEBRA A. WILLSIE, D.O.
UNIVERSITY OF MISSOURI–KANSAS CITY

Dysmorphology

Dysmorphology is the study of abnormal form in the human body. This relates to anatomy of patients who may have genetic and congenital birth defects. The pediatrician, endocrinologist, embryologist, and clinical geneticist, Dr. David Smith, first began this area of interdisciplinary study of medicine in the 1960s. At this time, clinical genetics were at their infancy. The study of dysmorphology involves observation and assessment of patients, the understanding of intricacies in the genetic disorder, and any relevant treatment measures available. When a physician confronts the patient and family issues relating to morphological birth defects and their genetic components, that physician is taking on the role of dysmorphologist.

In the developing world, a myriad of congenital birth defects remain underdiagnosed, poorly treated, and misunderstood. The social stigma, isolation, and lack of adaptation can lead to a loss of quality of life. A physician acting as dysmorphologist is able to identify these risks for defects and offer clinical support to the patient and family. The lack of access to this treatment and assessment in least developed nations throughout the world leads to patient suffering.

For example, the level of care that is expected for such assessments when the index of suspicion is high for any dysmorphology include nutrition; basic lifestyle and occupation and work details; medical, obstetric, and drug histories; if possible, genetic and biochemical data collection (difficult in the developing world); and overall assessment of clinical dysmorphology with a family history. Also, assessing a person's body proportion (the length of the arms and legs relative to the trunk) may provide information for further examination.

With a prolonged birth and breech presentation, congenital dislocation of the hip, clubfeet, and a flattened, elongated "breech head" can result. These morphological abnormalities are usually benign and can be corrected. However, a simple obstructed urethra causing a deficient volume of amniotic fluid leads to flattened facial features and fixed joints.

One minor malformation in the patient should not cause major concern, particularly if the feature is shared with a parent and does not affect daily life. As outlined by many clinical genetics protocols, three or more malformations, especially if associated with short stature, failure to thrive, a slower developed head and brain, or other developmental delay, should bring about further investigation in the newborn or infant. Much of these needs cannot be met in the developing world.

For example, abnormalities of the spine can be major malformations that are readily apparent at birth but poorly treated in developing nations. Some specific examples that plague developing countries without access to prenatal care as in the case of Africa and Asia are anencephaly (absent skull and brain), encephalocele (cranial defect with brain coming out into external sac), and spina bifida. All of the above dysmorphological disorders result in death to the child.

SEE ALSO: Adolescent Development; Beals, Rodney K.; Birth Defects; Brain Malformations; Genetic Testing/Counseling; Growth Disorders; Neural Tube Defects.

BIBLIOGRAPHY. "Basic Dysmorphology," http://www.usd.edu/med/som/genetics/curriculum/2EDYSMO5.htm (cited June 2007); Muin J. Khoury, et al., "The Interaction between Dysmorphology and Epidemiology: Methodologic Issues of Lumping and Splitting," *Teratology* (v.45/2, 1992).

JOHN M. QUINN V, M.P.H.
UNIVERSITY OF ILLINOIS AT CHICAGO

Dysphagia

Dysphagia is a condition of having difficulty swallowing. Two classifications exist: transfer dysphagia and esophageal dysphagia. Both are characterized by the complaints that foods and liquids are slow to go down and cling to the throat. Both can be either sporadic or chronic in nature. Additionally, both have certain triggers that help classify the disorder.

Transfer dysphagia is caused by disorders often stemming from strokes or neurological complications. In this case, a disruption of the motor sensors and controls prevents a patient from being able to trigger the swallowing mechanisms in an automatic fashion. The life span of transfer dysphagia is affected by what the underlying cause is. Patients who have had a stroke often experience weakness of one side of the mouth that makes the swallowing process difficult. This weakness, however, can be mediated with time and practice. Some neurological disorders, however, have a bleaker outcome and the life of the patient may be riddled with bouts of dysphagia.

Regardless of the underlying cause of transfer dysphagia, it is characterized as being triggered by the swallowing process rather than a certain type of food. Because the problem is with the swallowing action, a major concern for transfer dysphagia patients is that food or drink will enter the lungs or chest cavity, cause choking, or be expelled from the nose.

Unlike transfer dysphagia, esophageal dysphagia is typically caused by structural disorders in the throat. Tumors and lesions in the throat are very common to the esophageal dysphagia patient. The defining aspect between transfer dysphagia and esophageal dysphagia is that esophageal dysphagia is linked directly to food and not the act of starting to swallow. In esophageal dysphagia, the act of swallowing can be initiated with success, but the food or drink may be slow to go down the throat, or may cause a clinging sensation—a feeling that the food is clinging to the throat.

Esophageal dysphagia can be long lasting or may occur only a few times without a noticeable pattern. With that, esophageal dysphagia can start out weak and progress in severity, or start out in a very severe fashion and ease with time. The major factors at work in either case are the underlying conditions that are causing the esophageal dysphagia. Structural disorders such as a tumor may be slow to grow and will not block as much food as would occur in the later stages of growth. Conversely, a heavy impact to the throat or muscles surrounding the throat may cause a sudden challenge to swallowing, one that will soften with time.

Regardless of the cause, patients with esophageal dysphagia often experience comfort with regurgitation of the food. Regurgitation is typically better tolerated than trying to force the food to swallow, which may cause some additional discomfort. Complaints such as heartburn, sore throat, chest pain, and coughing up food are common to the esophageal dysphagia patient. Both transfer dysphagia and esophageal dysphagia are defined as difficulty swallowing. Transfer dysphagia is characterized by the physical act of initiating the swallow, while esophageal dysphagia is characterized by the food or drink not going down correctly.

SEE ALSO: Bell's Palsy; Cancer (General); Food Allergy.

BIBLIOGRAPHY. Elayne Achilles, *The Dysphagia Cookbook: Great Tasting and Butritious Recipes for People with Swallowing Difficulties* (Cumberland House, 2003); Lynn S. Bickley, ed., *Bates' Guide to Physical Examination and History Taking*, 8th ed. (Lippincott Williams and Wilkins, 2003).

WILLIAM J. HAMILTON
ARIZONA STATE UNIVERSITY

Dystonia

Dystonia is a movement disorder consisting of involuntary muscle contractions, which force certain parts of the body into abnormal, sometimes painful, movements or postures. This can affect any part of the body including the arms, legs, trunk, neck, eyelids, face, or vocal cords. This movement is not controlled by the patient and can be painful. Dystonia can be present in patients with cerebral palsy, Parkinson's disease, or other neurological problems. If dystonia causes any type of impairment, it is because muscle contractions interfere with normal body function. Features such as cognition, strength, and the special senses are usually normal. Dystonia is not fatal; however, it is a chronic disorder and prognosis is difficult to predict due to the different body systems involved. It is the third most common movement disorder after Parkinson's disease and tremor that affect more than 300,000 people in North America. Dystonia does not discriminate and it effects all races and ethnic groups the same way. In the developing world, diagnosis and treatment of dystonia can be elusive and complex as symptoms vary and neurological diagnostics are often nonexistent. The German neurologist, Dr. Hermann Oppenheim, of Berlin was interested in the variation in muscle tone seen in neurologic pathologies that he encountered in several young patients. In his papers, he used the term *dystonia* to indicate that muscle tone was hypotonic at one occasion and tonic spasm at another. Hypotonic means having less-than-normal tension in the muscle and tonic is continuous tension or nonstop contraction of muscles.

As the term *dystonia* has been widely accepted and has been used by neurologists and other physicians alike; other terms such as repetitive movement disorder and muscle twitch have also been used. These terms and concepts are directly related to muscle tone. This is the level of muscle contraction present during resting state. With increased tone, there is stiffness and rigidity, while with decreased tone, there is looseness of the limbs and trunk.

However, the definition of dystonia has grown with the levels of diagnosis and categories expanding. The major issue most diagnosticians have with these additions to dystonia is that by using only sustained postures for their definition, this allows many types of abnormal postures to be called dystonia, such as fixed postures that could develop from a stroke. Furthermore, these definitions do not take into account other types of abnormal neurological movements. In the early 1980s, a committee consisting of members of the Scientific Advisory Board of the Dystonia Medical Research Foundation developed the following definition: "Dystonia is a syndrome of sustained muscle contractions, frequently causing twisting and repetitive movements, or abnormal postures." This committee also proposed a classification schedule for dystonia. This scheme recommends three classifications: age at onset, parts of body affected, and etiology or the cause and origin of disease.

SEE ALSO: Aphasia; Bell, Charles; Bell's Palsy; Dysphasia; Movement Disorders; Muscle Disorders.

BIBLIOGRAPHY. Mitchell Brin, Cynthia Comella, and Joseph Jankovic, *Dystonia: Etiology, Clinical Features, and Treatment* (Lippincott Williams & Wilkins, 2004); Dystonia Medical Research Foundation, http://www.dystonia-foundation.org.

JOHN M. QUINN V, M.P.H.
UNIVERSITY OF ILLINOIS AT CHICAGO

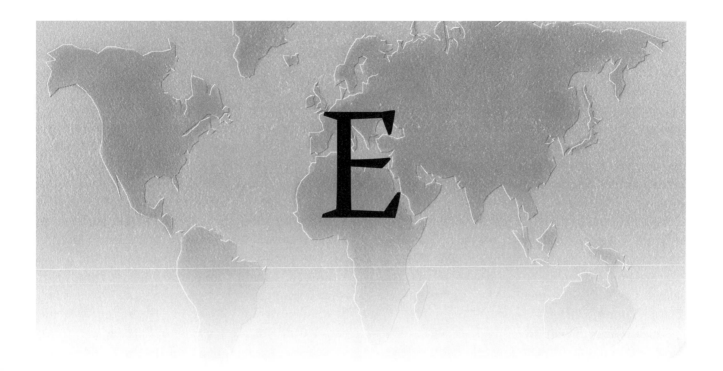

Ear Disorders

Ears are the organs that help humans hear. The ears modify sound input, communicate it through the cartilaginous tissue and ear canals, and send signals through nerves, and into the brain. In addition, ears participate in body systems assisting with balance. Ear disorders have a variety of causes. The ear, or auricle, has three separate areas: the external ear, the middle ear, and the inner ear. An otoscope is the tool medical practioners use to examine the ear. Often a pneumatic bulb is used as well.

The outer part of the ear is made of cartilage. This part of the ear collects sound through the air. The sound is then transmitted into the external canal, through the middle ear, and to the inner ear where hair cells send signals through the nerves to the brain. The layers of the skin around the ear and the canal have thin hairs and, cerumen, or ear wax, is produced. Sometimes cerumen can completely occlude the external ear canal and dampen sound. External ears have been decorated for thousands of years. In some cultures, earlobes have stretched and enlarged to signify importance within the community. Other cultures have traditionally pierced earlobes for decorative jewelry. Occasionally, superficial infections of the skin on the ear can occur, sometimes due to

these piercings or insect bites. Repeated injury to the cartilage sometimes does not allow the ear to heal correctly to its original shape; the normally soft and malleable cartilage becomes hard and lumpy. Thus, frequent trauma can distort the entire cartilage sometimes seen in "wrestler's ear" or "cauliflower ear." Foreign bodies may become lodged in this location of the ear, as well. Additionally, the external canal of the ear can become infected, a condition known as "otitis externa" or "swimmer's ear." This uncomfortable ailment is commonly treated with topical medications. Although rare, congenital external ear malformation can occur during embryologic development. Also, bony growths, called osteomas, may be in the external canal and uncommonly cysts and tumors will grow there. Anatomically, the external ear ends at the tympanic membrane, or eardrum.

The middle ear compartment begins behind the tympanic membrane. Sound is conducted through air in this compartment. The Eustachian tube connects the middle ear compartment to the posterior area of the pharynx. This tube helps to equalize pressure from the surrounding atmosphere to the middle ear cavity. Although the tube is normally closed, it opens up with swallowing and positive pressure. Increasing altitude in an airplane causes the air to expand and open the tube. However, upon descent, the volume of air shrinks and causes a vacuum in this closed system. Divers also experience this "Eustachian tube dysfunction" but for a different reason. In those cases, as divers go deeper, the external atmospheric pressure under water increases. This also causes a vacuum to occur. When the Eustachian tube is not working correctly, people will complain of a pressure sensation, or a popping and clicking sound in their ear. Active opening of the tube (by applying pressure to the nasal cavity) is sometimes necessary to open the Eustachian tube. An otoscope with the attached pneumatic bulb can help assess the movement of the tympanic membrane and assist with the examination of the middle ear and diagnosis. Sometimes, fluid can accumulate behind the ear drum. Clear, noninfected fluid is known as "serous otitis."

This may accumulate when the Eustachian tube is not functioning correctly, occasionally because of viral illnesses or seasonal allergies. When the fluid behind the ear drum becomes thicker appearing or discolored, it may be infected. The ear drum compensates for this fluid accumulation by bulging and reddening, and is called "otitis media." These painful occurrences may be either viral or bacterial, and antibiotics are not always required. Occasionally, a tympanic membrane ruptures. A spontaneous rupture may occur secondary to fluid accumulation and infection, behind the ear drum. Purulent drainage and blood then may become evident, as the discharge comes out of the middle ear and through the external ear canal and to the outside of the ear. Tympanostomy tubes are sometimes placed surgically, through the ear drums, to assist in the treatment of chronic ear infections. When the tube is functioning correctly, any fluid accumulating behind the ear drum will drain out.

Traumatic tympanic membrane ruptures may also happen from exposure to sudden loud sounds, severe pressure changes related to Eustachian tube dysfunction, or puncture wounds from foreign bodies placed in ears. A ruptured tympanic membrane is typically painful and impairs hearing until healing is complete. Scars become evident on the tympanic membrane from ruptures, and repeated scarring may chronically impair ability to hear. Rarely, a cholesteatoma may grow within the middle ear. This benign mass is typically skin tissue that may be locally destructive and have chronic drainage, causing hearing loss and nerve damage.

The inner ear is the third part of the ear. This area of the ear helps with hearing and balance through a se-

ries of bones, semicircular canals, hollow areas, fluid filled areas, different types of hair cells, and a cranial nerve sending signals to the brain. A common symptom might include dizziness due to a malfunction of the balance centers. Because physicians are unable to directly visualize the inner ear, it is more difficult to definitively diagnose these problems.

Hearing loss is a common disorder of ears. Hearing impairment is further categorized as conductive hearing loss (often pathology of the external ear, the middle ear, or both), sensorineural hearing loss (related to a problem with the inner ear or the nerves leading to the brain), or a mixed hearing loss which is both conductive and sensorineural. The loss may be sudden or chronic. A 512-Hz tuning fork may help with delineate the type of hearing loss. Softly striking the tuning fork and placing it midline on the patient's forehead is called the Weber's test. In patients with normal hearing, the sound remains midline. However, a conductive hearing loss causes the sound to be heard best in the affected ear and a sensorineural hearing loss causes the sound to be heard best in the normal ear. A Rinne test helps to assess air conduction and bone conduction. The 512-Hz tuning fork is softly struck. Patients should be able to hear the sound as it is placed on the mastoid bone. This assesses bone conduction. Once the sound is no longer appreciated by the patient, the tuning fork is then placed next to the ear canal to assess air conduction. The sound is appreciated through the air in patients with normal hearing or sensorineural hearing loss meaning air conduction is better than bone conduction. However, the sound is not heard in conductive hearing loss, implying bone conduction is better than air conduction.

Formal audiometry testing is indicated in patients with hearing loss. Furthermore, speech development is dependent upon ability to hear; many hospital nurseries now screen newborn children for congenital hearing loss with specialized mechanical equipment, just after delivery.

SEE ALSO: Deafness; Dizziness and Vertigo; Ear Infections; Infant and Toddler Development; Infant and Toddler Health; Piercings and Tattoos.

BIBLIOGRAPHY. *Clinical Practice Guideline–Diagnosis and Management of Acute Otitis Media* (American Academy of Pediatrics and American Academy of Family Physicians, 2004); Jon E. Isaacson, and Neil M. Vora, "Differential Diagnosis and Treatment of Hearing Loss," *American Family Physician*, (v.68/6, 2003); Robert Sander, "Otitis Externa: A Practical Guide to Treatment and Prevention," *American Family Physician* (v.63/5, 2001).

Ann M. Karty, M.D., Faafp
Kansas City University of Medicine
and Biosciences

Ear Infections

Ear infections, specifically infections of the middle ear, are common childhood infections in industrialized countries and the leading cause of outpatient antimicrobial treatment of children in the United States. Infections of the middle and inner ear can cause temporary or permanent loss of hearing and associated speech and language delays. The World Health Organization estimates that in developing countries, 51,000 children under 5 years of age die annually from complications of infections of the middle ear. There are three types of ear infections characterized by location in the ear.

Infection of the middle ear is known as otitis media and is characterized by infected fluid behind the eardrum. Otitis is the Latin word for inflammation of the ear. The eardrum separates the inner ear from the ear canal. Infections of the middle ear are defined by acute otitis media, a middle ear infection with both effusion, or fluid, and presence of signs or symptoms of an acute infection, or by otitis media with effusion, a middle ear infection with effusion and without signs or symptoms of an acute infection. Signs and symptoms of acute otitis media include pulling of the ear in an infant, irritability in an infant or toddler, discharge from the external ear, and fever. By 3 years of age, 50 to 85 percent of children in the United States have had acute otitis media with peak incidence between ages 6 and 11 months. Recurrent acute otitis media infections, defined as three or more episodes of infection, affect 10 to 20 percent of children by 1 year of age. Children with recurrent acute otitis media infections may have a surgical treatment, myringotomy, whereby a small tube is placed inside the affected ear by an otolaryngologist. Infections of the middle ear are caused

by Eustachian-tube dysfunction, bacterial infection, viral infection, or immune response to infection. Common bacterial infections include *Streptococcus pneumoniea*, *Moraxella catarrhalis*, and nontypeable *Haemophilus influenzae*. Risk factors for infections of the middle ear include young age (less than 2 years old), daycare attendance, having older siblings, fall and winter season, impaired immune system, genetic predisposition, and family history. Acute otitis media spontaneously resolves, without treatment, within 2 to 14 days in 80 percent of children between 2 and 12 years of age. Antibiotic treatment is recommended for children without improvement in symptoms following 48 to 72 hours of observation.

Infection of the outer ear is known as otitis externa and is characterized by infected fluid in the ear canal. Infection of the outer ear is also known as swimmer's ear. Infections of the outer ear are defined by acute or chronic forms. Acute otitis externa is generally diagnosed by signs and symptoms of a bacterial infection, such as an odorless secretion from the ear, itching, and pain. Chronic otitis externa is commonly due to a fungal infection or allergic reaction, generally due to an inflammation of the skin of the ear canal. Acute otitis externa affects 4 in 1,000 people annually in the United States, is most common in children 7–12 years of age, and is associated with high humidity, warmer temperatures, swimming, local trauma in the ear, and hearing aids. Chronic otitis externa affects 3 to 5 percent of the population in the United States. Treatments for infections of the outer ear include topical therapy and

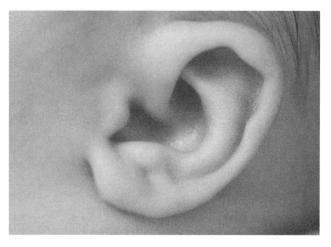

Ear infections are the leading cause of outpatient antimicrobial treatment of children in the United States.

amelioration of inciting factors. Twenty-five percent of individuals treated for otitis externa will also be given an antibiotic.

Infection of the inner ear is known as otitis interna or labyrinthitis. Inner ear infections can be caused by bacterial infections such as meningitis or syphilis (either congenital or acquired). Viral infections also cause infections of the inner ear through congenital infection, as part of a systemic viral illness, or an isolated involvement of the inner ear. Confirmed associations have been identified between infections of the inner ear and cytomegalovirus (congenital infections) and mumps (acquired). Cytomegalovirus is considered the most common congenital infection in the United States and the most common infectious cause of congenital deafness. Suspected pathogens associated with infection of the inner ear include rubella (congenital), rubeola, influenza, varicella-zoster, EBV, poliovirus, RSV, adenovirus, parainfluenza, and herpes simplex viruses. Congenital infection with the protozoa, toxoplasmosis, also leads to inner ear infections. Fungal infections of the inner ear are rare unless an individual is immunocompromised. Symptoms of infections of the inner ear include dizziness, vertigo, ringing in the ears, and hearing loss. Idiopathic sudden sensorineural hearing loss in an otherwise health individual is usually due to a viral inner ear infection. Approximately 30 to 70 percent of patients will have partial or complete recovery of hearing with proper treatment.

SEE ALSO: Bacterial Infections; Deafness; Hearing Problems in Children; Otolaryngologist; Viral Infections.

BIBLIOGRAPHY. J. David Osguthorpe and David R. Nielsen, "Otitis Externa: Review and Clinical Update," *American Family Physician* (v.74/9, 2006); Maroeska M. Rovers, et al., "Otitis Media," *Lancet* (v.363, 2004).

Rebecca Malouin, Ph.D., M.P.H.
Michigan State University

East Timor

Located in southeast Asia, East Timor was a Portuguese colony from 1702, and in 1951 became an overseas province of Portugal. In August 1975, there was a civil war, and soon afterward, Indonesia invaded East Timor, occupying it until 1999 when it was controlled by the United Nations. In May 2002, it finally gained independence.

During most of the period of Portuguese rule, the healthcare services were underdeveloped. Many of the health problems in East Timor were because of malaria and other insect-borne diseases, as well as poor hygiene. To improve these, J. Gomes da Silva was appointed to take over the running of medical services in East Timor, and found that the hospital was badly equipped, and all the Christian cemeteries were badly positioned, causing possible contamination of the water supply for Dili and other towns, and being a probable source of cholera. No action was taken on the report he made on the problems he found. In December 1940, José dos Santos Carvalho was appointed as the health delegate for the central and eastern parts of East Timor, remaining there during the Japanese Occupation, and writing the major work on the history of medicine in East Timor.

In 1948, there were four hospitals and six doctors in East Timor. The health problems at the time included malaria, pneumonia, elephantiasis, tuberculosis, cholera, and venereal diseases. Four years later, in 1952, the First National Congress of Tropical Medicine was held in the Portuguese capital, Lisbon. Annual congresses were held for the next few years where Portuguese colonial administrators coordinated their medical care programs, which at that stage were mainly for the Portuguese and other Europeans. By 1958, the congresses had become renamed the International Congress for Tropical Medicine and Malaria, and over the next few years the World Health Organization led campaigns to eradicate malaria which did affect many people in East Timor.

When Indonesia invaded East Timor in 1975, there was only one major hospital, located in Dili, the administrative capital of East Timor. Even though the vast majority of the population of East Timor opposed the Indonesian Occupation, many did accept that the Indonesians did massively improve healthcare in what became their 27th province. Indeed, prior to the Indonesian invasion, there was only one surgeon and one dentist covering the entire population of 610,000, although there were often a dozen doctors serving in the Portuguese army. From 1976 until 1999, the provision of healthcare in East Timor was much better than many other parts of Indonesia, with the Indonesian government eager to win over the population of the place. More hospitals were built, and clinics opened in many small towns. However, in 1999, in a referendum, the people voted heavily in favor of independence. After this, pro-Indonesian militia destroyed much of the government infrastructure in the place. This destruction saw the burning down of clinics and medical centers around the country.

Since 1999, there have been attempts to rebuild the East Timorese health services, and the presence of large numbers of United Nations and foreign soldiers and officials in the country, several hospitals were refurbished. Malaria still remains a major problem in the country, with problems over dengue fever, tuberculosis, and cholera.

SEE ALSO: Cholera; Dengue; Indonesia; Malaria.

BIBLIOGRAPHY. Geoffrey C. Gunn, *Timor Loro Sae: 500 Years* (Livros do Oriente, 1999); José dos Santos Carvalho, *Vida e morte em Timor durante a segunda Guerra mundial* (Livraria Portugal, 1972).

JUSTIN CORFIELD
GEELONG GRAMMAR SCHOOL, AUSTRALIA

Eating Disorders

Eating disorders are among the most lethal of the psychiatric diagnoses and generally occur in adolescent girls or young women. However, eating disorders do not exclusively affect females; men experience these illnesses at surprisingly high rates as well. An estimated five million Americans each year are affected by these multidimensional illnesses which can cause devastation to the individual's work, home, and personal life. While these illnesses are generally characterized by a serious eating disturbance accompanied by excessive concern about body weight and shape, each disorder has distinct clinical features. Anorexia nervosa (AN) is described as a refusal to maintain normal body weight for one's age and height, an intense fear of becoming fat, and a loss or disruption of menstrual periods, while bulimia nervosa (BN) is characterized by episodic binge eating followed by an engagement in compensatory behaviors such as vomiting or laxative misuse. The third and largest category is eating disorder not otherwise specified (EDNOS) which includes binge-eating disorder.

DIAGNOSTIC CRITERIA

The *Diagnostic and Statistical Manual of Mental Disorders*, 4th edition (DSM-IV), published by the American Psychiatric Association, establishes criteria used in diagnosing and distinguishing eating disorders.

AN is diagnosed according to four diagnostic criteria: a refusal to maintain body weight within a normal range for the person's age and height; an intense fear of gaining weight; a severe disturbance of body image in which body image becomes responsible for self-worth accompanied by a denial of the gravity of the illness; and in women past the age of menarche, an absence of more than three menstrual cycles (amenorrhea). Additionally, there are two currently recognized subtypes of AN: restricting (ANR) and bingeing/purging (ANBP). Individuals with ANR use constraint in their eating to reduce their weight and are, in general, more perfectionistic and restrictive in their eating behaviors. In contrast, individuals with ANBP may binge and use purging methods (i.e., vomiting, laxatives) to control their weight; the ANBP subtype is typically more categorically impulsive, older, and may be more likely to be suicidal or to have substance abuse problems.

The DSM-IV criteria for BN include recurrent episodes of binge eating accompanied by a feeling of a loss of control (binge eating constitutes a consumption of larger-than-normal quantities of food in a discrete period); recurrent compensatory measures to avoid gaining weight post-binge that either involve purging (e.g., self-induced vomiting) or nonpurging activities (e.g., excessive exercise or fasting); the bingeing and purging behaviors occur a minimum of two times a week for a duration of three months; self-evaluation is disproportionately influenced by body shape and weight. In addition, these disturbances do not occur during episodes of AN.

Also included in the DSM-IV is the category eating disorder not otherwise specified, which includes all clinically significant eating behaviors that do not fit neatly into the categories of AN or BN. Although it is referred only as a research diagnosis, binge-eating disorder falls into this category and is receiving much attention in the current contexts of the obesity epidemic as well as in the pending revisions to the DSM-IV. Binge-eating disorder's hallmark characteristic is binge eating (i.e., consuming in a discrete period a larger-than-normal amount of food for that particular time) at least two days a week for a duration of six months. These binges are similar to those that occur with BN, but in addition, meet at least three of the five following criteria: eating more rapidly than normal; eating until uncomfortably full; eating large amounts of food when not otherwise feeling physically hungry; eating alone out of embarrassment; or feeling disgusted with oneself or guilty after overeating.

EPIDEMIOLOGY, CAUSE, AND FEATURES

Epidemiological trends in eating disorders are difficult to characterize due to the complex nature of the illness and the manner in which they are conservatively self-reported. However, the majority of research studies indicate a growing trend in the emergence of anorexia and bulimia during the last half-century. Although eating disorders usually occur in adolescent girls or young women, a significant number of new cases are seen in boys and men.

The first nationally representative study of eating disorders in U.S. households found that the overall lifetime prevalence of eating disorders in 0.6 to 4.5 percent. This same population-based interview estimated the lifetime prevalence of AN to be 0.9 percent in women and 0.3 percent in men. BN also primarily affects women and tends to develop during late adolescence and early adulthood. Thus, prevalence rates for younger adolescents are generally lower than those reported by college students. Current lifetime prevalence rate for BN is 1.5 percent in women and 0.5 percent in men.

Although the range of disordered eating is broad outside a diagnosis of AN or BN, relatively little is known about EDNOS itself. Individuals who receive a diagnosis of EDNOS are often excluded from other treatment studies. It is estimated, however, that between 3 to 5 percent of women aged 15–30 in Western countries suffer from EDNOS. Its most studied disorder, binge-eating disorder, occurs more frequently in females, yet is also more evenly distributed across age, gender, and ethnicity than other eating disorders. The lifetime prevalence of binge-eating disorder is 3.5 percent in women and 2.0 percent in men.

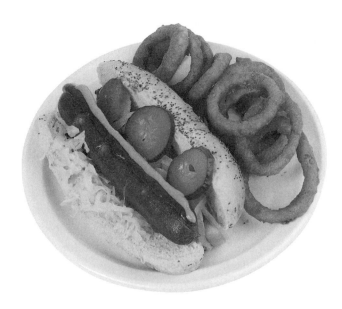

Eating disorders are are among the most lethal of the psychiatric diagnoses and affect an estimated five million Americans a year.

To date, the precise causes of eating disorders remain to be identified although neurochemical, genetic, developmental, psychological, family, and sociocultural factors have been implicated in various combinations. For example, societal ideals of thinness and harmful media images have received much attention for contributing to the development of body image disturbance. A causal relationship has been established between women who experience body dissatisfaction and media images, which in turn, can create a risk for development of disordered eating behaviors. A history of dieting in response to societal factors has also emerged as a predictor of eating disorders and disordered eating attitudes. Additionally, young women who engage in sports or artistic endeavors that emphasize thinness (such as ballet, modeling, or running) are observed to have a higher incidence of eating disorders.

The role of families in the social influence of eating disorders has been explored for causal factors of the illness. In a psychoanalytic model of family influence, eating disorders were interpreted as a fear of sexual maturity in young women, although these fears may not be exclusively associated with eating disorders. The psychodynamic model of family influences attributes eating disorders to an unresolved mismatch between parental and child needs, while a family systems model studies parental criticism and dysfunction. Another perspective further examines the observation that eating disorders run in families by asserting that disordered eating attitudes and weight concerns are, in fact, behaviors learned by children from their parents.

Cognition, behavior, and personality also contribute to the development of eating disorders. For example, AN has been associated with high levels of constraint and perfectionism, while BN is linked with impulsive behavior and poor emotional regulation. Negative emotionality is common to both disorders.

The etiology of eating disorders is multifactorial; traumatic experiences, including sexual violence, have been implicated as a risk factor in a number of studies. The results, however, are conflicting and reveal a complex yet nonspecific relationship between eating disorders and sexual assault. Several studies have found that a history of sexual trauma is more often reported by women with BN than by women with AN and that trauma-induced dissociation influences bulimic symptomatology.

There is incontestable evidence that biology contributes to the etiology of eating disorders. The role of neurochemical interactions that govern satiety is another area ripe for research. Neurotransmitters such as norepinephrine and serotonin may account, at least partially, for the cardiac and neuropsychiatric changes seen in individuals with AN. Also, genetics studies have concluded that women with first-degree relatives with eating disorders are at significantly higher risk for developing an eating disorder themselves. Current research on twins also shows increased heritability for eating disorders.

Individuals with AN typically display the following features upon examination in a clinical setting: a recent history of weight loss, dizziness, absence of menstrual periods (amenorrhea), low blood pressure (hypotension), feeling cold all the time (hypothermia), and slow heart rate (bradycardia). Other clinical findings characteristic of AN are constipation and feeling bloated after meals, fatigue, nausea, dry skin, development of fine hairs across the body (lanugo), yellowish or orange discoloration of the skin (hypercarotenemia), and bluish discoloration of the hands or feet (acrocyanosis). Additionally, she may demonstrate a distorted body image by claiming that she is overweight or deny that her extreme weight loss

is problematic. She may also engage in an excessive amount of exercise to control her weight.

Unlike individuals with AN, women with BN may not have a history of weight loss, as many who suffer from this disorder are able to maintain a normal weight in spite of the characteristic binge and purge behavior. She may admit to feeling "out of control" around food and attempting to control her weight by engaging in compensatory behavior (typically self-induced vomiting or laxative use) after a binge episode. Her relationship to food may have an addictive quality; she may also have a history of substance abuse or may be currently abusing other substances such as alcohol or cigarettes. A physical examination may reveal some swelling of the salivary glands and abrasions or calluses near the knuckles termed *Russell's sign* (caused by scraping against teeth during episodes of self-induced vomiting). She may also exhibit dental problems attributed to the erosion of enamel by stomach acid. Like women with AN, women who suffer from BN may experience interruptions in their menstrual cycle.

SCREENING FOR EATING DISORDERS

There are several screening tools of varying length that have been developed to detect eating disorders in individuals. The Eating Attitudes Test (EAT) is perhaps the most commonly used evaluative tool and has an accuracy rate of approximately 90 percent in diagnosing eating disorders according to DSM-IV criteria. Two shorter tools, the SCOFF questionnaire and the ESP, are also recognized for their efficacy in identifying individuals who might be at risk for an eating disorder although neither tool has been validated.

EATING DISORDERS, ETHNICITY, GENDER

Eating disorders were once thought to be an illness ascribed only to affluent, white women, but they are now an undiscriminating phenomenon; eating disorders are increasingly observed in various socioeconomic and ethnic minority groups. Although research currently is too limited to address variations in subgroups within the four main ethnic minority categories in the United States, there are both risk and protective factors inherent in each group's cultural values.

According to research, African-American women appear to be less likely to suffer from eating disorders than white women and, at a given weight, to be more satisfied with that weight. In contrast, rates of eating disorders in Hispanic women are very similar to those in white women although with more severe bingeing and greater body dissatisfaction in the former group. Although Asian women were found to be less likely to score high on eating disorders screening tools, there have been other studies that suggest Asian women did not differ from white women in levels of body dissatisfaction.

Studies on eating disorders in Native-American samples suggest an increased level of purging among girls in this group. Additionally, there are differences in clinical presentation of eating disorders among these ethnic minority groups. For example, in some Asian cultures, weight gain does not carry the stigma that it does in the United States, and women with anorectic symptoms instead may attribute their food refusal to a physical ailment (e.g., somatization).

The rate of men seeking treatment for eating disorders has increased in recent decades. Some studies have shown higher rates of eating disorders in men who participate in certain sports where weight is important (e.g., wrestling) and also in homosexual men compared to the general population; however, data concerning the latter are conflicting. On the whole, eating disorders in men closely resemble eating disorders in women, and more work is needed to understand why.

OUTCOME

The list of medical complications arising from these eating disorders is extensive. The American Academy of Pediatrics has issued a policy statement on the medical dangers of both bulimic and anorexic behaviors. Purging can result in severe electrolyte imbalances in the bloodstream, damage to the esophageal lining, poor dentition, enlarged salivary glands (which is erroneously interpreted by bulimic patients as having a "fat face"), calluses on the hands, and cardiac abnormalities. Severe caloric restriction as seen in AN can also lead to electrocardiographic and gastrointestinal abnormalities (e.g., mitral valve prolapse), anemia, amenorrhea, bone loss (osteopenia), seizures, amenorrhea, and difficulty in psychological functioning. Osteopenia is one of the most severe consequences of self-starvation and is often the most difficult to reverse. This bone loss can occur over even a short period and may lead to an increased risk for fracture of the hip and/or spine later in life. Eating disorders can be

fatal; the mortality rate for women with AN is 12 times greater than for women in the general population.

Studies indicate that about half of all patients with AN have "good" outcomes as measured by weight gain and return of menstrual cycles. A number of patients "cross over" into bulimia during their recovery phase, and overall, 32 to 70 percent of those with AN achieve full recovery at a 20-year follow-up.

Symptoms of BN appear to decrease over time as well, although about 30 percent of women who met the criteria for bulimia continued to engage in bingeing and purging behaviors for 10 years during follow-up. Strong fears of maturing and a low self-esteem emerged as predictors of outcome in AN and BN, respectively.

TREATMENT AND PREVENTION

Treatment of eating disorders is costly and can range from $10,000 to $20,000 per patient per year and varies by the type of eating disorder. Because they require medical as well as psychological treatment, women with AN spend more time and resources in an inpatient setting than women with BN. Moreover, most women with BN never seek treatment for their disorder. Symptom severity, psychosocial impairment, and psychological comorbidity are all predictors of increased treatment use.

Treatment for AN typically includes nutritional care, medical monitoring, and psychological treatment that may include cognitive behavioral therapy (relating thoughts and feelings to behavior) or family therapy. Effective treatment for those with BN may include cognitive behavioral therapy, other interpersonal therapy, antidepressant medication, and some combination of the three. For individuals with binge-eating disorder, dietary approaches in combination with psychotherapy and antidepressants have all been used with some success. Ideally, care for an individual with an eating disorder would employ a multidisciplinary team approach consisting of a medical provider, a dietitian, a mental health provider, and some form of nutritional therapy. However, for individuals with severe medical and/or psychological symptoms of their eating disorder, hospitalization may be required.

There are a range of treatment options for those seeking specialized care for their eating disorder. These options include inpatient treatment, residential treatment programs, and outpatient treatment. Inpatient treatment programs generally include medical monitoring, monitored meals, and group therapy sessions. Residential treatment programs, such as the renowned Renfrew Center, are similar to inpatient treatment programs and provide specialized, around-the-clock care exclusively for eating disorders. Outpatient programs are generally less expensive than inpatient or residential care and offer a high degree of flexibility in therapeutic intervention as well as offer controlled environment for mealtimes, depending on the type of program chosen, that is, day or evening.

Eating disorder patients may encounter various forms of psychotherapy during their treatment, but cognitive behavioral therapy remains the most effective for individuals with BN. Cognitive behavioral therapy aids the patient in linking thoughts and feelings to disordered eating, as well as in managing anxiety and developing coping strategies.

Pharmacotherapy for AN is limited, while use of antidepressants in treating BN is far more successful, particularly with the antidepressant fluoxetine (typically marketed as Prozac®). Similar success with antidepressants has been demonstrated in those with binge-eating disorder.

Efforts at prevention of eating disorders have demonstrated limited success in changing disordered eating behavior; however, improvements in both knowledge and attitudes are noted. The challenge remains to increase understanding of the risk factors that lead to eating disorders as well as to sustain the success shown immediately after the intervention.

SEE ALSO: Anorexia; Bulimia; Obesity; Psychiatry; Psychotherapy.

BIBLIOGRAPHY. Anne E. Becker, et al., "Eating Disorders," *New England Journal of Medicine* (v.341, 1999); Sara F. Forman, "Eating Disorders: Epidemiology, Pathogenesis, and Clinical Features," in B. D. Rose, ed., *UpToDate* (, 2007); Sara F. Forman, "Eating Disorders: Treatment and Outcome," in B. D. Rose, ed., *UpToDate* (, 2007); James I. Hudson, et al., "The Prevalence and Correlates of Eating Disorders in the National Comorbidity Survey Replication," *Biological Psychiatry* (v.61/3, 2007); Pamela Keel, *Eating Disorders* (Pearson Education, 2005).

LAREINA NADINE LA FLAIR, M.P.H.
HARVARD UNIVERSITY

Ecogenetics

Related to environmental sciences (particularly environmental health or biomedicine) and to molecular biology and genetics, ecogenetics is an emergent discipline in the interphase of these sciences. Ecogenetics initially attempted to study and understand how the genetic and environmental factors could together influence the organism's response to carcinogenic agents and other imposed stresses.

However, ecogenetics represents a growing science with many practical purposes, particularly in the field of prevention of environmentally related genetic diseases. Today, we could consider that understanding the play between heredity and environment and relating it to disease causation is the task of ecogenetics. The field of ecogenetics has emerged from the older area of pharmacogenetics and investigates how genetic polymorphisms may represent risk factors for a number of diseases associated with exposure to toxic chemicals and other environmental substances and factors.

In addition, the extrapolation that genetic variations would be expected to affect responses to any kind of environmental and xenobiotic agent, not just drugs, lead to "ecogenetics," by analyzing the critical genetic determinants that dictate susceptibility to environmentally influenced adverse health effects. Currently, it is postulated that many diseases are the result of environmental factors acting on genetically susceptible individuals. Many genetic conditions, including those involving hematological and liver diseases, serum proteins alterations, skin disorders, DNA repair diseases, and others have now been included in the study of diseases that are subject of ecogenetics.

This discipline is growing faster in the area of cancer ecogenetics, particularly with the objective of preventing or avoiding neoplastic diseases. This would be reached through the use of genetic markers. Although ecogenetics seeks to examine genetically mediated differences in susceptibility to environmental agents, researchers often examine the relationship between genetic markers and disease without regard to environmental determinants. By using epidemiologic definitions of genotype–environment interaction, it can be shown that the relative risk of disease for the genetic marker is a function of the frequency of exposure to the environmental agent, the strength of interaction between the genotype and the agent, and the specificity of the environmental effect vis-à-vis the genotype.

Currently, applications of ecogenetics to various types of diseases and some of its associated factors can be found in the biomedical literature, as the ecogenetics of some parasitic pathogens and its vectors (e.g., leishmaniasis, Chagas's disease, etc.).

Today, the field of the ecogenetics is, by far, more complex than some years ago, given the vast number of ethical, legal, and social issues related to the discipline. This is particularly important with studies investigating and evaluating genetic polymorphisms in human populations and should consider the impact of this emergent science on risk assessment, regulatory policies, and medicine and public health.

SEE ALSO: Environmental Medicine; Epigenetics; Genetics; Genetic Disorders; Genomics.

BIBLIOGRAPHY. Lucio G. Costa and David L. Eaton, *Gene-Environment Interactions: Fundamentals of Ecogenetics* (Wiley, 2006); Muin J. Khoury, "An Epidemiologic Approach to Ecogenetics," *American Journal of Human Genetics* (v.42/1, 1988); François Noireau, "Ecogenetics of Triatoma sordida and Triatoma guasayana (Hemiptera: Reduviidae) in the Bolivian Chaco," *Memórias do Instituto Oswaldo Cruz* (v.94/4, 1999).

Alfonso J. Rodriguez-Morales, M.D., M.Sc.
Universidad de Los Andes, Venezuela
Carlos Franco-Paredes, M.D., M.P.H.
Emory University

E. Coli Infections

Escherichia coli are bacteria of which the virulent strains can cause significant gastrointestinal morbidity and mortality. E. coli O157:H7 is the strain most well known to the general public for causing epidemics after ingestion of contaminated water and foods, including undercooked hamburgers, lettuce, and spinach. The Centers for Disease Control and Prevention estimates that over 73,000 cases of infection and 61 deaths occur in the United States annually because of E. coli O157:H7.

First isolated in 1982, E. coli O157:H7's virulence stems from its ability to produce several toxins. These toxins have the ability to invade the gastrointestinal mucosal surfaces, causing a range of symptoms including asymptomatic infections, severe abdominal cramps with or without fever, watery diarrhea, or grossly bloody diarrhea. More severe diseases may also occur. Hemolytic uremic syndrome causes a blood disorder, acute renal failure, and neurological symptoms, while thrombocytopenic purpura can cause low platelets. Among reported U.S. outbreaks, 23 percent of patients were hospitalized, 6 percent had hemolytic uremic syndrome or thrombocytopenic purpura, and approximately 1percent died from *E. coli* infections.

E. coli is ubiquitous around the world. The incidence and prevalence of *E. coli* infections remain underreported because many infected persons do not report to their physician when they are infected, the physician does not send the correct laboratory test for definitive diagnosis, or the physician does not report the infection to the proper authorities. Seasonally, *E. coli* infections occur more frequently in the summer, which may be due to the higher consumption of ground meats during outdoor barbeques.

Transmission of *E. coli* to humans occurs primarily through the contamination of the food and water supply. E. coli O157:H7 can be found in the intestines of cattle, deer, goats, and sheep. The meat may be contaminated through slaughter or through the process of grinding the meat. Additionally, *E. coli* can infect raw milk if the bacteria have colonized cows' udders. *E. coli* is also found in sprouts, salami, and unpasteurized milk and juice. Swimming or drinking sewage-contaminated water can also be a means of transmission. Handling infected stools or inadequate hand washing can also transmit *E. coli* rapidly, especially among toddlers and young children.

Once *E. coli* infection is suspected, the diagnosis can be confirmed by growing colonies of the bacteria and then assaying the colonies for the O157 antigen, the protein that causes the infection. Although it is recommended that all physicians screen for *E. coli*, only one-quarter of laboratories actually screen all stool specimens. Because the antigen declines steeply after six days of illness, it is imperative to culture stools early. Currently, rapid detection tests are being developed.

No specific treatment exists for *E. coli* infection. Most infected people recover from this self-limiting illness within five to 10 days. Studies have not found antibiotics to be effective, and in some cases, antibiotics have worsened the illness. Antimotility agents (i.e. Immodium) should not be used in infected patients. One study found that patients who used antimotility agents were at increased risk to develop hemolytic uremic syndrome. In terms of prevention, a safe food supply and better hygiene practices can help curb the incidence of *E. coli* infections. Physicians should counsel patients on proper handling of meat, including correct cooking temperatures, hand washing, using only treated water for cooking and drinking, and drinking only pasteurized liquids.

SEE ALSO: Bacterial Infections; Centers for Disease Control and Prevention (CDC); Digestive Diseases (General), Drinking Water; Food and Drug Administration (FDA); Food Contamination/Poisoning; Food Safety.

BIBLIOGRAPHY. T.G Boyce, D.L. Swerdlow, and P.M. Griffin, "Escherichia coli O157:H7 and the Hemolytic-Uremic Syndrome," *New England Journal of Medicine*(v.333/6, 1995); Centers for Disease Control and Prevention, "Escherichia coli O157:H7", www.cdc.gov (cited October 2006); C. Su, and LJ Brandt "Escherichia coli O157:H7 Infection in Humans." *Annals of Internal Medicine* (v.123/9, 1995).

LINDSAY KIM, MPH
EMORY UNIVERSITY SCHOOL OF MEDICINE

Ectoparasites

Parasites are organisms that feed, grow, or find shelter in or on a host organism without contributing to the survival of the host. Ectoparasites are parasites, usually insects, that reside on the exterior of the host organism, as opposed to endoparasites, which live inside organs, tissues, or cells. Human ectoparasites live on or in the skin and usually feed on blood or keratin from their human host. Most ectoparasites go through at least part of their life cycle on their host organism and are members of the insecta class of invertebrates—lice, fleas, and flies—or the arachnida class—ticks, scabies, and others.

Ectoparasites are very common and were responsible for transmitting the infectious agents that caused some of the worst plagues in human history. Today, they continue to cause significant morbidity and even mortality in many parts of the world. The human diseases caused by ectoparasites are due either to the infestation itself, or a virus, bacteria, or parasite carried by the ectoparasite vector.

Many ectoparasites are simply a nuisance, such as lice of the head, body, or pubic area. Lice cause itching, irritation, and occasionally secondary bacterial infections, but rarely any more serious disease. Other ectoparasites such as scabies and the tungiasis (tunga penetrans) flea cause disease when the female lays her eggs in the skin of human hosts. This causes intense itching and discomfort and can also lead to secondary infections. Similarly, certain tropical species of flies can intentionally or accidentally deposit their eggs under human skin. These eggs develop into larva which cause pain and irritation and eventually exit the skin, much to the surprise of the unsuspecting host. Scabies and lice are the most common ectoparasites encountered in North America and are a common cause for presentation to primary care providers.

Many other types of chiggers, mites, and blister beetles inhabit environments from mattresses to jungles, and have effects from allergic irritation to blistering and infection. Certain types of ticks can cause paralysis in children by injecting a potent neurotoxin into the blood as it feeds. Over several days, the effects of tick paralysis may present as a feeling of unsteadiness and progress to weakness in the limbs and possible respiratory failure. This type of tick paralysis is rare, but residents and visitors to tick-infested areas should be aware of the risks, and inspect their bodies for ticks after outdoor activities.

The most important route by which ectoparasites cause disease in humans is by acting as vectors for dangerous bacteria. For example, Lyme disease is caused by a bacteria transmitted in North America by the Ixodes ticks found primarily in New England states. Lyme disease presents initially as a bulls-eye rash, and if not treated, it may lead to nervous disorders, heart problems, or joint swelling and pain. Over 15,000 cases of Lyme disease are reported in the United States each year; while treatment is available and effective, many cases go unnoticed.

Another very important family of diseases transmitted by ticks are rickettsia (also known as Ehrlichia). These are very small bacteria that are responsible for a variety of diseases including the typhus group (murine typhus, epidemic typhus, and scrub typhus), the spotted fever group (Rocky Mountain spotted fever, rickettsial pox, and others), as well as Q fever and trench fever. Each of these diseases is carried by a different type of ectoparasite tick, louse, or mite, which is, in turn, normally carried by a mammal such as a mouse, dog, squirrel, or human. The diseases caused by rickettsia range from mild to life threatening, but all are treatable with antibiotics if properly diagnosed.

Ectoparasites, specifically ticks, can also carry and infect humans with viral infections. An example of this is tickborne encephalitis (TBE). The TBE virus is found in forested areas throughout eastern Europe and Asia. Most cases of TBE are subclinical and are not detected, but in certain cases, TBE can cause severe disease and death. There is a vaccine available for TBE and it is recommended for people who live or travel in high-risk areas for long periods.

While it is difficult to estimate the global impact of ectoparasite and ectoparasitically transmitted disease, there is no doubt that ectoparasites have been, and will continue to be, associated with human disease. Despite advances in hygiene-related prevention and antibiotic treatments, ectoparasites, like many other emerging and reemerging diseases, are increasingly resistant to the medical treatments available, including the safest insecticides and repellants. As human habitation encroaches farther into ectoparasite habitats and as humans live in more densely populated communities, it is likely that ectoparasite-related illness will only increase.

SEE ALSO: Lyme Disease; Parasitic Diseases.

BIBLIOGRAPHY. Eugene Braunwald, et al., eds., *Harrison's Principles of Internal Medicine*, 15th ed. (McGraw-Hill, 2001); J. H. Diaz, "The Diagnosis, Management, and Prevention of Common Ectoparasitic Infections," *Journal of the Louisiana State Medical Society* (v.158/2, 2006); J. H. Diaz, "The Epidemiology, Diagnosis, Management, and Prevention of Ectoparasitic Diseases in Travelers," *Journal of Travel Medicine* (v.13/2, 2006).

BARRY PAKES, M.D., M.P.H.
UNIVERSITY OF TORONTO

Ecuador

Ecuador is located on the northwestern edge of South America, with a coast on the Pacific Ocean. The famed Galapagos Island, part of Ecuadorian territory, lays 965 kilometers (600 miles) offshore. The country was a Spanish colonial possession until 1821 and has never really found political or economic stability. Economic disparity is wide in Ecuador, with most of the money and power in the hands of those of European ancestry, while mesitzos and indigenous peoples live in abject poverty.

The population of Ecuador is estimated at around 13,756,000 and growing at 1.55 percent annually. The birth rate is 21.91 births per 1,000, with a death rate of 4.21 deaths per 1,000 and a net migration rate of minus 2.16 migrants per 1,000. The population is mostly young: median age is 24 years, and 41 percent of the population is under the age of 18. Life expectancy at birth is currently 73.74 years for males and 79.63 years for females.

Ecuador has one of the most unequal distributions of wealth in the world. It is estimated that the richest 20 percent of Ecuadorians hold 50 percent of the nation's wealth, while the poorest 20 percent hold only 5 percent. A 2004 survey found that the majority of the urban poor subsist on $2.70 a day, while indigenous poor in the rural areas live on a mere $1.30. This inequality had heavy implications for public health within the country.

Ecuador still has a significant burden of communicable disease within its borders. Malaria is common through the country, as is dengue fever in the costal regions. Cases of Chagas disease began in the early 1990s. There have been occasional reports of jungle yellow fever over the past two decades. Rabies and other zoonotic diseases are endemic throughout the country. There are sporadic cases of leprosy. Acute respiratory disease affects thousands each year. Cholera cases dropped in the 1990s, but diarrhea and other gastrointestinal diseases are common. HIV/AIDS impacts 0.3 percent of the adult population, or an estimated 23,000 people. There have been about 1,000 AIDS-related deaths since the virus first emerged. Political problems have hampered the country's efforts to institute education and prevention programs, and only 34 percent of those in need are taking antiretroviral drugs. However, the Joint United Nations Programme on HIV/AIDS (UNAIDS) notes that there have been improvements in care in recent years, particularly for at-risk women and children.

Noncommunicable diseases and external issues also take their toll on the population. Cardiovascular disease is common, and often stems from other degenerative conditions, such as rheumatic fever. With 63 percent of Ecuadorians living in urban areas, accidents and violence are the frequent cause of hospital admissions. Its geographic location leads to death, disease and injuries from a variety of natural disasters, including floods, earthquakes, and volcanic eruptions.

Infant and child mortality dropped between 1990 and 2005, with 25 deaths per 1,000 for children aged 1 to 5 years and 22 deaths per 1,000 for those under the age of 1. Immunization rates have risen to 94 percent. Malnutrition remains an issue, particularly among indigenous children. Twelve percent of children are classified as underweight, with 26 percent showing signs of stunted growth from long-term poor nutrition. Approximately 5.5 percent of Ecuador's Gross Domestic Product goes to healthcare, and the country spends about $127 per capita. There is both a private and a public healthcare system. An estimated 18,000 doctors and 19,500 nurses work within the country, augmented by over 1,000 midwives. There are about 14 hospital beds for every 10,000 people.

SEE ALSO: Diarrhea; Malaria.

BIBLIOGRAPHY. "Ecuador," *CIA World Factbook*, www.cia.gov/library/publications/the-world-factbook/geos/ec.html (cited June 2007); "Ecuador—Overview—An inequitable society," UNICEF, www.unicef.org/ecuador/overview_2834.htm (cited June 2007); "Ecuador," UNAIDS: The Joint United Nations Programme on HIV/AIDS, www.unaids.org/en/Regions_Countries/Countries/ecuador.asp (cited June 2007); World Health Organization, "Core Health Indicators/WHO 2007," Core Health Indicators/WHO 2007, www.who.int/whosis/database/core/core_select.cfm (cited June 2007).

HEATHER K. MICHON
INDEPENDENT SCHOLAR

Edema

Edema is an increase in interstitial fluid in any organs and used to be called dropsy or hydropsy. It generally manifests itself in a swelling of the feet and the ankles, but can occur in any organ or tissue in the body. Technically, it can also appear in plants where plant organs swell after an excessive accumulation of water.

The production of interstitial fluid in the body is usually kept in balance but occasionally it can change through increased secretion of fluid into the interstitium or when there is impaired removal of the fluid. Edemas in some parts of the body are affected by gravity and this is known as peripheral edema or dependent edema. Gravity means that for people who spend much of their time upright, excess fluid often ends up in the ankles or feet, resulting in swelling there. However, for bedbound people, the first instance of edema can often be sacral edema.

The main causes of peripheral edema include the high hydrostatic pressure on the veins, which leads to general inflammation, a poor reabsorption of fluids, low oncotic pressure, or an obstruction to the system of draining the lymph glands. In the case of pressure on the veins, it may originate from long periods in the same position (such as on long-haul flights), or the use of tight knee pads, or the wearing of tight jeans. This might lead, in the most extreme cases, to deep vein thrombosis, resulting from venous obstruction, congestive heart failure, or varicose veins. Low oncotic pressure may result in cirrhosis, renal protein loss, or even malnutrition. The obstruction of the lymph glands usually leads to infections but can also lead to fibrosis after surgery, and even cancer. It is also possible that edema might lead to allergic conditions such as angioedema.

Although the symptoms of edema have been well known since ancient times, they were explained by the Greeks and the Romans by their belief in "humors" in the body, who saw an imbalance in them as the cause of swelling. Gradually, the knowledge of edemas increased with Herman Elwyn writing about it in 1929, and Cecil Drinker producing a major work in 1950.

SEE ALSO: Cirrhosis.

BIBLIOGRAPHY. Cecil K. Drinker, *Pulmonary Edema and Inflammation* (Harvard University Press, 1950); Herman Elwyn, *Edema and Its Treatment* (Macmillan, 1929); Alfred P. Fishman and Eugene M. Renkin, *Pulmonary Edema* (American Physiological Society, 1979).

JUSTIN CORFIELD
GEELONG GRAMMAR SCHOOL, AUSTRALIA

Egypt

Egypt is one of the oldest civilizations in the world and has the largest population (78,887,007) of all Arab countries. Today, the government is struggling to return Egypt to a position of economic viability. Health services and free education have deteriorated, resulting in a less healthy population where large segments are unemployable. A per capita income of $3,900 places Egypt 146th in world incomes. Some 32 percent of the population is involved in agriculture, much of it subsistence. Nearly 10 percent (9.5 percent) of the work force is unemployed. One-fifth of Egyptians live in poverty, and in some areas as many as 58 percent are severely impoverished. Three percent of Egyptians live on less than $1 a day. Some estimates place the number of Egyptians outside the healthcare system because of residency in informal areas at 48 million. In Cairo, around two million people live in squatter settlements or slums. It is believed that some 12 million Egyptians live in shacks, garages, mosques, and under staircases. Other impoverished Egyptians have taken up residency in the small one- and two-room houses built in cemeteries for temporary use by families visiting the dead. Income disparity also exists, and Egypt ranks 34.4 on the Gini index of inequality. The top 10 percent of the population claims a fourth of all resources while the bottom 10 percent share only 4.4 percent. The United Nations Development Programme's (UNDP) Human Development Report ranks Egypt 111th in the world in overall quality of life issues.

While health insurance is readily available to more affluent Egyptians, it is beyond the reach of many Egyptians, and the government has not been able to breech this divide. There is a major problem with the quality of healthcare received by poor Egyptians. Three percent of total government expenditures are directed toward healthcare. The government designates 5.8 percent of the total Gross Domestic Product (GDP) for healthcare, and $235 (international dollars) per capita are expended in this area. Government funding provides 42.6 percent of all healthcare funding; and 27.1 percent of that total is earmarked for social security, which provides monthly allowances to orphans, divorced individuals, the elderly, and the disabled. The private sector provides 57.4 of all healthcare expenditures, and 93.2 percent

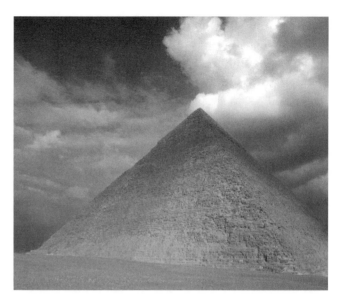

Health services in Egypt have deteriorated, resulting in a less healthy population where large segments are unemployable.

of private spending is out of pocket. There are 0.54 physicians, 2.00 nurses, 0.14 dentists, and 0.10 pharmacists per 1,000/ population in Egypt.

Ranking in the mid-range on life expectancy, Egyptians can expect to live 71.29 years. On average, women outlive men by five years. Literacy is relatively low in Egypt, at 57.7 percent, and there is an appreciable difference in male (68.3 percent) and female (46.9 percent) literacy. Egypt has limited fresh water resources outside the Nile area. However, all urban residents and 97 percent of rural residents have sustained access to safe drinking water. Less than 60 percent of rural Egyptians have access to improved sanitation as compared to 84 percent of urban residents.

Women produce approximately 2.83 children each in Egypt. Between 1970 and 1990, the fertility rate dropped from 6.1 to 4.3. This is due in great part to the fact that women are marrying later and 60 percent of Egyptian women now use birth control. Trained personnel are present at 69 percent of all births, and 69 percent of women receive antenatal care. The adjusted maternal mortality rate is 84 deaths per 100,000 live births. The rural mortality rate is almost double that of urban areas.

Infant mortality stands at 31.33 deaths per 1,000 live births, the 79th highest infant mortality rate in the world. However, some significant success has been made. Between 1990 and 2004, infant mortality plummeted from 76 to 26 deaths per 1,000 live births, and under-5 mortality declined from 104 to 36 deaths. Twelve percent of all infants are underweight at birth, and nine percent of under-5s fall into this category. Four percent suffer moderate to severe wasting, and 16 percent experience stunting. The government subsidizes all required vaccinations. Consequently, immunization rates are high, with 98 receiving diphtheria, pertussis, and tetanus (DPT1) and tuberculosis vaccines, and 97 percent receiving DPT3, polio, measles, and hepatitis B vaccinations. Around 29 percent of under-5s receive necessary oral rehydration therapy when needed.

Seventeen percent of Egyptian children are not enrolled in primary school. While 88 percent of males attend secondary school, only 82 percent of females do so. Six percent of children between the ages of 6 and 14 are in the labor force, and their presence is particularly prevalent in the cotton industry. Over half of Egyptian children suffer from anaemia, and a fifth of all children suffer from vitamin deficiencies. The health of Egypt's street children is particularly precarious. A joint United Nations Children's Fund (UNICEF) and World Food Program study revealed that 66 percent of these children suffer from substance abuse. Thirty percent of them have never attended school, and 70 percent have dropped out. Female genital mutilation/cutting is still common in Egypt, and 95 percent of urban and 99 percent of rural females undergo this procedure.

While Egypt is not experiencing HIV/AIDS to the same extent as many of the poorest African nations, the country has a 0.1 percent adult prevalence rate. Some 12,000 are living with the disease, and 700 have died. The first successful treatment of trachoma can be traced back to the ancient Egyptians, but the disease continues to affect modern Egyptians. It is the leading cause of blindness among rural Egyptians, and 36.5 percent of rural children are suffering from active trachoma. In one rural community, one out of every five adults is also afflicted with the completely preventable disease. The Carter Center of Emory University works with other international agencies to eradicate schistosomiasis and Guinea worm disease in rural Egypt. A major avian influenza epidemic hit Egypt in 2006.

SEE ALSO: Saudi Arabia; United Arab Emirates.

BIBLIOGRAPHY. Central Intelligence Agency, "Egypt," *World Factbook*, www.cia.gov; Commission on the Status of Women, "Egypt", www.un.org; Peter Kandela, "Alexandria: Oversupply of Doctors Fuels Egypt's Health-Care Crisis," *The Lancet* (v.352/9122, 1998); Helen Chapin Metz, ed., *Egypt: A Country Study* (Federal Research Division, 1991); Hania Sholkamy and Faha Ghannan, eds., *Health and Identity in Egypt: Shifting Frontiers* (American University in Cairo Press, 2004); Social Watch, "Egypt," www.socialwatch.org; Khalid F. Tabbara, "Blinding Trachoma: The Forgotten Problem," *British Journal of Ophthalmology* (v.85/12, 2001). UNICEF, "Egypt," www.unicef.org.

ELIZABETH R. PURDY, PH.D.
INDEPENDENT SCHOLAR

Ehlers-Danlos Syndrome

Ehlers-Danlos syndrome (EDS) is a collection of genetic diseases that cause instability of the collagen or its partner proteins, and therefore of connective tissue. Common features include joint hyperextensibility and elastic skin prone to tearing and bruising. One feature which may indicate EDS is the Gorlin sign, which is the ability to reach the tip of the nose with the tongue.

There are many disorders of the connective tissue. Some are genetic, some are environmental, and some are idiopathic, meaning they don't have a known cause. Genetic connective tissue disorders include Ehlers-Danlos syndrome, affecting collagen or the proteins that interact with collagen to provide stability to the connective tissue. EDS is panethnic and affects males and females equally. Overall, approximately one in 5,000 individuals has some form of EDS.

Several genetic diseases that result in defective collagen are classified as EDS. EDS can be caused by other genetic mutations as well, but the major ones identified so far have been grouped into six classes, each containing one or more 'types'. Initially there were eleven types of EDS; in 1997, scientists came together to simplify the system and combine like disorders into types. Today, former EDS types 1 and 2 are called Classical EDS. Classical EDS involves a mutation in type V or type I collagen, and results in joint hypermobility, dislocation or subluxation (partial or incomplete dislocation) of joints, highly elastic and velvety skin which readily bruises and tears, and often mitral valve prolapse, a cardiac condition. A woman with Classical EDS is at mortal risk if she becomes pregnant. Classical EDS is documented at a frequency of fewer than five in 100,000 patients.

Former type 3 EDS is called Hypermobility. These patients also have joint hypermobility, dislocation, and subluxation; and often have mitral valve prolapse. Hypermobility is caused by a dominant mutation in one of two autosomal (non sex-chromosomal) genes.

Former type 4 is called Vascular EDS. In Vascular EDS, the type 3 collagen gene (also autosomal) has a dominant mutation found in one in 100,000 people. Vascular EDS primarily affects the vasculature of individuals. Small blood vessels are weakened, as well as organ membranes, and people with Vascular EDS often do not live greater than 40 years. A common occurrence in people with this form of EDS is an aneurysm. Like other forms of EDS, Vascular EDS causes elastic, velvety skin which easily bruises and tears, and it can appear translucent. Women with Vascular EDS are also in mortal risk if they become pregnant.

Former type 5 is not a major class of EDS; former type 6 is called Kyphoscoliosis. These individuals develop progressive scoliosis due to a rare, autosomally recessive mutation in their lysyl hydroxylase gene. Former types 7A and 7B EDS are called Arthrochalasis, and are due to a defect in type I collagen. The most affected joint in Arthrochalasis is the hip; these individuals often develop osteoarthritis. Former type 7C is the rarest of the major EDS classes. It is called Dermatosparaxis, and results in elastic, fragile skin which becomes progressively more brittle with age.

There are five more types of EDS that are all classified as Other. These types are the former types 5, 8, 9, 10, and 11. Combined symptoms of these types include low blood pressure, frequent blood clotting, periodontal complications, and loose joints.

Currently, there is no known cure for EDS; rather, patients manage their disease with supportive treatment. A major management step is protecting the joints from damaging impacts or dangerous stretching. Too much impact or stretching could lead to arthritis as well as dislocation of the joints. People with EDS must be vigilant in their eye care as the whites of the eyes may be weakened. Additionally, the skin must be protected from the sun.

SEE ALSO: Cardiology; Connective Tissue Disorders; Marfan Syndrome; National Institutes of Health (NIH).

BIBLIOGRAPHY. Peter Beighton, ed., *McKusick's Heritable Disorders of Connective Tissue* (C. V. Mosby, 1993); Kenneth J. Carpenter, *The Official Patient's Sourcebook on Ehlers-Danlos Syndrome: A Revised and Updated Dictionary for the Internet Age* (Icon Health Publications, 2002); ICON Health Publications, *Ehlers-Danlos Syndrome: A Medical Dictionary, Bibliography, and Annotated Research Guide to Internet References* (ICON Health Publications, 2004).

CLAUDIA WINOGRAD
UNIVERSITY OF ILLINOIS

Ehrlich, Paul (1854–1915)

Born on March 14, 1854, in modern-day Poland (then part of Germany) to Ismar and Rose Weigert Ehrlich, Paul Ehrlich created the first-known cure for syphilis, a disease later treated by antibiotics, and he discovered the process of chemotherapy, using chemicals to combat disease. Furthermore, because of his blood sample research, hematology became a scientific discipline. In 1908, Ehrlich received the Nobel Prize for Physiology or Medicine with Ilya Mechnikov for his discoveries about the human immune system.

Ehrlich studied at the Universities of Breslau, Strasbourg, Freiburg-im-Breisgau, and Leipzig, earning his Ph.D. in medicine in 1878. He worked at the Berlin Medical Clinic, staining tissues with dyes, and discovering that all dyes were basic, acid, or neutral. Even today, the method for staining the tuberculosis bacteria is a derivative of Ehrlich's process. In 1882, Ehrlich became a professor at the University of Berlin.

In 1883, Ehrlich married Hedwig Pinkus, with whom he had two daughters. Contracting tuberculosis, possibly through his laboratory work, Ehrlich recuperated in Egypt, staying there from 1886 until 1888. In 1890, he began his breakthrough immunological studies at the new Institute for Infectious Diseases.

He collaborated with two bacteriologists to find a cure for diphtheria. In 1894, their antitoxins began being used on children. Through this process, they recognized the need for dyes that stained bacteria but not other cells to help them combat disease; as they sought out these dyes, Ehrlich discovered that arsenic helped people overcome syphilis.

In 1897, Ehrlich was chosen as the public health officer in Frankfurt-am-Main; in 1899, he became the director of the Royal Institute of Experimental Therapy and of the Georg Speyerhaus; there, he founded the basis of chemotherapy. He called these chemicals "magic bullets" for their ability to target disease in the human body. During the later years of his career, Ehrlich experimented with methods to defeat tumors.

The street where the Royal Institute was located was renamed Paul Ehrlichstrasse, which was reversed during the Hitler years in Germany. After World War II ended and the region became part of Poland, the street was named Ehrlichstadt. Ehrlich had a minor stroke in 1914. On August 20, 1915, he suffered a fatal one.

SEE ALSO: Chemotherapy; Diphtheria; Sexually Transmitted Diseases.

BIBLIOGRAPHY. "Paul Ehrlich," www.cartage.org.lb/en/themes/Biographies/MainBiographies/E/Ehrlich(cited July 2007); "Paul Ehrlich," *Nobel Lectures, Physiology or Medicine 1901–1921* (Elsevier, 1967); "Paul Ehrlich: The Nobel Prize in Physiology or Medicine 1908," nobelprize.org (cited July 2007).

KELLY BOYER SAGERT
INDEPENDENT SCHOLAR

El Salvador

El Salvador is located on the Pacific Coast of Central America, surrounded by Guatemala and Honduras. It is the smallest country in Central America, the most heavily industrialized, and the only one that does not have a coastline on the Caribbean. It is a mountainous country poetically called the Land of Volcanoes—a geological happenstance that leads to frequent earthquakes, while its geographical location makes it vulnerable to tropical storms and hurricanes. In 1998, the remnants of Hurricane Mitch dumped an enormous amount of rain on the country, leading to massive flooding that killed 300 and left at least 30,000 homeless. The country has not been free from man-made disasters either: A civil war from 1980 to 1992 took the lives of more than 75,000 Salvadorans before peace was declared.

El Salvador has a population of 6.82 million and is growing at 1.72 percent annually. The birth rate is 26.61 births per 1,000 people and the death rate is 5.78 per 1,000 people. The migration rate is minus 3.61 migrants per 1,000. An estimated 3.1 million Salvadorans are living outside the country.

Although the country has a well-developed industrial sector, the economy remains poor. Almost 17 percent of the Gross Domestic Product in 2005 came from remittances, money wired back into the country from emigrants. The agricultural sector has been hit by droughts, deforestation, soil erosion, and the collapse of world coffee prices.

Per capita income in $4,700 a year, but 32 percent of the population live below the poverty line. The country recently entered into the Central American Free Trade Agreement (CAFTA), which it hopes will revitalize the country's economy.

Average life expectancy at birth is 67.88 years for males and 75.28 years for females; healthy life expectancy is 57.2 for men and 62.36 for women. Infant mortality is 24 deaths per 1,000 live births. Another 28 of every 1,000 children die between the ages of 1 and 5. Maternal mortality is 150 deaths per 100,000 live births. Sixty-eight percent of women receive prenatal care and 92 percent have a trained attendant present at delivery.

The Salvadoran diet is based on rice and beans, and small cornmeal cakes called pupusas, which are filled with farmer's cheese, beans, and fried pork fat or other meats. Even with the addition of local fruits and vegetables, this diet lacks essential vitamins and nutrients.

A quarter of Salvadoran children are malnourished. There has been a concerted effort to increase childhood immunizations, and common diseases such as measles and polio have been all but eradicated in recent years. Civil war, natural disasters, and the search for work outside the country has led to 180,000 children under the age of 17 living as orphans.

About 82 percent of the population have clean water to drink and 63 percent have access to sanitary facilities. Nevertheless, common waterborne and communicable diseases are under control within El Salvador, with only sporadic outbreaks of illnesses such as cholera. Leprosy is becoming increasingly rare.

Salvadorans are more likely to die in accidents; from heart disease, cancer, and pneumonia; or in natural disasters than from an infectious disease. There is a nationwide monitoring network in place to deal with outbreaks; for example, dengue fever—both classic and hemorrhagic—broke out in 2006 and triggered a massive government response to stem the spread of the illness. Tuberculosis is on the rise, with 60 cases per 100,000 people. The HIV/AIDS rate is 0.7 percent, with 30,000 people living with the virus and 2,200 having died since it first emerged. Studies have shown that 89 percent of the cases were sexually transmitted, and the government has launched education campaign across the country.

The government allocates $84 per person on healthcare. It is making strides to increase access to both urgent and preventative care but remains hampered to some degree by the poor economy. The World Health Organization counted 7,938 physicians and 5,103 nurses working in the country in the year 2000.

SEE ALSO: Healthcare, South America.

BIBLIOGRAPHY. John R. Eriksson, Margaret Arnold, Alcira Kreimer, *El Salvador: Post-Conflict Reconstruction* (World Bank Publications, 2000); Aldo Lauria-Santiago, and Leigh Binford, *Landscapes of Struggle: Politics, Society, and Community in El Salvador* (University of Pittsburgh Press, 2004.)

HEATHER K. MICHON
INDEPENDENT SCHOLAR

Elbow Injuries and Disorders

Musculoskeletal injuries are the most frequently occurring medical conditions in the United States. Although elbow injuries are among the least common musculoskeletal problems, their impact on daily life and an individual's independence can be quite significant. The most common elbow injuries can be broken down into two main categories: overuse and trauma.

ANATOMY

In order to understand disorders of the elbow, an appreciation for the basic anatomy is required. The elbow joint consists of the articulation of the upper arm, or humerus, with the two bones of the forearm, the radius and ulna. The radius and ulna articulate with the lateral and medial portions of the humerus (termed *condyles*) in a manner allowing for hinge-like movement, as well as pivoting movements termed *pronation* and *supination*. The elbow joint movements are stabilized posteriorly by the olecranon process of the ulna bone, and laterally and medially by two major ligament complexes. Bursa, or fluid filled sacs, facilitate movement by reducing friction between elbow components.

OVERUSE

Humeral epicondylitis is the most common elbow problem and is a result of overuse of the elbow joint. The associated pain is a result of inflammation of the area where the forearm muscles attach to the humerus. The inflammation is more commonly on the lateral humerus (aka "tennis elbow"), but can also occur on the medial side (aka "golfer's elbow") or posteriorly around the triceps tendon. These conditions are most common between the age of 30 and 50 in those who perform repetitive hand or arm movements as a part of their profession.

Repetitive forceful extensions of the elbow can also cause bony collisions between the olecranon and the humerus, leading to a condition called posterior impingement syndrome. The bones will often thicken and or fragment in response to the trauma, leading to pain over the olecranon process, limited range of motion, and swelling.

Overuse of the elbow can also lead to inflammation of the bursa or muscle tendons, conditions termed *bursitis* and *tendonitis*, respectively. Bursitis most commonly involves the olecranon bursa, and tendonitis most commonly involves the biceps or triceps tendons.

TRAUMA

Trauma to the elbow joint can typically result in two types of injury: fracture or dislocation. Elbow dislocation often results from falling on an outstretched arm. Dislocation in any direction is possible, but posterior movement of the forearm bones is most common. A dislocated elbow will commonly be held at a 45-degree angle and will often have a clear deformity on or around the olecranon process. In children, a partial dislocation called radial head subluxation is possible. This occurs when a child's arm is forcibly pulled while in the extended position, causing the radial head to slip underneath the annular ligament (part of the lateral ligament complex that stabilizes the radial head articulation with the ulna).

Elbow fractures most commonly involve the radial head or olecranon process. Radial head fractures account for a third of elbow fractures, and often result from falling on a partially flexed but outstretched arm. Symptoms include point tenderness on the radial head, pain with pronation and supination, decreased range of motion, and possibly swelling. Olecranon process fractures generally result from direct trauma to the posterior elbow, often from falling backward. Alternatively, and less commonly, the olecranon suffers a stress fracture from forceful triceps muscle contraction while the arm is flexed, as in throwing a baseball. Much less commonly, the humerus may be fractured. Fractures above the condyles are termed *supracondylar fractures*, and are most common in kids under the age of 10. Although rare, condylar fractures can also occur.

It is important to consider that dislocations or fractures of the elbow can lead to secondary injury of the nerves or vessels that traverse the elbow joint. This includes the brachial, radial, and ulnar arteries, and the radial, ulnar, and median nerves. These structures target the forearm and hand, and injuries can thus lead to downstream deficits in sensation, motor function, or blood supply. One such syndrome resulting from ulnar nerve compression is called cubital tunnel syndrome, and causes tingling and weakness in the hand. This discussion of elbow disorders is not comprehensive, and elbow pain or dysfunction can be caused by numerous other factors such as arthritis, infection, or cancer.

SEE ALSO: Arthritis; Bursitis; Fractures; Occupational Injuries; Osteoarthritis; Rheumatoid Arthritis; Sports Injuries; Wrist/Arm Injuries and Disorders.

BIBLIOGRAPHY. B. Morrey, *The Elbow and Its Disorders*, 3rd ed. (Saunders, 2000); M. Pecina and I. Bojanic, *Overuse Injuries of the Musculoskeletal System* (CRC Press, 1993); C. K. Stone and R. L. Humphries, *Current Emergency Diagnosis and Treatment*, 5th ed. (McGraw-Hill, 2004).

DAVID J. LUNARDINI
UNIVERSITY OF VIRGINIA

Elder Abuse

Elder abuse is any act or lack of appropriate act whose consequences are harm or distress to an elderly person. In the United States, it is estimated that each year 1 million elderly Americans are abused by their relatives, and with the aging of the population worldwide, elder abuse will naturally increase if not prevented. Abused seniors are at higher risk for depression and death compared to nonabused seniors.

There is currently enough evidence to affirm that elder abuse is a worldwide problem, and the various existing studies have found a surprisingly high incidence of it, ranging from 3 to 6 percent of people above 65 years of age being abused annually. That puts elder abuse in the present developmental agenda.

The perpetrators of elderly abuse are generally spouses or adult children, although they can be other family members and even informal or paid caregivers. While some behaviors are clearly abusive, the line that separates abuse from normal behavior may be tenuous. For example, people often cross this line when intending to control daily activities and schedules of their lucid but frail senior relative who could well decide upon his or her activities and maintain autonomy even if dependent on others to perform them. In that sense, caregivers for elderly persons who have chronic medical problems may not realize abusive behaviors or may be isolated enough to lose contact with other people and other caregivers, losing insight of what is normal. The harmful effects of caregiver burden are well studied and there are many options to relieve this burden, from services of care to the patients to services of care to the caregivers.

RISK FACTORS
There are known risk factors for elder abuse. For the victim, they include impairment (physical, functional, and cognitive impairments) and social isolation. On the abuser's side, they include substance abuse, psychiatric disorders, history of violence, stress, and dependence on the victim.

A very common example of abuse includes administering medication by force. Abandoning a dependent elder or leaving him or her unattended so as to endanger his or her life is also a very common form of abuse.

Approximately 60 percent of elder abuse is toward women, as is the majority of elder homicides, which suggests that domestic violence in old life may be a continuation of wife abuse in the past.

TYPES OF ELDER ABUSE
Elder abuse may be classified in neglect, for example, when a person is denied food, basic medication, heat,

clothing or comfort; rights abuse, when civil and constitutional rights of mentally capable elderly people are denied; financial, when the senior's property, money, or other valuables are used illegally or with no authorization of the elderly person; physical, as in direct physical aggression, restraining or providing wrong medication or dosage; psychological, such as shouting at an elderly person, humiliating or frightening him or her in any way; and sexual, for example, by forcing the elderly person to engage in any nonconsensual sexual activity.

One form of elder abuse must be stressed: doing any action or having the senior do any action that requires his or her consent in the case where the elderly person is not able to consent because of mental incapacity is to be considered elder abuse. It may fall into any of the above categories and can include transferring of power of attorney, changing heirs in one's will, transferring property, engaging in sexual activities, and so on.

DIAGNOSIS AND TREATMENT

Social isolation is commonly linked to elder abuse and can make the suspicion difficult, as abused elders tend to visit their health professionals less frequently, but also because the abuser often controls the victim's access to other people and it is estimated that only one in 14 cases are revealed. Professional unawareness and lack of specific training may contribute to that picture; but even though symptoms and signs of abuse may be confounded with disease, certain clinical situations are suggestive of elder abuse and may be recognized by the experienced health professional. This is important because the physician or other healthcare practitioner may be the only person other than the abuser that the victim may be able to have contact with, and the American Medical Association has published guidelines for the identification of elder abuse. Maintaining a high level of suspicion is also important for its detection.

The complexity of the situation makes a wide interdisciplinary approach essential, as is determining if the mistreatment was an isolated event or part of a chain of abusive actions. If the patient is mentally competent, he or she must be informed of the available options and decide what to do. If the patient is mentally incapable, then it is up to the healthcare team to decide what to do.

A nonabusing caregiver of a victim of abuse may also require assistance: the psychological hazards of

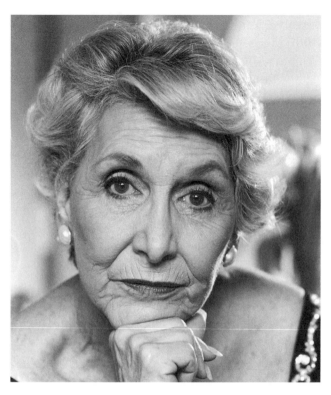

Studies have found an incidence of elder abuse ranging from 3 to 6 percent of people above 65 years of age annually being abused.

family violence are high, possibly constituting even a physical health menace in older caregivers.

Ideal treatment recognizes the multidimensionality of causes and consequences of elder abuse and, thus, the patient would be ideally treated by an interdisciplinary team, which may include physicians, nurses, social workers, psychologists and other therapists, lawyers, and law enforcement officials. Any previous failure should be investigated in order to improve any further intervention's chance of success.

ETHICAL DILEMMAS

Physicians and health workers worldwide are in general traditionally bound to keep secret the information gathered during their practices and respect the patient's right to decide if some information is disclosed to the public. The importance of elder abuse, however, has prompted the issuing of protective laws in different countries that compel anyone aware of elder abuse to notify a competent agency. Finally, in many countries, such agencies are still incipient and incapable of handling the problem to its real extent. This situation may put health workers in an ethical dilemma in cases where the abused senior does not want to turn the situation public: while the professional rules command them to respect those wishes, the law obliges them to report the abuse. Another problem in many countries is that the services for abused elderly people are very incipient and not enough for every case, and reporting the abuse may only cause the victims to loose access to the health service where the abuse was reported.

Elder abuse is an important public health issue; as the percentage of elderly within the populations increase all over the world, its incidence is expected to grow despite any effort already made to prevent it. While the incidence of elder abuse has varied between 3 to 6 percent a year on those above 65 years in different studies, the real picture may be even worse because many cases may not be reported at all. Elder abuse is often difficult to detect for many health professionals and may be perpetrated even without the intention of the aggressor to do so. If health professionals need continuous education for better detection of the problem, the entire society must discuss what solution to give to those cases already identified.

SEE ALSO: Child Abuse; Geriatrics.

BIBLIOGRAPHY. American Medical Association, *Diagnosis and Treatment Guidelines on Elder Abuse and Neglect* (American Medical Association, 1992); C. McCreadie, G. Bennett, and A. Tinker, "General Practitioners' Knowledge and Experience of the Abuse of Older People in the Community: Report of an Exploratory Research Study in the Inner London Borough of Tower Hamlets," *British Journal of General Practice* (v.48, 1998); K. Pillemer and D. Finkelhor, "The Prevalence of Elder Abuse: A Random Survey," *Gerontologist* (v.28, 1988).

THIAGO MONACO, M.D., PH.D.
UNIVERSITY OF SÃO PAULO MEDICAL SCHOOL, BRAZIL

Electromagnetic Fields

Electromagnetic fields (EMFs) are physical fields that are produced by electrically charged objects. Electric fields are produced by stationary charges and magnetic fields are created when electric current flows. These fields interact with close-by charged objects thus affect-

ing their condition. EMFs can be viewed as the combination of an electric field and a magnetic field and are defined by their frequency and wavelength. The frequency simply describes the number of oscillations or cycles per second, while the term *wavelength* describes the distance between one wave and the next.

Electromagnetic fields include static fields such as the Earth's magnetic field and fields from electrostatic charges, electric and magnetic fields from the electricity supply at power frequencies, and radio waves from television, radio and mobile phones, radar, and satellite communications.

It is important to separate two types of EMFs: Some electromagnetic waves carry so much energy that they have the ability to break bonds between molecules and these are called ionizing radiation. Fields whose energy is insufficient to break molecular bonds are called non-ionizing radiation and include visible light, infrared, and radio waves.

Due to the increase in the human use of technologies using EMFs, this is an area that has know an exponential growth, which has also lead to new complaints and concerns. One of the most common is connected with the association between power lines and cancer. Research results are still controversial, but some studies point to an increase in the numbers of early cancer in people living downwind of power lines. Although there is no certain explanation for this higher rate (some even believe it might be just a "statistical artifact"), one that has recently known more supporters has to do with "corona ion" effects. Researchers have proposed that the air immediately surrounding a high-voltage power line becomes ionized by the electric field, thus combining with pollutants in the air, giving rise to charged airborne particles. If inhaled by someone closely exposed, they may be deposited in the lungs and eventually develop cancer.

Other sources of electromagnetic fields that have spawned controversy are mobile phones. No conclusion has been reached when assessing whether the radiation arising from mobile phones and base stations is connected to disease.

Other common sources of EMFs are wireless solutions, which are being implemented throughout the environment. Its impact is still to be assessed.

On the account of this increase in exposure, a number of individuals have reported a variety of health problems that they relate to exposure to EMFs. This has been known as "electromagnetic hypersensitivity" and symptoms range from mild to severe, including skin redness, tingling, and burning sensations to fatigue, dizziness, nausea, heart palpitation, and digestive disturbances. The World Health Organization is currently conducting research to determine prevalence and ways to lower the impact of EMFs on those with this condition.

SEE ALSO: Childhood Cancers; Environmental Health; Leukemia; Radiation Exposure.

BIBLIOGRAPHY. BBC News, "Cancer Rise Linked to Power Lines," news.bbc.co.uk/2/hi/science/nature/933678.stm (cited September 2000); Independent Expert Group on Mobile Phones, "Stewart Report," www.iegmp.org.uk/ (cited May 2000); World Health Organization, "Electromagnetic Hypersensitivity," www.who.int/mediacentre (cited December 2005).

RICARDO MEXIA, M.D.
INDEPENDENT SCHOLAR

Electrophysiology

Electrophysiology is a study of the electrical properties that exist within biological cells and tissues, and this has developed to include the ability of these cells to react to electrical current. To do this, researchers have had to measure the change of voltage and also the flow of electric current covering a variety of scales, ranging from places such as the heart to single-ion channel proteins.

The origin of electrophysiology goes back to the research of the German, Emil Heinrich Du Bois-Reymond, from Berlin who, during his work at the University of Berlin, decided to concentrate on electrical activity in nerve and muscle fibers. His initial work was on fish and that they were capable of generating electrical currents on their own. From this, he turned to researching electrical conduction along muscle and nerve fibers which led him into work on electrical stimulation of muscles. His work on nerve and muscle stimulation led to the two-volume work *Untersuchungen über thierische Elektricität* (Researches on Animal Electricity), the first volume being published in 1848, and the second volume was not published until 1884. The books are still regarded as pioneers in the field of scientific electrophysiology. Du Bois-Reymond collaborated with Hermann von Helmholtz, Carl Ludwig, and Erich von Brücke; and his work was continued and developed by French physician Jacques-Arsène D'Arsonval from the University of Poitiers, Limoges, and Paris. D'Arsonval started to use electricity to treat skin and mucous membranes with his work being known as D'Arsonvalization.

Traditionally, electrophysiology has involved the placing of electrodes on various biological tissues. These electrodes may range from needles and discs, and then to printed circuit boards, and even hollow tubes such as glass pipettes filled with electrolytes. The last of these, if small enough, have been used to pass electricity to a single cell, although sometimes it is has been found that it is not necessary for the electrode tip to physically touch the cell. The biological tissues can also vary considerably, ranging from living organisms, excised tissue, cells removed from excised tissue, artificially grown cells or tissue, or hybrids of these preparations.

The main drawback of these traditional (or classical) practices has been that these techniques have only allowed electrophysiologists to observe the effect of an electrical current at a single point within the volume of the tissue. This has led to the development of optical electrophysiology with practitioners eager to overcome that drawback. This, in turn, resulted in work on a variety of related fields such as electroantennography (covering the olfactory receptors in arthropods), electrocardiography (for treatment of the heart), electroclography (for treatment of eyes), electrocorticography (for treating the cerebral cortex), electroculography (for treatment of the muscles), electroencephalography (for treatment of the brain), and electroretinography (for treatment of the retina of eyes).

Electrophysiology relies on the accuracy of intracellular recording whereby scientists measure the voltage or current which crosses the membrane of the cell being treated. Research in this field resulted in Alan Lloyd Hodgkin, Andrew Fielding Huxley, and Australian Sir John Carew Eccles winning the Nobel Prize in Physiology or Medicine in 1963. Their research was largely conducted on the Atlantic squid, *Loligo pealei*, using the voltage clamp technique. Huxley was later knighted for his services to science, as was Alan Hodgkin. In

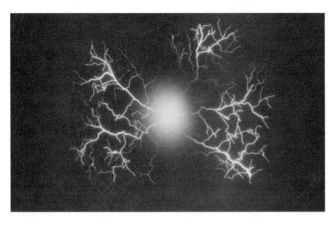

Electromagnetic fields include magnetic fields from the electricity supply at power frequencies, and radio waves.

1967, Finnish-born Swedish physiologist, Ragnar Arthur Granit, and Americans George Wald and Haldan K. Hartline won the Nobel Prize for their work on the internal electrical changes which take place when the eye is exposed to light, the work on the chemistry of vision and the neurophysiological mechanisms of vision, respectively. Further work on electrophysiology has helped with a greater understanding of it.

SEE ALSO: Electromagnetic Fields.

BIBLIOGRAPHY. John R. Heckenlively and Geoffrey B. Arden, eds., *Principles and Practice of Clinical Electrophysiology of Vision*, 2nd ed. (MIT Press, 2006); Lynn Snyder-Mackler, *Clinical Electrophysiology: Electrotherapy and Electrophysiologic Testing* (Williams & Wilkins, 1989); Natalie Virag, Olivier Blanc, and Lukas Kappenberger, *Computer Simulation and Experimental Assessment of Cardiac Electrophysiology* (Future Publishing, 2001).

JUSTIN CORFIELD
GEELONG GRAMMAR SCHOOL, AUSTRALIA

Emphysema

Emphysema is a chronic and irreversible lung condition which affects 4.7/100,000 persons in the United States. The primary cause of emphysema is tobacco smoking; other causes include chronic exposure to toxins and fumes. Some patients are more susceptible to the effects of tobacco smoking than others, suggesting a genetic predisposition to develop chronic obstructive pulmonary disease (COPD).

PHYSIOLOGY/PATHOPHYSIOLOGY

Emphysema is one of a group of conditions called COPD; these diseases obstruct airflow.

During inspiration, air enters the lungs through the trachea (windpipe) to reach air passages known as bronchi. Bronchi repetitively branch into progressively smaller and smaller branches (envision an upside-down tree, without the leaves) until finally reaching thin-walled structures called alveoli (tiny air sacks). The walls of the alveoli interface with the bloodstream (capillaries) where oxygen crosses over the alveolar-capillary membrane to enter the circulation. Oxygen is needed by all organs for normal function; when oxygen transfer ceases to occur, organs die.

In emphysema, destruction of the alveoli occurs through repetitive exposure to toxins such as tobacco smoking; stimulation of inflammation and the action of enzymes (e.g., elastase), cause destruction of the alveolar supporting structures. Without the supporting structures, the alveoli balloon out and oxygen is unable to cross over to enter the bloodstream. The net effect of this is low oxygen in the blood stream, called hypoxemia. Administration of supplemental oxygen can be successful early on in helping to overcome low oxygen levels in the bloodstream, but eventually, as emphysema progresses, this may not be adequate to allow for maintenance of life.

Alpha-1 antitrypsin deficiency is an inherited condition estimated to be responsible for only 1 to 2 percent of all cases of emphysema. These patients lack adequate amounts of the protein responsible for keeping an enzyme called elastase in check; left unchecked, elastase destroys healthy lung tissue. Alpha-1 antitrypsin is a protein produced by the liver; deficiency of this protein leads to development of emphysema and cirrhosis of the liver. Screening for alpha-1 antitrypsin should be undertaken in all patients with emphysema as recognition of genetic deficiency of this protein should cause the practitioner to carefully evaluate whether or not the patient should receive artificial supplementation.

In addition, development of pulmonary hypertension (elevated blood pressure in the pulmonary blood vessels) commonly develops in patients with emphysema. This is often irreversible and can be quite debilitating, leading to failure of the right side of the heart (also called cor pulmonale). This is a common cause of death in patients with emphysema.

SIGNS AND SYMPTOMS OF EMPHYSEMA

Signs and symptoms of emphysema include shortness of breath (also called dyspnea). Dyspnea is often initially noted only on exertion (i.e., walking, running) however, with progression, eventually will be present at rest. Coughing, with or without phlegm production are frequently noted, as is wheezing (a musical noise sounding similar to a deflating accordion, noted on exhalation). Because patients with emphysema are predisposed to recurrent infections in the lungs, the first time a patient is diagnosed with emphysema may be following development of a chest infection.

DIAGNOSIS

Diagnosis of emphysema begins with suspicion. Emphysema is traditionally diagnosed by the performance of pulmonary function testing (also called spirometry or PFTs). Spirometry is the first test performed and confirmation of the results of spirometry is required; in such cases, patients are typically referred to pulmonary function laboratories for additional testing including lung volumes.

Emphysema causes reduced lung function and in particular, air trapping. As opposed to asthma, which, during an acute exacerbation, also leads to typically temporary air trapping, the air trapping associated with emphysema is very much less likely, and typically does not, substantially resolve with bronchodilators.

Bronchodilator challenge is performed when evidence of airway obstruction is noted on PFTs. Patients with asthma will typically demonstrate at least a 12 percent improvement in one or both parameters (FEV1 [forced expiratory volume in 1 second] and FVC [forced vital capacity]), whereas the great majority of patients with emphysema will not substantially improve with bronchodilator therapy. Patients with emphysema will also demonstrate an elevated residual volume (consistent with air trapping) and a reduced diffusion capacity for carbon monoxide (DLCO).

All patients with emphysema should be evaluated for hypoxemia; this includes performance of either an arterial blood gas or oximetry at rest and with exertion. When discovered, hypoxemia must be treated with oxygen supplementation as this is the only treatment shown to reduce mortality in emphysema.

Patients with emphysema may require oxygen supplementation only with exertion. Patients with emphysema who plan to travel by airline or visit areas of high altitude, should consult with their physicians, as oxygen supplementation may be required during those periods, even if the patient has no documented need for oxygen supplementation otherwise. All patients with emphysema should undergo screening for alpha-1 antitrypsin, particularly when there is a family history of emphysema, or emphysema is diagnosed at an early age. The test for alpha-1 antitrypsin deficiency is a blood test; abnormal results should be confirmed by repeat testing.

Chest X-rays performed in patients with emphysema, particularly advanced emphysema, typically demonstrate air trapping (enlarged lungs), and may show the presence of blebs. Other tests sometimes done in emphysema patients include computed tomography (CT) scans, and arterial blood gas (done to check for low oxygen levels).

TREATMENT

All patients with emphysema or at risk for emphysema, and who smoke should be aggressively counseled and assisted with smoking cessation programs. The most effective programs are those that are multidisciplinary including use of counseling along with nicotine supplementation (in the form of gum, nasal sprays, patches, or tablets). Few patients who quit "cold turkey" (sudden discontinuation of smoking without behavioral or pharmacologic intervention) will be successful long term.

The mainstay of therapy of existing emphysema is the use of bronchodilators. Evidence-based treatment guidelines such as the GOLD guidelines provide a guide for the treatment of emphysema and include information for both patients and care providers. These guidelines were developed by the World Health Organization in collaboration with world experts in COPD and are updated frequently.

Patients who are documented to have severe deficiency of alpha-1 antitrypsin should be evaluated for administration of supplementation. This therapy is costly and benefits versus risk and cost must be considered. Surgical intervention for very severe emphysema may include lung volume reduction surgery (where stapling and removal of large, non-functional portions of the lung is undertaken) and lung transplantation. Both of these interventions are associated with increased morbidity (complications) and mortality (death) compared to medical therapy. Patients being considered for either of these therapeutic interventions should be evaluated by a recognized center of excellence.

SEE ALSO: Chronic Obstructive Pulmonary Disease (COPD);.

BIBLIOGRAPHY. Centers for Disease Control and Prevention, www.cdc.gov/nchs/fastats/emphsema.tm (cited July 2007); *Emphysema—A Medical Dictionary, Bibliography, and Annotated Research Guide to Internet References* (ICON Health Publications, 2004).

Sandra K. Willsie, D.O., FACOI, FACP, FCCP
Kansas City Uiversity of Medicine
and Biosciences

Empiric Risk

Empiric risk refers to the chance that a particular event or disease will occur in a person, family, or population, based on experience or observation (*empeira* = experience), as opposed to predicting risk based on theoretical considerations or conjecture.

For example, the empiric risk can be calculated for relatives of inflammatory bowel diseases (IBDs) sufferers based on observed population statistics. Among Ashkenazi Jews, the age-corrected empiric risk estimates for IBDs are 8.9 percent to offspring, 8.8 percent to siblings, and 3.5 percent to parents. These estimates can be used for both genetic counseling and genetic modeling. Empiric risk can also be expressed as a risk ratio. For example, first-degree relatives of prostate carcinoma patients have a summary recurrence risk ratio of 2.53.

The concept of empiric risk is used to investigate multifactorial traits and events such as cancer. The empiric risk is not calculated but is an observed population statistic used to predict recurrence of a multifactorial trait in a family. The empiric risk increases with severity of the trait, the number of affected relatives, their sex, and degree of relatedness to the affected individual.

SEE ALSO: Genetic Testing/Counseling.

BIBLIOGRAPHY. M. P. Roth, et al., A Familial Empiric Risk Estimates of Inflammatory Bowel Disease in Ashkenazi Jews," *Gastroenterology* (v.96/4, 1989).

Barry Pakes, M.D., M.P.H.
University of Toronto

Employment Retirement Income Security Act (ERISA)

Passed in 1974, the Employee Retirement Income Security Act (ERISA) is a federal law that sets minimum standards for most voluntarily established pension and health plans in private industry to provide protection for individuals in these plans. It requires plan administrators—the people who run plans—to give plan participants in writing the most important facts they need to know about their retirement and health benefit plans including plan rules, financial information, and documents on the operation and management of the plan. Some of these facts must be provided to participants regularly and automatically by the plan administrator. Others are available upon request.

One of the most important documents participants automatically receive when becoming a participant of an ERISA-covered retirement or health benefit plan or a beneficiary receiving benefits under such a plan, is a summary of the plan, called the summary plan description (SPD). The summary plan description gives participants details with regard to what their plan provides and how it operates, such as the manner in which benefits are calculated, when benefits become vested, and how claims are filed. In addition to the summary plan description, the plan administrator must automatically give participants a copy of the plan's summary annual report each year. This is a summary of the annual financial report that most plans must file with the Department of Labor. The summary annual report is available at no cost. To learn more about the plan assets, participants may ask the plan administrator for a copy of the annual report in its entirety.

There have been a number of amendments to ERISA, expanding the protections available to health benefit participants and beneficiaries. One important amendment, the Consolidated Omnibus Budget Reconciliation Act (COBRA), gives workers and their families who lose their health benefits the right to choose to continue group health benefits provided by their group health plan for limited periods of time under certain circumstances such as voluntary or involuntary job loss, reduction in the hours worked, transition between jobs, death, divorce, and other life events. Qualified individuals may be required to pay the entire premium for coverage up to 102 percent of the cost to the plan. COBRA generally requires that group health plans sponsored by employers with 20 or more employees in the prior year offer employees and their families the opportunity for a temporary extension of health coverage (called continuation coverage) in certain instances where coverage under the plan would otherwise end.

COBRA outlines how employees and family members may elect continuation coverage. It also requires employers and plans to provide notice. Another amendment to ERISA is the Health Insurance Portability and Accountability Act (HIPAA), which provides rights and protections for participants and beneficiaries in group health plans. HIPAA includes protections for coverage under group health plans that limit exclusions for preexisting conditions; prohibit discrimination against employees and dependents based on their health status; and allow a special opportunity to enroll in a new plan to individuals in certain circumstances. HIPAA may also gives individuals the right to purchase individual coverage if they have no group health plan coverage available, and have exhausted COBRA or other continuation coverage.

SEE ALSO: Health Insurance Portability and Accountability Act (HIPAA); Health Maintenance Organization (HMO).

BIBLIOGRAPHY. Melody A. Carlsen, "Will COBRA Begin to Strike Employers Again?," *National Underwriter Property & Casualty-Risk & Benefits Management* (March 30, 1992); Hinda R. Chaikind, et al., eds., *The Health Insurance Portability and Accountability Act (HIPAA): Overview and Analyses* (Novinka Books, 2004); United States Department of Labor, www.dol.gov. (cited October 2006).

BEN WYNNE, PH.D
GAINESVILLE STATE COLLEGE

Endemic

The term *endemic* should be defined according the context, an endemic plant or animal means that they are native or restricted to a specific geographic area. Whereas, in an epidemiological context it is defined as the continuous presence of a disease in a specific geographical area or population with relatively low to moderate level of prevalence and incidence compared to other areas or populations, without exhibiting extreme fluctuations over time. It may also indicate that the infection can persist in that area or population for a long period of time without the need of being reintroduced from an external source. The definition of hyperendemic is similar to that of endemic but the prevalence or incidence rates are persistently high.

Endemic diseases are present all over the globe. Some are old diseases such as malaria and measles, and others are newly discovered such as HIV/AIDS or re-emerging (e.g. multidrug resistant tuberculosis). Although the historical roots of the term *endemic* was related mostly to communicable diseases, some noncommunicable diseases fall under the category of endemic disease. A good example of these is endemic goiter that occurs among populations of communities with iodine-depleted soil.

Endemic diseases may lead to severe effects on populations and countries suffering from such diseases. The range of effects includes various aspects such as the economic and social aspects and is not limited to the medical aspects and human suffering. Malaria, for example, is an endemic disease in large areas of the African continent. In addition to 300 million acute cases taking place globally every year, resulting in more than a million deaths, of which 90 percent occur in Africa. The economic cost is estimated to be above $12 billion of lost Gross Domestic Product (GDP) of African countries.

Another disease which is endemic in some African regions is HIV/AIDS which had devastating effects on the social fabric of some communities where the levels of HIV/AIDS related mortality was so high among adults leaving many children without parents to provide required care for them. This phenomenon was called the AIDS orphans. In 2005, it was estimated that the number of orphans because of AIDS in South Africa was 1,200,000, while in Zimbabwe 77 percent of the number of orphans in the same year was because of AIDS. In the sub-Saharan Africa it is predicted that there will be 15.7 million AIDS orphans by the year 2010.

The above-mentioned information testifies to the need for directing efforts toward controlling and preventing endemic diseases. The first step in that direction is to establish an efficient surveillance system that provides the needed information for monitoring the trends of disease occurrence including endemic diseases. This will give public health professionals information about the levels of endemic diseases and whether the endemicity is stable or fluctuating. It will also be helpful in detecting epidemics where the occurrence of a certain disease in a community or population group becomes clearly in excess of expected levels.

A disease can be endemic in one place and epidemic in another. A classical example of that is smallpox in the early 17th century. While, smallpox was endemic among children in Europe, it caused a devastating epidemic in 1633 among indigenous Indians living at the Massachusetts Bay killing all the population in some plantations.

With the recent advances in the fields of technology, communication and transport (traveling) the whole notion of endemic diseases should be readdressed. Infections and infectious agents do not know borders and can move quickly from one place to another. An infectious agent can arrive from a continent to another in a matter of hours. The recent bird's flu and SARS epidemics are clear proofs of that fact. Some diseases such as HIV/AIDS became endemic in almost the entire globe. This shows the need for global cooperation in the field of disease control and prevention.

SEE ALSO: Epidemiology; Epidemic.

BIBLIOGRAPHY. AVERT, "AIDS Orphans" www.avert.org (cited December, 2006); Centers for Disease Control and Prevention, "Protecting the Nation's Health in an Era of Globalization: CDC's Global Infectious Disease Strategy," www.cdc.gov/globalidplan (cited December, 2006) Leon Gordis, *Epidemiology* (W.B. Saunders, 2004); John Last, *A Dictionary of Epidemiology* (Oxford University Press, 2000); Roll Back Malaria- World Health Organization, "Malaria in Africa," www.rbm.who.int (cited December 2006).

ABDULLATIF HUSSEINI
BIRZEIT UNIVERSITY-PALESTINE

Endocrine Diseases (General)

Endocrine diseases are those that affect the human endocrine system which are the group of ductless glands used to regulate the human body processes by secreting chemical substances called hormones, which are then carried to a number of specific target organs and tissues by the bloodstream. The diseases or disorders result in too much hormone secretion or too little hormones being secreted, or from problems within the body which prevent the hormone to be used effectively.

From the early 20th century, medical researchers have been involved in cataloging the various endocrine diseases and other disorders of the endocrine system. The first of these was disorders of the adrenal system. These include problems with adrenal insufficiency such as Addison's disease, congenital adrenal hyperplasia (sometimes called adrenogenital syndrome), and mineralocorticoid deficiency. Other adrenal problems include Conn's syndrome, Cushing's syndrome, pheochromocytoma, and adrenal-cortical carcinoma.

Another range of problems with the endocrine system can be categorized as glucose homeostasis disorders, such as diabetes mellitus, and hypoglycemia, which include idiopathic hypoglycemia and insulinoma. Metabolic bone diseases include osteoporosis, osteitis deformans (sometimes called Paget's disease of bone), and rickets and osteomalacia.

There were also a large number of pituitary gland disorders such as diabetes insipidus, hypopituitarism (and panhypopituitarism), and pituitary tumors. The last includes pituitary adenomas, prolactinoma (and hyperprolactinoma), acromegaly, and Cushing's disease. Other disorders include those affecting the parathyroid gland and the thyroid gland: hyperparathyroidism, pseudohyperparathyroidism primary hyperparathyroidism, secondary hyperparathyroidism, and tertiary hyperparathyroidism—some connected with Graves-Bassedow disease.

The other endocrine diseases involve sex hormones, including disorders of sexual development, and intersex disorders, such as hermaphroditism, gonadal dysgensis, and androgen insensitivity syndromes; hypogonadism such as gonadotropin deficiency, Kallman syndrome, Klinefelter syndrome, ovarian failure, testicular failure, and Turner syndrome.

The earliest evidence of medical practitioners becoming aware of the endocrine system was the Chinese, who, as early as 3000 B.C.E. started diagnosing some endocrinologic disorders and working out some effective treatments. One of the most obvious of these disorders was goiter which involved an enlargement of the thyroid gland, which rapidly becomes noticeable on sufferers. It was discovered that eating seaweed could help reduce the problem, but it was not until the 19th century that it was found that the cause was iodine deficiency and the cure was effective as seaweed was rich in iodine.

The creation of eunuchs in the ancient world in Egypt, China, and elsewhere led to direct endocrinologic intervention, although this was not realized at the time. In Europe from the Middle Ages until as late as the 18th century, some boys were castrated to preserve their treble voices for singing in cathedral choirs. It was, curiously, the system of castration that led to some early surgeons to begin to study the endocrine system, even though it did not have that name at the time. A Scottish surgeon and anatomist, John Hunter, practicing in London, managed to successfully transplant the testis (testicle) of a rooster into the abdomen of a hen.

His work was followed by that of French physiologist and neurologist Charles-Édouard Brown-Séquard, who concluded that he believed the testicles contained a substance that had rejuvenation properties. In 1889, he injected himself with fluid from the testicles of freshly killed dogs and guinea pigs, to which he had added water. His work helped pioneer the studies of endocrinology, and hence helped others start work on describing, then diagnosing endocrine diseases. The work of the French physiologist Claude Bernard came up with the concept of humans—and, indeed, other living organisms—having what he described as the *milieu intérieur* (internal environment). This led to Walter Bradford Cannon, the American physiologist, using the homeostasis for the first time.

SEE ALSO: Endocrinology.

BIBLIOGRAPHY. J. E. Griffin and S. R. Ojeda, *Textbook of Endocrine Physiology* (Oxford University Press, 2000); V. C. Medvei, *A History of Endocrinology* (MTP Press, 1982).

JUSTIN CORFIELD
GEELONG GRAMMAR SCHOOL, AUSTRALIA

Endocrinology

Endocrinology is a branch of medicine that deals with the disorders of the endocrine system and also deals with specific secretions called hormones. This involves disorders such as diabetes mellitus, hyperthyroidism, and other similar problems.

The origins of endocrinology come from the discovery that all multicellular organisms need to have a system to regulate and integrate the functioning of cells. To do this, especially in higher animals, the nervous system and the endocrine system are both used. For the latter, the body releases, usually into the blood, chemical agents that are essential for the proper development and function of organisms. This was first realized by some thinkers of the classical world such as the Greeks, Aristotle and Hippocrates, and the Romans, Lucretius, Celsus, and Galen. However, these tended to emphasize the influence of "humors," and it was not until the 19th century that pathologists and others came up with a more detailed knowledge of the endocrine system. As a result, the branch of medicine known as endocrinology was developed whereby doctors and medical researchers deal with biosynthesis, storage, body chemistry, and the physiological function of hormones and with the cells of the endocrine glands and also tissues that secrete hormones into the glands.

The development of research into endocrinology has seen researchers being involved in the diagnostic evaluation of a large number of symptoms and variations that occur between different people, and tabulate these to work out a long-term management of disorders which come from either a deficiency or an excess of a particular hormone. The most common field in which endocrinologists are involved is that of treating people with diabetes mellitus, first in diagnosing the presence of the disorder and then working out the most suitable way that people can manage it.

An early French endocrinologist was Antoine Lacassagne who studied under Marie Curie, and worked heavily with radium. However, the study of it on a scientific level began with Arnold Adolph Berthold in the 1840s, and was developed by Charles Edouard Brown-Séquard. The pioneer of endocrinology in the United States was Harvey Williams Cushing (eponym of Cushing's syndrome) who was involved in the removal of a portion of the anterior lobe of the pituitary, being shown to be a successful way of treating acromegaly. In

1916, P. E. Smith and Bennet Allen reported separately about the fact that pituitary surgery could result in a diminished growth rate and reduce the function of the thyroid gland. As interest in endocrinology mounted, it was decided to form what became the Endocrine Society. It was founded on June 4, 1917, as the Association for the Study of Internal Secretions. The certificate of incorporation was filed on January 13, 1918, and the society gained its present name on January 1, 1952. It has held annual meetings since 1916 (with the exception of 1943 and 1945), and has published *Endocrinology* since January 1917. It has also published the *Journal of Clinical Endocrinology*, which predates the society, having published its first issue in 1914. On January 1, 1952, it became *The Journal of Clinical Endocrinology and Metabolism.*

There are currently between 7,000 and 8,000 endocrinologists in the United States, and these include Edwin B. Astwood who introduced the use of thiouracil in the treatment of thyrotoxicosis; Gerald Auerbach who isolated the parathyroid hormone; Paul Bell who elucidated the molecular weight of ACTH; Drs. A.H. Hersch and E. C. Kendall who treated rheumatoid arthritis with cortisone; and pioneers R. D. Evans, S. Hertz, A. Roberts, and J. G. Hamilton who worked with radioactive iodine. Other endocrinologists include Solomon A. Berson and Rosalyn S. Yalow who introduced the technique of radioimmunossay; Franciszek Kokot; Zvi Laron; Stafford Lightman; and Bernhard Zondek, a pioneer of reproductive endocrinology. Some recent endocrinologists have been involved in research that has massively helped other fields of medicine with Elwood V. Jensen, president of the Endocrine Society from 1980–81, winning the 1980 Charles F. Kettering Prize of the General Motors Cancer Foundation for his work on "discovering the steroid receptor protein present in certain mammary cancers and for developing a method for determining which breast cancers were hormonally sensitive and thereby responsive to endocrine therapy."

SEE ALSO: Endocrine Diseases (General).

BIBLIOGRAPHY. Endocrine Society, www.endo-society.org; J. E. Griffin and S. R. Ojeda, *Textbook of Endocrine Physiology* (Oxford University Press, 2000); V. C. Medvei, *A History of Endocrinology* (MTP Press, 1982); J. D. Wilson, "Charles-Edouard Brown-Séquard and the Centennial of Endocrinology," *Journal of Clinical Endocrinology and Metabolism* (v.71, 1984).

JUSTIN CORFIELD
GEELONG GRAMMAR SCHOOL, AUSTRALIA

Engram

Especially throughout the 20th century, philosophers, psychologists, and neurologists have tended to fiercely disagree about whether the brain and mind are modular and functions are localized (as in the caricature of 19th-century phrenologists) or whether it is more uniform and acts more globally, with its functions diffusely represented.

One contested aspect of brain function is memory: When one has a new memory, what changes in the brain? Where does the memory "go" in the brain? The engram (or "trace") is the putative particular brain locus for memories. Based on the failure of his own lesion studies to find any such entity, the American neuropsychologist Karl Lashley, in his famous 1950 essay, "In Search of the Engram," sides against localization and concludes that the engram is represented broadly throughout the brain.

One alternative explanation we may consider is that this difficulty in locating memories in the brain exists because memories are encoded in an immaterial mind and therefore would not alter the brain at all. This Cartesian dualistic notion is easily refuted by examples of patients who have changes in memory functioning by physical damage to their brains, or by the example of (physical) drugs that are given and subsequently alter the ability of a person to form or retrieve memories.

Modern scientific methods have allowed a more nuanced position than the either/or of the Lashley era and the dualism pervasive since Descartes, or possibly even earlier via the 11th century Islamic philosopher Ibn Sina. In contrast, the 2000 Nobel Prize in Medicine was given partially to Eric Kandel for his work demonstrating the molecular mechanisms of memory storage at neuronal synapses. These basic learning mechanisms seem to, in fact, be conserved among all animals. Further evidence that memories are created, stored, and retrieved by the actions of functionally differentiated brain regions was provided by the increasing evidence from the neuropsychology clinic. The famous patient H. M. had his medial temporal lobes removed (most importantly, his hippocampus) and subsequently could no longer form new long-term declarative memories. Additional evidence has shown that procedural memories (e.g., learning how to throw a curveball) are created and stored in a manner separate from declarative memories (e.g., remembering a phone number).

With the advance of modern cellular, molecular, and recombinant genetic methods of neurological research, the debate has somewhat resolved. Memory seems to have both definitive aspects of functional localization as well as diffuse representation: certain cortical and subcortical areas are absolutely crucial for nonpathological memory functioning, and yet many diffuse projections and interconnections exist between memory and other relevant brain regions.

SEE ALSO: Memory; Neuroscience; Psychology.

BIBLIOGRAPHY. Darryl Bruce, "Fifty Years since Lashley's 'In Search of the Engram': Refutations and Conjectures," *Journal of the History of the Neurosciences* (v.10/3, 2001); A. Casadio, et al., "A Transient Neuron-Wide Form of CREB-Mediated Long-Term Facilitation Can Be Stabilized at Specific Synapses by Local Protein Synthesis," *Cell* (v.99, 1999); Karl Lashley, "In Search of the Engram," in *Society of Experimental Biology Symposium No. 4: Physiological Mechanisms in Animal Behaviour* (Cambridge University Press, 1950); W. B. Scoville and B. Milner, "Loss of Recent Memory after Bilateral Hippocampal Lesions," *Journal of Neurology, Neurosurgery and Psychiatry* (v.20, 1957).

OMAR SULTAN HAQUE
HARVARD MEDICAL SCHOOL

Environmental Health

Environmental health is the subfield of public health that is concerned with assessing and controlling the impacts of people on their environment (including vegetation, other animals, and natural and historic landmarks) and the impacts of the environment on them. The environment is a vital tool that has been used by human beings for centuries. The environment has provided food, shelter, and energy, but because of industrialization, technology has been drawing from and consuming more resources, causing adverse effects not only to the environment but also to people.

Environmental pollution affects the people around it by contaminating the air and water with foreign material, causing widespread disease. Manmade chemicals used in the environment can infect the human body through inhaling pollutants in the air or drinking the one found in the water. Not only can the chemicals have long-standing effects on the individual exposed to them, but they can also have hereditary effects on the progeny of that person. Many herbicides have caused irreversible damage to the environment and the surrounding people (the most notable example of this is Agent Orange, which was developed by the United States and used in Vietnam). Every human being on the planet depends on the environment, so when it becomes contaminated, the environment has the potential to cause disease among people. Awareness of the effects people have on the environment is the most important factor in dealing with pollution because the best way to prevent the spread of disease through pollution is to eliminate its source.

Herbicides are created to kill certain kinds of plants (mostly weeds) and are typically used by farmers. The chemicals in these herbicides are toxic to humans, so adequate warning is often provided when an area is to be sprayed to avoid human exposure to it. However, in some instances, a warning is not given. During the Vietnam War, the U.S. government developed an herbicide designed to destroy the foliage used by the Vietcong to hide the movement of their troops and set up ambushes. The herbicide was code named Agent Orange after the orange stripe on the barrels containing the herbicide. Although Agent Orange fulfilled its objective by destroying the plant life, the damage it caused has taken decades to recover from and will take many more. Furthermore, it has affected the soldiers and Vietnamese by causing several different health effects. People exposed to Agent Orange had a higher chance to contract liver problems, chances of cancer, and immune system disorders. Also, birth defects were more prevalent in children born from Vietnam veterans who were exposed to Agent Orange.

Contamination of a water supply is dangerous because it spreads rapidly and affects every person in the area. In 2005, residents of New Delhi, India, dealt with a cholera contamination in the water supply. A survey of water samples in 15 resettlement colonies and slums in the capital by Hazard Centre, a technical consultancy firm, revealed that 90 percent of those were contaminated. In the developing countries, the fact that human excreta often mix with drinking water supplies plays a central role in public health. Water quality is an important facet of the environment and must be a constant concern in the minds of humanity. Without taking the appropriate measures to cleanse water supplies, especially those used for drinking and bathing purposes, diseases such as cholera will continue to infect the world. In addition to its existence from sources such as human excreta, water pollution comes from waste water discharges from factories. Two plants located on the Xinqiang River, a drinking water source for central China's Hunan Province, were accused of discharging waste water directly into the tributary; the arsenide content of the waste water was more than 1,000 times higher the national average.

Air pollution shares the same dilemma as water pollution, because once started, the pollution spreads quickly and is almost impossible to contain. The Gansu Province of China had dealt with a severe lead poisoning incident. Residents of Xinsi and Mouba villages were poisoned by a lead smelting plant that continued to operate in summer 2006 after being told to cease production but has since been demolished.

In an effort to eliminate air pollution, the U. S. Environmental Protection Agency banned the use of lead in gasoline. Lead poisoning affects children in a much harsher manner than adults. The chance of full recovery is lesser for children than for adults. Adults usually recover from mildly elevated levels, but children can suffer permanent impairment of their intelligence. People who survive severe toxic lead levels are likely to suffer some permanent brain damage.

The health of the people is directly related to the health of the environment. Because pollution affects the air we needed to breathe and the water we needed to drink, people must be aware of the condition of the environment. It is because of this dependency on the environment that humanity must be conscious of environment's status to prevent pollution before it starts. As long as people depend on the environment, its deteriorating condition due to the pollutants from automobiles and factories will continue to affect the health of the people. Even the herbicides created for agricultural or military means can cause people to be poisoned, the effects of which may be passed down to the progeny in the form of ailments and diseases. The environment provides many resources vital to people. However, in an effort to extract these resources the environment can become contaminated, which in turn contaminates the people. This cycle must end before the environment is completely destroyed and humanity is left with no more resources and widespread disease.

SEE ALSO: Environmental Protection Agency (EPA); Lead Poisoning; Pollution.

BIBLIOGRAPHY. L. Hodges, *Environmental Pollution* (Holt, Rinehart and Winston, 1977); L. Hui, "250 Kids Hospitalized in Gansu after Lead Poisoning," news.xinhuanet. com/(cited December 6, 2006); N. Khanna, "Water Contamination: Cholera Cases on the Rise," http://www.ndtv. com/ (cited December 6, 2006); D. W. Moeller, *Environmental Health* (Harvard University Press, 1992); L. Vancil, "Agent Orange," www.vvvc.org cited October 16, 2006).

DeMond Shondell Miller
Joel C. Yelin
Rowan University

Environmental Medicine

A new biomedical science related to the study of short-, but also, long-term effects of environmental factors (physical, biological, and chemical) on human health. Although the concept and general application of environmental medicine is certainly older and well known, its vision was only focused to environmental health. In the past, this discipline, indeed, only dealt with solving of existing environmental problems at urban or rural ecosystems that could lead to problems in public health (e.g., contamination of rivers, lakes, wetlands, and other water sources). Currently, this concept is wider. Environmental medicine currently encompasses a plethora of preventive aspects, even considering the importance of the environmental health surveillance. This emergent discipline originated due to the growing number of links between environmental factors and human diseases. Environmental medicine is also called clinical ecology. Adverse effects of the environment on human health have become a major issue throughout the world during the last several decades. This issue is influenced not only by such events as Love Canal, Seveso, and Chernobyl, but also by recognition of the harmful effects of industrial emissions and, for example, worldwide waste problems. In most developed countries with established healthcare systems, environmental medicine has evolved as a special area with sources in the public health sector (environmental hygiene) and also in the individual care for patients with health problems linked to adverse environmental conditions.

Currently, environmental medicine is closely related to different biomedical and environmental sciences such as public health, epidemiology, environmental epidemiology, toxicology, ecology, ecoepidemiology, ecogenetics, global health, tropical medicine, medical geography, medical geology, wilderness medicine, agricultural medicine biometeorology, medical demography, and occupational medicine, among others.

A new important concept was introduced in this field few years ago: the concept of primary environmental care, related in its essence to the methodical principles of the primary healthcare, but in this case oriented to the environment, in which a person is interacting. Primary environmental care is a strategy of environmental action, basically preventive and participative at the local level, that recognizes the right of the human being to live in a healthy and proper environment and to be informed about the risks of the environment for the health, well-being and survival, but at the same time defining responsibilities and duties in regard to the protection, conservation, and recovery of the environment and the health.

With this concept, it is important to add that environmental medicine is also related to public education about the interaction between humans and their environment, as well as to promote optimal health through prevention and effective treatment of the causes of illness.

Other visions and concepts are currently in development; the model of environmental medicine is based on the growing appreciation that the human body is constantly coping with its dynamic environment by means of a number of inherited, built-in, complexly interacting, and usually reversible biologic mechanisms and systems. These systems are designed to maintain overall homeostatic mechanisms among all biological mechanisms. Their ongoing adjustments are unique to the individual and change continually over time.

In the terminology emerged from the environmental medicine science, adverse consequences that result when interactions among biological functions are compromised by external or internal stressors are called the environmentally triggered illnesses. The stressors may range from severe acute exposure to a single stressor, to cumulative relatively low-grade exposures to many stressors over time. The resultant dysfunction is dependent on the patient's genetic makeup, his or her nutrition and health in general, the stressors, the degree of exposure to them, and the effects of seven fundamental biological governing principles: biochemical individuality, individual susceptibility, the total load, the level of adaptation, the bipolarity of responses, the spreading phenomenon, and the switch phenomenon.

The environment could be considered in a broader sense today. The task of this science is related to the study of the health risks posed by contaminants and other factors at home, in the workplace, and in the ambient environment. Although incipient yet, some authors consider that this will also include the aerospace as an environment where a person could suffer diseases and generate conditions for human illnesses (which will be in relation to the aerospatial medicine).

In the current scenario of global change, environmental medicine is today more important than yesterday; and jointly with occupational medicine, this new specialty is encouraged to be strategic rather than tactical to optimize its value in the core business of industry-related medical needs. Because employers, governments, and workers bear major costs, they have a strategic interest in outcomes. Strategic opportunities exist for reduction of the impact of occupational injury and disease; stewardship of the environment, product, and process; the reduction of nonoccupational healthcare costs; for having occupational and environmental health and safety follow best business practices and be prominent in the leadership of change; for optimizing human relations/labor policies and practices; and for meeting regulatory requirements. The strategic position of the specialty can be strengthened through discussion, dialogue and vision development, role definition, establishment and use of performance indicators, improved career structures and training, and a proactive approach to qualify initiatives, research, marketing, and development of strategic alliances.

In the study of environmental medicine, one of the oldest and more important disciplines contributing substantially to the knowledge of this science is the toxicology. Chemical compounds ubiquitous in our food, air, and water are now found in every person. The bioaccumulation of these compounds in some individuals can lead to a variety of metabolic and systemic dysfunctions, and in some cases outright disease states. The systems most affected by these xenobiotic compounds include the immune, neurological, and endocrine systems. Toxicity in these systems can lead to immune dysfunction, autoimmunity, asthma, allergies, cancers, cognitive deficit, mood changes, neurological illnesses, changes in libido, reproductive dysfunction, and glucose dysregulation. Chemicals and their effects on these systems should be reviewed inside the frame of environmental medicine. Additionally, a focus on therapeutic regimens to combat the toxic effects of these and other compounds need also to be considered. Chemicals known as solvents are part of a broad class of chemicals called volatile organic compounds. These compounds are used in a variety of settings, are ubiquitous, and off-gas readily into the atmosphere. As a result of their overuse, they can be found in detectable level in virtually all samples of both indoor and outdoor air. Certain of these compounds are detectable in adipose samples of all U.S. residents. Once in the body, they can lead to a variety of neurological, immunological, endocrinological, genitourinary, and hematopoietic problems. Some individuals also have metabolic defects that diminish the liver's clearing capacity for these compounds. Supplementation may be of benefit to help clear these compounds from the body and to prevent adverse health effects.

EXTERNAL CONTAMINANTS

Other important aspect that deserves to be studied in the field of environmental medicine is the problem with pesticides. Although the use of pesticides has doubled every 10 years since 1945, pest damage to crops is more prevalent now than it was then. Many pests are now pesticide resistant due to the ubiquitous presence of pesticides in our environment. Chlorinated pesticide residues are present in the air, soil, and water, with a concomitant presence in humans. Organophosphate and carbamate pesticides—the compounds comprising the bulk of current pesticide use—are carried around the globe on air currents. Municipalities, schools, churches, business offices, apartment buildings, grocery stores, and homeowners use pesticides on a regular basis. Pesticides are neurotoxins that can cause acute symptoms as well as chronic effects from repeated low-dose exposure. These compounds can also adversely affect the immune system, causing cell-mediated immune deficiency, allergy, and autoimmune states. Certain cancers are also associated with pesticide exposure. Multiple endocrine effects, which can alter reproduction and stress-handling capacity, can also be found. Limited testing is available to assess the toxic overload of these compounds, including serum pesticide levels and immune system parameters. Treatment for acute or chronic effects of these toxins includes avoidance, supplementation, and possibly cleansing.

In spite of this, new contributions of recent medical advances have been introduced in the artillery of research tools for environmental medicine, particularly those related to geographical sciences and to molecular biology disciplines. A revolution in biology and medicine is taking place as a direct consequence of rapid developments in the field of molecular biology. The tremendous advances in our knowledge of basic molecular genetics and cell biology have opened the door for new methods of diagnosis, assessment of individual susceptibility to disease, and elucidation of the pathogenesis of disease. These advances will have a profound impact on the practice of occupational and environmental medicine. The core value guiding the work of physicians and health workers, including those in environmental and occupational epidemiology and medicine and injury prevention, is to protect the health of the public, especially its most vulnerable individuals. In these fields, we emphasize teaching the use of epidemiology, the core discipline of public health, as a tool for early detection and prevention of disease and injury, as well as an instrument for hypothesis testing. The classic core topics are toxic and physical exposures and their effects, and strategies for their prevention; emerging issues are child labor, mass violence, and democide. In environmental health, students need to be prepared for the reality that the most important and severe problems are often the most difficult to investigate, solve, and evaluate. The following are some recommendations for producing graduates who are effective in protecting communities from environmental hazards and risks: 1.) Teach the precautionary principle and its application; 2.) Evaluate programs for teaching environmental and occupational health, medicine, and epidemiology in schools of public health by their impact on the World Health Organization (WHO) (http://www.who.int/) health indicators and their impact on measures of ecosystem sustainability; 3.) Develop problem-oriented projects and give academic credit for projects with definable public health impact and redefine the role of the health officer as the chief resident for Schools of Public Health and Community Medicine; 4.) Teach the abuses of child labor and working conditions of women in the workplace and how to prevent the hazards and risks from the more common types of child work; 5.) Upgrade teaching of injury prevention and prevention of deaths from external causes; 6.) Teach students to recognize the insensitivity of epidemiology as a tool for early detection of true risk; 7.) Teach the importance of context in the use of tests of statistical significance; 8.) Teach the epidemiologic importance of short latency periods from high exposures as sentinel events for later group risk for cancer and stating the case for action; 9.) Protect students and colleagues who are whistle-blowers in environmental health from harassment and punishment; 10.) Develop curricula and workshops that promote the use of epidemiologic tools for preventing genocide, democide, and their precursors. Schools of Public Health and Community Medicine are at the interface between the resources of academic power and the major problems of community health. Implementing the above recommendations will strengthen academic investigation and impact.

SEE ALSO: Environmental Health; Environmental Protection Agency (EPA); Environmental Toxicology; Epidemiology; Toxicology.

BIBLIOGRAPHY. Gordon Cook and Alimuddin Zulma, *Manson's Tropical Diseases* (Saunders, 2003); Walter J. Crinnion, "Environmental Medicine, Part One: The Human Burden of Environmental Toxins and Their Common Health Effects," *Alternative Medicine Review* (v.5/1, 2000); Walter J. Crinnion, "Environmental Medicine, Part Two: Health Effects of and Protection from Ubiquitous Airborne Solvent Exposure," *Alternative Medicine Review* (v.5/2, 2000); Walter J. Crinnion, "Environmental Medicine, Part Three: Long-Term Effects of Chronic Low-Dose Mercury Exposure," *Alternative Medicine Review* (v.5/3, 2000); Walter J. Crinnion, "Environmental Medicine, Part 4: Pesticides—Biologically Persistent and Ubiquitous Toxins," *Alternative Medicine Review* (v.5/5, 2000); J. J. Krop, "Clinical Ecology and Its Role in Diagnosis of Chronic Diseases Caused by Environmental Pollution. Indoor Air Pollution as a Major Factor," *Folia Medica Cracoviensia* (v.34/1–4, 1993); R. K. McLellan, "Clinical Ecology," *Journal of the American Medical Association* (v.269/13, 1993); A. J. McMichael, et al., *Climate Change and Human Health: Risks and Responses* (WHO/WMO/UNEP, 2003).

ALFONSO J. RODRIGUEZ-MORALES, M.D., M.Sc.
UNIVERSIDAD DE LOS ANDES, VENEZUELA
CARLOS FRANCO-PAREDES, M.D., M.P.H.
EMORY UNIVERSITY

Environmental Protection Agency (EPA)

The United States Environmental Protection Agency (EPA) is responsible for protecting the public health of Americans and for safeguarding the environment. EPA activities are frequently carried out in conjunction with state, local, and tribal governments. Major EPA efforts include guaranteeing that air is safe and healthy throughout the country; that drinking water is clean and safe to drink; that rivers, lakes, wetlands, aquifers, and coastal and ocean waters are protected; that foods are free of unsafe pesticide residues; and that wastes are stored, treated, and disposed of safely and in accordance with the natural environment. Furthermore, EPA is charged with reducing environmental risks from climate change, stratospheric ozone depletion, and other threats to a healthy global environment.

EPA national headquarters is located in the Ariel Rios Building, 1200 Pennsylvania Avenue, NW, Washington, D.C. 20460. In addition to several other offices headquartered in the capital, the Environmental Science Center is located in Forte Meade, Maryland.

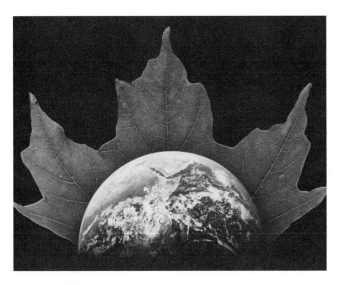

The EPA works to reduce environmental risks from climate change, and other threats to a healthy global environment.

General information on EPA may be accessed by telephone at (202) 272-0167 and through the 10 regional offices. Detailed information is available on the EPA Web site (http://www.epa.gov/), which also provides a listing for various telephone hot line numbers (http://www.epa.gov/epahome/hotline.htm). EPA libraries distributed throughout the country have traditionally served as valuable resources for information on the environment and the agency; however, the future of these libraries is in jeopardy due to proposed cuts by the George W. Bush administration.

The EPA was created in 1970 in response to rising concern about environmental issues. Today, the Agency employs around 18,000 individuals in various offices and laboratories. Over half of those employees are engineers, scientists, and policy analysts. Other professionals include specialists in legal matters, public affairs, financial planning, information management, and computer technology. The remaining employees make up the EPA's support team. The EPA also maintains Research Triangle Park (RTP) in North Carolina where research is conducted on various pollutants and how humans react to them. Programs instituted under the Clean Air Act are encompassed in RTP, which also houses the EPA National Computer Center. Other EPA research facilities are located throughout the country, including Montgomery, Alabama; Denver, Colorado; Athens, Georgia; Las Vegas, Nevada; Narragansett, Rhode Island;

Gulf Breeze, Florida; Duluth, Minnesota; Corvallis, Oregon; Cincinnati, Ohio; Ada, Oklahoma; Edison, New Jersey; and Ann Arbor, Michigan.

The administrator of the EPA, who is appointed by the president of the United States, is responsible for leading the agency in fulfilling its mission. The following EPA offices make up the Office of the Administrator: Administrative Law Judges, Children's Health Protection, Civil Rights, Congressional and Intergovernmental Relations, Cooperative Environmental Management, the Environmental Appeals Board, Environmental Education, the Executive Secretariat, Executive Services, Homeland Security, Policy Economics, and Innovation, Public Affairs, the Science Advisory Board, and Small and Disadvantaged Business Utilization.

Other offices that answer to the administrator include the Office of Administration and Resources Management, which is responsible for managing EPA's human, financial, and physical resources; the Office of Air and Radiation, which carries out air and radiation protection activities; American Indian Environmental Office, which works with tribal leaders to enhance environmental efforts among the native population; the chief financial officer, who has the responsibility for managing and coordinating budget, analysis, and accountability within EPA; the Office of Enforcement and Compliance Assurance, which focuses on community pollution prevention; the Office of Environmental Justice, which protects predominately minority communities and low-income populations; and the Office of Environmental Information, which focuses on innovative ways to use information to promote EPA mission.

Additional offices that come under the direction of the administrator are the History Office, which archives materials and provides relevant information to the public; the Office of General Counsel, which houses the EPA legal team; the Office of Inspector General, which audits and investigates EPA programs; the Office of International Affairs, which serves as a liaison between the United States and the international community; the Office of Prevention, Pesticides, and Toxic Substances, which is responsible for the control of toxins and alerting the public about potential risks; the Office of Waste and Emergency Response, which oversees waste management and disposal and manages the Superfund Program created to fund cleanup of toxic waste sites; and the Office of Water, which regulates the quality of drinking water and provides oversight for all other water sources. The deputy administrator chairs the Science Policy Council, which liaises with the media, other federal programs, and researchers involved in cross-disciplinary issues that affect environmental policy.

The EPA's strategic goals include promoting clean air and global climate change, ensuring that water remains clean and safe, land preservation and restoration, producing healthy communities and ecosystems, and improving compliance and environmental stewardship. The EPA's research activities are carried out under the Office of Research and Development, which partners with academicians involved in environmental research through research grants and fellowships. These research programs focus on a variety of topics crucial to a healthy environment. The Environmental Monitoring and Assessment Program (EMAP) monitors and analyzes trends in ecological research. The Lake Michigan Mass Balance Study, carried out through the Great Lakes National Program Office, involves the study of toxic chemicals found in Lake Michigan and records observations of how those toxins interact with the large-scale ecosystem of the lake. The EPA is also involved in the research of such agencies as the Human Exposure Research Division of the National Exposure Research Laboratory, the National Center for Environmental Assessment, the National Center for Environmental Economics, the National Center for Environmental Research, the National Environmental Scientific Computing Center, and the Office of Science and Technology of the Office of Water.

SEE ALSO: Drinking Water; Pollution.

BIBLIOGRAPHY. Mark Allen Eisner, *Governing the Environment: The Transformation of Environmental Regulation* (Lynne Rienner, 2007); Environmental Protection Agency, www.epa.gov; *Major Management Challenges and Risk: Environmental Protection Agency* (Government Accounting Office, 2003); Brent M. Haglund and Thomas Still, *Hands-On Environmentalism* (Encounter, 2005); Daniel E. Harmon, *The Environmental Protection Agency* (Chelsea House, 2002); Kenneth J. Meier and Laurence J. O'Toole Jr., *Bureaucracy in a Democratic State: A Government Perspective* (Johns Hopkins University Press, 2006); Robert Repetto, ed., *Punctuated Equilibrium and the Dynamics of U.S. Environmental Policy* (Yale University Press, 2006); Dennis D. Riley, et al., *Bureaucracy and the Policy Process: Keeping the Promises* (Rowman & Littlefield, 2006).

ELIZABETH R. PURDY, PH.D.
INDEPENDENT SCHOLAR

Environmental Tobacco Smoke

Environmental tobacco smoke (ETS, also known as secondhand smoke or involuntary or passive smoking) is a worldwide phenomenon affecting people in all countries and communities. It has been linked to multiple health effects in both children and adults. Policies requiring smoke-free environments are the most effective measure of decreasing ETS exposure.

ETS is a mixture of the smoke released from the burning end of a cigarette, pipe, or cigar (sidestream smoke) and the smoke exhaled by smokers (mainstream smoke). It contains over 4,000 chemicals, of which over 40 substances are known to be cancer causing (carcinogenic). In 1992, the U. S. Environmental Protection Agency (EPA) classified ETS as a group A carcinogen, based on evidence linking it as the cause of over 3,000 lung cancer deaths in humans each year.

According to a report by the U. S. Department of Health and Human Services in 2006, more than 126 million nonsmoking Americans are exposed to secondhand smoke in their daily lives, both at home and work. Children are even more exposed to passive smoking than adults. Nearly 30 percent of U. S. children in the age group 3–11 years are exposed to ETS. About 25 percent of children live with at least one smoker, in contrast to only about 7 percent of nonsmoking adults. Although there has been a decline in the exposure to ETS in the United States over time, passive smoking continues to be a common and preventable public health hazard worldwide.

There are several significant short-term effects of exposure to ETS. Tobacco smoke is a known allergen, causing exacerbation of symptoms in both allergy sufferers and asthmatics. Even in those without any known allergies, compared to when breathing smoke-free air, nonsmokers may experience multiple symptoms in the presence of smoke, such as cough, headache, nausea, and fatigue. Even though these short-term effects terminate immediately after exposure, repeated exposure is believed to cause many significant long-term effects.

There is comprehensive scientific evidence linking ETS to multiple long-term health effects in both adults and children. Nonsmokers who live with a smoker increase their risk of developing lung cancer by 20 to 30 percent. In addition, through the exposure of ETS in the workplace, a nonsmoker has a 16 to 19 percent increased risk of developing lung cancer. Secondhand smoke reduces the lung function of nonsmokers and causes irritation to the lining of the lungs, leading to coughing, excess phlegm, and chest discomfort. It can also irritate the eye, nose, and throat. In addition, daily exposure to ETS increases the risk of developing heart disease by 25 to 30 percent in nonsmokers.

With their developing lungs, higher breathing rates than adults, and lack of control over their indoor environments, children are particularly vulnerable to the effects of secondhand smoke. Children exposed to ETS are at an increased risk for sudden infant death syndrome (SIDS), acute respiratory infections, ear problems, and more severe asthma. Newborns, whose mother smoked while pregnant or who were exposed to secondhand smoke after birth, develop weaker lungs than unexposed infants.

According to EPA reports, in children younger than 18 months, ETS exposure causes between 150,000 and 300,000 lower respiratory tract infections (including pneumonia and bronchitis), leading to 7,500 to 15,000 hospitalizations each year. Passive smoking also causes a buildup of fluid in the middle ear of the exposed child, resulting in numerous middle ear infections. Asthmatic children who are exposed to secondhand smoke are especially at risk. The EPA estimates that the number, severity, and frequency of asthma exacerbations increases significantly with exposure, affecting between 200,000 to 1 million children annually. In nonasthmatic children exposed to ETS, there is an increased risk of developing lung disease.

As a result of the clear scientific evidence of the effect of ETS on nonsmokers, in 2003, the World Health Organization (WHO) passed a resolution encouraging all countries to implement smoke-free policies in workplaces and indoor public buildings. The WHO recognizes that every person has the right to breathe air free of tobacco smoke. Several studies have indicated that there is no risk-free level of exposure to secondhand smoke. Completely eliminating smoking in indoor areas has been shown to fully protect nonsmokers from exposure to ETS. Simply separating smokers from nonsmokers, cleaning the air, or ventilating buildings cannot effectively eradicate the effects of passive smoking. As such, several countries (including Sweden and Ireland) and many parts of the United States (including the states of Florida, California, Ohio, and New York) have passed smoking bans, regulating smoking in public areas. Even though it is largely disputed by the hospitality industry, these bans have not been shown to have an impact on restaurant or bar revenues.

There have been several disputes from the tobacco industry criticizing the validity of the research showing a link between ETS and health effects. However, a review of this research found that the only factor affecting the results was the presence of funding from the tobacco industry.

SEE ALSO: Environmental Toxicology; Smokeless Tobacco; Smoking and Youth; Smoking Cessation.

BIBLIOGRAPHY. California Environmental Protection Agency's Office of Environmental Health Hazard Assessment, "Health Effects of Exposure to Environmental Tobacco Smoke," www.oehha.ca.gov (cited February 2007); U. S. Department of Health and Human Services, "The Health Consequences of Involuntary Exposure to Tobacco Smoke: A Report of the Surgeon General," www.cdc.gov/tobacco/sgr (cited February 2007).

SHANNON GEARHART, M.D.
INDIANA UNIVERSITY SCHOOL OF MEDICINE

Environmental Toxicology

Environmental toxicology refers to the poisoning of the environment either accidentally or deliberately, leading to the term *ecotoxicology* being coined by R. Truhart in 1969. The idea of poisoning an environment dates back to the ancient world with the much-highlighted story of the Romans sowing salt over the fields of their defeated enemy Carthage following the destruction of that city in 146 B.C.E. The salinity was to ensure that no crops would grow there, but historians now doubt that the Romans would have done this, owing to the vast cost of salt in the ancient world and the fact that Carthage was refounded as a Roman city soon afterward. However, there remains the possibility that the Romans might have used seawater to destroy some of the fertile fields around Carthage.

Biological warfare has been considered early during the 20th century; however, the concept goes back to medieval and early modern times when there were attempts to pass the bubonic plague to enemies, especially in Renaissance Italy. There were also instances of the poisoning of waterholes by American and Australian settlers to kill indigenous people in their respective countries. The destruction of their food supplies, such as the killing of the vast bison herds which provided much food for the Native Americans, and the kangaroos in the case of the Australian aboriginals, are further examples of environmental destruction. During the Vietnam War, the use of Agent Orange and other defoliants with the specific aim of destroying rainforests where Vietcong guerrillas were hiding, is the most widespread recent use of poisons to deliberately destroy entire ecosystems.

However, the concept of environmental toxicology in the modern era largely came from *Silent Spring* by Rachel Carson. The book was published in 1962 despite attempts by pesticide companies to prevent its publication. Carson highlighted the accidental side effects from the use of toxins, especially DDT, and fertilizers, which were used by farmers and had the result of killing large amounts of wildlife. She concentrated on researching the side effects from these, which some felt might have led to higher levels of cancer in humans. First alerted to the threat of DDT by a bird sanctuary in Massachusetts whose wildlife had been killed by DDT from an aerial spraying of crops nearby, Carson was able to show that pollutants used in one area could quickly affect another neighboring area, and the destruction of a particular part of the food chain upsets the "balance of nature" and can quickly lead to the destruction of an ecosystem. Chemical companies felt that Carson's work unfairly attacked their products and a few tried to pressure the publisher to stop the book coming out.

Since Carson's book, work by people such as Dr. R. Truhart led to the establishment of the field of eco-toxicology which has been defined as the branch of toxicology which is concerned with the study of the toxic effects, caused either by natural or synthetic pollutants, to the constituents of ecosystems, animals and humans, vegetables and microbial life.

This has focused attention on industrial pollution and discharge from the mines, both deliberate and accidental. The result has been seen near many gold mines where there has been widespread use of cyanide, which has led to the poisoning of the environment, including the water table. The effects have become noticeable around some mines such as those at Kalgoorlie in Western Australia. There had also been much pollution at the Panguna Copper Mine in Bougainville, leading to the local people, including some workers at the plant, to stage a revolt and eventually take control of the island to close down the mine.

Environmental toxicology has also came about from accidents, the largest of which were clearly during the nuclear accident at Chernobyl and the chemical gas poisoning from the Union Carbide factory at Bhopal, the former resulting in a very high level of cancer in Ukraine and also neighboring areas, with large parts of the agricultural heart of the former Soviet Union being made uninhabitable; and the latter in the deaths of about 3,000 people on the night of December 3, 1984, and with injuries sustained by as many as 50,000 more.

There have also been other accidents that have poisoned entire ecosystems such as the running aground of the Exxon Valdez on Prince William Sound, Gulf of Alaska, on March 24, 1989, and accidents by many other oil tankers which have resulted in massive oil slicks killing fauna and flora, and contaminating the shoreline. This also took place following the deliberate discharge of oil into the Persian Gulf by Iraqis in Kuwait just prior to the start of fighting between the United States and the Iraqis in the Gulf War of 1991. Other environmental toxicology has come from the dumping, deliberately or accidentally, of medical and nuclear waste around the world.

SEE ALSO: Environmental Health; Environmental Medicine; Environmental Protection Agency (EPA).

BIBLIOGRAPHY. Rachel Carson, *Silent Spring* (Houghton Mifflin, 1962); Inge F. Goldstein and Martin Goldstein, *How Much Risk? A Guide to Understanding Environmental*

Health Hazards (Oxford University Press, 2001); Lester B. Love, *Toxic Chemicals, Health and the Environment* (Johns Hopkins University Press, 1987).

JUSTIN CORFIELD
GEELONG GRAMMAR SCHOOL, AUSTRALIA

Enzyme-Linked Immunosorbent Assay (ELISA)

Enzyme-linked immunosorbent assay (ELISA) is a biochemical procedure that is used in scientific research and as a clinical tool. The basis of this technique is the ability of antibodies to bind specifically to their cognate antigens. ELISA is quite sensitive and specific, as well as relatively inexpensive, and therefore, is useful as a preliminary diagnostic tool. It is widely utilized in human immunodeficiency virus (HIV) testing and similar applications.

During ELISA, an antibody is mixed with the antigen it recognizes, creating antibody–antigen complexes. A second antibody is then added that binds to these complexes—via either the antigen or the antibody component. This second antibody is coupled to an enzyme. When the enzyme's substrate (the substance it modifies) is added, the enzyme will convert it into a light-releasing product. The result of the ELISA is that the presence of the original antigen–antibody complexes is detected as a fluorescent signal.

ELISA is utilized to evaluate the presence of an antigen in a sample, or conversely, to detect the presence of an antibody. In the first case, an antibody specific for the antigen is used to coat a surface, and sample possibly containing the antigen is added. In the second case, the surface is coated with the antigen and the sample to be tested for the presence of antibody is added. In either scenario, an enzyme-linked secondary antibody is then used to detect the formation of antigen–antibody complexes.

USE OF ELISA IN HIV TESTING

The first step in HIV testing is usually an ELISA. When an individual becomes infected with HIV, the immune system will attack the virus and produce antibodies specific for viral components. Rather than testing directly for HIV proteins, the ELISA tests for these anti-HIV antibodies. The assay is performed as follows: first, HIV viral proteins are coated on a surface (usually a plastic 96-well plate). Then, serum from a patient is added to the well. Excess serum is washed away and a second, enzyme-linked antibody is added that recognizes the anti-HIV antibodies. Excess antibody is washed away, and the enzyme's substrate is added. If this results in a sufficiently strong fluorescent signal, the person is most likely infected with HIV. If there is little or no signal, the individual does not have anti-HIV antibodies.

CAVEATS OF ELISA

According to the U.S. National Institute of Allergy and Infectious Diseases (NIAID), ELISA is reliable nearly 99.9 percent of the time. However, this means that the assay will give an incorrect result—either false-positive or false-negative—for approximately 1 in every 1,000 individuals tested. False-positives occur when an individual is not infected with HIV but his or her serum contains antibodies that cross-react with components of the HIV antigen mixture. False-negatives usually occur when an individual becomes infected with HIV a short time before the test, and his or her immune system has not yet produced antibodies against HIV.

Because of the shortcomings of ELISAs, it is important to be tested periodically and to confirm positive results by ELISA retesting and by performing more specific and reliable assays such as a Western blot or polymerase chain reaction (PCR).

SEE ALSO: AIDS; Immune System and Disorders; Immunology; Polymerase Chain Reaction (PCR).

BIBLIOGRAPHY. U.S. National Institute of Allergy and Infectious Diseases, "Tests for HIV Infection," http://www.niaid.nih.gov/dir/labs/lir/hiv/packet1.htm (cited March 1999).

KEVIN SHENDEROV
NEW YORK UNIVERSITY

Epidemic

A sudden and great increase of new disease cases in a given human population from a common source. This can also understood as an increase in incidence of a disease in a given population. Incidence is the number of new disease cases or patients found or diagnosed over a given period of time. The Greek translation is understood as: *epi-* "upon" and *demos* or people. The rise in new cases with the disease is faster than what is to be expected in that given population from what is currently known about the disease and about the population. If the outbreak of disease affects the whole world it is refereed to as a pandemic: *pan-* all and *demos-* people. This is an important concept in global health as epidemics have decimated populations with malaria, tuberculosis, and many other communicable diseases. In a globalizing world, epidemics spread fast and efficiently from country to country and region to region devastating populations and quality of life.

An outbreak refers to an increase in disease quickly to a small village or town whereas epidemic is an increase in disease for a specific region in the world or nation. Epidemics involve infectious disease and are detrimental to the communities they affect. Epidemics affect the health and well-being of millions throughout the developing world each year and many are preventable disease that can be avoided with simple measures such as vaccines, hygiene education, and public awareness.

TYPES OF EPIDEMICS

Epidemics are classified based on origin and pattern of transmission of disease. Epidemics can involve a single exposure to a disease or pathogen, multiple, or continuous exposures to disease causing agents. The disease involved in an epidemic can be transmitted by a vector (disease carrying agent) like a rat that carries bubonic plague, from person to person transmission (lack of hand washing or cramped living conditions), or from a common source such as contaminated water or food source.

For example, a common water supply with cholera caused an epidemic in London in the middle of the 19th century. Many London citizens had uncontrollable diarrhea and other symptoms that used this water source. However, concluding the water source as the main point of transmission of disease was not so easy. To combat this epidemic, a large-scale epidemiological study was performed by a medical pioneer in this field, Dr. John Snow. His systematic methods used to study outbreaks and epidemics are the basis for epidemiological study used today.

Epidemics such as influenza, cholera (mentioned above), malaria, tuberculosis and most recently avian influenza virus, or bird flu, have inflicted millions across the globe. These diseases are preventable and their infection rate increases in the developing world with too few treatment measures. It is important to realize that not just the region or area that has the epidemic is affected—the whole world population feels ripple effects of these epidemics in a myriad of ways. These recent epidemics are able to move quickly transmitting from person to person in smaller communities and then moving across the globe passing socioeconomic barriers and inadequate treatment measures. For example, the affects of HIV/AIDS has graduated from epidemic to pandemic as new cases are growing and no population or community are immune. Indeed, everyone is negatively affected across the globe with this pandemic—medically, socially, economically, living standards, and in many other unforeseeable ways—HIV/AIDS affects everyone. However, the regions hardest hit with HIV/AIDS are sub-Saharan Africa, central Asia, and Latin America.

Epidemics can spread and become pandemics as seen with HIV/AIDS. However, epidemics are usually contained to a specific community or geographical region as the incidence rises over time. For example, the bubonic plague or "Black Death" swept across the European continent by rats and more patients were getting the disease than any one city or area could adequately deal with—causing more disease to spread. This concept is arguably more recently observed with how bird flu has traveled across the globe on a much smaller scale inflicting less people but with lethality. The concept of globalization and easy connection of many people through trade, travel and the effects of war (forced migration and displacement), common markets, and mass transportation further enable transmission of disease across regions. This is epidemic in the 21st century.

Sudden and major environmental changes can easily give rise to epidemics where populations are not suited to deal with such change and are resource poor (i.e., developing nations such as sub-Saharan Africa, the Middle East, Asia, and South America). One such example is malaria. There have been many spikes of malaria throughout the world in recent history and most centralized in Africa in the second half of the 20th century.

THE MALARIA EPIDEMIC

Malaria has affected millions throughout human history. Prevention and treatment of malaria are readily known and not readily available to those regions that need it most. Various factors have prevented the public health community from eradicating the disease altogether. Environmental changes in weather and climate, irrigation and man-made standing waters where mosquitoes may breed, and people living in closer proximity to one another all enable the disease to infect many populations fast and efficiently. Furthermore, evolutionary changes in the malaria microbe and in mosquitoes, malarias vector, and human behavior toward the disease have all contributed to the durability of this epidemic.

Malaria is a tropical parasitic disease that infects between 300 to 500 million people and kills nearly 3 million people annually. Furthermore, there has been an increase in multidrug-resistant parasitic strains that conventional medicine cannot treat. As a disease, malaria is transmitted through a mosquito bite that carries the parasite. If the disease is quickly diagnosed and properly treated, malaria is curable. Most countries that have the largest risk to contract malaria lack the resource to quickly diagnose or treat it—hence, the ongoing epidemic with a preventable and treatable disease.

EPIDEMIC AND EPIDEMIOLOGY

Epidemiology is the study of disease across populations and tries to conclude on disease as it will affect many people. This is different than clinical medicine where the individual is the focus of study and not a population or community. An epidemic affects populations and communities with disease and oftentimes an epidemiologist aids in the investigation and work to curb the spreading disease—like Dr. John Snow mentioned above in this entry. The epidemiologist will study the disease by looking at the physical and social environments where disease occurs. For example, malaria in Africa and government resource to combat epidemics and the lack of access the given country may have to disease prevention, quick diagnosis and effective treatment. Epidemiology involves all of this study material.

Many doctors, nurses, and public health workers across the globe apply epidemiologic principles to better understand and prevent epidemics. The Centers for Disease Control and Prevention (CDC) is a U.S. federally funded agency that attacks epidemics globally. The CDC, based in Atlanta, Georgia, currently monitors the world for emergence of disease and epidemics. The CDC looks for health risks and promotes the prevention and treatment of global health risks and epidemics. Currently, the CDC is working with many other governments to curb epidemics and prevent further illness. Epidemics will never be eradicated from the health experience, but they can be caught quickly, treated, and prevented from future human suffering.

SEE ALSO: AIDS; Bird Flu; Centers for Disease Control and Prevention (CDC); Cholera; Endemic; Epidemiologist; Epidemiology; Incidence; Malaria; Malariology.

BIBLIOGRAPHY. Rob Desalle, *Epidemic! The World of Infectious Disease*, (Norton, 1999); K. Kemm, Roger Bate and Lorraine Mooney, eds., *Malaria and the DDT Story–Third World Problems–First World Preoccupations, Chapter 1* (Butterworth Heinemann, 1999); Sheldon Watts, *Epidemics and History: Disease, Power, and Imperialism* (Yale University Press, 1999).

JOHN MICHAEL QUINN V, M.P.H.
UNIVERSITY OF ILLINOIS AT CHICAGO

Epidemiologist

An epidemiologist is someone who studies diseases in populations in order to attribute factors that may be associated with a specific disease or a set of diseases with the end goal of finding methods of prevention and/or harm reduction. Epidemiologists may collect and analyze data attributed to an outcome of interest or use previously collected data, such as hospital records, in order to achieve their goals. Epidemiologists also play an instrumental role in designing observational and experimental studies involving human beings.

One of the most cited pioneers in the field of epidemiology was an English physician in the 1850s named John Snow. During his time, the overall belief among the medical community was that cholera was transmitted through miasma, a concept that was usually described as "bad humors." During a cholera epidemic in London in 1853, he observed that cases tended to

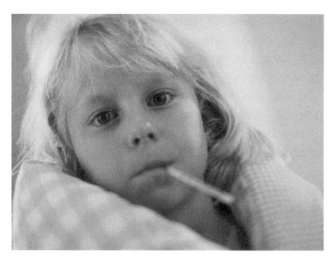

Epidemics such as influenza, cholera, malaria, tuberculosis have inflicted millions across the globe.

losophy (PhD). The most common places to employ epidemiologists are governmental health departments, academic and research institutions, as well as private corporations such as pharmaceutical companies.

SEE ALSO: Epidemiology.

BIBLIOGRAPHY. Dana Asher, *Epidemiologists: Life Tracking Deadly Diseases* (Rosen Publishing Group, 2003); Viet Thanh Nguyen, et al., *Cholera, Chloroform, and the Science of Medicine: A Life of John Snow* (Oxford University Press, 2003).

JOSE S. LOZADA
CASE WESTERN RESERVE UNIVERSITY

be clustered. He eventually recorded cases on a map and concluded that most cases of cholera had used the same water pump on Broad Street as their main water source. In a somewhat maverick approach, he removed the pump's handle and observed an overall reduction in the number of new cases of cholera. His findings were first rejected by the medical community but eventually received recognition for his findings.

Some other famous epidemiologists are Richard Doll, Austin Hill, Robert Frost, and Jonathan Lister. Dr. Doll and Dr. Hill were instrumental in linking the dangers of cigarette smoking and risks for lung cancer. Dr. Frost was well known for his work in tuberculosis as well as founding the first epidemiology program in the United States. Dr. Lister is renowned both for his work with infection transmission and control as well as for Listerine®, the antiseptic mouthwash. In more recent times, individuals who have aided in the evolution and education of the field include Leon Gordis, Kenneth Rothman, Sander Greenland, Robert Elston, James Robins, and David Kleinbaum.

Epidemiology began as a specialty within the medical profession, but epidemiologists are now trained independently of medical training in postgraduate programs, either in schools of public health or schools of medicine. The most common degrees awarded to individuals who wish to train in epidemiologic theory and practices are a master's of science or master's of health sciences (MS, MHS), master's in public health (MPH), a doctor of public health (DrPH), and a doctor of phi-

Epidemiology

In the strictest sense, epidemiology is the study of epidemics. However, a broader definition is accepted today—epidemiology is the branch of medicine that specializes in studying the causes of disease, its distribution, and ways of controlling its spread in populations. Following its origins in the early 1800s, epidemiology has evolved through distinctive eras. These are characterized by its initial focus on sanitary conditions, then infectious diseases, and after World War II, heightened focus on chronic diseases. Epidemiological research has traditionally been quantitative and concerned with the incidence and prevalence of disease. Epidemiology has been criticized for focusing too narrowly on individual-level risk factors at the expense of political, economic, and social factors that underlie patterns of morbidity and mortality. The discipline may be entering a new era, characterized by multilevel research projects which incorporate molecular, individual, and societal levels of analysis.

THE DEVELOPMENT OF EPIDEMIOLOGY

The work of John Snow in 1854 shaped the development of epidemiology. Working to understand an outbreak of cholera in the Soho district of London, Snow mapped the geographical location of victims and investigated what they may have had in common. One factor was that they were drinking water that originated in a common and contaminated pump. Snow closed the pump and was able to contribute toward stopping the epidemic. Importantly, he achieved this without knowledge of the bacterial mechanisms underlying the disease, and his methods influenced subsequent epidemiological research. This marked the first era of epidemiology, wherein sanitary conditions were the primary focus of research. This was followed by an infectious disease era (late 19th century to mid-20th century) and the development of germ theory. After World War II and coinciding with the growing prevalence of chronic diseases, epidemiological research increasingly focused on individual-level risk factors and "healthy lifestyles." This era was marked by an increasing acceptance of a "web of causality" model, in which no single causal agent would be expected to explain patterns of disease. In contrast, epidemiological research often operated within a "black box" paradigm, where associations could be theorized and investigated as causal without an understanding of biological mechanisms. This was a strength of epidemiology, for it could expand its research into areas not yet studied by other branches of science. However, it was also an important weakness, and criticisms have been made that associations without plausible underlying biological mechanisms do little to advance knowledge of public health concerns and may lead to false-positive (spurious) findings.

THE TOOLS OF EPIDEMIOLOGY

In practice, epidemiology is a very diverse field, and it is practiced by social scientists, physicians, demographers, biologists, and a wide range of other specialists in both the social and natural sciences. The central concept in epidemiology is a case, which can denote an episode of a disorder or illness, or an event, such as death. Epidemiologists study rates of incidence, or the number of new cases during a specific period of time, as well as rates of prevalence, or the total number of cases in a given period of time. Prevalence is often reported as a measure of point prevalence (at a specific point in time, such as a day), period prevalence (during a specific period of time, such as a year), and lifetime prevalence (reflecting the number of people expected to have a particular disorder at least once in their lifetime). Central to the work of epidemiologists is also the notion of a rate. This can be a crude rate, reflecting the number of cases per population, for example, infant mortality per 1,000 live births. Adjusted rates are also used to examine the effects of specific variables or social characteristics, for example, age-adjusted mortality rates.

THE CRITIQUE OF EPIDEMIOLOGY

A focus on identifying individual-level risk factors has led to a criticism of epidemiology for neglecting the political, economic, and social factors that underlie patterns of disease. For example, the growing literature on the social determinants of health suggests that in order to better understand the fundamental causes of disease, researchers need to expand their theoretical models of causality to not only include individual-level risk factors, but also include large-scale social factors such as income inequality. An even more radical critique has developed from political economy, which suggests that researchers need to examine a society's system of commodity production and distribution. From this perspective, health, like income inequality, is a consequence of macroeconomic forces governed by the structure of the economic system.

CHALLENGES AND OPPORTUNITIES

A key challenge for epidemiology is to sustain a sense of coherence in light of increasing specialization; indeed, in recent decades, myriad branches of the discipline have developed, including pharmacoepidemiology, social epidemiology, genetic epidemiology, and molecular epidemiology. A successful integration of these subdisciplines, and awareness that, increasingly, health issues are global issues, may signal a new paradigm, which Mervyn Susser and Ezra Susser have labeled "eco-epidemiology." This era would be characterized by a multilevel approach to the study of disease, wherein advances at the molecular, individual, and societal levels of study would be integrated.

SEE ALSO: Disease and Poverty; Epidemiologist; Medical Geography.

BIBLIOGRAPHY. Nancy Krieger, ed., *Embodying Inequality: Epidemiologic Perspectives* (Baywood, 2005); Mervyn Susser and Ezra Susser, "Choosing a Future for Epidemiology: I. Eras and Paradigms," *American Journal of Public Health* (v.86/5, 1996).

FERNANDO DE MAIO, PH.D.
SIMON FRASER UNIVERSITY

Epigenetics

The DNA in cells carries the blueprints, or genes, that code for the proteins necessary for cellular structure and function via the processes of transcription and translation. The double-stranded DNA is divided into several large, discrete components within the cell called chromosomes, and distinct chromosomes carry specific genes. An entire set of chromosomes is called a genome. Epigenetics refers to the study of changes in the genome of an organism that do not alter the actual sequence of nucleotides in that organism's DNA, but do modify the DNA structure in other ways, by adding other chemical groups or by binding regulatory proteins to the DNA backbone. An epigenetic change affects the phenotype, the appearance, physiological functioning, or physical construction of that organism, rather than the genotype, the actual DNA sequence of the gene, the genes found on each chromosome, and the number of chromosomes. Thus, epigenetic changes are distinct from genetic mutations, which alter the DNA sequence of nucleotides.

Despite not affecting the gene itself, epigenetic changes are heritable, meaning that they can be passed on from one cellular generation to the next as cells divide and replicate. Furthermore, although it was previously believed that epigenetic changes could not be passed from one organism to another via the sexual reproduction of multicellular organisms, new evidence indicates that epigenetic changes to gametes, or sexual reproduction cells, can also remain stable from one generation to the next. Epigenetic changes are less permanent than alterations to the genetic code, however, and can often be reversed, thus allowing cells more flexibility in adapting to environmental conditions than genetic mutations alone would allow.

There are many cellular processes that lead to epigenetic changes. Some of these involve differential gene expression at the cellular level. One of these is differential ribonucleic acid (RNA) splicing, whereby the nascent messenger RNA (mRNA) transcript coded from the same gene in two different types of cells is patched together differentially to lead to two different types of protein products. Another involves the preferential transcription of certain genes in certain cells via the use of transcription factors, molecular 'tags' that encourage RNA polymerase to copy some genes more often than others. 'Maternal effect' epigenetic changes

can occur during fetal gestation, as the embryo inherits RNA and transcription factors from the maternal oocyte during the process of fertilization. Unlike genetic mutations, however, epigenetic changes do not generally affect the sequencing of the amino acids that make up the normal protein found in a specific cell.

Gene expression is also controlled at the chromatin level, and other epigenetic processes alter the physical structure (although not the nucleotide sequence) of DNA such that some genes are more readily transcribed and translated than others. Histone modification, the process of altering the proteins that bind and compact strands of DNA chromatin into chromosomes, can alter gene expression. Methylation of histone proteins will inactivate a gene, while acetylation of histones will make a gene more readily available to the cellular machinery that transcribes DNA. In human females, one copy of the X chromosome is often randomly inactivated via methylation.

Epigenetics changes are important in somatic cellular differentiation, the process by which cells in different parts of a multicellular organism, all of which have the same genome, take on their unique characteristics and distinct abilities to function in certain ways. Thus, epigenetic changes are what allow human liver cells, for instance, to carry out different processes than stomach cells, despite having identical genomes. Almost all mammalian cells undergo this process of terminal differentiation, that is, once they have differentiated, they have "memory" of epigenetic changes and can only reproduce other similarly differentiated cells. Only stem cells retain totipotency, the ability to form any type of cell.

Epigenetic changes can cause disease. Because one copy of a gene is often methylated or "silenced," an individual inheriting a single copy of a recessive disease allele can show symptoms of the disease, even though that individual possesses a healthy allele. These individuals are said to be "hemizygous" for that trait or disease, which does not exhibit normal Mendelian inheritance patterns. This process of inactivating one copy of a gene, also called "imprinting," often distinguishes the maternally inherited chromosome from the paternally inherited copy; some genetic diseases in humans are more likely to be caused by a disease allele on a specific parent's chromosome. Epigenetic responses to carcinogens can alter regulation of the cell cycle, leading to cancerous tumor growth, even if these carcinogens are not mutagens; that is, they do not alter the DNA sequence of a gene.

SEE ALSO: DNA; DNA Repair.

BIBLIOGRAPHY. Vincenzo E. Russo, Arthur D. Riggs, Robert A. Martienssen (Eds), *Epigenetic Mechanisms of Gene Regulation* (Cold Spring Harbor Laboratory Press, 1996). David Stewart (Editor), Bruce Stillman (Editor), *Epigenetics: Cold Spring Harbor Symposia on Quantitative Biology, Vol. 69*, (Cold Spring Harbor Laboratory Press, 2004);

ANNIE DUDE
UNIVERSITY OF CHICAGO

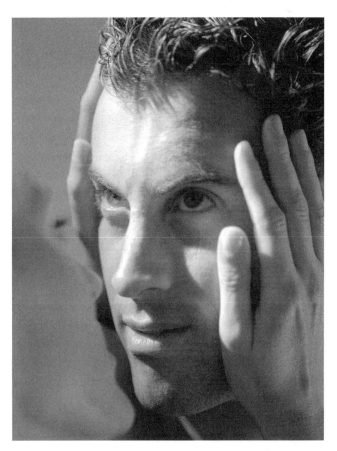

For most people with epilepsy, experiencing seizures is sporadic, but the psychosocial consequences continually influence quality of life.

Epilepsy

Epilepsy is one of the most common neurological disorders and affects people of any age, gender, race/ethnicity, social class, and geographic location. It is a chronic condition influencing brain function characterized by discharge of excessive levels of neurons, resulting in seizures that vary in frequency, severity, and type. The causes of epilepsy vary as much as the people affected by the illness. For most people with epilepsy, experiencing seizures is sporadic, but the psychosocial consequences continually influence quality of life. Advances in medicine and specific research on the underlying causes of the disease, the reasons for spontaneous seizures, diagnostic measures, as well as the psychosocial impact on patients, families and communities have led to more effective treatments.

WHAT IS EPILEPSY?

Epilepsy appeared in Indian and Babylonian medical texts dating back to 4500 B.C.E., with its name coming from the Greek word *epilambanein* meaning "to attack/seize." The experience of a seizure was believed to be the result of supernatural forces, cycles of the moon, or spiritual possession. In modern times, the causes of epilepsy although not well understood include genetics, brain disease, substance abuse, parasites, febrile illness, and head injury/trauma.

Not until the 17th and 18th centuries was epilepsy viewed as a medical disorder, and not until the establishment of the field of neurology was it thought of as a brain disorder. Epilepsy affects the brain through excessive release of neurons causing seizures that take on various forms based on the location and size of the area(s) affected. Generalized/grand mal seizures are characterized by loss of consciousness and muscle stiffness and contraction. A variation on this are petit mal seizures usually with shorter periods of unconsciousness. The second type of seizure is partial or focal, which start in one part of the brain and can spread to other parts, leading to generalized seizures. Partial seizures may result in brief losses of attention or longer periods of mental absence. The third type, status epilepticus is characterized by frequent seizures without recovery, which if not treated can lead to brain damage or death. It is not well understood why people experience certain types of seizures, but triggers for their onset have been identified, including flashing lights, physical exertion, lack of sleep, or stress.

EPIDEMIOLOGY OF EPILEPSY

Although epilepsy does not discriminate based on sociodemographic characteristics, most diagnoses occur among infants, adolescents, and older adults. According to the World Health Organization (WHO), approximately 8.2 per 1,000 (50 million) people currently live with active epilepsy (experience reoccurring seizures or are in need of treatment). Developing nations have a much higher incident rate with 100 per 100,000 compared to 50 in developed nations. People with epilepsy have an increased risk of mortality attributed to underlying brain disease (i.e., tumor), having seizures at dangerous times (i.e., while swimming, driving, etc.), status epilepticus, respiratory failure during seizures, and suicide.

PSYCHOSOCIAL CONSEQUENCES

The psychosocial consequences of living with epilepsy can drastically influence a person's quality of life. The psychological consequences include increased rates of mood and anxiety disorders, with the most common being depression and dysthymia. The underlying reasons for this are not well understood and have been attributed to the influence of epilepsy on the brain, anti-epileptic medications, disruptions in sleep, social factors, or various combinations. Anxiety is also more prevalent among people with epilepsy, characterized by feelings of fear, dread or uneasiness, and sometimes tied to the seizure experience or the result of not knowing when the next seizure will occur.

A common social consequence of epilepsy is the restriction on driving, which can limit a person's independence. People with epilepsy are also more likely to be on disability and not allowed to enter certain occupations where losses of consciousness could be dangerous (i.e., operating heavy machinery). Stigma, also a major consequence of living with epilepsy, can greatly alter social interactions. Moving toward a medical understanding of the disease along with increased public awareness have led to decreased levels of stigma, but it still exists. Stigma may especially be detrimental to children who may feel outcast by peer groups or reluctant to engage in activities out of fear of having a seizure. Studies have also documented the detrimental effect of epilepsy on education levels and marital status. Efforts made by groups such as the Global Campaign Against Epilepsy are essential to increase the quality of life among those with epilepsy by raising public awareness and helping to reduce misunderstandings and stereotypes.

RESEARCH AND TREATMENT

Increased knowledge about epilepsy is due to advances in understanding the brain and neurological function. Research on epilepsy generally falls into three areas including basic science (i.e., function of the brain and genetics), clinical (diagnosis and treatment), and psycho-social (i.e. how the experience of living with epilepsy influences quality of life). Treatment options are available depending on where you live (developed versus developing nation) and the ability to pay for it, and include pharmacotherapy (involving one or more anti-epileptic medications) or brain surgery. According to WHO, 70 percent with epilepsy respond to treatment, and are able to control their seizures through these means, but nearly three-quarters of people in developing nations are unable to afford treatment.

SEE ALSO: Seizures, Brain Diseases, Neurology

BIBLIOGRAPHY. Thomas R. Browne and Gregory L. Holmes, *Handbook of Epilepsy*, 3rd ed. (Lippincott Williams & Wilkins, 2004); Melissa A. Carran, et al., "Marital Status after Epilepsy Surgery," *Epilepsia* (v.40/12, 1999); Epilepsy Foundation, "Mood," www.epilepsyfoundation.org/about/related/mood/types.cfm (cited June 2007); World Health Organization, "Epilepsy," www.who.int/topics/epilepsy/en/ (cited July 2007).

NOAH J. WEBSTER, M.A.
CASE WESTERN RESERVE UNIVERSITY

Equatorial Guinea

Equatorial Guinea, on the western coast of Africa, is smaller than the State of Maryland, has the smallest population of any country on the continent, and is the smallest Spanish-speaking nation in the world. Significant oil reserves were discovered in 1996, producing 420,000 barrels a day by 2005. On paper, Equatoguineans have the third highest per capita income in the world, just behind Luxembourg and Bermuda. In reality, the people see little evidence of these huge oil revenues, most of which goes directly into the pockets of the leadership.

President Teodoro Obiang Nguema has ruled the country as a semidictatorship since seizing power in a military coup in 1979. In recent years, Equatorial Guinea has become "one of the most paranoid, suspicious and xenophobic countries in Africa," according to John Vidal, a Western journalist who made a rare trip inside the country in 2004. This apparently stems from Obiang's fear that outside forces are plotting to steal the country's oil reserves. This institutional paranoia makes assessing the health of Equatoguineans difficult.

The population is estimated at approximately 540,000, with a annual growth rate of 2.05 percent. The birth rate stands at 35.59 births per 1,000 people and the death rate is believed to be 15.06 per 1,000. There is little migration. Fifty percent of the population live in urban areas.

Life expectancy at birth is 48 years for males and 51 years for females, with healthy life expectancy at 45 years for men and 46 years for women.

The fertility rate is 5.9 births per woman; maternal mortality rates stand at 880 deaths per 100,000 live births. Infant mortality is 103 deaths per 1,000, and 205 deaths per 1,000 for children aged 1–5. Both infant and child mortality rates have actually risen since 1990.

Malaria, cholera, and yellow fever remain serious problems in Equatorial Guinea. (The regional strain of malaria has reportedly grown resistant to chloroquine, usually the most effective form of treatment.) With little potable water available to Equatoguineans, gastroenteritis and parasitic diseases are endemic.

AIDS statistics are hampered by what the Joint United Nations Programme on HIV/AIDS (UNAIDS) calls "irregular" surveillance. It estimates the adult prevalence rate at 3.2 percent, with 8,900 adults currently infected. There are little data on treatment rates or attempts by the government to quell the spread of the virus.

Increased government revenues have not gone into medical care; per capita spending on healthcare is estimated at $65. There are still limited hospital facilities throughout the small country. The U.S. Department of State notes that payment is usually required up front for any medical services, and that patients are often required to provide their own bed linens and, frequently, their own bandages and dressings. In 2004, there were 153 physicians, 228 nurses, and 43 midwives working in the country.

SEE ALSO: Healthcare, Africa.

BIBLIOGRAPHY. *Encyclopedia of the Nations*, http://www.nationsencyclopedia.com/Africa/Equatorial-Guinea-HEALTH.html (cited July 2007); World Health Organization, "Equatorial Guinea." http://www.who.int/countries/gnq/en/ (cited July 2007); "Equatorial Guinea—Health."

HEATHER K. MICHON
INDEPENDENT SCHOLAR

Eritrea

Eritrea is a small country on the eastern coast of Africa, bordering on the Red Sea. Endlessly at war with its southern neighbor Ethiopia and mired in drought, Eritreans have faced many hardships in recent years, many of them having an impact on the general health and welfare of the people.

The total population is approximately 4,790,000 and growing at a rate of 2.47 percent annually. The birth rate is 34.33 per 1,000 and the death rate is 9.6 per 1,000; there is little or no migration. Life expectancy at birth is 58 years for males and 62 years for females, with healthy life expectancy at 49 years for men and 51 years for women. Eritrea is overwhelmingly rural, with just 21 percent of the population living in urban areas. Most Eritreans are subsistence farmers. Gross national income is $145 annually.

Eritrea has had to cope with back-to-back disasters since the late 1990s. Between 1998 and 2000, more than 1 million Eritreans were displaced by war with Ethiopia, with another 70,000 to 100,000 reportedly killed. (There are an estimated 70,000 still living in refugee camps around the country.) In 2000, a severe drought led to a total crop failure. Recent years have seen crop yields rebound slightly, but not enough to stave off persistent food insecurity. In 2005, the United Nations estimated that 2.2 of 3.8 million Eritreans lacked adequate food supplies.

Access to potable water is limited to about 44 percent of the population and only 9 percent use sanitary facilities—a mere 3 percent in rural areas. Malaria, tuberculosis, human immunodeficiency virus (HIV)/AIDS, and malnutrition account for 60 percent of all outpatient cases and 40 percent of inpatient admittances in 2003. These four conditions were responsible for 56 percent of the deaths among inpatients in

2003, a figure which increased in 2004. Acute respiratory infections are also a problem, accounting for more than 17 percent of hospital cases.

Immunization rates among children are good in most areas, although not good enough in some regions to prevent localized measles epidemics. Infant mortality is 50 per 1,000 and child mortality is 78 per 1,000. Under-5 mortality has been cut in half since 1990.

Eritrean women face many challenges. Child marriage is widely practiced, with about 60 percent of rural teens wed before the age of 16 (as are 31 percent of urban children). Female genital mutilation (FGM) is widespread, with a 1997 survey finding 90 percent of women reporting they had undergone some type of FGM in youth. In many areas, the cutting is performed in infancy, and in most of Eritrea, is rarely performed after the age of 7. The most radical form, type III or infibulation (including the removal of the clitoris and labia and sewing shut of the vaginal area) is performed mainly in the northern regions of the country, while type I (clitoridectomy) or type II (removal of the clitoris and labia minora) are spread throughout the country.

Early marriage and childbearing contributes to a high maternal mortality rate of 630 per 100,000 live births. Seventy percent of all births happen at home, with just 28 percent under the supervision of a trained attendant. An uncounted number suffer from obstetric fistula, an injury of childbearing that leaves an open hole in the birth canal which leads to chronic fecal and urinary incontinence. Only 8 percent of Eritrean women have access to birth control. Women account for more than half of all HIV/AIDS cases within the country. The adult prevalence rate for HIV/AIDS is estimated at 2.4 percent. There are 59,000 Eritreans living with HIV/AIDS, 31,000 of them women. Ongoing internal and cross-border instability has made it difficult for the government or international organizations to craft a national plan to combat the spread of the virus or other sexually transmitted diseases.

Delivery of healthcare services is uneven at best. Hospitals are understaffed, poorly equipped, and lacking in critical drug inventories. There are about 215 physicians and 2,500 nurses working within the medical system (excluding those working with nongovernmental organizations). With so much of the population living outside the cities, the sick or injured often face long treks to the nearest health centers. Once they reach care, they must try to find the money to pay for services: patients are responsible for 100 percent of medical expenditures. Per capita spending on healthcare by the government amounts to about $4 a year.

SEE ALSO: Healthcare, Africa.

BIBLIOGRAPHY. World Health Organization, "Eritrea," http://www.who.int/countries/eri/en/ (cited July 2007); "Teenage Childbearing and Child Health in Eritrea, *RePEc* (Research Papers in Economics), http://ideas.repec.org/p/dem/wpaper/wp-2005-029.html (cited June 2007).

HEATHER K. MICHON
INDEPENDENT SCHOLAR

Esophageal Cancer

Esophageal cancer is a malignant (cancerous) growth which occurs in the muscular tube connecting the throat to the stomach. The main function of the esophagus is to aid in the passage of food and liquids from the throat to the stomach. The occurrence of cancer in this part of the body interferes with these normal functions. The two most common types of esophageal cancer are squamous cell carcinoma (also known as epidermoid carcinoma) and adenocarcinoma.

Together, these account for over 95 percent of all esophageal cancers. Typically, the former occurs in the upper to middle portion of the esophagus, whereas the latter usually affects the lower third of the esophagus. Unfortunately, early-stage esophageal cancer often goes unnoticed because the individual typically does not suffer from symptoms of this disease until it has progressed to a later stage. This, alongside the lack of a serosal barrier makes the prognosis for esophageal cancer generally poor. The method of treatment and prognosis for esophageal cancer depends very much on the stage the cancer is classified as once identified. Both squamous cell carcinoma and adenocarcinoma each have their own etiologies (causes), and are therefore often studied separately by researchers in this respect. Common to both esophageal squamous cell carcinoma (SCC) and adenocarcinoma (AC), factors such as sex, race, economic status, as well as geographical location have been found to play a role in the risk of developing one type of esophageal cancer over another, making this disease a global health phenomenon.

Although the causes of SCC and AC are very different, the symptoms are often similar. For instance, persons who are diagnosed with esophageal cancer frequently describe symptoms that include progressive difficulty with swallowing foods and/or liquids (a medical condition referred to as dysphagia), hoarseness, chest pain, and significant weight loss. Common symptoms of a more advanced stage of esophageal cancer includes painful swallowing (also known as odynophagia) and regurgitation, which are often the result of a large tumor causing an obstruction within the esophagus.

A barium swallow (a type of X-ray test) is most often used to identify whether an individual potentially has esophageal cancer. If further investigation is required, typically an endoscopy (the use of a lighted, flexible instrument called an endoscope, to examine the inside of certain parts of the body such as the esophagus) accompanied by a biopsy (the removal and examination of a sample of tissue) are used to better identify the disease. The cancer can be classified from stage I (small, localized, and usually curable cancer) to stage IV (cancer which has spread and is inoperable). There is also the TNM (**t**umor, **n**ode, **m**etastases) system which can be used to classify solid tumors.

Generally, late-stage esophageal cancer (i.e., stage III or IV) makes treatment options such as surgery, chemotherapy, and radiation to be palliative (to alleviate symptoms relating to the disease) rather than curative (to eliminate the disease). Photodynamic therapy (PDT) has also been administered as both a palliative and curative treatment method. The former has been used in advanced cancers to alleviate dysphagia and the latter has been used in early-stage esophageal cancer (i.e., a precancerous lesion).

There are two well-documented conditions that have been found to contribute to the development of *esophageal AC*, these include 1.) gastroesophageal reflux disease (GERD) and 2.) Barrett's esophagus (BE). The symptoms associated with GERD include frequent episodes of heartburn and reflux (gastric contents splashing back up into the esophagus) particularly after the consumption of certain foods or proceeding certain movements (i.e., laying down,

sitting up, etc.). GERD causes a degree of damage to the esophageal mucosa which may become a serious problem if it manifests into a chronic condition. Chronic GERD, or an inflammation of the esophagus (esophagitis) can result in BE, which is a precursor for esophageal AC. BE is a condition where the cells in the lower end of the esophagus have undergone an abnormal change in cells (metaplasia) either resembling the lining of the stomach or of the intestines. Two different online books edited by Holzheimer and Mannick, and Thomson and Shaffer provide chapters specifically dedicated to the esophageal conditions, disorders, symptoms, and the treatment of esophageal neoplasms; these sources are recommended for further reading.

Other documented risk factors of AC include hiatal hernia, being overweight, reduced lower sphincter pressure, diet, and to some degree, tobacco and alcohol consumption. There are a number of aspects relating to diet that have been associated with SCC, these are particularly relevant to high-risk regions of China and in some African and Far East countries. Poor dietary habits (i.e. consumption of high starchy foods and a diet low in fresh fruits and vegetables) as well as the occurrence of Plummer-Vinson syndrome (a complex vitamin deficiency) are amongst these. The consumption of dietary carcinogens such as nitrosamines (which have been detected in various foods and drinking water) and n-nitroso compounds (found in pickled or moldy foods) have also been implicated for their role in SCC occurrence.

Chronic irritation and inflammation of the esophagus have also been found to be of major importance in the etiology of SCC. For instance, the consumption of scratchy foods as well as the practice of eating food rapidly without sufficient mastication are qualities amongst those with SCC in the high-risk region of Northern Iran. Additionally, the consumption of foods and drinks (particularly hot mate tea) at extremely high temperatures, chronic esophagitis, previous lye-induced injury, and exposure to silica fibers and other occupational exposures and fumes, have also been suspected in SCC's etiology. Other possible risk factors include disorders such as achalasia (an abnormal function of esophageal nerves and muscles which make swallowing difficult), esophageal diverticulum (an outpocketing of the esophageal wall), and tylosis (a genetic disorder), and human papillomavirus."

Most esophageal cancers that occur in the world are SCC. The highest rates of SCC occur in poor regions of the world and equally affect males and females. In the Western world this is not the case; AC is more common than SCC. Nevertheless, SCC that occurs in the Western world disproportionately affects men (especially those that are single) and certain races. For instance, rates were elevated almost four to five times higher for black women and men in comparison to white women and men with SCC.

The occurrence of esophageal cancer is infrequent before 40 years of age, with the exception of some regions found within the "esophageal cancer belt" region of the world. The esophageal cancer belt, located in central Asia, "is an area that stretches eastward from Iran through Turkmenistan, Northern Afghanistan, Uzbekistan, and Kazakhstan into Northern China and Mongolia" (Kuska, 2001). Recent studies have provided evidence that the geographical limits of the esophageal cancer belt has been extended southwest to Quetta, Balochistan, located in Pakistan (Roohullah, et al., 2001; Bhurgri, et al., 2002). There have been other documented high-risk areas in the world (unrelated to the esophageal cancer belt region); among some of these are regions within France, Uruguay, and Transkei.

Over the past two decades, AC has been on the rise throughout North America and parts of Europe, especially among white men. A number of hypotheses have been put forth to explain this increase by identifying possible risk factors for this disease. Some of the main explanations suggested for this increase, and warranting further research, have been succinctly noted by J. Lagergren to include (1) the increased frequency of GERD, (2) an increase in the use of medication which contributes to reduced sphincter pressure, and (3) an increase in the rate of obesity (which is thought to increase intraadominal pressure). Some studies have examined the role of workplace exposures in relation to increasing AC trends and the male predominance only to report minor to no influence in this regard (Jansson, et al., 2006; Jansson, et al., 2005; Engel, et al., 2002). Nevertheless, several researchers have noted the possibility of environmental exposures as the culprits for this dramatic increase.

Numerous studies have been conducted which examine the various causes of esophageal cancer as de-

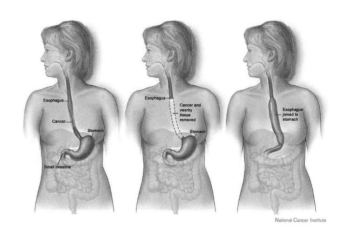

A drawing of esophageal cancer surgery, where the cancer and nearby tissue are removed and the stomach is joined to the esophagus.

scribed above. Amongst these, several studies have found some association with occupational exposures in relation to esophageal cancer, particularly those associated with exposures to silica dust and chemical solvents or detergents (Yu, et al., 2005; Cucino and Sonnenberg, 2002; Tsuda, et al., 2001; Sullivan, et al., 1998; Ruder, et al., 1994). In North America, esophageal cancer still disproportionately affects males, and those of certain races. For instance, in a report written by the U.S. Cancer Statistics Working Group in 2005, it was found that in the United States (based on 17 Surveillance, Epidemiology, and End Results Program [SEER] areas) esophageal cancer incidence ratios per 100,000 for the years 2000-2003 were 10.8:3.3 for black men in comparison to black women. Further, 7.8:1.9 incidence ratios for white men in comparison to white women were reported. Socioeconomic class has also been found to play a role in esophageal cancer incidence in much of the literature, with the exception of a study conducted by Bossetti, et al., (2001) in Italy which showed that there was a disappearance of the social gradient amongst esophageal cancer (and other upper digestive tract cancers) in the 1990's that was once identified amongst this population in the 1980's. Allen Pickens and Mark B. Orringer provide an overview of the geographical distributions and racial disparities of esophageal cancer.

As evidenced by global statistics provided by Ferlay and colleagues (2004), worldwide esophageal cancer not only disproportionately affects more males than females, its highest incidence rates can be found in certain areas of the world; amongst these are Eastern and Southern Africa and Eastern and South-Central Asia. These rates are consistent with those previously reported by Ferlay, et al., (2001). The only drastic changes between the global statistics reported for esophageal cancer in 2001 in comparison to those reported in 2004 are those pertaining to Fiji. Esophageal cancer incidence rates for Fiji were reported at more than nine times higher for males and more than four times higher for females compared to rates reported in 2001. However, these rates should be interpreted with caution since issues related to registry collection may be to blame for this increase (i.e. a change in compliance in reporting; a change in resources required to retrieve data, etc.,). Therefore, these reported increased rates may not necessarily be the result of an actual increase in risk over the years. In order to better understand the underlying issues and implications surrounding the incidence of esophageal cancer, further investigation of discrepancies which exist amongst sex, race, economic status as well as geographical location are necessary."

SEE ALSO: Cancer (General); Surveillance, Epidemiology, and End Results Program (SEER).

BIBLIOGRAPHY. Y. Bhurgri, et al., "Cancer Patterns in Quetta (1998–1999)," *The Journal of the Pakistan Medical Association* (v.52/12, 2002); William J. Blot, et al., "Rising Incidence of Adenocarcinoma of the Esophagus and Gastric Cardia," *Journal of the American Medical Association* (v.265/10, 1991); C. Bosetti, et al., "Changing Socioeconomic Correlates for Cancer of the Upper Digestive Tract," *Annals of Oncology* (v.12/3, 2001); Linda Morris Brown, et al., "Excess Incidence of Squamous Cell Esophageal Cancer among U.S. Black Men: Role of Social Class and Other Risk Factors," *American Journal of Epidemiology* (v.153/2, 2001); Linda Morris Brown, et al., "Chapter 1: Epidemiology of Esophageal Cancer," in M. C. Posner, E. Vokes, R. Weichselbaum, eds., *Cancer of the Upper Gastrointestinal Tract* (Decker, 2002); Claudia Cucino and Amnon Sonnenberg, "Occupational Mortality from Squamous Cell Carcinoma of the Esophagus in the United States during 1991–1996," *Digestive Diseases and Sciences* (v.47/3, 2002); Lawrence S. Engel, et al., "Occupation and Risk of Esophageal and Gastric Cardia Adenocarcinoma," *American Journal of Industrial Medicine* (v.42/1, 2002); Jacques Ferlay, et al., *GLOBOCAN 2000: Cancer Incidence, Mortality and Prevalence Worldwide, Version 1.0, IARC Cancer Base No. 5* (IARC Press, 2001); Jacques Ferlay, et al., *GLOBOCAN 2002: Cancer Incidence, Mortality and Prevalence Worldwide IARC CancerBase No. 5. Version 2.0* (IARC Press, 2004), http://www-dep.iarc.fr/ (cited October 2006); P. Ghadirian, "Food Habits of the People of the Caspian Littoral of Iran in Relation to Esophageal Cancer," *Nutrition and Cancer* (v.9/2–3, 1987); P. Ghadirian, J. Vobecky, and J. S. Vobecky, "Factors Associated with Cancer of the Oesophagus: An Overview," *Cancer Detection and Prevention* (v.11/3–6, 1988); P. Ghadirian, J. M. Ekoe, and J. P. Thouez, "Food Habits and Esophageal Cancer: An Overview," *Cancer Detection and Prevention* (v.16/3, 1992); René G. Holzheimer and John A. Mannick, "Surgical Treatment: Evidence-Based and Problem-Oriented," http://www.ncbi.nlm.nih.gov/books/bv.fcgi?rid=surg (cited October 2005); Catarina Jansson, et al., "Socioeconomic Factors and Risk of Esophageal Adenocarcinoma: A Nationwide Swedish Case Control Study," *Cancer Epidemiology, Biomarkers and Prevention* (v.14/7, 2005a); Catarina Jansson, et al., "Occupational Exposures and Risk of Esophageal and Gastric Cardia Cancers among Male Swedish Construction Workers," *Cancer Causes and Control* (v.16/6, 2005b); Catarina Jansson, et al., "Airborne Occupational Exposures and Risk of Oesophageal and Cardia Adenocarcinoma," *Occupational and Environmental Medicine* (v.63/2, 2006).

ANN NOVOGRADEC, PH.D.
YORK UNIVERSITY, TORONTO

Esophagus Disorders

The esophagus is the second part of the digestive tract, following the mouth and preceding the stomach. It is a tube that propels food down to the stomach, via rhythmic wave-like contractions called peristalsis.

There are many esophageal disorders, but most have two particular symptoms. The first symptom is general chest or back pain. The second symptom is a difficulty in swallowing, called dysphagia. Esophageal disorders can be caused by an injury or an obstruction, or esophageal bleeding or cancer. Other disorders may affect peristalsis; these disorders are called propulsion-related esophagus disorders.

In order to keep oral and gastric contents out of the esophagus while a person is not swallowing, the esophagus is flanked by two muscular sphincters. As a normal part of aging, these sphincters become weaker and sometimes cannot keep acidic stomach contents from entering the esophagus. This condition is called presbyesophagus, with the prefix 'presby' signifying the condition's relationship to old age. Some younger people experience periodic gastric acid reflux, another example of the acidic stomach chyme entering the esophagus abnormally. The healthy esophagus is protected by a thick layer of tough cells which line the esophagus. These epithelial cells are of the squamous cell type. A person with chronic acid reflux may have a weakened or damaged esophageal lining. People suffering from bulimia who force themselves to vomit also damage their esophageal lining.

Any cell population that is continuously replenishing itself and therefore undergoing genetic replication is at an elevated risk for developing cancer. The continuous genetic replication cycles can promote a mutation that might otherwise be inconsequential. Forced vomiting or acid reflux disease, add undo stress to the cells lining the esophagus, leading to an enhanced rate of cellular division while the esophagus tries to repair itself. This enhanced division rate also increases the risk of developing esophageal cancer.

Esophageal cancer begins in the innermost cell layer lining the esophagus. In the past, esophageal cancer was difficult to treat and survival was rare. Today, a precancerous condition known as Barrett's esophagus can be recognized early, when cancer treatment is most effective. Barrett's esophagus is a result of acid reflux disease. Smoking and drinking in excess can also strain the esophagus and predispose it to cancer. Other risk factors include age above fifty-five years, male gender, being African American, being overweight, eating a diet poor in fruits and vegetables, and working in professions with exposures to certain chemicals such as dry cleaning solutions and construction materials, and other toxins or irritants such as during mining.

Crohn's disease is a chronic disorder of the digestive tract that often affects the large intestine, though it can affect the tract from the esophagus to the rectum. It is an inflammatory disorder that may be auto-immune. It may have genetic components, but often the cause is idiopathic, meaning it is unknown. The inflammation can result in pain and difficulty in eating. Crohn's patients can attempt to keep the disorder in check by following a diet regimen that avoids aggravating foods while maintaining proper nutrition, taking corticosteroids and antibiotics if necessary, and painkiller medications. A supplement of vitamin E may need to be added to the diet, as Crohn's patients may not absorb enough vitamin E from a regular diet. The disease typically inflames during periods of high stress or after exerting physical activity.

Developmental disorders and physical malformations can also lead to dysphagia. Loss of coordination in the normally rhythmic contractions of the musculature encircling the esophagus can lead to difficulties with swallowing, food regurgitation, or choking. Other causes of esophageally located dysphagia that are not directly due to the esophagus include movement disorders such as Parkinson's disease or Huntington's disease. Certain medications and other drugs may also cause dry mouth, which will affect the ability of food to travel down the esophagus.

In the United States, the primary funding source for scientific investigations into disorders of the esophagus is the National Institute of Diabetes and Digestive and Kidney Diseases, part of the National Institutes of Health.

SEE ALSO: Acid Reflux; Bulimia; Esophageal Cancer; Gastroenterologist, Gastroenterology; National Institute of Diabetes and Digestive and Kidney Diseases (NIDDK); National Institutes of Health; Otolaryngologist; Otolaryngology.

BIBLIOGRAPHY. Antonio Carminati, *New Research on Esophageal Cancer (Horizons in Cancer Research)* (Nova Science Publishers, 2006); Randi E. McCabe MD, Traci L. McFarlane MD, and Marion P. Olmsted PhD, *Overcoming Bulimia: Your Comprehensive, Step-by-Step Guide to Recovery (New Harbinger Self-Help Workbook)* (New Harbinger Publications, 2004); Tracie M. Dalessandro MS RD CDN, *What to Eat with IBD: A Comprehensive Nutrition and Recipe Guide for Crohn's Disease and Ul-*

cerative Colitis (iUniverse, Inc., 2006); Thomas Murry and Ricardo Carrau, M.D., *Clinical Management of Swallowing Disorders* (Plural Publishing, 2006); Henry Parkman and Robert S. Fisher, *The Clinician's Guide to Acid / Peptic Disorders and Motility Disorders of the Gastrointestinal Tract (The Clinician's Guide to GI Series)* (Slack Incorporated, 2006); Richard E. Sampliner, Ajay Bansal, Jacques Bergman, and Navtej Buttar, *Barrett's Esophagus and Esophageal Adenocarcinoma* (Blackwell, 2006).

CLAUDIA WINOGRAD
UNIVERSITY OF ILLINOIS

Estonia

Since the dissolution of the Soviet bloc, Estonia has maintained strong ties with the West. The economy is largely dependent on the electronics and telecommunications sectors and on trading relations with Finland, Sweden, and Germany. With a per capita income of $17,500, Estonia ranks 58th in world incomes. The Gini coefficient for Estonia is 37.2. The richest 10 percent hold 29.8 percent of the country's wealth while the poorest 10 percent share only three percent. Unemployment stands at 7.9 percent and inflation at 4.1. Although Estonia has a low external debt, the budget deficit draws needed resources away from social programs. The United Nations Development Programme's (UNDP) Human Development Report ranks Estonia 40th among 177 countries on overall quality of life issues.

During the transition to a market economy, the government attempted to turn Estonia into a social welfare state, implementing the Estonian Healthcare Project (1995–98) according to World Health Organization guidelines to improve the quality of healthcare. In 2001, the Health Services Act set quality controls on healthcare and established the Healthcare Board. A social tax designed to generate funding for health services, pensions, and child benefits was also implemented. Despite good intentions, the government could not absorb the costs of the program, so benefits were reduced. Local governments were assigned the responsibility for administering social assistance, and living and housing allowances were abolished. The elderly were disproportionately affected by the changes.

Between 1993 and 2004, Estonia spent an average of 16 percent of the budget on healthcare. The government now commits 5.3 percent of the Gross Domestic Product (GDP) to healthcare, allotting $682 (international dollars) per capita. Government funding provides 77.1 percent of total health expenditures, and 84.9 percent of that amount is earmarked for social security. In Estonia, social security is a combination of social insurance and mandatory individual accounts. Employees do not pay for the program, but the self-employed pay one-third of the minimum salary, and employers are required to contribute one-third of payrolls. The program covers the elderly, the disabled, and survivors.

The private sector furnishes 22.9 percent of healthcare costs, and 88.30 percent of private provisions are derived from out-of-pocket expenses. When out-of-pocket expenses are high, the poorest segment of the population may be unable to afford healthcare or may be impoverished by meeting healthcare costs. Household budget surveys have indicated that the number of households spending more than one-fifth of their capacity to pay for healthcare rose steadily between 1995 and 2002. Again, the elderly who are require constant care and large amounts of medication are disproportionately affected. There are 4.48 physicians, 8.50 nurses, 0.34 midwives, 1.28 dentists, and 0.42 pharmacists per 1,000 population in Estonia.

Estonia's population of 1,324,333 has a life expectancy of 72.04 years. The gap between male (66.58 years and female (77.83 years) is wider than in most countries. Literacy is virtually universal at 99.8 percent. While 99 percent of children attend primary school, enrollment drops slightly at the secondary level. Seventy percent of Estonian women use birth control, giving birth to an average of 1.4 children each. All births are attended by trained personnel. However, Estonia's adjusted maternal mortality rate of 63 deaths per 100,000 live births is relatively high.

The current infant mortality rate is 7.73 deaths per 1,000 live births. Between 1990 and 2004, Estonia cut infant and under-five mortality in half, reducing rates from 12 to six deaths per 1,000 live births and from 16 to eight deaths per 1,000 live births, respectively. Four percent of all infants experience low birthweight. In most cases, immunization rates are high in response to government and international commitment. Ninety-nine percent of infants are immunized against tuberculosis; 98 percent against diphtheria, pertussis, and tetanus (DPT1) 96 percent against measles; and 95 percent against polio. Other immunization rates are lower, and the percentage of infants receiving DPT3 vaccinations drops to 94 percent, and only 90 percent receive hepatitis B vaccinations. The lowest immunization rate is found among infants inoculated against *Haemophilus influenzae* type B (27 percent).

Air and water pollution became major issues in Estonia during the socialist decades, but the government has been successful in precipitating a steady decline, reducing emissions by 80 percent between 1980 and 2000. At the same time, levels of untreated waste being discharged into water sources were reduced by one-twentieth. HIV/AIDS poses threat to Estonians, with a 1.1 percent adult prevalence rate. Around 7,800 people are living with the disease, and some 200 have lost their lives.

SEE ALSO: Finland; Sweden; World Health Organization (WHO).

BIBLIOGRAPHY. William H. Berqquist, *Freedom: Narratives of Change in Hungary and Estonia* (Jossey-Bass, 1994); Central Intelligence Agency, "Estonia," *World Factbook*, www.cia.gov/cia/publications/factbook/geos/en.html; Jarno Habicht, et al, "Detecting Changes in Financial Protection: Creating Evidence for Policy in Estonia," *Health Policy and Planning* (November 2006); Martin A. Levin and Martin Shapiro, eds., *Transatlantic Policymaking in an Age of Austerity: Diversity and Drift* (Georgetown University Press, 2004); Kaja Polluste, et al., "Quality Improvement in the Estonian Health System Assessment of Progress Using an International Tool," *International Journal for Quality in healthcare* (v.18/6, 2006).

ELIZABETH R. PURDY, PH.D.
INDEPENDENT SCHOLAR

Estrogen Replacement Therapy (ERT)

Estrogen is a group of hormones present in women that regulate sexual characteristics, including growth, maturation, and reproduction. Estrogen production declines during menopause, when the body moves into a stage in which pregnancy and childbirth are no longer possible, although other functions continue as normal.

This occurs on average between the ages of 45–55 in women in developed countries. The lack of estrogen causes a number of symptoms which can be troublesome to quality of life, including hot flushes, emotional disturbance, and sleeplessness, while also representing an often unwelcome constant reminder to the woman of the change of physical status she is undergoing. Within the woman, the ovaries cease to produce estrogen and the same effect can be produced by surgery, for example as a result of a hysterectomy. In some cases, therefore, medical practitioners may prescribe estrogen replacement therapy (ERT) as a means of controlling these symptoms. ERT is a subset of hormone replacement therapy (HRT), which also includes the replacement of other types of hormones for a variety of medicinal purposes.

Postmenopausal women may suffer from the demineralization of bones and related conditions, including osteoporosis and atrophic vaginitis. Estrogen replacement may be effective in countering these threats and so may be prescribed, either through an orally or dermally administered procedure. The hormone may also be administered through the vagina. Estrogen administered alone ("unopposed") is effective in treating postmenopausal symptoms, reduces osteoporosis threat, and has other benefits, but it has not been established how quickly this works on an individual basis and in the level of dosage required.

However, there are negative side effects associated with unopposed estrogen replacement, not least of which is the elevated threat of various kinds of cancer, which is a threat that may persist beyond using ERT treatments. More research is necessary to determine which forms of estrogen pose higher risks than others, what is the time scale involved, and which groups of women may be at higher levels of risk than others, as well as explaining why that might be. As a result of this, medical practitioners now generally recommend using estrogen in combination with other substances, in a format known as "opposed." It is most common for estrogen to be combined with progestin in this way; progestins are another type of hormone which are involved with regulating the maintenance of pregnancy.

Estrogen combined with progestin make up the oral contraceptive. Unfortunately, the combination of opposed estrogen also produces often-distressing and uncomfortable side effects, including bloating, bleeding, and depression.

Additionally, the long-term effects of the treatment are not clear and there is research exploring the link between opposed and unopposed ERT and the elevated incidence of breast cancer, coronary disease, and Alzheimer's disease, especially among older women. It seems clear that women do respond differently to different regimes of estrogen and progestin and that important factors include age and the presence of an intact womb or otherwise. Medical advice should be sought to determine what is considered most appropriate in the individual case. Researchers continue to experiment with varied doses and dosage protocol to shed further light on these issues.

Generally, the levels of estrogen recommended have decreased over time. Daily dosage is now commonly set at 0.625 mg per day, which is only one-quarter of doses recommended in the past. ERT became particularly popular—or at least more commonly prescribed—in the 1960s and 1970s in the United States and then declined as emergent risks became known. Currently, some 15 to 20 percent of American women will use ERT in one form or another. Some reject the idea because of the belief that synthetic products should not interrupt natural processes or because of fear of side effects or because of lack of good-quality information. Given the continuing lack in specific knowledge in particular, important areas of knowledge, as well as the need to balance benefit and risk in the case of individual patients, it would be prudent to seek individualized advice before deciding whether the benefits outweigh the risks for women suffering from symptoms specified above.

SEE ALSO: Hormones; Menopause.

BIBLIOGRAPHY. Lynn Rosenberg, "Hormone Replacement Therapy: The Need for Reconsideration," *American Journal of Public Health* (v.83/12, 1993); Ronald K. Ross, et al., "Effect of Hormone Replacement Therapy on Breast Cancer Risk: Estrogen versus Estrogen plus Progestin," *Journal of the National Cancer Institute* (v.92/4, 2000); Richard L. Tannen, et al., "Estrogen Affects Post-Menopausal Women Differently than Estrogen plus Progestin Replacement Therapy," *Human Reproduction* (v.22/3, 2007), published online ahead of print publication.

JOHN WALSH
SHINAWATRA UNIVERSITY

Ethiopia

Ethiopia, on the eastern edge of Africa, is an ancient land. For centuries, it served as the crossroads of Arab and African culture. It is the second oldest Christian country; its rich artistic and cultural heritage is undeniable. Virtually alone among its neighbors, it managed to remain independent during decades of European imperialism. However, the final decades of the 20th century and the first years of the 21st century have not been easy for the people of Ethiopia, bringing widespread famine, war, and disease that killed millions of people.

With 74,800,000 residents, Ethiopia is the second most populous country in Africa after Nigeria. The population is growing at a rate of 2.31 percent annually. Only 16 percent of Ethiopians live in urban areas. Eighty percent live on less than $2 a day; per capita income is below $100 a year. Agriculture and subsistence farming is the linchpin of the economy.

Life expectancy at birth is currently 49 years for males and 51 years for females, with healthy life expectancy at 41 years for men and 42 years for women. Infant mortality rates have dropped slightly since 1990, now standing at 109 deaths per 1,000 live births. Mortality for children between the ages 1–5 has also edged down, dropping from 204 per 1,000 in 1990 to 164 per 1,000 in 2005. Maternal mortality is high, with 850 deaths per 100,000 live births. Only 28 percent of women receive any kind of prenatal care, and 6 percent have a trained attendant present at birth. Fifteen percent have access to birth control. As it is across the Horn of Africa, female genital mutilation (FGM) is widely practiced in Ethiopia. Sanitation and clean water access is scarce, with 22 percent of Ethiopians able to use potable water and 13 percent using sanitary facilities (figures drop significantly outside the cities, where only 11 percent have clean water and 7 percent have safe latrines). This leads to a high risk of food- and waterborne illness such as bacterial and protozoal diarrhea, hepatitis A, and typhoid fever.

Malaria, meningitis, and malnutrition are among the biggest health issues in Ethiopia today, with human immunodeficiency virus (HIV)/AIDS and tuberculosis following closely behind. Malaria cases have grown from 1.1 million in 1995 to 6.1 million in 2003. There were widespread outbreaks of meningitis in 2000, 2001, and 2002. A 2005 survey found 38 percent of the population underweight and 47 percent showing signs of stunting from long-term malnutrition. In the Somali region, almost 24 percent of the population were found to suffer from acute malnutrition. About 2.5 million were in need of supplemental food aid in 2006 alone.

The adult prevalence rate for HIV/AIDS is estimated at 2.8 to 6.7 percent of the population, with between 950,000 and 2.3 million Ethiopians currently infected. Five thousand new cases are contracted every week. The Ministry of Health counted just under 25,000 people receiving antiretroviral medications in 2005; the estimated number of patients in need was 211,000. There are about 400 testing sites spread across a country two-thirds the size of Alaska.

Government expenditures on healthcare works out to about $3 per capita. The U.S. Department of State describes medical facilities in Addis Ababa as "limited," and virtually nonexistent outside the city. Doctors are generally well trained but hampered by poor hospital facilities, out-of-date equipment, and inadequate drug inventories. There were 1,936 physicians and 14,900 nurses working in the country in 2004.

SEE ALSO: Healthcare, Africa.

BIBLIOGRAPHY. Helmut Kloos and Zein Ahmed Zein, eds. *Health, Disease, Medicine and Famine in Ethiopia: A Bibliography* (Greenwood Press, 1991); World Health Organization, "Ethiopia," http://www.who.int/countries/eth/eth/en/ (cited June 2007).

HEATHER K. MICHON
INDEPENDENT SCHOLAR

European Association for Cancer Research (EACR)

Established in 1968, the European Association for Cancer Research (EACR) is made up of over 5,000 members and is dedicated to the advancement of cancer research throughout Europe. Membership is open to those who possess an academic degree or the equivalent and have held an appointment or worked actively in cancer research for at least two years. Different membership levels include active, student, emeritus, honorary, distinguished, and sustaining members. The first five categories of membership are open to individual scientists as well as members of scientific societies engaged in cancer research.

The last category is open to organizations in recognition of regular contributions to the aims and activities of the Association. Members are elected according to the EACR's bylaws. The Association strives to foster communication with laboratory, translational, and clinical cancer researchers in all areas of oncology from basic research to prevention, treatment, and care. The Association also promotes opportunities for collaborative research with and within other Member Societies of the Federation of European Cancer Societies (FECS), of which EACR is a founder member, including the European Society for Medical Oncology (ESMO), European Society of Surgical Oncology (ESSO), European Society for Therapeutic Radiology and Oncology (ESTRO), European Branch of the International Society of Pediatric Oncology (SIOP), and European Oncology Nursing Society (EONS). To promote the efforts of new generations of healthcare professionals, the EACR sponsors education and training for the young cancer researcher through free membership for postgraduate students, and fellowships to promote technical exchange.

The EACR also gives awards for lectures and posters at meetings, and sponsors special programs to assist researchers in eastern Europe, and promotes Young Investigators Forums to generate ideas for developing and enhancing the EACR. The General Assembly, as the supreme governing body of the Association, is composed of the membership of the EACR. The Executive Committee conducts the affairs of the Association and is advised by the Council which consists of elected representatives from each major European country. *The European Journal of Cancer* is the official journal of the EACR, the European Organization for Research and Treatment of Cancer (EORTC), the European School of Oncology (ESO), the FECS and the European Society of Mastology (EUSOMA). It is an international comprehensive oncology journal that publishes original research, editorial comments, review articles, and news on experimental oncology, clinical oncology (medical, pediatric, radiation, surgical), and cancer epidemiology and prevention. The Journal's editorial board is made up of some of Europe's leading professionals in various fields of cancer research. The EACR also produces newsletters and a number of reports to disseminate useful information to its membership and each year sponsors a number of regional meetings as well as a major annual conference.

SEE ALSO: Cancer (General); American Cancer Society (ACS).

BIBLIOGRAPHY. British Association for Cancer Research, www.bacr.org.uk (cited September 2006); European Association for Cancer Research, www.eacr.org (cited September 2006); Federation of European Cancer Societies, www.fecs.be/emc.asp (cited September 2006); Joseph G. Sinkovics and Joseph Horvath, eds., *Viral Therapy of Human Cancers* (Informa Healthcare, 2004).

BEN WYNNE, PH.D
GAINESVILLE STATE COLLEGE

European Association for the Study of Obesity (EASO)

The European Association for the Study of Obesity (EASO) was founded in 1988. It is headquartered in London and currently has more than 2,500 members from 27 different countries. Members represent a wide range of professions including sports specialists, dieticians, physicians, and scientists. EASO promotes research into obesity, facilitates contact and collaboration between organizations and individuals, and seeks to educate professionals and the public on the epidemic of obesity. The Association has created a number of task forces including those specifically aimed at Public Health and Prevention, Obesity Management, and Childhood Obesity. The overall goals of EASO revolve around enhancing the understanding and treatment of obesity in Europe; improving the quality of obesity education across Europe; developing a coherent approach to obesity management throughout Europe; forging European and global links between individuals and organizations concerned with the study of obesity; connecting active researchers from diverse disciplines who contribute to the development of a European perspective on obesity; and providing optimal input at the international level from a European perspective. In 1988, the EASO sponsored the first European Congress on Obesity (ECO), and since then, this annual meeting has been held in major cities throughout Europe. It routinely draws thousands of international delegates who meet to discuss the latest research and trends related to the study of obesity. As part of its mission, EASO also supports Young Investigators United (YIU) to facilitate the networking of young Europeans scientists and provide an arena for the exchange of ideas between leading experts and future leaders in the field. The YIU hold an annual meeting in conjunction with the EASO national conference.

EASO sponsors a number of publications, including *Obesity Reviews*, a review journal that publishes papers from all disciplines related to the study of obesity. *Obesity Reviews* is designed to appeal to all professionals with an interest in obesity, such as endocrinologists, cardiologists, gastroenterologists, obstetricians, rheumatologists, and healthcare professionals working in general medicine or surgery. In addition, the Journal contributes to education and interprofessional development by publishing a variety of diverse opinions dealing with current controversies in the field.

The *International Journal of Obesity* is a journal for clinicians and researchers working in obesity, diabetes and related disorders, dietetics, psychology, psychiatry, epidemiology, metabolic function, biochemistry, physiology, molecular biology, and genetics. In addition to periodicals, the Association regularly publishes various reports and position papers related to the study of obesity, including an annual survey on obesity throughout Europe. Related organizations include the United Kingdom Association for the Study of Obesity (ASO), the Hellenic Medical Association for the Study of Obesity (HMAO), the Netherlands Association for the Study of Obesity (NASO), and the Czech Society for the Study of Obesity (CSS).

SEE ALSO: North American Association for the Study of Obesity (NAASO); Obesity.

BIBLIOGRAPHY. European Association for the Study of Obesity (EASO), www.easoobesity.org (cited September 2006); Hellenic Medical Association for the Study of Obesity, www.hmao.gr (cited September 2006); Aileen Robertson, ed., *Food and Health in Europe: A New Basis for Action* (World Health Organization, 2004); United Kingdom Association for the Study of Obesity, http://www.aso.org.uk (cited September 2006).

BEN WYNNE, PH.D
GAINESVILLE STATE COLLEGE

European Food Safety Authority (EFSA)

The European Food Safety Authority (EFSA) was created by a European Parliament and Council Regulation and adopted in January 2002. The regulation established the basic principles and requirements of food law and stipulated that EFSA would be an independent source of scientific advice, information, and risk communication in the area of food and food safety issues. The impetus for the creation of the Authority was a series of food scares in the late 1990s that undermined consumer confidence in the safety of food and of the ability of governmental authorities to adequately deal with the problem.

Ultimately, this led the European Union institutions to conclude that there was a need to establish a new scientific body charged with providing independent and objective advice on food safety issues associated with the food chain. The administrative offices of the Authority moved from Brussels, Belgium, to Parma, Italy, in 2005.

Four distinct bodies make up the EFSA: the Management Board, the Executive Director and staff, the Advisory Forum, and the Scientific Committee and Panels. The EFSA Management Board includes 14 members appointed from across the European Union and an additional representative from the European Commission. The Board's primary responsibilities include implementing internal rules and regulations, drafting budgets and work programs, and in general ensuring that the EFSA functions efficiently. The Executive Director is the legal representative of the authority and is charged with handling daily management responsibilities for all staff matters. The Advisory Forum is the EFSA's consultative body. It advises the Executive Director on scientific matters and is an important forum for exchange on risk assessment and food safety issues.

Numbering eight in total, the Scientific Committee and Panels are made up of independent scientific experts in various fields who are dedicated to providing the authority with the latest scientific information available related to food and food safety. Through the work of its Scientific Committees and Expert Panels, EFSA's Department of Science provides risk assessment on all matters linked to food safety, including animal health and welfare and plant protection. The EFSA actively communicates with the public concerning its activities and recommendations.

The Authority's scientific opinions provide interested parties and the general public with objective, reliable, easily understood information through the dissemination of press releases, newsletters, and other communication tools designed to reach a broad audience. With a circulation of well over 10,000, the *EFSAnews* is the EFSA newsletter, which provides information relating to EFSA's activities, ranging from its core scientific work to its corporate events, Web site developments, and publications. Editions of *EFSAnews* are available in several languages and in print or electronic versions. Each year, EFSA sponsors an annual meeting as an opportunity for industry, farming groups, consumer groups, and other non-governmental organizations such as those working on environmental issues to informally share knowledge and exchange views on food and food safety with EFSA staff.

SEE ALSO: Food and Drug Administration (FDA); Food Safety.

BIBLIOGRAPHY. European Food Safety Authority, www.efsa.europa.eu/en.html (cited September 2006); Food Safety from the Farm to the Fork, ec.europa.eu/food/food/biotechnology/index_en.htm (cited September 2006); Food Standards Agency, www.food.gov.uk (cited September 2006).

BEN WYNNE, PH.D
GAINESVILLE STATE COLLEGE

European Public Health Alliance (EPHA)

The European Public Health Alliance (EPHA) was established in 1993 as an international nonprofit association registered in Belgium. The organization came into being amid concerns by a number of groups that while many European Union (EU) policies had an impact on public health, the EU at times did not directly recognize or address many of the public health issues involved. The Alliance hopes to promote and protect the health interests of all individuals living in Europe and to strengthen dialogue between EU institutions, the general public, and nongovernmental entities. The EPHA promotes the idea that the problems and concerns related to public health are international in character and therefore require solutions based on international cooperation. As a result, the EPHA supports an "open Europe" larger than the EU itself and enriched by the diversity and perspectives of an ever-expanding trans-European horizon. Among the specific goals of the organization include the introduction and implementation of policies that promote health in all areas of European policy; the promotion of the rights of all citizens to participate in decisions involving their own health and healthcare; ensuring cooperation among existing European organizations related to public health, health promotion, patient care, citizens rights and human rights; monitoring developments within the EU in the field of public health and providing a regular flow of information to and between members; influencing EU institutions and other relevant bodies in Europe and internationally to promote and evaluate effective public health policies: and seeking a greater role for public health and health promoting associations in the formulation and management of EU health policies. The EPHA operates on democratic principles and therefore facilitates communication and participation between and among member organizations and those EU institutions involved in policy development and program implementation. From year to year, the Alliance also aids many nongovernmental agencies in their advocacy work and in information dissemination, particularly in newer EU countries.

Since its creation, the EPHA has grown dramatically in size and represents more than 100 organizations with an interest in health issues. As a result, the Alliance has developed into a broad-based organization with a significant and growing influence on public policy. The EPHA's membership consists of organizations, associations, and other groups at the local, regional, national or international level that in turn represent the interests of a broad, diverse cross section of society.

There are two levels of membership. Full members are nongovernmental organizations that are active in the public health sector while associate members are other nonprofit organizations, professional bodies, academic institutions and local or regional authorities. The activities of the Alliance are governed by the Annual General Assembly, which convenes the membership once a year to discuss and evaluate policy. The Assembly elects an Executive Committee to oversee the overall day-to-day work of the organization and consultation and seminars are held with member organizations throughout the year as needed. The administrative offices of the EPHA are located in Brussels, Belgium.

SEE ALSO: Healthcare, Europe; Global Health Council.

BIBLIOGRAPHY. European Public Health Alliance, www.epha.org (cited September 2006); EU Business, www.eubusiness.com (cited September 2006); EUractiv.com, www.euractiv.com/en (cited September 2006); EUobserver.com, www.euobserver.com (September 2006); European Voice, www.european-voice.com (cited September 2006).

Ben Wynne, Ph.D
Gainesville State College

European Public Health Association (EUPHA)

Founded in 1992, the European Public Health Association (EUPHA) serves as an umbrella organization for health associations in Europe. It is an international, multidisciplinary scientific association that brings together more than 10,000 public health experts for professional exchange and collaboration. The organization includes almost 50 members and three associate members from 38 European countries and is governed by an elected Executive Council. The EUPHA's mission revolves around being a proactive platform for public health professionals in research and practice and providing a medium to link theses concerned parties and policy-makers. The Association seeks to promote and strengthen public health research and practice in Europe; improve communication between researchers, practitioners, and policy-makers, provide a platform for the exchange of information, experience and research; and encourage and promote effective European joint research and other activities an the field of public health research and health services research in Europe. In accomplishing its mission and goals, the EUPHA has created specific sections to explore individual healthcare themes and bring together public health professionals working in the same or closely related fields.

These sections are open to all EUPHA members, and among the themes are food nutrition, epidemiology, social security and health, child and adolescent health, public health practice and policy, migrant health, health services research, infectious disease control, utilization of medicines, and public health genetics. Each year, the EUPHA sponsors a number of meetings including a major national convention of researchers, practitioners, and policy-makers that focuses on the factors that cause diseases, disease control and cure, and the ongoing need to promote positive lifestyle changes for individuals. The International Scientific Research Committee of the EUPHA selects from hundreds of proposals those papers that will be presented and chooses topics for a wide variety of workshops.

Since its inception, the Association has also worked with other groups to promote a wide rage of projects, programs, and initiatives. Along with the Open Society Institute (OSI), the EUPHA has established a major initiative for the support of public health associations as key links between governments, the scientific community, and the general population in central and eastern Europe. In addition, the Association regularly collaborates with the American Public Health Association (APHA), the Association of Schools of Public Health in the European Region (ASPHER), the European Health Management Association (EHMA), the International Union of Health Promotion and Education (IUHPE), the World Federation of Public Health Associations (WFPHA), and the World Health Orga-

nization/Regional Office for Europe (WHO/EURO). Six times a year, the EUPHA publishes the *European Journal of Public Health*, a peer-reviewed journal that includes original research articles and provides a forum for discussion and debate on current international health issues with a focus on Europe.

SEE ALSO: Healthcare, Europe; European Public Health Alliance (EPHA).

BIBLIOGRAPHY. Association of Schools of Public Health in the European Region, www.aspher.org (cited September 2006); Wilhelm Kirch, ed., *Public Health in Europe* (Springer, 2004); World Federation of Public Health Associations www.wfpha.org (cited September 2006); World Health Organization, *The European Health Report 2005: Public Health Action for Healthier Children and Populations* (World Health Organization, 2005); European Public Health Association, www.eupha.org (cited September 2006).

BEN WYNNE, PH.D
GAINESVILLE STATE COLLEGE

Evidence-Based Medicine

Evidence-based medicine (EBM) is a process clinicians can use to integrate current research and personal clinical expertise to make informed diagnostic, prognostic, therapeutic, and preventive decisions. At its ideal, EBM is a process of self-directed learning that provides clinicians with a lifelong method of updating clinical knowledge in a targeted, patient-centered fashion. The increasing organization and availability of up-to-date research on a broad range of topics makes EBM important and possible for all practitioners.

STEPS OF EBM

EBM processes can be broken down into five steps:

1) Formulate a question relevant to the elements found in the mnemonic PICO: patient, intervention, comparison, and outcome.
2) Identify the current best sources of reliable evidence.
3) Evaluate the evidence.
4) Apply evidence.
5) Evaluate performance.

Step one, formulating a focused clinical question, is critical, as the structure of the question guides the subsequent steps. The ideal question considers the elements of the mnemonic PICO: patient and the patient's condition (P), describes the specific intervention (I), or more broadly, considers questions of etiology, diagnosis, treatment, prognosis, or cost-effectiveness, asks about comparison (C) intervention when appropriate, and considers the desired outcome (O).

Step two is accomplished ideally through targeted search strategies in appropriate databases. The quantity of information has expanded, particularly with greater accessibility on the internet. Important sources of information directed at EBM include the Cochrane Library, the American College of Physicians Journal Club, and MEDLINE. The Cochrane Library is the product of an international collaboration between clinicians, consumers, and researchers whose primary purpose is to promulgate systematic reviews that serve as an authoritative summation of the medical literature on topics relevant to clinical practice. The American College of Physicians Club and the *British Medical Journal* serve as sources of up-to-date medical research.

In step three, studies are evaluated according to two criteria, the first being "levels of evidence" that assign different levels of strength to research based on methodology and study design. This is determined by the type of question and by the rigor of the study design and subsequent statistical tests. The second criteria is importance of the evidence to the clinician's specific question.

In step four, the clinician evaluates the situation, his or her clinical knowledge, and patient preferences to integrate the evidence to answer the initial question. In step five, the clinician evaluates his or her ability to carry out these four steps to reflect on his or her performance.

EBM IN DEVELOPING COUNTRY SETTING

In a developing country setting, obstacles to implementing evidence-based medicine include unreliable access to information, including electronic repositories of information, may make implementation of EBM difficult. However, it has been suggested that inculcating healthcare workers with the skills and philosophy of EBM may improve not only medical practice but also the quality of evidence in these settings.

SEE ALSO: Case-Control Study; Cohort Study; Randomized Control Trial.

BIBLIOGRAPHY. Center for Evidence Based Medicine, http://cebm.net/; Antonio Dans and Leonila Dans, "The Need and Means for Evidence-Based Medicine in Developing Countries," *Evidence Based Medicine* (v.5, 2000); David Sackett, *Evidence-Based Medicine: How to Practice and Teach EBM* (Churchill Livingstone, 1988); Laura Zazowski, Christine Seibert, and Selma VanEyck, "Evidence-Based Medicine: Answering Questions of Diagnosis," *Clinical Medicine & Research* (v.2/1, 2004).

CONSTANCE W. LIU, M.D.
CASE WESTERN RESERVE UNIVERSITY

Exercise for Children

Exercise is a subcategory of physical activity (an umbrella term meaning any bodily movement produced by skeletal muscles that leads to anexpenditure of energy above the basal level, including work and leisure) that is planned, structured, repetitive, and aims to improve or maintain to a greater or lesser extent our physical fitness. It is well-known that physical exercise brings about many well known physical, psychological and social benefits to children. In comparison to adults and adolescents, exercise in children requires specific adjustments in terms of both type of exercise and load, requires an active involvement and supervision on behalf of parents, and most importantly, children should see it as a fun activity to do rather than an obligation.

HEALTH BENEFITS OF EXERCISE

Active children have higher levels of muscle and bone strength, a smaller risk of developing type 2 diabetes as well as a tendency toward lower blood pressure and cholesterol levels.

Exercise also helps children develop social skills such as sharing, taking turns, cooperation, sense of belonging and learning about winning and losing. It also enhances physical skills like eye–hand coordination and ball skills. Furthermore, it may help foster stress coping strategies, as exercise may help children overcome difficulties with sleep, concentration, socializing, or with any emotional challenges of the daily routine,

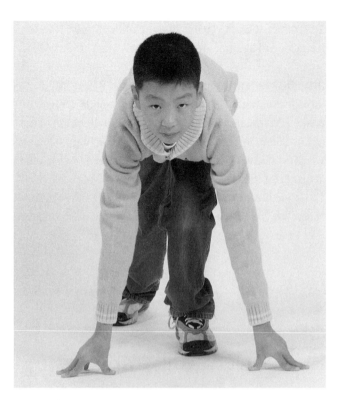

Exercise for children has many benefits including improved health and fostering social skills.

such as running to catch a bus or studying for a test. It also makes them have a better outlook on life.

On the other hand, developing regular exercising habits in children, in combination with healthy eating patterns is a good way to achieve weight control and to avoid becoming overweight and obese in this age group. Moreover, it should be noted that young children should avoid prolonged periods of inactivity (no more than one hour unless they're sleeping or two hours in case of school-age children).

Children are more likely to be motivated and stick to a certain type of exercise or sport if their families engage actively in that sort of activity and act as role models. The family should also not forget that, above all, exercise in children should be a fun activity. However, there is the danger of trespassing a threshold of healthy involvement when families become overinvolved and competitive and try to push their children into attaining goals and pursuing levels of exercise they are not ready or interested to pursue.

Overexercising can cause similar effects to those of anorexia nervosa, such as weight loss, overuse injuries and hormonal imbalances like amenorrhoea. On the other hand, many children with anorexia nervosa also overexercise.

TYPES OF EXERCISE
The ideal type of exercise for children depends on the age group. Children are normally not ready for competitive sport until around age 8 or 9. Suitable activities for children under about 8 years include walking, cycling, kicking, throwing and hitting balls, using playgrounds, water activities, dancing, gymnastics, martial arts at a noncompetitive level, or taking pets for a walk or run.

AMOUNT OF EXERCISE
The American Heart Association recommends that children age 2 and older undergo at least 30 minutes of enjoyable, moderate-intensity activities on a daily basis, as well as 30 minutes of vigourous physical activities at least three to four days each week to achieve a good level of cardiovascular fitness. A suitable alternative is to split those 30 minute periods into two 15- or three 10-minute periods during the day.

The National Association for Sport and Physical Education (NASPE) states that for infants, there are no specific exercise requirements, and that exercise should encourage motor development. As for toddlers, it advocates one and a half hours of minimum daily activity, namely 30 minutes of planned physical activity and 60 minutes of unstructured physical activity (free play). As far as preschool children are concerned, it recommends two hours of minimum daily activity, including 60 minutes of planned physical activity and 60 minutes of unstructured physical activity. Finally, it calls for one hour or more broken up into bouts of 15 minutes or more. Even though children tend to spend a lot of time in sedentary activities such as television, computer games, the internet, and homework, time allocated to exercise should come at the expense of reducing these sedentary activities. Even if children are involved in competitive sport, they need to be protected from injury. Thus, it is important to incorporate warm-up and cool-down exercises, as well as to wear protective gear such as knee pads or helmets.

SEE ALSO: Exercise for Seniors; Exercise/Physical Fitness; Sports Injuries.

BIBLIOGRAPHY. National Association for Sport and Physical Education, www.aahperd.org/naspe/ (cited October

2006); U.S. Department of Health and Human Services, www.healthierus.gov/dietaryguidelines (cited September 2006); KidsHealth, www.kidshealth.org/parent/nutrition_fit/fitness/exercise.html (cited September 2006).

TIAGO VILLANUEVA
CENTRO HOSPITALAR DE LISBOA-ZONA
CENTRAL, PORTUGAL
KARIM KHAN
INDEPENDENT SCHOLAR

Exercise for Seniors

Exercise changes the body's chemistry. Seniors benefit by improving quality of life, slowing the processes of deterioration, maintaining overall fitness leading to greater independence in later years. The long-term Harvard Nurses' Health Study indicated specific benefits of mild-to-moderate exercise. Just getting moving is the first step. Including any activity to increase movement, from gardening to golf or dancing, allows a person to start expending energy, allows the muscles to work.

Benefits from exercise include physical, psychological, and quality of life. Physical benefits include fewer fatal heart attacks, diminished risk for stroke, reduced risk for some cancers, and maintained bone density. Psychological benefits include the release of endorphins acting as antidepressants, decreased stress and improved coping skills, better mood, improved feeling of well-being, and better attitude. Quality-of-life benefits include increased energy and endurance, improved sleep, and better sexual function. Existing medical conditions are not an excuse to keep from exercising. Exercise can provide improvement. For arthritis, professionals recommend low impact, starting slow, and paying attention to the body's signals like additional pain to stop. For those people with diabetes or diabetes risk factors, exercise improves the body's ability to convert blood sugar to energy and has a stabilizing effect on blood sugar.

While many professionals suggest 30 minutes of exercise every day is ideal, studies have shown that one to two hours every week provides some improvement. The important message is to get regular exercise.

During middle age, muscles begin to shrink, and joints begin to stiffen with diminished joint flexibility.

Building muscles creates strong muscles and bones, tones the muscle to do the work it is intended to do, supporting the body and providing strength to perform daily activities. The most effective muscle workout is to exercise major muscle groups. Allow the muscles to recuperate for 48 hours before repeating. Don't do the same exercise every day; vary the routine to allow muscles the time needed to recover and to work different muscle groups.

Using light weights, dumbbells, or resistance bands to work the eight major muscle groups needing attention include chest, back, abdominals, biceps, triceps, shoulder, buttocks, and hips and legs, improves muscle tone. Push ups, sit ups, and squats are all strength exercises and work by lifting the body's own weight. Consulting a professional before beginning a weight program or performing the exercises under professional supervision decreases the risk of injury and improves the efficiency of the exercise.

STRETCHING AND BALANCE

Aging adults experience slower reaction times and diminished sense of body position. Stretching and balance exercises improve the body's ability to know when it is off balance and take action to remedy the situation. Stretching may reduce the risk of injuries from falls. Books, videos, and television programs provide a variety of stretching exercises designed for seniors; some can even be done while sitting. Pilates and the martial arts disciplines all involve stretching and bending. Seniors can find a stretching program suitable to their interest and abilities.

AEROBIC EXERCISE

Continuous, uninterrupted, gentle exercise that encourages deep breathing but doesn't allow the senior to get out of breath burns fat for energy, requires oxygen and engages heart and lungs increasing lung capacity, improving heart function. To get out of breath means the exercise is anaerobic and is burning glycogen instead fat as the main source of energy. The longer a person goes without exercising, fat burning enzymes diminish leading to fat deposits and being overweight. Aerobic exercise can be from mild to moderate to strenuous. Walking is an example of a mild aerobic exercise. Bicycling is an example of a moderate exercise. Running is an example of a strenuous or vigorous exercise. Seniors have numer-

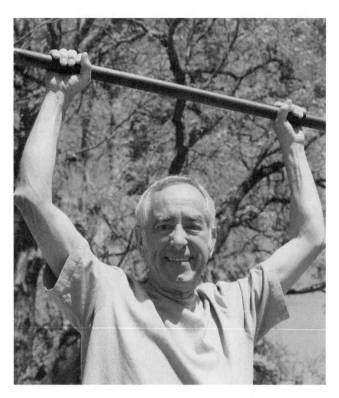

Physical benefits for seniors include fewer fatal heart attacks, diminished risk for stroke, and maintained bone density.

ous aerobic exercises to choose from including dancing, swimming, rowing, cross-country skiing, skating, racket sports, and aerobic classes.

SAFETY AND INJURY PREVENTION

Sports injuries common to older exercisers are pulled muscles, torn ligaments and tendons, dislocated joints, and broken bones. To prevent these injuries, it is imperative to exercise within personal physical limits.

Seniors beginning an exercise program should consult with their physician to determine their capabilities and limitations. Physicians may perform a stress test to see how much pressure the heart muscle can take and also the maximum heart rate and target heart rates during exercise. Sports literature provides a quick heart rate formula adjusted for age: 220 minus age equals the maximum heart rate and suggests working out at 65 to 80 percent of maximum heart rate will proved the aerobic zone. Keep in mind the formula is based on average and everyone is an individual with individual needs. A stress test will determine the individual maximum heart rate. They will also help the patient choose exercise option geared to the patient's diagnosis and

risk factors. Women at risk for osteoporosis and the potential of fractures from falls may find the most benefit from tai chi and strength training with resistance bands. Men at risk for heart disease may achieve better overall health benefit from aerobic exercise.

Exercise should start slow and increase gradually. Include a five minute warm-up with stretching to help prevent injuries by supplying blood flow and oxygen to muscles. Wear protective gear appropriate to the sport, for example, helmets for biking; helmets, knee pads, elbow pads, and wrist protection for rollerblading. Take advantage of the professional assistance to make sure exercises are done with the proper form. Remember to do cool-down exercises after strenuous exercise to allow the heart rate to return to normal gradually, reduce lactic acid in the muscle tissue (lactic acid causes cramping, sore muscles, and pain), and prevent blood from pooling in the lower extremities.

SEE ALSO: Gerontology.

BIBLIOGRAPHY. Theodore Berland, *Fitness for Life* (American Association of Retired Persons, 1986); Edward L. Schneider, and Elizabeth Miles, *Ageless Take Control of Your Age and Stay Youthful for Life* (Rodale, 2003); C. Bree Johnston, William L. Lyons, and Kenneth E. Covinsky, "Geriatric Medicine" in *Current Medical Diagnosis & Treatment 2004* (Lange, 2004).

LYN MICHAUD
INDEPENDENT SCHOLAR

Exercise/Physical Fitness

Exercise is a means of combating one of the greatest dilemmas facing many developed countries. This issue is the consequences that arise from being overweight. This excess weight stresses our body's systems. Additionally, when extra weight is present, quality of life also diminishes. Ultimately, many of us are not living to our full potential. Although this description sounds grim, the battle of the bulge can be won. All of us have the ability to fight back and win. There are two parts of the equation to fight this battle: diet and exercise. Essentially, a healthy diet includes eating in moderation a variety of good foods from the food pyramid.

The second part of the equation is exercise. Although diet is important to our health and well-being, we will focus on exercise. Good old-fashioned exercise, of just moving your body, is a part of the solution to either target excess weight or maintain a healthy weight.

Exercise is not a bad word. Exercise or physical activity is as simple as the major shoe brand ad "Just Do It," or is it? Yet if just doing physical activity is so easy, then why do the developed countries suffer from obesity? So "just doing it" must be more complex than what the shoe ad claims.

REASONS TO EXERCISE

One of the main reasons is that cardiovascular disease is the number one killer in the United States. The American Heart Association (AHA) Web site lists 10 risk factors for cardiovascular disease: age, heredity, smoking, alcohol, high cholesterol, high blood pressure, excess weight, diabetes mellitus, stress, and lack of activity. Because we know that we are getting older and we cannot change our heredity, these risk factors will not be mentioned further. The remaining eight risk factors are controllable, meaning we can do something about them. Of these eight risk factors, let us focus on lack of activity. If we were to change lack of activity to physical activity, then how does that change the remaining seven risk factors? Physical activity is known to decrease high cholesterol. Specifically, low-density lipoprotein (LDL), which is considered the "bad" cholesterol, decreases; and high-density lipoprotein (HDL), which is the "good" cholesterol, increases. Exercise allows our body to use the HDL to help clean our blood vessels of the bad cholesterol. This change makes it easier for the heart to pump. Next, exercise causes a decrease in blood pressure. Exercise causes blood pressure to drop by strengthening the heart so that it can pump more efficiently while also improving the stretchiness of the blood vessels themselves. Physical activity also decreases weight. Not only does the actual physical activity burn calories, but continual exercise increases muscle mass. An increase in muscle mass allows the body to burn more calories at rest. The symptoms of diabetes mellitus are decreased or even completely eradicated as a result of physical activity. Many of the symptoms diabetics suffer from such as tingling/pain in the extremities and cuts healing slowly are a direct result of poor circulation. Again, exercise improves the heart's ability to pump and the vessels' ability to distribute the blood; therefore, the cells of the body, such as nerve cells or skin cells, get the necessary oxygen and nutrients from the blood that they need to function and repair themselves. Another major problem of diabetics is the ability of their cells to respond to insulin. Exercise directly improves the cells' ability to respond to insulin. Last, physical activity decreases stress. Physical activity does not remove the stressors from your life, but it makes you feel more in control and focused, essentially better equipped to handle the stressors of life. Hence, by changing one risk factor, you have decreased or removed another five risk factors.

Physical activity has other benefits as well. Increasing activity will also decrease the risk of certain types of cancer. Previous research has shown that regular exercise can decrease the risks of colorectal and lung cancer. Specifically important for men, exercise can also reduce the risk of prostate cancer. Additionally, the risks of getting breast and endometrial cancer are reduced by regular physical exercise. Beneficial to men, but of particular importance to older women, is the fact that activity increases bone density which decreases the risk of osteoporosis. Physical activity in children has the same benefits as it does in adults. When children exercise, it improves their cardiovascular system as well. Of note to the parents, children who are physically active sleep better. For parents of teenagers, physical activity helps with stress, especially during puberty. Puberty can be a very stressful and uncertain time for teenagers. Physical activity, again, helps teenagers cope with everyday stresses and helps build their self-esteem. Both of these points are crucial during puberty. Maintaining an active lifestyle during pregnancy helps decrease the discomforts of expectant mothers. We now know that maintaining and even starting (under the guidance of a physician) an exercise regime during pregnancy is safe and beneficial to the mother and baby. Exercise during pregnancy helps a woman maintain agility so she can continue with her everyday activities throughout the pregnancy. Exercise also decreases the pains associated with pregnancy. Exercise also improves her self-esteem. Additionally, labor and delivery times decrease. For the elderly, activity slows down the aging process. For people of any age, exercise gives you more confidence and improves your self-esteem. Another important benefit of physical activity is energy. For those who feel exhausted and tired all the time, exercise helps. Although exercise cannot make up for a lack of sleep, it does give you an energy boost. In this way, it is true that exercise is a paradox; if you want energy, then you need to use energy. If you use your energy being physically active, then you will gain more energy from it. Exercise is great for the body and can be done at any age and stage of life.

REASONS FOR NOT EXERCISING

Besides, these numerous benefits of exercise, most people still do not do it. To really get people moving, we need to truly understand why we are not active. The five main reasons people do not exercise are embarrassment, unable to exercise vigorously, do not enjoy it, lack of time, and money. Whether you have an extra 15 pounds or 150 pounds or more, most people who need to lose weight (and from the figures, statistical and otherwise, this is most people), we feel insecure about exposing our skin and fat.

Most people have a "fear" of being seen wearing shorts and a T-shirt. Then mentioning the idea of going to a public place (i.e., around your block or a gym) in shorts, most people will not do it even if their doctor tells them they must for health reasons. Now, besides being overweight and embarrassed by being seen exposed in shorts and a T-shirt, we have to try to figure out how to use all of these new machines which look like some ancient torture devices—it's no wonder many people cannot break out of the "fat mold." For most people, the embarrassment factor is too great for them to overcome. Additionally, many people do not begin exercise because they are unable to move. For people so overweight that they have lost mobility, it is not only embarrassing but physically difficult to move their body.

For these individuals, the idea of exercising vigorously is not possible. Another reason most people are not physically active is because they simply do not enjoy exercise. For many people, walking on a treadmill, for example, is extremely boring. Even if a physician tells you to exercise, if you do not enjoy it, why would you start doing it and keep doing it. Simply put, most people do not voluntarily do something for 30 or more minutes, three or more times per week if they find it boring. Despite our many technological advances to help us save time, it is a real challenge to find the time to exercise. People, in general, work at least eight hours a day, then have numerous activities they or their families are involved in which occupy all of their time. People are so busy with work, clubs, committees, and driving their children to sports that they cannot find time to be physically active. Last, many people do not exercise because of the additional expense. In order to lose weight, many people will join a gym or fitness center which is very costly. Especially for people with middle- to lower-class incomes who need to lose weight, they cannot justify the cost of gym membership for their health. There are many valid areas that need to be addressed to get people moving and to keep them active for years to come.

GETTING STARTED

To address these issues and to get people moving, remember to CARE. This acronym stands for Commit, Accountable, Realistic, and Excite. First of all, we need to commit today. We need to first commit to doing 10 minutes of activity three times every week. This can be done by making an appointment either mentally in your daily schedule or physically

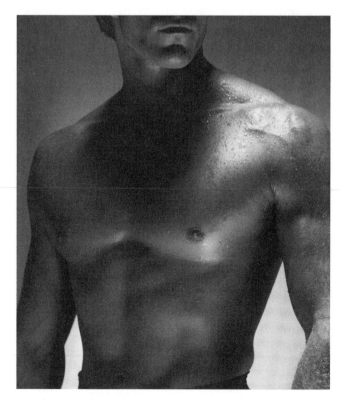

Exercise is a part of the solution to either target excess weight or maintain a healthy weight.

write it in your day planner. The first step affirms a commitment to living healthier. Next, it is crucial to be accountable to someone to keep this appointment. If someone is a disciplined person, then once he or she makes an appointment or plan, he or she will follow through no matter what. Many people are not this disciplined; therefore, it is crucial to enlist a friend, coworker, boyfriend/girlfriend, or husband/wife. Be honest to determine the type of accountability needed. Once accountability is established to help achieve the task of maintaining physical activity, then set a goal and a starting point. The goal and starting point must be realistic. Depending on a person's initial fitness level, the starting point may be to walk the length of the house or apartment three times for three days.

The physical activity does not need to start at a vigorous pace for the beginner; this is something that can be changed later. If this is the case, then the first goal would be to be active 10 minutes a day for three days of the week. Once this goal is achieved, then the next goal would be 30 minutes of activity for three times per week. If possible, continue to add time until the activity lasts for 40 minutes, and then add days of activity with six days being the maximum. During this process of adding time or days, changing the intensity level, or how hard you work, is a great way to improve health. Next, and one of the most important points, is experiment with what is exciting. People will continue to be active if they enjoy what they are doing! To find what is exciting, the key is experiment with different types of aerobic activities: biking (outside or stationary), hiking, rowing, swimming, aerobics classes (step aerobics, jazzercise, tae bo, etc.), walking (outside or on a treadmill), or a strength training circuit.

The local public library is a valuable source of exercise videos that can be checked out for free. This resource will help people experiment with what is exciting and can be done at home to avoid feeling embarrassed. Because these videos are free at the public library, the cost of beginning an exercise regime is just time. Last, add an S to the acronym CARE to get CARES. One of the most important principles is "something is better than nothing." Based on the physics principle of inertia (objects in motion tend to stay in motion and objects at rest tend to stay at rest), the most difficult part of exercising is starting. So, get up and do something today. After starting the first day, it will get easier every time thereafter. Because he or she CARES, we will start moving today.

EXERCISE PRESCRIPTION

Now that we know what needs to be done to get started, what is the ultimate goal suggested by the AHA for decreasing cardiovascular risk factors. The AHA suggests 30 to 40 minutes of vigorous physical activity three to six times per week. However, this can be spread throughout the day into three 10-minute sessions, for example. Remember, most people will not start at this level, but this may be a long-term goal to achieve after months or years. The AHA states that even walking at a slow pace for one hour per week reduces the risks of cardiovascular disease for women in half. Additionally, the AHA's Web site suggests a strength and flexibility component. To reiterate, the strength component of an exercise program helps build muscle mass which will increase the calories burned at rest. The flexibility component of exercise helps prevent injury to the joints during exercise and during normal daily activities. This exercise "prescription" is to decrease the cardiovascular risk factors. A person's initial fitness level will determine the intensity of the activity. The harder the intensity of exercise will cause the cardiovascular system to work harder, thus increasing the heart rate. Therefore, the intensity of exercise can be determined by heart rate (HR). To determine if the exercise is at the intensity of choice, one must calculate target HR. Target HR is just that— the pulse (or heart rate) that one aims to reach during the physical activity. There are numerous ways to determine HR; below are two different formulas:

$$[(HRmax - HRrest) \times \% \text{ intensity}] + HRrest$$
$$(HRmax - Adjuster) \pm 5 \text{ bpm}$$

To determine HRmax, one of the following formulas can be used. Target HR will vary slightly depending on the formula used, but this will be a good start. To find HRrest, take a pulse for one minute first thing in the morning (waking up without an alarm clock) while still in bed. This is done by placing your index and middle finger gently on the inside of the wrist (thumb side). A general guide for intensity level is low/light 50 to 60 percent, medium 60 to 70 percent, hard/high 70 to 80 percent, and elite >80 percent. For the equation, move the decimal point after the 0 over two spots to the left (i.e., 50 percent becomes 0.50). A quick check on intensity that does not involve math is the "talk test." The intensity is too easy if a person can talk easily. Conversely, the intensity is too hard if a conversation is not possible. By using these principles, a person can determine if he or she is exercising at an appropriate level.

Determining target HR is important for knowing the level of intensity of exercise. However, even if the level of intensity is light, the ultimate goal to achieve numerous health benefits is 30 minutes a day, three times per week. This goal can be achieved by Committing, being Accountable, setting Realistic goals, experimenting with what is Exciting, and by doing Something. While working toward this goal, do something exciting at a comfortable pace and place. Ultimately, these changes will decrease the cardiovascular risk factors. Decreasing these risk factors enables the cardiovascular system to function more effectively and for the rest of the body to feel good.

SEE ALSO: Exercise for Children; Exercise for Seniors.

BIBLIOGRAPHY. Peter Brukner, Karim Khan, and John Kron, *The Encyclopedia of Exercise, Sport and Health* (Allen & Unwin, 2004); Frank J. Cerny and Harold W. Burton, *Exercise Physiology for Health Care Professionals* (Human Kinetics, 2001).

LINDA MAY
KANSAS CITY UNIVERSITY OF MEDICINE
AND BIOSCIENCES

Exercise Treadmill Test

An exercise treadmill test (ETT) is an real-time evaluation of the heart while under cardiovascular stress. A primary care provider or well-trained professional performs ETTs in the outpatient setting. The testing is performed with a treadmill or bicycle and the heart's electrical activity (electrocardiogram, EKG), blood pressure, heart rate, and pain levels are measured. Individuals undergoing this exam have typically exhibited unclear chest discomfort or signs of myocardial ischemia and have significant risk factors for coronary artery disease (CAD). The ETT aims to reproduce any chest discomfort or electrical changes in the heart for an evaluation of worsening disease. ETTs are most beneficial in symptomatic men, older than 45 years old with risk factors for CAD, and are least predictive of disease in women, and individuals less than 35 years old.

Although there are numerous acceptable protocols to complete an ETT, the overall goal remains consistent. The intensity of the treadmill increases until the patient reaches approximately 85 percent of his or her predicted maximum heart rate for his or her age group. If any type of pain occurs prior to reaching this goal, the testing may be terminated early. Interpretation of ETTs involve monitoring the EKG, heart rate, and blood pressure values for changes indicative of worsening ischemia, decreased exercise capacity, or arrhythmias. Following the results, a clinician may determine that this patient is a candidate for angioplasty, a procedure involving the unblocking of the heart's coronary arteries.

ETT is relatively safe, but as myocardial infarctions occur in 1 of 2,500 tests, clinical discretion of which patients are most appropriate for testing is imperative. Patients with cardiac arrhythmias, electrical conduction blocks, a recent heart attack, or uncontrolled heart failure represent absolute contraindications. Patients who are overly obese, have difficulty walking, have significant pulmonary disease, or have central nervous system disorders may have limitations preventing testing completion; thus, other testing modalities may need to be performed. ETT can be combined with further imaging including ultrasound (echocardiography), to visualize the heart's wall motion, or with nuclear imaging to measure heart muscle perfusion.

SEE ALSO: American Heart Association (AHA); Cardiologist; Coronary Disease; Heart Attack; Heart Diseases (General); Heart Disease—Prevention.

BIBLIOGRAPHY. "ACC/AHA 2002 Guideline Update for Exercise Testing," www.americanheart.org (cited July 2002); Sharonne N. Hayes and Patrick McBride, "Diagnosing Coronary Heart Disease: When to Use Stress Imaging Studies," *The Journal of Family Practice* (v.52/7, 2003).

STEPHANIE F. INGRAM
UNIVERSITY OF SOUTH FLORIDA COLLEGE OF MEDICINE

Extragonadal Germ Cell Tumor

Extragonadal germ cell tumor (EGCT) originates from developing cancerous sperm or egg cells traveling from gonads to other parts of the body. The term *extragonadal* means *outside of the gonads* (reproductive organs). Germ cells refer to the reproductive cells such as the sperms and the eggs which are initially located in the yolk sac outside of the embryo. During development, the germ cells migrate to the embryo into the pelvis to become ovarian cells or into the scrotal sac as testicular cells. EGCT develops when these germ cells migrate to other parts of the body and begin to grow. EGCTs are rare among germ cell tumors and can be either benign (noncancerous) or malignant (cancerous). Benign EGCTs are called benign teratomas, which are often large and more common than malignant EGCTs. The great majority of these tumors is benign and can be treated with surgery alone; most of these benign tumors occur in children.

Although benign tumors do not spread, they may cause other problems such as pressing on nearby organs. On the other hand, malignant EGCTs can be divided into two types: nonseminoma (e.g., embryonal carcinoma, yolk sac tumor, and mixed germ cell tumors) and seminoma (or germinoma in females). Although they are much more common in males with the malignant form, extragonadal tumors can also occur in females with equal frequency as in males for the benign type. Nonseminomas tend to grow and spread more quickly than seminomas. As a result, they usually are large and cause symptoms. If untreated, malignant EGCTs may metastasize to the lungs, lymph nodes, bones, liver, or other parts of the body.

EGCTs can be diagnosed via a variety of tests and investigations such as biopsy (removing a sample of tumor for examination under microscope), complete blood count and other blood tests, and medical imaging such as computed tomography (CT) scan, magnetic resonance imaging (MRI), X-ray, and ultrasound. In addition, EGCTs often produce proteins, sometimes known as tumor markers, that can be measured from the blood. These markers are alpha-fetoprotein (AFP) and human chorionic gonadotrophin (HCG), and their levels are checked in the diagnosis of EGCT as well as monitored throughout treatment.

There are different treatments available for EGCT patients and several factors need to be considered when designing a treatment plan: whether the tumor is nonseminoma or seminoma, size and location of the tumor, levels of tumor markers in the blood, extent of metastasis, initial response to treatment, and recurrence. Typically, patients with nonseminoma EGCT-carrying tumor in the back of the abdomen with slightly higher tumor marker levels in the blood and no spread of tumor to other organs are given good prognosis. In contrast, patients with nonseminoma EGCT-carrying tumor in the chest with high level of tumor markers and metastasis of tumor cells to organs other than the lungs have poor prognosis. There are three standard treatments available: radiation therapy, chemotherapy, and surgery. For seminoma, treatments often involve radiation therapy for small tumors in one area. Chemotherapy is administered if the tumors are larger or have spread, and surgery might be required if there is large tumor remaining after chemotherapy. For nonseminoma, chemotherapy followed by surgery is often performed to remove any remaining tumor.

SEE ALSO: Cancer; Chemotherapy; Chemoradiotherapy; Childhood Cancers; Liver Cancer; Lung Cancer.

BIBLIOGRAPHY. Mark H. Beers, Robert S. Porter, and Thomas V. Jones, eds., *The Merck Manual of Diagnosis and Therapy*, 18th ed. (Merck Research Laboratories, 2006); Raymond E. Lenhard Jr., Robert T. Osteen, and Ted Gansler, eds., *Clinical Oncology* (American Cancer Society, 2001).

STEPHEN CHEN
UNIVERSITY OF TORONTO

Eye Cancer

The eye is anatomically complex. It has three major parts: the globe, the orbit, and the adnexal structures. From anterior to posterior, the globe contains the cornea, the uvea, the lens, and the retina. The uvea is comprised of the choroid, the iris, and the ciliary body. Cancers that affect the globe, or eyeball, are called intraocular (within the eye) cancers. The orbit consists of the tissues surrounding the globe. This includes the extraocular muscles that are responsible for moving the globe and the nerves attached to the eye. Cancers affecting these tissues are referred to as orbital cancers. The adnexal (or accessory) structures include the eyelids and tear glands. Cancers in this area are called adnexal cancers.

INTRAOCULAR CANCERS

Intraocular cancers can be either primary or secondary. Secondary intraocular cancers are cancers that have spread to the eye from another part of the body. Breast and lung cancers are among the most common cancers to spread to the eye, usually to the uvea. In contrast, primary cancers originate inside the globe. Melanoma is the most common primary intraocular cancer in adults, followed by lymphoma. Melanomas of the eye are classified as anterior when arising in the iris and posterior when arising in the choroid or ciliary body. Ninety percent of intraocular melanomas are posterior choroidal, with nearly the remaining 10 percent being melanomas of the iris. Posterior choroidal melanoma arises from melanocytes in the choroid. The incidence in the United States is approximately six cases per 1 million and is highest around age 55, although this figure varies in regions with more or less sun exposure.

Choroidal melanoma commonly results in partial or complete visual loss in the affected eye due to either tumor destruction of ocular tissues or as a consequence of treatment. It is associated with a mortality rate of 30 to 50 percent within 10 years, owing to its highly metastatic nature. There is currently no effective treatment for intraocular melanomas, although enucleation (removal of the eye while sparing orbital contents) and irradiation are potentially life saving. Primary intraocular lymphoma is the next most common intraocular malignancy in adults but remains exceedingly rare. An intraocular lymphoma is considered extranodal and is always of the non-Hodgkin type (as opposed to Hodgkin's lymphoma). The elderly and patients with human immunodeficiency virus (HIV)/AIDS have a propensity for this cancer, likely due to their immunocompromised state. Over 80 percent of patients develop cerebral involvement, which is associated with a much poorer prognosis. Randomized treatment trials are scarce owing to the rarity of this cancer, but case reports support external beam radiation as an effective treatment.

In children, retinoblastoma is the most common primary intraocular cancer, followed by medulloepi-thelioma. Retinoblastoma is a tumor of the retinal photoreceptor precursor cells. It occurs due to mutations in the RB1-gene, although only 5 percent of patients who develop the disease have a positive family history. It has an incidence of approximately 11 per 1 million children worldwide. It occurs mostly in children younger than 5 and accounts for three percent of all neoplasms in children under 15. Retinoblastoma can be unilateral or bilateral and is usually first detected by leukocoria (a white papillary reflex replaces the normal red-light reflex). Visual disturbances are often noted because of the intrinsic retinal involvement of this cancer. Management varies per patient and includes radiation, neoadjuvant chemotherapy, and surgery. The most important prognostic factor remains early detection, resulting in survival rates of approximately 86 to 92 percent. Extraocular extension through the sclera or along the optic nerve is associated with higher mortality. Unfortunately, highly advanced cases of retinoblastoma are still seen in the developing world. This can be attributed to neglect, poverty, cultural beliefs, politics, health-seeking behavior, and so forth.

ORBITAL AND ADNEXAL CANCERS

Cancers of the orbit and adnexa are not unique to the eye. They develop from muscle tissue, nerve fibers, and skin, similar to neoplasms found elsewhere in the body. The most common orbital malignancy in adults is a cavernous hemangioma, representing 4.3 percent of all orbital neoplasms. Cavernous hemangioma is a benign, slow-growing, highly vascular lesion. It presents as a painless, unilateral, progressively proptotic eye. Unless visual acuity or field loss is appreciated, conservative management is all that is recommended. The tumor has a predilection for the intraconal space (between the optic nerve and the extraocular muscles); as a result, complications such as compressive optic neuropathy and mortality from intraoperative bleeding can occur. Novel surgical and laser techniques for the management of cavernous hemangiomas are being investigated. A lymphoid tumor is the second most common orbital tumor in adults. Orbital lymphoma is a painless, slow-progressing malignant neoplasm. A past medical history of non-Hodgkin's lymphoma is common. Patients note extraocular motility problems and proptosis as the initial symptoms. The tumor can be diagnosed by biopsy and is managed with focal radiation. Chemotherapy is reserved for those patients with systemic involvement.

The most common orbital tumors in children are capilliary hemangioma, dermoid cyst, and rhabdomyosarcoma. Capilliary hemangioma is a benign vascular lesion that manifests at birth or by 6 months of age. It is characterized as a rapidly enlarging red spongy mass that usually appears in the upper eyelids. The growth phase is normally followed by spontaneous regression beginning at 1 year and is 75 percent complete by 7 years. Due to its size, capilliary hemangiomas have been associated with refractive error and possible ambylopia. There is also a rare association with Kasabach-Merritt syndrome, where platelets are entrapped within a large capilliary hemangioma, causing thrombocytopenia (low platelets) and bleeding diathesis. The most accepted treatment modality is to administer slow and careful intralesion steroid injections. An orbital dermoid cyst is also a benign orbital tumor. It is an example of a choristoma—a tumor that originates from aberrant primordial tissue. They are most commonly found at the junction of cranial sutures, specifically the frontozygomatic suture. Orbital dermoid cysts can grow large enough to displace the globe and compress the extraocular muscles and optic nerve, leading to diplopia and vision loss. Malignant orbital tumors can occur in childhood, the most common being rhabdomyosarcoma. Rhabdomyosarcoma is a cancer of striated muscle origin. Approximately 9 percent of all rhabdomyosarcomas occur in the orbit, with a predilection for the superior nasal orbit. The average age of onset is about 6 years, with a male-to-female ratio of 1.5:1. These tumors grow very rapidly and may infiltrate bone and adjacent tissues and produce marked proptosis. Prognosis is more favorable for orbital rhabdomyosarcoma than for rhabdomyosarcoma elsewhere in the body; however, management remains complex. A biopsy is required for diagnosis, but surgical excision of the tumor is usually limited due to its infiltrative nature. Radiation and chemotherapy comprise the initial treatment regimen.

The most common adnexal tumor is basal cell carcinoma (BCC), followed by squamous cell carcinoma (SCC), melanoma, and sebaceous carcinoma, all involving the eyelid. BCC is described as having a waxy, pearly appearance with a crater-like depression. The tumor is slow growing and is usually secondary to ultraviolet (UV) light exposure. Over 60 percent occur in the lower lid. The tumor rarely metastasizes, but excision with appropriate margins and lid reconstruction is recommended. SCC typically appears as a red, scaly patch with ulceration, crusting, and central keratinization. It is more aggressive than BCC and has been associated with UV light exposure or hereditary diseases such as xeroderma pigmentosa. Unlike BCC, SCC metastasizes often, spreading to the orbit, sinuses, and lacrimal system via direct extension or along nerve sheaths, lymph channels, and blood vessels to more distant sites. It is associated with a mortality of 0 to 30 percent, making early surgical excision with a frozen pathological specimen crucial. Exenteration is necessary when SCC invades the orbita. Melanoma of the eyelid is a different entity than the previously discussed intraocular melanoma. It is most common in elderly whites and represents 1 percent of all lid tumors. Missing eyelashes near a suspicious lesion is a common clinical finding. Over 40 percent of melanomas in the eyelid are amelanotic, making a biopsy warranted when clinical suspicion exists. The depth of invasion is used to stage this highly metastatic tumor; it will also guide the extent of surgical excision required. Cryotherapy should never be used for the treatment of melanoma. Sebaceous carcinoma is one of the most lethal eyelid tumors. Lymph node metastasis occurs in 17 to 23 percent of the cases. The mortality rate increases to 76 percent when orbital extension occurs (6 to 16 percent of the time). Clinically, these tumors have a higher incidence in Asians. They manifest as a painless or irritating enlarging mass, with patients often presenting with a history of recurrent chalazion refractory to treatment. Diagnosis requires properly prepared tissues with a special oil-red O stain. The management of sebaceous carcinoma is multidisciplinary and physicians familiar with this malignancy should be consulted. In addition, wide surgical excision with radical neck dissection and possible radiation is recommended.

SEE ALSO: Eye Care; Eye Diseases (General).

BIBLIOGRAPHY. J. A. Borden, "Treatment of Tumors Involving the Optic Nerves and Chiasm," *Ophthalmology* (v.17/1, 2002); D. Bouvier and C. V. Raghuveer, "Aspiration Cytology of Metastatic Chordoma to the Orbit," *American Journal of Ophthalmology* (v.131/2, 2001); "Cavernous Hemangioma," http://www.emedicine.com/oph/topic216.

htm (cited May 14, 2007); S. J. Chawda and I. F. Moseley, "Computed Tomography of Orbital Dermoids: A 20-Year Review," *Clinical Radiology* (v. 54/12, 1999); "Collaborative Ocular Melanoma Study Report no. 10: The Collaborative Ocular Melanoma Study (COMS) Randomized Trial of Pre-enucleation Radiation of Large Choroidal Melanoma II: Initial Mortality Findings," *American Journal of Ophthalmology* (v.125/6, 1998); J. J. Dutton, "Clinical and Surgical Orbital Anatomy," *Ophthalmology Clinics of North America* (v.9/4, 1996); R. C. Eagle, *Eye Pathology: An Atlas and Basic Text* (Saunders, 1999).

Jared Daniel Ament, M.D., M.P.H.
Harvard Medical School
Harvard School of Public Health

Eye Care

Eye care is a global health issue that holds significant impact on people's lives, yet it has the potential for vast improvement given the proper resources and commitment. While the most common eye care problems are low visual acuity and disorders such as cataract, glaucoma, and diabetic retinopathy, several other issues such as ocular infections and childhood blindness also need to be addressed. As with many global health problems, there is a strong link between poor eye health and poverty or lack of education. While encouraging measures such as Vision 2020 are significantly improving eye health, much more still needs to be done to address this critical, yet relatively easily, health issue.

MAJOR EYE CARE PROBLEMS

It is estimated that there are 259 million people with visual impairment worldwide, including people with refractive error. Of this number, 42 million people are blind, while 217 million have less severe visual impairment. Uncorrected refractive error from problems such as myopia (nearsightedness) or hyperopia (farsightedness) is the major cause of visual impairment worldwide, but can be addressed through measures as simple as prescription eyeglasses. Aside from refractive error, several common eye disorders significantly contribute to visual impairment. Cataract is responsible for approximately half of all blindness worldwide; fortunately, surgery and im-

plantation of a synthetic lens can correct the problem and restore proper visual function to millions. Much of blindness is caused by chronic disorders such as glaucoma (12 percent), diabetic retinopathy (5 percent), and age-related macular degeneration (9 percent), all of which progress slowly and thus difficult to notice. Because these disorders damage nerve cells of the retina, their detrimental effects on vision are largely irreversible. Infectious eye diseases such as trachoma (4 percent) and onchocerciasis (1 percent) used to be major causes of blindness but are now more controlled thanks to coordinated international efforts by the World Health Organization (WHO) and partners. Childhood blindness due to disorders such as amblyopia and congenital (birth) defects affects 1.4 million children worldwide and comprises nearly 4 percent of worldwide blindness. However, because nearly half these cases can be prevented or treated through known measures, there is huge potential for improvement in this area.

Visual impairment undoubtedly harms people's lives through many ways, the most obvious of which is loss of productivity. Even when taking into account the success of the Vision 2020 initiative, unaccommodated blindness alone is responsible for a $44 billion productivity loss every year. The blind and visually impaired face much greater susceptibility to accidents and death, especially in the poorest of nations. Stigma, isolation, and inability to lead normal lives are unquantifiable, yet significant, detriments to quality of life.

RISK FACTORS

There is an undeniable link between poverty and poor eye care. Over 90 percent of the world's blind live in developing countries. Africa is home to 18 percent of the world's blind, while southeast Asia and the western Pacific region are home to 32 percent and 25 percent of global blindness, respectively. Old age is the biggest risk factor for visual impairment; over 82 percent of the world's blind are over age 50. With current trends of increasing longevity, the prevalence of age-associated disorders such as cataract, glaucoma, diabetic retinopathy, and age-related macular degeneration is expected to increase even more in coming years. Social and environmental conditions such as malnutrition, poor hygiene or sanitation, lack of access to early treatment, and lack of knowledge regarding eye care are all major contributors to blindness and visual impairment.

MEASURES TO IMPROVE EYE CARE

In recent years, measures have been taken to improve global eye health. The most significant of these is the Global Initiative for the Elimination of Avoidable Blindness, or Vision 2020—the Right to Sight. This partnership between the WHO and the International Agency for the Prevention of Blindness began in 1999 and aims to eliminate the causes of preventable blindness by the year 2020. Furthermore, Vision 2020 hopes to prevent the projected doubling of worldwide cases of unavoidable visual impairment between 1999 and 2020. In 2006, a monitoring committee evaluated the progress of Vision 2020 and concluded that while the program was lessening increases in blindness and was lowering cases of avoidable blindness worldwide, significant further action was needed in order to meet the program goals.

Recommendations included providing more financial resources for the program, contributing to the underlying problems of socioeconomic stagnation and lack of health awareness, increasing the quality and quantity of human resources through more training, addressing glaring inequities of health access in rural or underserved areas, improving infrastructure and supply storage and delivery, encouraging formation of national-level programs to address eye care, and strengthening coordination among all the partners involved in Vision 2020.

The encouraging feature of global eye care is how certain inexpensive, easily delivered treatments can lead to profound improvement in the lives of millions. In the 1970s, the WHO led an international movement to eliminate xerophthalmia (night blindness) caused by vitamin A deficiency. Simple measures such as the administration of oral drops and dietary supplements were sufficient to cure the disorder. Today, with around 70 nations actively addressing the problem, xerophthalmia is no longer the widespread, debilitating cause of blindness that it once was. When cataract surgery first became widespread, most poor patients could not afford intraocular lens implantation and were forced to use thick glasses in order to see again. The introduction of increasingly efficient cataract operations and inexpensive intraocular lenses now restores normal sight to millions of cataract patients within days after surgery. Much more needs to be done to improve eye care. Such measures will undoubtedly need to address basic health issues such as poverty, hygiene, awareness, and access to timely care. However, given the proper investment, coordination, and dedication, the prospects for systemic improvement in eye care may indeed look hopeful.

SEE ALSO: Amblyopia; Cataract; Cornea and Corneal Disease; Eye Diseases (General); National Eye Institute (NEI); Optometrist; Ophthalmologist; Ophthalmology.

BIBLIOGRAPHY. Lalit Dandona and Rakhi Dandona, "What Is the Global Burden of Visual Impairment?" *BMC Medicine* (v.4, 2006); A. Foster and S. Resnikoff, "The Impact of Vision 2020 on Global Blindness," *Eye* (v.19 , 2005); Kevin D. Frick, "The Magnitude and Cost of Global Blindness: An Increasing Cost that Can Be Alleviated," *American Journal of Ophthalmology* (v.135/4, 2003).

Nakul Shekhawat
Vanderbilt University

Eye Diseases (General)

There are a variety of ocular diseases and pathology that may affect a person's vision. Some common eye diseases and conditions are reviewed here.

REFRACTIVE ERROR

People with emmetropic vision have no refractive error. In these patients, the cornea, which provides two-thirds of refractive power, and the lens, which provides the remaining one-third of refractive power, perfectly focus an image on the retina. By contrast, people with ametropic vision require corrective lenses in order for the image to be in proper focus.

COLOR BLINDNESS

Color blindness is usually an X-linked recessive condition affecting retinal photoreceptors that affects about 10 percent of the male population. There are several forms of color blindness, ranging for asymptomatic types to the most common type where the patient may confuse red with green. Cone dystrophy can also induce diminished color vision. Physicians commonly use the Ishihara or Hardy-Rand-Rittler pseudoisochromatic color vision plates to assess color vision of each eye individually.

DIPLOPIA

Diplopia, or double vision, can be divided into two subtypes—monocular or binocular—and can be intermittent or constant. In monocular diplopia, patients have double vision when closing one eye. In binocular diplopia, patients have double vision only with both eyes open, and closing one eye causes the double vision to disappear. Some causes of monocular diplopia include corneal irregularities, astigmatism, cataracts, and refractive error. A common cause of binocular diplopia is strabismus (misalignment of the eyes) or neuromuscular disorders.

COMMON DISORDERS OF THE EYELIDS

A hordeolum, commonly referred to as a sty, is an infection of the hair follicles or meibomian glands, usually due to *Staphylococcus aureus*. A chalazion is a chronic, granulomatous inflammation of a meibomian gland, which unlike a hordeolum, does not have acute inflammatory signs. Treatment consists of warm compresses and antibiotic ointment, and surgical drainage and excision if unresponsive to medical treatment.

Blepharitis, or inflammation of the eyelid margin, is a very common condition that can be subdivided into anterior and posterior blepharitis. Patients with blepharitis usually have symptoms of burning, itching, redness, and tearing. Anterior blepharitis can be further subdivided into staphylococcal or seborrheic blepharitis. Usually, both types of blepharitis are present. Posterior blepharitis is usually secondary to meibomian gland dysfunction, and patients may have frothy or greasy tears.

A xanthelasma is a common lesion that affects the upper eyelid more often that the lower eyelid. This lesion, while sometimes associated with elevated lipids, can also be found in patients with normal serum lipids.

DRY EYE SYNDROME

In patients with dry eye syndrome, they may have a foreign body sensation with sandy, scratchy, burning, or red eyes. Some of the many causes of dry eye syndrome include hypofunction of the lacrimal gland due to congenital, acquired, infectious, traumatic, or medication-induced causes; mucin deficiency due to chemical burns, medications, chronic conjunctivitis, and Stevens-Johnson syndrome; lipid deficiency due to blepharitis; or defective spreading of the tear film secondary to eyelid abnormalities, lagophthalmos, proptosis, or conjunctival abnormalities. Some diagnostic measures include Schirmer test and assessing tear film breakup time with a slit-lamp examination. Fluorescein staining and slit-lamp examination will show the corneal irregularities present.

Other conditions that can cause foreign body sensation include corneal abrasions, trichiasis (this occurs when eyelashes grow in the wrong direction, touching the conjunctiva), and corneal foreign bodies.

CONJUNCTIVITIS

Conjunctivitis, also referred to as pink-eye, is a common condition that prompts patients to see their physician. Conjunctivitis can be allergic in nature, and can also be caused by many different bacterial and viral infections. The infection can induce redness, tearing, itching, and discharge. While allergic conjunctivitis almost always causes itching, infectious conjunctivitis usually induces discharge. Viral conjunctivitis is more common than bacterial conjunctivitis, and of the viral cases, adenovirus is the most predominant. Patients with conjunctivitis must remember to frequently wash their hands and avoid rubbing their eyes. Treatment is determined by the etiology.

CATARACTS

A cataract is a clouding of the natural lens of the eye. People with cataracts usually experience glare or halos, and symptoms are worse at night. Cataracts can be caused by multiple factors, including normal aging, trauma, or congenital syndromes. People who use chronic steroids are predisposed to both cataract formation and glaucoma. Cataracts are commonly divided into nuclear sclerosis, cortical cataracts, and posterior subcapsular cataracts. All forms of cataracts that are visually significant can be treated with surgery. Surgical correction entails removing the cataract in its entirety and replacing it with a silicone or acrylic lens implant. This lens implant then functions to allow the eye to focus and see clearly after cataract extraction. Patients may or may not need glasses after surgery to maximize their visual potential. Technological advances in the treatment of cataracts has made this one of the most common and successful surgeries of all time.

GLAUCOMA

Risk factors for glaucoma include a family history of glaucoma, age, high blood pressure, African-American descent, and chronic steroid use. There are two types of glaucoma: acute and chronic. Acute glaucoma, also called angle closure glaucoma, causes sudden pain and an acute increase in intraocular pressure. This is an emergency in which the patient needs to be immediately seen by an ophthalmologist. Chronic, or open-angle glaucoma, is significantly more common that acute glaucoma, and is characterized by increased intraocular pressure, increased optic cup to disk ratio, and visual field defects on testing. In order to minimize peripheral vision loss, close monitoring and compliance with treatment is important.

RETINAL DETACHMENT

Patients with retinal detachment may present with sudden onset of flashes of light, floaters, decreased vision, and a "shadow or curtain" over their visual field. A dilated examination of the retina is required for diagnosis. Early presentation to a retina specialist for retinal detachment repair offers the patient the best change of maximal restoration of vision. Visual prognosis is variable, and depends on a variety of factors. Some common causes of a retinal detachment are trauma and traction from the vitreous. A rhegmatogenous retinal detachment is due to a tear or break in the retina. Subretinal fluid enters through this break and accumulates under the retina, further propagating the detachment. In serous and tractional retinal detachment, there is no retinal break.

AGE-RELATED MACULAR DEGENERATION

Age-related macular degeneration (ARMD) can be divided into two subtypes: wet, or exudative ARMD and dry, or nonexudative ARMD. Dry ARMD is characterized by drusen in the macular region and retinal pigment epithelial atrophy. Wet ARMD is characterized by choroidal neovascularization or retinal pigment epithelial detachment in addition to the findings of dry AMD. In both types of macular degeneration, central vision is first affected. There are a wide array of treatment modalities to help slow down progress and also treat active disease. Patients should monitor their vision with an Amsler grid, and regular follow-ups with an ophthalmologist are important.

TEMPORAL ARTERITIS

In patients over the age of 50 who present with headache and associated symptoms, temporal arteritis should be suspected. This condition is also known as giant cell arteritis and anterior ischemic optic neuropathy. Associated symptoms include jaw claudication, visual loss, fever, malaise, weight loss, eye pain, and polymyalgia rheumatica. This vasculitis can lead to irreversible visual loss, which is why early treatment is essential. Erythrocyte sedimentation rate (ESR) and c-reactive protein (CRP) are usually elevated in these patients, and definitive diagnosis can be confirmed by a temporal artery biopsy. High-dose steroids should be administered as soon as the physician suspects temporal arteritis. Early diagnosis and treatment can offset involvement of the second eye.

OCULAR MANIFESTATIONS OF SYSTEMIC DISEASES

Ocular disorders associated with systemic diseases are vast and various. Hypertension is one such disease that has a major impact on the ocular system, in particular the retina. The earliest pathologic feature of hypertensive retinopathy is narrowing of a major arteriole. As the disease progresses in severity, the narrowing of many other arterioles occurs. In younger patients, if the disease progresses rapidly, more dramatic changes may be seen such as occlusion of the arterioles causing blood loss, infarction, to the retina resulting in "cotton-wool spots" or mini-ischemic areas in the retina. Yellow hard exudates, due to lipid deposition deep in the retina and arising from leaking retinal vessels, also develop. Optic disk edema is a prominent feature of severe hypertensive retinopathy called papilledema. Vision is disturbed as a result of these changes. In contrast to the vascular response exhibited by younger patients, elderly patients do not seem to suffer the same retinal changes. The vasculature is often plagued by atherosclerosis, hardening of the arteries due to accumulation of cholesterol and lipids. The vessels are not as vulnerable to injury because of their rigid structure. With successful management of the hypertension, the retinopathy is irreversible. Treatment for the elderly population is not as successful as the atherosclerotic changes are irreversible.

Diabetic retinopathy is the leading cause of blindness in American adults, accounting for one-fourth of blind registrants in the Western world. Approximately 6.6 percent of the population between the ages of 20 to 74 has diabetes and approximately 25 percent of the diabetic population has some form of diabetic retinopathy. Diabetic retinopathy accounts for

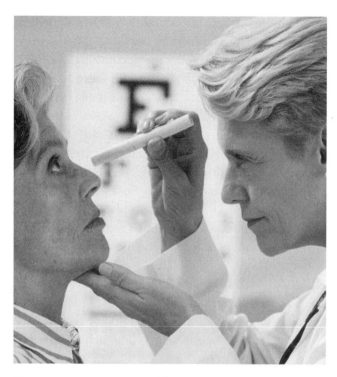

The most common eye care problems are low visual acuity and disorders such as cataract, glaucoma, and diabetic retinopathy.

approximately 10 percent of new cases of blindness each year. There are two major types of retinopathy: nonproliferative and proliferative. Nonproliferative diabetic retinopathy is marked by microaneurysms of the blood vessels, that can bleed into the retina. These hemorrhages may be seen as flame shaped or dot shaped. Macular edema, swelling, is the most common cause of visual loss and can be seen at any stage of the disease. This is caused by progressive weakening of the vasculature of the retina with resultant either focal or diffuse leakage. Proliferative

diabetic retinopathy can eventually progress and is the most severe consequence of ocular involvement of diabetes mellitus. With the progressive ischemia to the retina, there is stimulation of the growth of new vessels. These new vessels are friable and may cause extensive hemorrhaging in the eye if not treated early. They may grow near the optic disk, iris (rubeoisis iridis), or into the vitreous. The vitreous may eventually detach from the retina once the vessels begin to proliferate. This tractional pulling of the vitreous away from the retina may also cause the retina to detach. Treatment options consist of laser photocoagulation for proliferative retinopathy and also for the macular edema. If laser treatment is not successful, vitrectomy retinal surgery must be performed to treat the proliferative changes and the hemorrhaging in the eye.

SEE ALSO: Blepharitis; Cornea and Corneal Disease; Glaucoma; Ophthalmologist.

BIBLIOGRAPHY. Mark Beers and Robert Berkow, "Retinal Disorders," *Merck Manual* (v.17, 1999); Mark Dambro, "Retinopathy, Diabetic," *Griffiths 5 Minute Clinical Consult* (v.14, 2006); "Diabetes Mellitus," in *Harrison's Principles of Internal Medicine* (McGraw-Hill, 2005); Robert Hardy and Debra Shetlar, *Retina* (Lange Medical Books/McGraw-Hill, 2004); Peter K. Kaiser, Neil J. Friedman, and Roberto Pineda II, *The Massachusetts Eye and Ear Infirmary Illustrated Manual of Ophthalmology* (Saunders, 2004).

Komal Bharat Desai, M.D.
Sweta Tarigopala, M.S.
Jessica Winn, M.S.
Independent Scholar

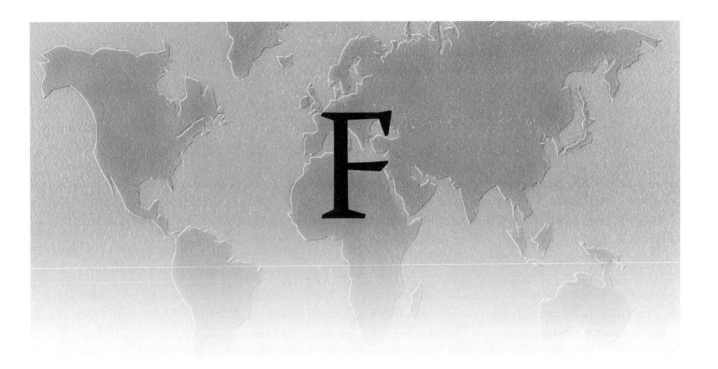

Facial Injuries and Disorders

Facial trauma, also referred to medically as maxillofacial injuries, encompass any injury to the mouth, face, and jaw. Almost everyone has experienced such an injury, or knows someone who has. Most maxillofacial injuries are caused by a sports mishap, motor vehicle accident, on-the-job accident, act of violence, or an accident in the home.

A craniofacial disorder refers to an abnormality of the face and/or the head. Craniofacial differences can result from abnormal growth patterns of the face or skull, which involves soft tissue and bones. A craniofacial condition may include disfigurement brought about by birth defect, disease, or trauma.

At the hospital, patients will most likely be seen by several medical personnel, one of whom will probably be an oral and maxillofacial surgeon. Oral and maxillofacial surgeons, surgical specialists of the dental profession, are specifically trained to repair injuries to the mouth, face, and jaw. After four years of dental school, oral and maxillofacial surgeons complete four or more years of hospital-based surgical residency training that may include rotations through related medical fields, including internal medicine, general surgery, anesthesiology, otolaryngology, plastic surgery, emergency medicine, and other medical spe-

cialty areas. At the conclusion of this program, oral and maxillofacial surgeons are prepared to perform the full scope of the specialty, which includes emergency care for the teeth, mouth, jaws, and associated facial structures.

FACIAL INJURY

One of the most common types of serious injury to the face occurs when bones are broken. Fractures can involve the lower jaw, upper jaw, palate, cheekbones, eye sockets, and combinations of these bones. These injuries can affect sight and the ability to breathe, speak, and swallow. Treatment often requires hospitalization.

Extensive maxillofacial fractures are often accompanied by other medical problems. A thorough physical examination, including neurologic examination, is necessary following a detailed history. Of particular importance are signs of raised intracranial pressure, other cranial nerve dysfunction, or pupillary abnormalities. The head and neck also require careful attention. Numerous neuralgias have been described as causes of facial pain. Neuralgia is defined as paroxysmal pain in the distribution of a particular nerve. The pain is typically maximal at onset and may be described as lancinating, "electric shocks," or as "jabbing." There may be a single sharp pain or repetitive pains in succession. The pain can last a fraction of a second or for several seconds. There may be a refractory period after the severe pain during which pain will not occur. Some neuralgic conditions have trigger zones (areas that when stimulated provoke an attack) or other triggers. The oral and maxillofacial surgeon coordinates treatment with other medical specialties to return the patient to his or her normal activities as soon as possible. The principles for treating facial fractures are the same as for a broken arm or leg. The parts of the bone must be lined up (reduced) and held in position long enough to permit them time to heal. This may require six or more weeks depending on the patient's age and the fracture's complexity.

During the healing period when jaws are wired shut, the oral and maxillofacial surgeon prescribes a nutritional liquid or pureed diet, which will help the healing process by keeping the patient in good health. After discharge from the hospital, the doctor gives the patient instructions on continued facial and oral care.

While not all facial injuries are extensive, they are all complex because they affect an area of the body that is critical to breathing, eating, speaking, and seeing. Even in the case of a moderately cut lip, the expertise of the oral and maxillofacial surgeon is indispensable. If sutures are needed, placement must be precise to bring about the desired cosmetic result.

Because avoiding injury is always best, prevention includes the use of automobile seat belts, protective mouth guards, and appropriate masks and helmets for everyone who participates in athletic pursuits at any level. New innovations in helmet and mouth and face guard technology have made these devices comfortable to wear and very effective in protecting the vulnerable maxillofacial area. New synthetic materials and advances in engineering and design have produced mouth guards that are sturdier yet lightweight enough to allow the wearer to breathe easily. Mouth guards can vary from the inexpensive "boil and bite" models to custom-fabricated guards made by dentists, which can be adapted to the sport and are generally more comfortable.

There are five criteria to consider when being fitted for a mouth protector. The device should be fitted so that it does not misalign the jaw and throw off the bite, lightweight, strong, easy to clean, and should cover the upper and/or lower teeth and gums. By encouraging sports enthusiasts at every level of play to wear mouth guards and other protective equipment,

oral and maxillofacial surgeons hope to help change the "face" of sports.

Trauma does not only result from major events such as combat or automobile accidents. Childhood injuries caused by skateboards, sports, or bicycle accidents frequently involve dental or maxillofacial trauma. Younger children often sustain damage to teeth or supporting structures from falls. Various safe and effective sedation techniques can be employed to deliver prompt, comfortable, and successful treatment in the office setting.

IMPACTED TEETH

A tooth that fails to emerge or fully break through the gum tissue is, by definition, "impacted." While this is a common problem associated with third molars, or wisdom teeth, as they are the last teeth to develop and erupt into the mouth, other teeth can also become impacted. Typical symptoms associated with impacted teeth are pain, swelling, and signs of infection in the surrounding tissues. An impacted tooth has the potential to cause permanent damage to adjacent teeth, gum tissue, and supporting bone structure. Impacted teeth are also associated with the development of cysts and tumors that can destroy large portions of the jaw. Many times, impacted wisdom teeth are not treated until symptoms are present; however, a recent study conducted by the American Association of Oral and Maxillofacial Surgeons and the Oral and Maxillofacial Surgery Foundation indicates that third molars should be removed by the time the patient is a young adult in order to prevent related gum disease or other problems.

FACIAL INFECTIONS

Infections in the maxillofacial region can develop into life-threatening emergencies if not treated promptly and effectively. Pain and swelling in the face, jaws, or neck may indicate an infection of dental or related origin.

TEMPOROMANDIBULAR JOINT DISORDERS (TMJ) AND FACIAL PAIN

A common cause of facial pain and headache is disease or dysfunction of the TMJ. Located where the lower jaw and skull meet, the TMJ is the ball and socket joint that enables the lower jaw (mandible) to move and function. TMJ disorders display a number of symptoms that may include earaches, headaches, and a limited range of movement. Patients may also complain of clicking or grating sounds in the joint, or pain when opening or closing their mouths.

Causes of TMJ disorders can be degenerative (osteoarthritis), traumatic (cartilage displacement or injury), inflammatory (rheumatoid arthritis), or stress related. Some patients experience a combination of muscle and joint problems. In order to properly diagnose and treat the problem, a clinical examination and a number of diagnostic procedures, including imaging studies (radiograph, computed tomography, magnetic resonance imaging) are utilized. Usually, nonsurgical management (soft diet, antiinflammatory drugs, physical, and/or bite splint therapy) is the first step. For certain conditions, joint surgery may be an appropriate option.

Lysis and lavage and arthroscopic joint surgery are minimally invasive procedures that have proven effective in resolving certain conditions involving TMJ pain and dysfunction. These procedures can be done under general anesthesia on an outpatient-surgery basis at a hospital or ambulatory surgery center. More complex joint surgery may be indicated for advanced conditions.

ORAL PATHOLOGY

Dental pathology is a common cause of facial pain. Specific inquiry regarding prior dental procedures should be made of all patients with facial pain. The presence of provocative factors such as chewing or heat or cold sensitivity may provide useful clues. Trigeminal neuralgia also has been associated with ipsilateral dental pathology. Cancer is a rarer cause of facial pain. Extracranial bony or soft tissue metastases may impinge upon cranial and upper cervical nerves causing headache or facial pain. In addition, occult lung neoplasms may cause referred pain in the periauricular region. Facial pain due to cancer is discussed in detail separately. If indicated, biopsies and other tests can be performed to diagnose the problem and develop an appropriate treatment plan. Early detection and treatment of oral lesions greatly improve the patient's prognosis. Lesions may be managed medically and/or surgically.

ORAL AND FACIAL DEFORMITIES

Differences in skeletal growth between the upper and lower jaws may lead to both functional and psychological difficulties. Functional difficulties may include problems with chewing, swallowing, speech, or TMJ performance.

Patients may also exhibit psychological difficulties stemming from aesthetic and social concerns. Some abnormalities may only involve misaligned teeth and can be corrected orthodontically with braces or other appliances. Serious growth disturbances, however, require surgery to realign the upper and lower jaws into a more normal relationship. Common dentofacial deformities, including under- or overdevelopment of the jaws (prognathia, micrognathia, retrognathia), or misaligned teeth (overbite or underbite), can make it difficult to eat, swallow, speak, and breathe. Corrective jaw surgery can be performed to produce a more balanced, functional skeletal relationship for the patient. Often performed in conjunction with treatment by an orthodontist and restorative dentist, corrective jaw surgery is usually performed in a hospital or ambulatory surgical center under general anesthesia.

Congenital deformities such as cleft lip and palate occur when all or a portion of the oral-nasal cavity does not grow together during fetal development. Cleft lip and/or palate is a separation of the parts or segments of the lip or roof of the mouth, which are usually joined together during the early weeks in the development of an unborn child. A cleft lip is a separation of the two sides of the lip and often includes the bones of the maxilla and/or the upper gum. A cleft palate is an opening in the roof of the mouth and can vary in severity. A cleft palate occurs when the two sides of the palate do not fuse as the unborn baby develops. A team of healthcare specialists play an important role in the carefully orchestrated, multiple-stage correctional program for these patients. The goal is to help restore the jaw and facial structures, leading to normal function and appearance. Care and treatment must consider function, appearance, nutrition, speech, hearing, and emotional and psychological development.

BURNING MOUTH SYNDROME (BMS)

BMS is defined as burning pain in one or several oral structures. Affected patients often present with multiple oral complaints, including burning, dryness, and taste alterations. Burning mouth complaints are reported more often in women, especially after menopause. Typically, patients awaken without pain but note increasing symptoms through the day and into the evening. Usually, no obvious etiology is found, but several possibilities exist that can be divided into local and systemic causes. A careful history and oral cavity examination assist in diagnosing the cause of BMS, which locally may include allergy, denture irritation, oral habits, infection (e.g., oral candidiasis), and reflux esophagitis. Systemic causes include vitamin and mineral deficiency, diabetes mellitus, and chemotherapy.

SEE ALSO: Accidents; American Dental Association (ADA); Birth Defects; Child Dental Health; Cleft Lip and Palate; Dental Health; Ear Infections; Oral Surgeon.

BIBLIOGRAPHY. E. Bohm and R.R. Strang, "Glossopharyngeal Neuralgia," *Brain* (v.85, 1962); C. Feinmann, "Idiopathic Orofacial Pain: A Multidisciplinary Problem," in *Pain: An Updated Review* (IASP Press, 1996); C. Feinmann, "The Long-Term Outcome of Facial Pain Treatment," *Journal of Psychosomatic Research* (v.37, 1993); J.E. Horgan, et al., "OMENS-Plus: Analysis of Craniofacial and Extracraniofacial Anomalies in Hemifacial Microsomia," *Cleft Palate-Craniofacial Journal* (v.32, 1995); D. Mock, W. Frydman, and A.S. Gordon, "Atypical Facial Pain: A Retrospective Study," *Oral Surgery, Oral Medicine, and Oral Pathology* (v.59, 1985); E.J. Ratner, et al., "Jawbone Cavities and Trigeminal and Atypical Facial Neuralgias," *Oral Surgery, Oral Medicine, and Oral Pathology* (v.48, 1979); J.G. Rushton, J.C. Stevens, and R.H. Miller, "Glossopharyngeal (Vagoglossopharyngeal) Neuralgia: A Study of 217 Cases," *Archives of Neurology* (v. 38, 1981); P. Tessier, "Anatomical Classification Facial, Cranio-Facial and Latero-Facial Clefts," *Journal of Maxillofacial Surgery* (v.4, 1976); L.P. Tourne and J.R. Fricton, "Burning Mouth Syndrome. Critical Review and Proposed Clinical Management," *Oral Surgery, Oral Medicine, and Oral Pathology* (v.74, 1992).

BARKHA GURBAN, B.A.
UNIVERSITY OF CALIFORNIA, LOS ANGELES

Failure to Thrive

Failure to thrive is a term traditionally associated with pediatrics, describing a weight gain and physical growth delay that can impair a child's development and maturation. The term has been borrowed into geriatric literature to describe a situation where elderly people fail to maintain functional and nutritional status disproportionally to their health conditions.

PEDIATRIC FAILURE TO THRIVE

Children are said to fail to thrive when presenting with clear underweight or failing to gain weight without an obvious reason. Different medical, psychological, environmental, and social factors are known that can impair normal growth in children.

Medical disorders, notably but not exclusively affecting the digestory tract, may affect food intake, retention, digestion, or absorption. Parental abuse may impair a child's appetite and different environmental and social factors may prevent the child from getting adequate nutrition. These include family's environment and financial status—the regularity and quality of a child's feeding directly reflect his or her development.

The diagnosis is made when a child's weight or rate of growing is far from what it should be by comparison with previous measures or height-weight charts and the treatment is based on eliminating the underlying cause. Nutritional supplementation is always offered and severe cases are treated in the hospital.

Because the first year of age is crucial in brain development, failure to thrive during this time may result in a permanent mental deficit from mild to severe. The best way to avoid this is based on the early identification and treatment of failure to thrive.

GERIATRIC FAILURE TO THRIVE

Geriatric failure to thrive is a syndrome and a diagnosis of exclusion in older people. It is defined by weight and function loss and it can lead to death in a short time. This condition has a prevalence of 10 to 20 percent after 65 years of age and may be caused by either organic disease or nonorganic problems, such as psychological, functional, or social problems.

Failure to thrive is characterized by progressive loss of physical functioning, weight, and lean body mass. Malnutrition, characterized by a loss of fat mass and visceral protein, is an important risk factor and so is low muscle mass, because it relates to physical function. Failure to thrive as a medical diagnosis is acceptable when its causes cannot be made clear. Almost all chronic systemic diseases and some medications can cause failure to thrive in very old people. Nonorganic causes of failure to thrive are usually linked to inability to get food, lack of interest in food or anorexia, or inability to consume available food. Depression is the most common psychological risk factor. Eating is a social event and it is not a surprise that social isolation also may lead to decreased food intake and failure to thrive. Poverty is also an important risk factor.

Abuse also may cause failure to thrive in the elderly, especially on those more frail and incapable of self-defense. The clinical picture of geriatric failure to thrive due to abuse is nearly identical to the effects of abuse-related pediatric failure to thrive.

The treatment of the potential causes is the basis of treatment of geriatric failure to thrive and dietary supplementation is also important and cost-effective in all cases. Geriatric failure to thrive is often treatable, with a positive impact on an older person's health.

SEE ALSO: Elder Abuse; Geriatrics; Nutrition; Pediatrics.

BIBLIOGRAPHY. Edmund Duthie, *Practice of Geriatrics*, 3rd ed. (Saunders, 1998); S.D. Krugman and H. Dubowitz, "Failure to Thrive," *American Family Physician* (v.68/5, 2003); R.G. Robertson and M. Montagnini, "Geriatric Failure to Thrive," *American Family Physician* (v.70/2, 2004).

THIAGO MONACO
UNIVERSITY OF SÃO PAULO MEDICAL SCHOOL,

Fainting

Fainting (medically known as syncope) is a sudden brief loss of consciousness and postural tone. The most common presentation of fainting is a person who was standing or sitting upright and then suddenly began to feel uneasy and uncomfortable. The person may sway, become anxious, or develop a headache; he or she often becomes pale or his or her face will turn a gray color. Before fainting, the skin will be damp and cold from sweat. Other symptoms include salivation, stomach upset, nausea, vomiting, ringing in the ears, and vision that may dim or close in concentrically. Patients attempt to suppress these symptoms by deep breathing, yawning, and sighing. Some fainting episodes can be suppressed by lying down. However, when an episode occurs, the patient typically collapses to the ground and is motionless (this differs from a seizure, which typically causes patients to exhibit convulsive movements). The skeletal muscles typically remain fully relaxed, and the patient retains control over bowel and bladder function. The fainting episode usually lasts a few seconds to minutes, but it is rarely longer than five minutes.

CLASSIFICATION AND CAUSES

There are three main types of fainting: neurogenic, orthostatic, and cardiogenic. All three are associated with a temporary significant reduction in blood flow to the brain. Systolic blood pressure is decreased, typically to less than 60 mm Hg.

Neurogenic faints are of several different types. The most common of these is vasovagal fainting. Vasovagal fainting occurs mainly in young patients and people in good health. It is not suggestive of any underlying disease. There is also evidence of a familial predilection. The reason for the faint is a block of the normal sympathetic nervous system reaction to bodily stress. For instance, physical and emotional stresses normally cause an increase in sympathetic nervous system activity. This is reflected by an increase in heart rate, blood pressure, and the volume of blood pumped by the heart each minute (cardiac output). A variety of situations can trigger a vasovagal faint. These include bodily pain or injury (especially involving the internal organs), exercise, strong emotions, and situations that cause dilation of peripheral blood vessels (such as a hot, crowded room, particularly when a person is fatigued or has ingested alcohol).

Carotid sinus hypersensitivity is another type of neurogenic fainting. The carotid sinus is a dilated portion of the carotid artery, which is one of the major arteries supplying blood to the head. The sinus has nerve endings and senses changes in blood pressure. It sends feedback to the vasomotor center in the medulla—this is an area of the brainstem that controls blood pressure and heart rate. For patients with carotid sinus hypersensitivity, compression of the sinus by everyday activities such as turning one's head to the side, shaving, wearing a seatbelt, or tightening a necktie can cause the patient to faint. There are two abnormal responses that take place simultaneously: a vagal response and a vasodepressor response. The vagal response is a reflex action by the body which slows the heart rate (bradycardia) and causes a pause in the heartbeat (asystole) for greater than three seconds. The vasodepressor response is a decrease in the systolic blood pressure by more than 50 mm Hg without causing a significant change in heart rate. Carotid sinus hypersensitivity is most common in elderly men and patients with ischemic heart disease, hypertension, and head or neck tumors. Fainting typically occurs suddenly and while the patient is standing. The patient may have small convulsive movements during the episode. The faint rarely lasts longer than 30 seconds.

Neurogenic fainting also includes situational reflex syncope. This type of fainting includes a variety of conditions with physical stimuli that can trigger an abnormal autonomic response. Examples include micturition, swallowing, exercise, and coughing. Micturition fainting mainly affects elderly men, typically at night when they awake to use the bathroom. The faint usually occurs at the end of voiding. The physiology behind this type of fainting is that the patient will awaken with a full bladder and associated vasoconstriction of the abdominal and pelvic blood vessels. When the bladder is emptied, the vessels dilate and consequently the patient becomes hypotensive. During sleep, the heart rate and resistance in the peripheral blood vessels are low, and this adds to the body's delay in being able to correct the low blood pressure. Factors that increase the risk of micturition fainting include fatigue, hunger, upper respiratory infection, and alcohol ingestion. Fainting can also occur after difficulty swallowing in patients with esophageal disease. It is thought that an increase in intrathoracic and/or intraabdominal pressure may cause a decrease in blood flow to the brain, thus precipitating a faint. A similar mechanism is thought to be the cause of fainting after sudden vigorous coughing. Coughing also increases the intracranial pressure, further limiting cerebral blood flow. Exercise-induced fainting typically occurs with aerobic exercise, such as running. It is associated with nausea and is thought to be a familial condition. Medications, such as beta-blockers, may be helpful for these patients. When considering exercise as a possible trigger for fainting, it is important to first rule out heart disease or abnormality.

Orthostatic fainting is another type of fainting. It is a result of orthostatic hypotension—a decrease in the systolic blood pressure greater than 20 mm Hg when a person suddenly rises from a supine or seat-

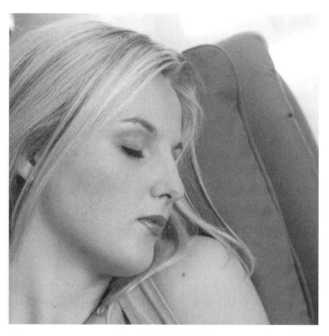

The most common presentation of fainting is a person who was standing or sitting upright and then suddenly began to feel uneasy.

ed position to standing or when someone is standing for an extended period of time. These patients have an inability to adjust their blood pressure for changes in position. For instance, upon standing for a long time, the blood pools in their legs (due to gravity), and there is constriction of the vessels in abdomen and upper extremities. Since a large volume of blood rests in the legs, less blood is able to be pumped to the brain. Fainting usually occurs within three minutes of being upright. The most common reasons for orthostatic hypotension and consequent fainting are a depletion of the central or total blood volume and the effects of medications (particularly antihypertensives and antidepressants). The underlying etiology may also involve impaired autonomic reflex control, the circulation of vasodilators (such as in a patient with carcinoid syndrome), or returning to activity after a period of prolonged bed rest, fasting, or alcohol use. Diabetes, alcoholism, pernicious anemia, and degenerative diseases of the nervous system (i.e., Parkinson's disease) have all been linked to orthostatic fainting.

Cardiogenic syncope is the third main type of fainting. The faints occur due to a sudden significant decrease in cardiac output. The symptoms that a patient experiences depend on the presence of cerebrovascular atherosclerotic disease and the nervous system's ability to compensate for the decline in cardiac output. The underlying cause may be electrical or mechanical. Electrical causes are more common, of which dysrhythmia is the most frequent diagnosis. Atrioventricular (AV) heart block is the dysrhythmia most likely to cause fainting. In healthy individuals, the body can normally adjust to maintain cerebral blood flow when the heart rate in between 40 and 185. However, patients with dysrhythmias have a decreased tolerance to changes in heart rate, and this is particularly evident in patients with premorbid cerebrovascular disease, coronary artery disease, and valvular disease. Fainting due to dysrhythmias is sudden and usually lasts less than three seconds. There are rarely any warning symptoms. Mechanical causes of cardiogenic fainting include outflow obstructions of the left and right ventricles, congenital heart defects with shunting, and acute massive myocardial infarction. Cardiac output is not sufficient to meet the body's demands, particular during periods of high stress such as exercise. Symptoms tend to occur during physical exertion, but may also be precipitated by medications or heat stress.

EVALUATION

A detailed history and physical examination provides a strong foundation for evaluating a patient who has fainted. The majority of cases will be able to be diagnosed based on the history and physical alone, without additional testing. A chronological account of the fainting episode—including the events and symptoms preceding it—is essential to the evaluation. The physician will ask about the patient's posture or positioning, the environment they were in, the activity they were doing at the time, and the presence of any seizure activity. It is also important to know the patient's past medical history and any medications they are taking (prescription and over the counter). With regard to the physical exam, attention is directed at the cardiovascular and neurologic systems. Patients are examined for orthostatic hypotension, hypertension, cardiac rhythm abnormalities, heart murmurs, signs of congestive heart failure, neurologic deficits, and signs of peripheral neuropathy.

If patients have symptoms of carotid sinus hypersensitivity or if elderly patients have had multiple fainting episodes, a procedure called carotid sinus massage is often helpful in diagnosis. One sinus is massaged for

five seconds and then the heart rate and blood pressure are monitored for changes. If there is a pause in the heartbeat for more than three seconds or if the blood pressure decreases more than 50 mm Hg without a significant decline in heart rate, this is suggestive of carotid sinus hypersensitivity. Carotid sinus massage is repeated on the other side to complete the evaluation.

An electrocardiogram (ECG) is the test of choice for patients who have had a fainting episode. It is commonly done in all patients but is crucial in the evaluation of patients whose diagnosis is not clear from the history and physical examination. The ECG is helpful in identifying cardiogenic causes of syncope such as heart block, ventricular tachycardia, or myocardial infarction.

For cases in which the history, physical exam, and ECG are not conclusive, other diagnostic tests can be done. These include echocardiogram, ambulatory ECG, exercise ECG, electrophysiologic studies, and cardiac catheterization. If all of these tests are negative, head-up-tilt testing is done with hemodynamic monitoring.

TREATMENT

The treatment of fainting is directed toward correcting the cause of decreased cerebral blood flow and preventing future episodes. Patients who are seen while fainting or after losing consciousness should be positioned so that cerebral blood flow is maximized. The head should be lowered between the knees or the patient should be placed in the supine position with both legs elevated. The head should be positioned so that the tongue is not at risk for falling into the back of the throat. Any tight clothing should be loosened. It is important that the patient does not try to stand or sit up until the sense of weakness resolves.

Prevention of fainting episodes depends on the particular type of fainting. Patients who have vasovagal episodes are encouraged to avoid physically and emotionally stressful environments. Beta-blockers, particularly acebutolol, have been used with success.

Education is important for patients with carotid sinus hypersensitivity. Patients should be told of ways to decrease the risk of fainting. These include wearing a loose shirt collar and turning one's whole body to look from side to side rather than just turning the head. Atropine has been effective in helping patients who have profound decreases in blood pressure and/or heart rate. Patients who do not respond to preventive measures or medications may be eligible for pacemaker placement.

Patients with orthostatic hypotension are advised to exercise their legs for a few seconds and sit at the edge of their beds before standing. If these patients know they will be standing for an extended period of time, crossing their legs forcefully can help to prevent a faint. Alternative medications can also be used for patients using antihypertensives and antidepressants if it is believed that medications are playing a role.

Elderly patients with recurrent fainting episodes are at significant risk of falls, fractures, and trauma. Preventive measures are recommended for around the home in order to decrease risk of injury. This includes covering the bathroom floor and bathtub with mats and increasing carpeting in the home. These patients are encouraged to walk on soft ground when outdoors and avoid standing in place for long periods. Padded hip protectors can also be worn for protection.

SEE ALSO: Cardiology; Coronary Disease; Stress; Stroke.

BIBLIOGRAPHY. "Orthostatic Hypotension and Syncope," in Mark H. Beers and Robert Berkow, eds., *The Merck Manual* (Merck, 1999); Sumanth Prabhu, Robert A. O'Rourke, and J. Donald Easton, "Faintness and Syncope: Pathophysiology," in Jay H. Stein, comp., *Internal Medicine* (Mosby, 1998); Allan H. Ropper and Robert H. Brown, "Faintness and Syncope," *Adams and Victor's Principles of Neurology* (McGraw-Hill, 2005).

STACY A. FRYE
MICHIGAN STATE UNIVERSITY

Falls

A very large number of admissions to hospitals come from falls which are defined as movement of people because of gravity. The vast number of personal injuries, both small and very serious and even fatal, is particularly common in elderly people where their vision and muscles are weakened. In addition, some elderly people taking multiple prescription medication may also lose balance, which combined with slower reaction times often prove serious, with their bones often being more susceptible to major damage. Although large numbers of children and adolescents are also involved in falls, their simple injuries often heal relatively easily; however, others have sustained serious injuries through risky behavior. According to figures for 2002 issued by the World Health Organization, some 392,000 people died from falls that year. Although many falls have resulted in deaths, others result in breakages of bones, bone fractures, or muscle and/or tendon injury or sprain.

Throughout history, there have been many people who have been injured from or died as a result of falls. In Greek mythology, Icarus fell from the skies after flying too close to the sun, and the heat from the sun melted the wax which held his wings together. Although falling over, falling off a cliff or other natural formation, have always led to medical problems, falls by rulers have sometimes been seen as ill omens. Duke William of Normandy fell in the sand when he landed on the beach at Pevensey, on the south coast of England on September 28, 1066, prior to the Battle of Hastings. While his men thought it was a portent of disaster, William rose with his hands clutching sand claiming it represented his seizure of England. Julius Caesar, suffering from epilepsy, also fell to the ground on some occasions, but suffered no injuries. U.S. President Gerald Ford also became famous for two public falls.

Until recently, falls from horses have led to large numbers of deaths and injuries, and still cause death and injury. Ptolemy VI "Philometor" of Egypt died after falling from his horse during battle and Alexander III of Scotland died when his horse fell over a cliff. Some of the important historical characters who have died from falling from horses include Pippin III, father of Charlemagne; John I, king of Aragon and his cousin John I, king of Castile; and James, Earl of Cardigan, who led the British cavalry at the Charge of the Light Brigade in 1854. William III of Orange, King of England died from injuries sustained after his horse tripped over a mole hill, leading to his enemies, the Jacobites, toasting "the little man in black." Many jockeys have been killed or injured by falling from horses during races. People have also been injured or killed falling from trains, buses, and occasionally even from cars, usually when hanging on to them. The biggest fall from which someone survived was by Vesna Vulovi who, in 1972, survived a fall from 33,000 feet without a parachute.

Some people engaged in high-risk activities have also been killed in falls. Mountaineer Francis Maitland Balfour, founder of embryology, died from a fall from

Mont Blanc, and British Everest mountaineer George Mallory almost certainly died from a fall while climbing Mount Everest. Circus acrobat Karl Wallenda died from a fall from a tightrope in San Juan, Puerto Rico, and many circus performers have been injured in falls during trapeze or other acts.

There have also been many people who have been killed or injured by falls from buildings. Some opponents of the Medicis in Renaissance Italy were thrown from the Palazzo Vecchio into the Piazza della Signoria in Florence, and the Thirty Years War in 1618 began with the defenestration by the people and the burghers of Prague when two royal deputies and a secretary were thrown from the window of the royal castle of Hradcany in Prague on May 23, 1618. In the incident at Prague, the three survived. One of Napoleon's marshals, Louis-Alexandre Berthier, Prince of Wagram, died from a fall from a window, in suspicious circumstances; U.S. writer Constance Fenimore Woolson died from a fall from her apartment in Venice; several stock brokers died after falling from tall buildings in Wall Street during the stock market crash in 1929; James V. Forrestal, the first U.S. Secretary of Defense, fell from the Bethesda Naval Medical Center, Maryland, while suffering from depression; and many others, less famous, have fallen from buildings.

SEE ALSO: Fractures; Sprains and Strains.

BIBLIOGRAPHY. Rose Anne Kenny, ed., *Syncope in the Older Patient: Causes, Investigations and Consequences of Syncope and Falls* (Chapman & Hall Medical, 1996); National Health and Medical Research Council (Australia), *Falls and the Older Person: Report of the Health Care Committee Expert Panel for Health Care of the Elderly* (National Health and Medical Research Council, 1994).

JUSTIN CORFIELD
GEELONG GRAMMAR SCHOOL, AUSTRALIA

False Negative

This type of error involves the acceptance of the null hypothesis when it is actually false; in other words, it represents a failure to detect a real effect. It is also known as a Type II error or β error. These errors are particularly common in studies with relatively small sample sizes. In medicine, false-negative findings are cases in which a test fails to detect a condition when it is actually present. This is often studied within the framework of receiver operating characteristics (ROC) curves, which graphically represent the trade-off between false-negative and false-positive findings for a particular test or set of tests.

SEE ALSO: Diagnostic Tests; False Positive.

BIBLIOGRAPHY. David De Vaus, *Surveys in Social Research* (Routledge, 2002); A. Rolfs, *PCR: Clinical Diagnostics and Research* (Springer-Verlag, 1997).

FERNANDO DE MAIO, PH.D.
SIMON FRASER UNIVERSITY

False Positive

This type of error involves the rejection of the null hypothesis when it is actually true. It is also known as a Type I error or α error. The null hypothesis, a statement of equality, always asserts that there is no relationship between the independent variable and the dependent variable. It is this assertion that forms the basis of inferential statistics, which can be used to determine our level of confidence that our findings (based on data from a random sample) represent true patterns in the population. A statistical test's level of significance (α, or alpha)

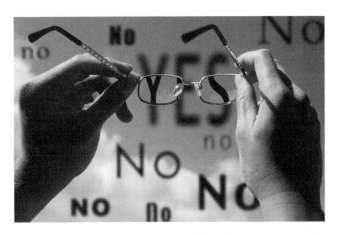

A false positive involves the rejection of the null hypothesis when it is actually true, and is also known as a Type I error.

indicates the risk of a false-positive finding. A level of significance of 0.05 is normally accepted in social science; this indicates that we accept a 5 percent chance of making a false-positive error. At more demanding significance levels, such as 0.01 or 0.001, the probability of making false-positive conclusions are lower.

For example, consider a study that observes a 2.5-point difference in mean body mass index between groups A and B. A researcher may use a t-test to examine the statistical significance of that difference in mean scores. If the resulting test has a significance value of less than 0.05, the researcher would conclude that the difference between the groups is real. However, if the significance value of the t-test was greater than 0.05, the likelihood of a false-positive finding would be too great and the researcher would conclude that the groups do not differ in body mass index score (even though their results indicated a 2.5-point difference).

SEE ALSO: Diagnostic Tests; False Negative.

BIBLIOGRAPHY. David De Vaus, *Surveys in Social Research* (Routledge, 2002); A. Rolfs, *PCR: Clinical Diagnostics and Research* (Springer-Verlag, 1997).

FERNANDO DE MAIO, PH.D.
SIMON FRASER UNIVERSITY

Farmer, Paul (1959–)

Dr. Paul Farmer is a medical anthropologist, a physician, and a professor of Medical Anthropology at Harvard University. Dr. Farmer is also a founding director of Partners in Health, an international organization that provides direct healthcare services, research, and advocacy for those who are sick and living in poverty in resource-poor areas. Dr. Farmer specializes in infectious disease control in resource-poor areas and has pioneered novel approaches to community-based strategies for infectious disease control, including HIV/AIDS and multidrug-resistant tuberculosis. He has published numerous works capturing his experiences in Haiti and detailing his view of the socioeconomic factors of disease progression.

Dr. Farmer first worked in Haiti in 1983 before he began medical school at Harvard University. His work in Haiti is based upon a multifaceted approach to address the healthcare needs in Haiti and other resource-poor areas. Dr. Farmer fostered his deep commitment to work in Haiti to address healthcare issues and moved forward to found Partners in Health (PIH) in 1987. The mission statement of PIH is "whatever it takes" and captures Dr. Farmer's dedication to his work. Working with colleagues, Dr. Farmer created a model of community-based healthcare that provides healthcare, food, clean water, housing, education, and other social services. This PIH model is based upon his belief that illness is caused by various socioeconomic factors that renders a patient vulnerable to disease. PIH has initiated a model of community-based care that proved that infectious diseases could be successfully treated. PIH has since become a worldwide health and social justice organization. Dr. Farmer has moved forward with an agenda to develop a system of healthcare that will continue to reach millions of afflicted poor in Haiti, Peru, Russia, Mexico, Guatemala, Rwanda, and Boston's inner city.

BEYOND PIH

Dr. Farmer is a course director at Harvard University, and also guest lectures at universities throughout the world. Dr. Farmer is a key player pushing forward AIDS/tuberculosis global agendas. He continues to train medical students and colleagues at Brigham and Women's Hospital in Boston. Dr. Farmer has received numerous prestigious awards for his dedication in securing healthcare for the sick in resource-poor areas.

PUBLICATIONS

Dr. Farmer has authored and coauthored over 100 articles, authored 6 books, and is the focus of another book that narrates his experience in Haiti.

SEE ALSO: AIDS; Haiti; Tuberculosis.

BIBLIOGRAPHY. Harvard Medical School, Department of Social Medicine, "Paul Farmer, MD, PhD," http://www.hms.harvard.edu/dsm/WorkFiles/html/people/faculty/PaulFarmer.html (cited July 2007); Brigham and Women's Hospital, "Social Medicine & Health Inequalities," http://www.brighamandwomens.org/socialmedicine/aboutfarmer.aspx (cited August 2003).

SUDHA R. RAMINANI, M.S.
THE FENWAY INSTITUTE

Federal Emergency Management Agency (FEMA)

Since the beginning of the 19th century, the federal government has responded to disasters which include hurricanes, earthquakes, tornadoes, floods, fires, hazardous material spills, and terrorism. The roots of the Federal Emergency Management Agency (FEMA) can be traced to the Congressional Act of 1803 when Congress authorized a federal response to a fire that destroyed much of a New Hampshire town. Subsequently, Congress passed over 100 laws to authorize assistance on a piecemeal basis. In the 1930s, the Reconstruction Finance Corporation was authorized to offer loans to repair public facilities after disasters struck. In 1934, the Bureau of Public Roads assumed responsibility for repairing public roads and bridges damaged by national disasters.

The Federal Disaster Assistance Administration was subsequently established under the auspices of the Department of Housing and Urban Development (HUD) in response to a series of disasters that included Hurricane Carla (1962), the Alaskan earthquake (1964), Hurricane Betsy (1965), Hurricane Camille (1969), Hurricane Agnes (1972), and the San Fernando earthquake (1971). The National Flood Insurance Act was passed in 1968. In 1979, President Jimmy Carter consolidated existing disaster-related responsibilities into FEMA. Statutory authority for FEMA activities can be traced to the Disaster Relief Act of 1974 and the Robert T. Stafford Disaster Relief and Emergency Assistance Act of 1988.

After the terrorist attacks on the United States on September 11, 2001, which caused the deaths of nearly 3,000 people, the Department of Homeland Security (DHS) was created by the Emergency Supplement Act (PL-107-38) to oversee counterterrorism activities and to plan responses to potential future attacks. On March 1, 2003, in the biggest government reorganization since the end of World War II, FEMA became part of DHS. Congress then appropriated billions of dollars to FEMA to be used in preparing the nation for potential attacks by terrorists. FEMA's mission has remained the same, and agency officials describe FEMA activities as a "disaster life cycle" in which the agency tries to prevent emergencies and disasters from occurring while preparing to deal with all eventualities. Whenever emergencies and disasters do occur, FEMA responds, assists in recovery, mitigates effects, and reduces risk of loss. As part of that responsibility, FEMA trains first responders and oversees the National Flood and Crime Insurance programs.

Today, FEMA employs more than 2,600 full-time workers distributed among the national and regional offices and the Mount Weather Emergency Operations Center. Some 4,000 standby employees are attached to the National Emergency Training Center, located in Emmitsburg, Maryland. The national headquarters of FEMA is located at 500 C Street, SW, Washington, D.C. 20472. Additional information on FEMA is available by phone (1-800-462-7595) or on the internet (http://www.fema.gov/). Requests for disaster aid are channeled through a hot line (1-800-621-FEMA). The agency Web site serves as a resource for disaster information on chemicals, dam failure, earthquakes, fires, floods, hazardous materials, heat, hurricanes, landslides, nuclear disasters, terrorism, thunderstorms, tornadoes, tsunamis, volcanoes, wildfire, and winter storms.

The director, who is answerable to the director of Homeland Security, serves as the head of FEMA. The FEMA director is supported by the chief of staff and the director of operations. The agency is divided into three divisions according to responsibilities: Mitigation, Recovery, and Response. The internal structure of FEMA is subdivided into the Office of Equal Rights, the Office of the Executive Secretariat, the Office of General Counsel, the Office of National Security Coordination, the Office of Plans and Programs, the Office of Policy, the Office of International Affairs, the Office of Intergovernmental Affairs, the Office of Legislative Affairs, and the Office of Public Affairs. Ten regional offices provide direct support for designated geographic areas. Puerto Rico and the Virgin Islands are covered by Region II, along with New York and New Jersey; and Region IX bears responsibility for American Samoa, Guam, the Commonwealth of the Northern Marian Islands, the Republic of the Marshall Islands, and the Federated States of Micronesia, along with Arizona, California, Hawaii, and Nevada.

When a disaster occurs, the governor(s) of the affected state(s) may request assistance from FEMA through regional offices. FEMA responds by conducting a preliminary disaster assessment. The presi-

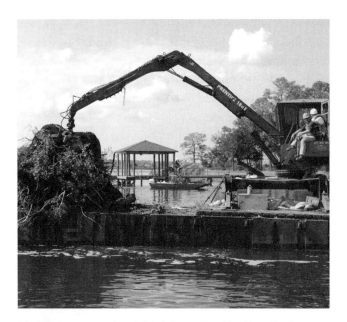

Workers remove marine debris leftover from Hurricane Katrina. FEMA funds wet debris removal, which the Coast Guard oversees.

dent may subsequently authorize federal assistance on the basis of emergency declarations or major declarations. In the first case, assistance is capped at $5 million per event and takes the form of emergency services and mitigation. Additional funding may be authorized by Congress. In the case of major declarations, the president determines that the resources of state and local governments are inadequate to respond to natural events such as hurricanes, floods, and earthquakes, thereby authorizing the entire range of federal assistance programs.

As part of its response efforts, FEMA officials work with state and local officials to deal with various aspects of the disaster. Postemergency assistance is available to individuals, communities, businesses, nonprofit organizations, and local emergency workers. This assistance often takes the form of grants, such as those awarded for specific disasters, environmental and historic preservation, hazard-related disasters, and nondisasters. The Repetitive Flood Claims Programs, which assists states and communities in areas that have filed one or more claims, is scheduled to close. FEMA grants may also be awarded for preparedness disaster training for specific groups such as firefighters and first responders. Direct assistance may take the form of loans, legal services, crisis counseling, unemployment assistance, emer-

gency food and shelter, and public assistance. FEMA also funds the National Urban Search and Rescue Response System to assist communities in the purchase, maintenance, and storage of rescue equipment and with training exercises and facilities. FEMA agents are available to conduct preparedness and response training for individuals, emergency workers, government personnel, businesses, farmers, teachers, tribal representatives, and volunteer agencies.

When Hurricane Katrina stuck America's Gulf Coast on the night of August 29, 2005, it set off a chain of events that tested FEMA's ability to respond to disasters to the limit. Subsequent testimony revealed that FEMA Director Michael Brown had informed the Bush administration that New Orleans, which is situated 20 miles below sea level, was extremely vulnerable to flooding if the outdated levees were breached. Requests for federal funding to update the levee system had previously been denied. On September 30, the levees broke, and 37 billion gallons of water poured into New Orleans. Thousands of people who had not been able to leave the city were stranded in public buildings without food, water, sanitary facilities, medicine, or other necessities. When television cameras brought the plight of the city to national attention, the public responded with outrage. FEMA was harshly criticized for its belated response, and criticism continued even after Brown resigned. Some critics believe the Bush administration's decision to strip FEMA of its independence led to the poor national response to Katrina. In 2006, a bipartisan Senate report, *Hurricane Katrina: A Nation Still Unprepared*, maintained that FEMA was beyond repair and recommended that the agency be dismantled and replaced with a newly created National Preparedness and Response Authority.

SEE ALSO: Disasters and Emergency Preparedness.

BIBLIOGRAPHY. Ronald J. Daniels, et al., eds., *On Risk and Disaster: Lessons from Hurricane Katrina* (University of Pennsylvania Press, 2006); Federal Emergency Management Agency (FEMA), http://www.fema.gov/; FEMA, *Disaster Assistance: A Guide to Recovery Programs* (FEMA, 2005); Spencer S. Hsu, "Senate Report Urges Dismantling of FEMA," Washington Post (April 27, 2006); Roger L. Kemp, *Homeland Security Handbook for Citizens and Public Officials* (McFarland, 2006); Roger L. Kemp, *The McGraw-Hill Security Handbook* (McGraw-Hill, 2006);

Kenneth J. Meier and Laurence J. O'Toole Jr., *Bureaucracy in a Democratic State: A Government Perspective* (Johns Hopkins University Press, 2006); James F. Miskel, *Disaster Response and Homeland Security: What Works, What Doesn't* (Praeger Security International, 2006); Dennis D. Riley, et al., *Bureaucracy and the Policy Process: Keeping the Promises* (Rowman & Littlefield, 2006); Louis Rowitz, *Public Health for the 21st Century: The Prepared Leader* (Jones and Bartlett, 2006); William M. Thaler, ed., Emerging Issues in Homeland Security (Nova Science, 2005).

ELIZABETH R. PURDY, PH.D.
INDEPENDENT SCHOLAR

Fee-for-Service

Traditionally, fee-for-service is a payment structure in which healthcare providers are paid a specified amount for each service they provide, including office visits, diagnostic tests, and medical procedures. Indemnity refers to insured individuals directly paying healthcare providers for a service, submitting bills to their insurance company, and then subsequently being reimbursed or indemnified for incurred costs. While fee-for-service and indemnity have inherently different meanings, the two terms are now often used interchangeably.

Fee-for-service or traditional indemnity health insurance plans typically allow patients the freedom to choose any physician or hospital as well as allow patients to self-refer to specialists. This is unlike most forms of managed care in which patients choose a primary care physician from a panel of doctors their health plan has contracted with to provide services. This physician then manages his or her patient's care by coordinating services and making appropriate specialist referrals. With fee-for-service plans, freedom of choice and flexibility come at a significant price. Insured individuals must pay a monthly fee or premium to their insurance company, an annual deductible, and coinsurance in which, for example, a patient pays 20 percent of his or her healthcare bill and the insurer pays 80 percent. Most fee-for-service plans do, however, have a cap or limit on how much an individual has to pay in out-of-pocket expenses for the year. Once this cap is reached, the insurance company pays for all subsequent costs.

There are undoubtedly advantages as well as disadvantages to the fee-for-service payment structure. Under fee-for-service plans, insured patients are at liberty to choose any physician, specialist, or hospital they wish. In addition, they do not require pre-authorization for services or referrals for specialist care. It has been argued that fee-for-service systems provide superior customer service—patient access to healthcare providers is prompt and direct. In addition, fee-for-service systems preserve physician autonomy. Physicians are left alone to decide what care their patients should receive and what prices should be charged. Despite such advantages, fee-for-service coverage also has apparent disadvantages. The financial burden in fee-for-service systems is high. Patients have higher monthly premiums as well as higher out-of-pocket expenditures. In addition, coverage only pays for reasonable and customary medical expenses. If healthcare providers charge more than the defined average in their area, patients must pay the difference. Fee-for-service systems also carry a significant paperwork burden. Patients or their healthcare providers must file claims for every insurance company reimbursement. Finally, it has been suggested that fee-for-service structures create perverse incentives for physicians. Physicians have a financial incentive to overtreat their patients because they are paid for every service they provide. In addition, physicians profit from sicker patients needing more services and this inherently creates a disincentive for preventive care and health promotion.

Advocates for fee-for-service and managed care systems are currently divided. However, both sides would undoubtedly agree that, as American Medical Association economist Carol Kane notes, "hopefully, as markets evolve and as we continue to learn about payment mechanisms, we will tend toward those arrangements where physicians are fairly and appropriately compensated for focusing on patient needs."

SEE ALSO: Health Maintenance Organization (HMO); Insurance; Managed Care; Point of Service (POS); Preferred Provider Organization (PPO).

BIBLIOGRAPHY. David M. Eddy, "Balancing Cost and Quality in Fee-for-Service versus Managed Care," *Health Affairs* (v.16/3, 1997); *Health, United States*, www.ahcpr.gov (cited September 2006); *Managed Care* Magazine online, www.

managedcaremag.com/archives/9904/9904.capvsffs.html (cited October 2006).

SANGEETA PATEL
UNIVERSITY OF ILLINOIS AT CHICAGO COLLEGE
OF MEDICINE

Female Circumcision

Often used synonymously with the terms *female genital cutting* or *female genital mutilation*, female circumcision refers to the removal of any part of the female external genitalia for a nonmedical purpose. The United Nations and the World Health Organization prefer the term *genital mutilation* to emphasize the often negative health and sexual consequences for women who have undergone the procedure, as well as to draw a clear distinction between removal of female genitalia from removal of the male foreskin, a procedure which carries fewer negative health consequences.

Female circumcision is a blanket term that refers to many related but distinct practices. Most involve removing at least some genital tissue, although in some instances, the ritual is symbolically simulated with a knife or needle but no tissue is removed. A clitoridotomy involves the removal or splitting of the clitoral hood; cliteridectomy means the partial or complete removal of the external part of the clitoris; and infibulation replaces the entire vulva with an intact layer of flesh from pubis to the anus, apart from a small hole for urine and menstrual blood. The labia are sewn together following excision and will heal as scar tissue. The opening is cut prior to childbirth and then resewn.

Although performed by trained medical personnel in some locales, female circumcision is often performed without anesthesia and using nonsterile equipment, which can cause a great deal of bleeding and pain. Girls and women are prone to infection following the procedure, following sexual intercourse, and following childbirth. Infibulation can also cause infections due to blocked passage of urine or menstrual blood, sometimes leading to infertility.

Female circumcision is often justified by citing religious texts or cultural norms, and is often carried out by females on their own younger relatives. Most human rights organizations deplore any form of female genital alteration, especially as it is often performed on girls too young to give consent, most commonly when they are aged between 4 and 8. Although the practice was legal in the United States until 1996, it is now illegal although still practiced clandestinely among some immigrant groups. Female genital alteration is still common in many countries, especially in the Middle East and Africa, where rates can exceed 95 percent. Views among people living in these countries are naturally quite variable, although a small but growing number of people are rejecting the practice for their own children.

SEE ALSO: Infertility; World Health Organization (WHO).

BIBLIOGRAPHY. Rogaia Mustafa Abusharaf, ed., *Female Circumcision: Multicultural Perspectives* (University of Pennsylvania Press, 2007); Ellen Gruenbaum, *Female Circumcision Controversy: An Anthropological Perspective* (Johns Hopkins University Press, 2000).

ANNIE DUDE
UNIVERSITY OF CHICAGO

Fetal Alcohol Syndrome

Fetal alcohol spectrum disorders are a continuum of alcohol-induced fetal malformations. The severe end of this spectrum is a specific pattern of malformations in the developing fetus termed *fetal alcohol syndrome.* The Centers for Disease Control and Prevention (CDC) estimates that the incidence of fetal alcohol syndrome in the United States is between 0.2 and 1.5 cases per 1,000 live births in the various regions of the country. The incidence of all fetal alcohol spectrum disorders is estimated to be several times higher still.

The actual mechanism of embryonic and fetal malformation due to maternal alcohol consumption is not known. It is thought that alcohol or its by-products may interfere with placental transfer of essential minerals and amino acids. The incidence of the fetal alcohol phenotype is directly related to the level of alcohol exposure. Approximately 30 percent of infants born to heavy drinkers have congenital anomalies compared to approximately 15 percent of those born to moderate drinkers.

Fetal alcohol syndrome is characterized by abnormal facial features, growth deficiency affecting length, weight, and head circumference, and central nervous system anomalies including developmental delay, mental retardation, and attention deficit disorder. The characteristic faces of the infant or child with fetal alcohol syndrome includes a thin upper lip, short palpebral fissures (the space between the margin of the eyelids), and an abnormal philtrum (the midline groove between the upper lip and the nose). Associated malformations that are not required for diagnosis but are, nonetheless, frequently seen include cardiac defects, particularly of the septum, and minor limb and joint anomalies.

Fetal alcohol syndrome is one of the leading causes of preventable birth defects and mental retardation. While affected children may benefit from special education initiatives and psychosocial support, there is no specific treatment for the syndrome. The syndrome is, however, 100 percent preventable by eliminating alcohol consumption during pregnancy. There is no known "safe" level of alcohol consumption during pregnancy and damage may occur during any trimester. All healthcare professionals should educate women of childbearing age regarding the deleterious effects of alcohol on their growing child and women who are pregnant should be specifically counseled to stop consumption of alcohol and be given appropriate support to do so. It is important for health professionals to not limit preventative interventions solely to the mother but to also recognize the role of fathers and other family members in preventing the occurrence of fetal alcohol syndrome.

SEE ALSO: Alcohol Consumption; Birth Defects; Mental Retardation.

BIBLIOGRAPHY. Centers for Disease Control and Prevention, "Fetal Alcohol Spectrum Disorders," http://www.cdc.gov/ncbddd/fas/ (cited January 14, 2007).

CLAIRE K. NGUYEN
JOHNS HOPKINS BLOOMBERG SCHOOL OF PUBLIC HEALTH

Fever

Fever, or pyrexis, is a condition in which body temperature rises above the normal. Mild fevers are associated with loss of liquid and chills, while more extreme fevers can lead to convulsion and even death. Generally, a fever is caused as a result of infection by virus or bacteria and results from the body's natural ability to produce more pyrogens than normal and these affect the brain's ability to detect temperature changes. It is possible that fever can be a beneficial response by the body to an infection and helps in resistance and recovery from it. However, this has not yet been fully established and some controversy surrounds the issue. Nevertheless, the elevated temperatures stimulate the production of white blood cells and may inhibit the growth of invading organisms.

During the course of a typical day, the internal temperature varies little and generally remains within one or two degrees of its average of 37.2 degrees C in the mouth; increases in temperature beyond this range are, therefore, defined as fever and temperature rises of above 40.5 degrees represent severe fevers; should the temperature reach 42.2 degrees or higher, then a genuine threat of death exists. Mild fevers generally feature increased sweating and reduced blood and urine production.

Although fever is generally associated with viral infection, it can also come about as a result of coronary trouble or in response to extreme physiological stress. In general terms, treating fever should be approached by treating the underlying causes of the fever, although this may be accompanied by measures to reduce any discomfort the patient might be feeling as a result of high temperature. Consequently, aspirin might be used as an antipyretic agent and other pharmaceuticals used to tackle the cause and nature of the infection or other cause.

A wide range of conditions are referred to as a form of fever, not always accurately. The name of the fever generally relates to its cause; for example, Rift Valley fever is caused by the bite of mosquitoes in the Rift Valley of Kenya and subsequently more widely; meanwhile, blackwater fever is a form of malaria in which the urine turns black. Hay fever is a condition in which an allergic reaction to pollen or similar item leads to flu-like symptoms, although strictly speaking this is not a fever at all. In many parts of the world, fevers continue to represent a serious threat to health. Dengue fever, for example, and hemorrhagic fever kill tens of thousands of people annually. Increases

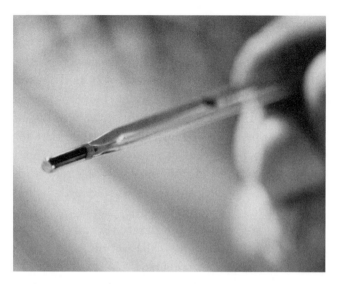

Fever is caused as a result of infection by virus or bacteria and results from the body's natural ability to produce more pyrogens.

in public health technical capacity and resources in affected countries would help to reduce these numbers. However, as climate change continues to cause migration of living creatures into different locations, vulnerability will spread beyond areas where those problems have previously been experienced.

SEE ALSO: Dengue.

BIBLIOGRAPHY. Centers for Disease Control Division of Vector-Borne Infectious Diseases (CDC-DVBID), "Dengue Fever Publications," http://www.cdc.gov/ncidod/dvbid/pubs/dengue-pubs.htm (cited January 2007); Duane J. Gubler, "Dengue and Dengue Hemorrhagic Fever," *Clinical Microbiology Reviews* (v.11/3, 1998).

JOHN WALSH
SHINAWATRA UNIVERSITY

Fiji

Fiji is an island nation in the Pacific Ocean, west of Tonga and south of Tuvalu. The nation is comprised of 322 islands (106 of them inhabited) and 522 islets. Almost 90 percent of the population lives on the two main islands of Viti Levu and Vanua Levu. A popular tourist destination for nearly 500,000 people a year,

Fijians have seen cycles of economic stagnation and political turmoil over the past 30 years. The nation has endured four military coups in the past 20 years, the latest in 2006. The population is 906,000, making it the most populous of the South Pacific's island nations. However, the annual rate of growth is just 1.4 percent, due to a low birth rate and increased emigration.

Many of those who leave the island are Indo-Fijians, descendents of Indian workers brought in by the British during a century of colonization. Once Fiji won independence in 1970, native Melanesians began to pass exclusionary laws against those of Indian heritage. Today, many Indo-Fijians suffer from racial discrimination and unequal access to public services, including education. Despite an overall literacy rate of 93 percent, a 1996 survey showed that only 14 percent of Indo-Fijian woman and 8 percent of men had received formal education.

Life expectancy rates have risen sharply since the 1960s, now standing at around 67 for males and 72 for females. Infant and child mortality has fallen to relatively low levels, with 16 infant deaths per 1,000 and 18 deaths per 1,000 for children aged 1–5. Mothers receive adequate prenatal care, and maternal mortality is rare.

While a variety of communicable diseases have been brought under control since the 1960s, problems do remain. The figures are not complete, but the World Health Organization estimates that at least 25 percent of Fijians live below the poverty line. Clean water and sanitation is spotty in some areas. Most child deaths are caused by acute respiratory diseases, meningitis, parasitic diseases, and anemia.

Noncommunicable, chronic lifestyle diseases such as diabetes and hypertension are also beginning to put an increasing burden on the health of Fijians. Like their island neighbors, Fijians have moved toward a more sedentary lifestyle and adopted a more westernized diet, leading to a rise in obesity levels. Smoking is also common. A 2002 survey indicated that the adult prevalence rate for diabetes was 12 percent, and the prevalence rate for hypertension was 19 percent. A third of all deaths in Fijians aged 40–59 were attributable to circulatory diseases.

Unlike most of the Pacific Islands, Fiji has a human immunodeficiency virus (HIV)-positive population, with 219 reported cases as of December 2006. Because HIV testing in Fiji is voluntary, the virus could be much more widespread; the Ministry of Health estimates that up to 4,000 Fijians could be undiagnosed. Other sexually transmitted diseases have also spiked up. Fiji contributes less of its Gross Domestic Product to total health expenditures than any Pacific nation, around 3 percent annually or $104 per capita. Little money has been allocated to hospital infrastructure or drug procurement. There are 24 general hospitals and 74 primary care centers to serve the population; the Ministry of Health counted 339 doctors, 1,682 nurses, and 1,435 other healthcare staff in 2003.

SEE ALSO: Healthcare, Asia and Oceania; Tonga; Tuvalu.

BIBLIOGRAPHY. Richard and Renee S. Katz, *The Straight Path of the Spirit: Ancestral Wisdom and Healing Traditions in Fiji*, (Inner Traditions International, 1999); "Fiji," World Health Organization, http://www.who.int/countries/fji/en/.

HEATHER K. MICHON
INDEPENDENT SCHOLAR

Filariasis/Elephantiasis

Currently affecting at least 120 million people in over 80 countries, lymphatic filariasis has for thousands of years been a leading cause of permanent and long-term disability worldwide. Its primary form, called *Wuchereria Bankcrofti*, is transmitted between humans by the bites of infected mosquitoes, mainly *Anopheles* and *Aedes* species in endemic parts of Africa and Asia, respectively. People living in areas of poor sanitation, where mosquitoes often breed, are at high risk for infection.

BIOLOGICAL IMPACT

Lymphatic filariasis is caused when several, threadlike parasitic worms invade the human lymph system, which fights infections and regulates the body's fluid balance. The microscopic worms live in the lymph vessels for five to seven years, often causing permanent damage. An impaired lymph system results in the swelling of arms, legs, and even genitals, often to several times the normal size, usually termed *lymphedema*. Lymphedema makes it difficult to fight infections and those affected typically have severe fungal and bacterial diseases that thicken and harden the skin, which is called elephantiasis.

SOCIAL IMPACT

As a chronic infection, lymphatic filariasis inflicts severe social problems upon its victims. People with the disease often suffer pain, disfigurement, and sexual disability. Communities frequently shun women and men disfigured by the disease, many of whom never marry or become rejected by spouses. Their families and communities are further affected as people disabled by the disease are frequently unable to work.

PREVENTION, TREATMENT, AND CONTROL

Prevention and control measures against lymphatic filariasis include sleeping under mosquito nets, with or without insecticide treatment, and the use of mosquito repellents. However, given the long life cycle of the filarial worms, even these mosquito control efforts have failed at eradicating the disease. Thus, in 2000, the World Health Organization launched a global program to eliminate lymphatic filariasis by mass drug administration (MDA) of at-risk populations with medicines, including diethylcarbamazine, ivermectin, and albendazole, known to kill the worms.

Such efforts have yielded promising results in endemic areas, such as in Egypt, where research suggests that filariasis can be eliminated after five rounds of MDA. The goals of this global campaign are to eliminate lymphatic filariasis as a public health problem and alleviate the social and economic hardships in individuals suffering from lymphatic filariasis-induced disability.

SEE ALSO: Healthcare, Africa; Healthcare, Asia and Oceania; Lymphatic Diseases; Parasitic Diseases.

BIBLIOGRAPHY. Division of Parasitic Diseases at the Centers for Disease Control and Prevention, "Lymphatic Filariasis," www.cdc.gov/Ncidod/dpd/ (cited October 2006); The Global Alliance to Eliminate Lymphatic Filariasis, "Global Alliance History," www.filariasis.org (cited October 2006); R.M. Ramzy, et al., "Effect of Yearly Mass Drug Administration with Diethylcarbamzine and Albendazole on Bancroftian Filariasis in Egypt: A Comprehensive Assessment," *Lancet* (v.367/9515, 2006).

RAJESH PANJABI, MPH
DEPARTMENT OF MEDICINE, UNIVERSITY OF NORTH
CAROLINA–CHAPEL HILL
JOHNS HOPKINS SCHOOL OF PUBLIC HEALTH

Finland

With a per capita income of $31,000, Finland is the 22nd richest nation in the world. The government provides a strong safety net; and according to the United Nations Development Programme's (UNDP) Human Development Report, Finland has the 11th highest standard of living. Income is relatively well distributed, and Finland is ranked 26.9 percent on the Gini index of inequality. The richest 10 percent of the population holds 21.6 percent of the country's wealth while the poorest 10 percent share 4.2 percent. Poverty is virtually nonexistent in Finland, but the government has been forced to deal with persistent unemployment (currently 8.4 percent).

Municipalities are responsible for providing health insurance in Finland, and local governments may choose to provide coverage themselves or to join municipal boards or turn to outside agents. As the aging population expands, government resources have become strained. Consequently, families and communities have taken on a greater share of the responsibility for caring for the elderly. While most Finns enjoy easy access to healthcare, people who live in remote areas are sometimes cut off from health services. The government addressed this need in a 2003 report, which introduced a plan in which central and municipal governments work with nongovernmental organizations (NGOs) to make healthcare affordable and accessible to all Finns. Targeted areas included restructuring the healthcare system and strengthening financing methods. Long-term health goals were laid out in Health 2015, which encouraged healthier lifestyles across the population. Goals for different age groups were established such as improving women's and children's health, curtailing alcohol and drug abuse among adolescents, slashing the rate of accidental and violent deaths among adult males, and meeting the needs of the aging population.

Finland spends an average of 3 percent of the total budget on health care. At present, 7.4 percent of the Gross Domestic Product (GDP) is designated for health-related programs, with $2,108 (international dollars) allotted per capita. The government provides 76.5 percent of all healthcare expenditures, and 21.5 percent of that amount is earmarked for social security. Social security in Finland covers the elderly, the disabled, and survivors. The system is financed by workers (4.4 percent of earn-

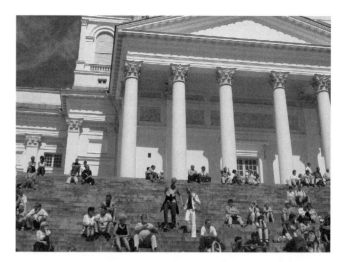

Finland is the 22nd richest nation in the world with a per capita income of $31,000.

ings), the self-employed (21.1 percent of earnings), and employers (from 1.3 to 4.45 percent of payroll) and supplemented by the government. The private sector furnishes 23.5 percent of total healthcare expenditures, and 81.20 percent of private funding is derived from out-of-pocket expenses. There are 3.16 physicians, 14.33 nurses, 0.76 midwives, 1.28 dentists, and 1.12 pharmacists per 1,000 population in Finland.

The population of 5,231,372 enjoys a life expectancy of 78.5 years, the 39th highest in the world. Women outlive men an average of seven years. Literacy is universal in Finland, and all of the relevant population attends primary and secondary school. All Finns have sustained access to safe drinking water and improved sanitation. The use of birth control is widespread (77 percent), and Finnish women give birth at a rate of 1.73 children each. All births are attended by trained personnel, and all new mothers receive antenatal care. The adjusted maternal mortality rate of six deaths per 100,000 live births is among the lowest in the world.

Finland has the sixth lowest infant mortality rate among the world's nations at 3.55 deaths per 100,000 live births. Between 1990 and 2004, infant mortality was cut in half, dropping from six to three deaths per 1,000 live births. At the same time, mortality for children under the age of five fell from seven to four deaths per 1,000 live births. Although Finnish children are remarkably healthy, four percent of infants are underweight at birth. Immunization rates are predictably high, and 98 percent of infants are immunized against diphtheria, pertussis, and tetanus (DPT1 and DPT3) and tuberculosis; 97 percent against measles; and 96 percent against polio and *Haemophilus influenzae* type B.

HIV/AIDS does not present a major problem in Finland, and the current adult prevalence rate is less than 0.1 percent. Around 1,500 people are living with the disease, and it has proved fatal to less than 100. In May 2000, meningococcal disease was identified in Finland, and the country experienced outbreaks of influenza in 2003 and 2004. Severe acute respiratory syndrome (SARS) surfaced in spring 2003. The leading causes of death in Finland are cardiovascular disease, alcoholism-related conditions, and accidents. High cholesterol and obesity are also of grave concern.

SEE ALSO: Childhood Immunization; Obesity.

BIBLIOGRAPHY. Central Intelligence Agency, "Finland," *World Factbook* www.cia.gov/cia/publications/factbook/geos/fi.html; Commission on the Status of Women, "Finland" www.un.org/womenwatch/daw/Review/responses/FINLAND-English.pdf (cited April 2007); Spencer Di Scala, *Twentieth Century Europe: Politics, Society, Culture* (McGraw-Hill, 2004); Sandra Halperin, *War and Social Change in Modern Europe: The Great Transformation Revisited* (Cambridge University Press, 2004); Martin A. Levin and Martin Shapiro, eds., *Transatlantic Policymaking in an Age of Austerity: Diversity and Drift* (Georgetown University Press, 2004); Jeremy Rifkin, *The European Dream: How Europe's Vision of the Future Is Quietly Eclipsing the American Dream* (Jeremy P. Tarcher/Penguin, 2004); Social Security Administration, "Finland" www.ssa.gov/policy/docs/progdesc/ssptw/2002-2003/europe/finland.html (cited April 2007); Eric Solsten and Sandra W. Meditz, *Finland: A Country Study* (Federal Research Division, LOC, 1990); Peter Taylor-Gooby, *New Risks, New Welfare: The Transformation of the European Welfare State* (Oxford University Press, 2004).

ELIZABETH R. PURDY, PH.D.
INDEPENDENT SCHOLAR

Flea Bites

A flea bite is the resulting injury from a flea sting, which could produce a local inflammatory reaction, or after an incubation period, a flea-borne disease, such as plague, endemic typhus fever, dipylidiasis, and hymenolepiasis, among others, but most species of flea do not transmit pathogens.

Fleas belong (taxonomically) to the order *Siphonapetra*, with two important families for human and animal health: *Pulicidae* and *Tungidae*. The above-mentioned diseases are transmitted by members of family *Pulicidae* (*Pulex*, *Ctenocephalides*, and *Xenopsylla*).

In history, *Xenopsylla cheopis* represented the most important vector of an ancient disease previously known as the Black Death (plague), one of the worst natural disasters in history. Plague or Black Death is an infection of rodents caused by *Yersinia pestis* and accidentally transmitted to humans by the bite of infected fleas. Plague has three forms: bubonic plague (infection of the lymph glands), septicemia plague (infection of the blood), and pneumonic plague (infection of the lungs). Pneumonic plague can spread from person to person. Fortunately, this disease is treatable with antibiotics if detected early. Prevention consists of controlling rodent fleas, educating the public and the medical community in places where plague occurs, and using preventive medicines and vaccines as appropriate.

Endemic typhus fever or typhus (also called flea-borne typhus and murine typhus) is a disease caused by small bacteria called *Rickettsia*. Dipylidiasis is a common tapeworm infection of dogs and cats caused by *Dipylidium caninum*. Arthropods serve as intermediate hosts for this parasite, including then the fleas which include the dog flea (*Ctenocephalides canis*), the cat flea (*C. felis*), and the dog louse (*Trichodectes canis*). The risk to human beings to acquire this disease is low, because this occurs by ingestion of arthropod intermediate hosts which harbor the cysticercoid larvae. The hymenolepiasis, caused by the dwarf tapeworm or *Hymenolepis nana*, is the most common tapeworm infection diagnosed in the world. Although it is not the most common form of transmission, fleas could vectorize this disease in animals and may be in humans. People get infected by accidentally ingesting tapeworm eggs, by ingesting fecally contaminated foods and water, by touching the mouth with contaminated fingers, or by ingesting contaminated soil.

Another important infection directly caused by fleas is the tungiasis which is a common health problem in economically depressed communities in South American and sub-Saharan African countries, but it should be considered in the increasing number of international travelers to tropical destinations. The causative ectoparasite,

Tunga penetrans (a flea of approximately 1 millimeter of size), penetrates into the skin of its host, undergoes a peculiar hypertrophy, expels several hundred eggs for a period of less than three weeks, and eventually dies. Besides the human, this flea could infect cattle, sheep, and horses.

SEE ALSO: Medical Entomology; Medical Helminthology; Parasitic Diseases; Tick Bites.

BIBLIOGRAPHY. Harold Brown, *Clinical Parasitology* (Appleton-Century-Crofts, 1983); Albert Camus, *The Plague* (Penguin, 1970); Gordon Cook and Alimuddin Zulma, *Manson's Tropical Diseases* (Saunders, 2003); Hermann Feldmeier, "Severe Tungiasis in Underprivileged Communities: Case Series from Brazil," *Emerging Infectious Diseases* (v.9/8, 2003); Becerri Flores and Romero Cabello, *Medical Parasitology* (McGraw-Hill, 2004); David Heymann, *Control of Communicable Diseases in Man* (APHA/PAHO/WHO, 2004).

ALFONSO J. RODRIGUEZ-MORALES, M.D., M.SC.
UNIVERSIDAD DE LOS ANDES, VENEZUELA
CARLOS FRANCO-PAREDES, M.D., M.P.H.
EMORY UNIVERSITY

Fluoride

Fluoride is the ionic form of the element fluorine, and there are organic and inorganic compounds containing fluorine which form fluorides. Some of these are found naturally in low concentrations in drinking water and in tea and other foods, and indeed, the ocean itself has an average concentration of fluoride compounds of 1.3 parts per million. In industry, hydrofluoric acid is used for the etching of glass and also for the making of integrated circuit boards and other industrial applications. However, generally, in terms of healthcare, it is used to deal with prevention of tooth decay. In a very concentrated form, it can be a prescription drug as a part of drug molecules to resist the detoxification in the liver by the Cytochrome P450 oxidase.

Fluoride has been used for a long time in the treatment of teeth to prevent tooth decay, and is found in toothpaste. In 1951, Joseph C. Muhler and Harry G. Day of Indiana University reported that their research on stannous fluoride was an effective means of preventing tooth decay, and the university sold the research findings to Procter & Gamble who started using it in their Crest® toothpaste. Nowadays, fluoride is found in most toothpastes, and it is possible to use fluoride although care must be taken not to use too much, otherwise dental fluorosis could occur through overexposure.

In addition, there has been much debate over water fluoridation with some parts of the world introducing it into water supplies to help reduce the level of tooth decay in children. This has led to widespread debate around the world with the World Health Organization and the American Dental Association recommending increasing the level of fluoride in water to between 0.7 and 1.2 parts per million. Opponents of water fluoridization claims that an increase in fluoride could weaken the human immune system, and this could lead to increased prevalence of certain diseases and disorders.

However, most international health service agencies recognize that the benefits involved in the prevention of dental decay hugely outweigh the concerns that some people have expressed regarding the side effects. Articles on the role of fluoride and it possible side effects have been published in the *British Medical Journal* and also in forums such as *The Journal of Fluorine Chemistry*. This has not stopped politicians in many countries opposing the fluoridization of water, some of which involved several marathon debates in the British House of Commons, the latest of which was in November 2003.

SEE ALSO: Dental Health.

BIBLIOGRAPHY. L. L. Demos, et al., "Water Fluoridation, Osteoporosis, Fractures—Recent Developments," *Australian Dental Journal* (v.46/2, 2001); M.S. McDonagh, et al., "Systematic Review of Water Fluoridation," *British Medical Journal* (v.321, 2000); G.M. Whitford, "Fluoride in Dental Products," *Journal of Dental Research* (v.66/5, 1987).

JUSTIN CORFIELD
GEELONG GRAMMAR SCHOOL, AUSTRALIA

Folic Acid

Folic acid, whose chemical name is pteroylmonoglutamic acid, was first isolated in 1945. Folic acid is B vitamin found in leafy greens, animal proteins, fruits, and vegetables. Humans absorb this vitamin from the proximal small intestine and store folate primarily in the liver and red blood cells (RBCs). Folate is indirectly responsible for the synthesis of DNA. Many etiologies exist for folate deficiency including infection, pregnancy, malabsorption/starvation syndromes, certain cancer medications, and antibiotics. With low levels of folic acid, RBCs tend to enlarge in volume, a term known as *macrocytosis*. With this enlargement, RBCs are not able to routinely carry enough oxygen to tissues creating a scenario known as megaloblastic anemia. Megaloblastic anemia can be diagnosed by measuring the mean volume of RBCs, examining peripheral blood smears of RBCs, measuring serum folate levels, and by examining bone marrow.

Another major cause of megaloblastic anemia is vitamin B12 deficiency. The distinction between the two disease states is important in terms of treatment. If the cause of the anemia is due to vitamin B12 deficiency, increasing the dietary folate levels may improve the anemia temporarily but will not prevent the neurologic decline that occurs with vitamin B12 deficiency. Similarly, in the case of malabsorption syndromes, increasing the folate intake will not improve the ultimate source of the vitamin loss.

Among the general public, folic acid is most well known for its importance in preventing neural tube defects (NTDs). The incidence of these ailments affecting proper development of the brain and spinal cord are significantly reduced by as much as 70 percent with the minimum daily dietary intake of 400 µg. The mechanism by which folate is able to prevent NTDs is not completely understood and the involvement in NTD development is possible even in the first week of pregnancy when a woman may be unaware she is pregnant. Thus, all women of childbearing age are especially encouraged to incorporate folic acid into their diets.

In the United States, most flour and grain products are supplemented with folic acid in order to decrease the number of infants born with NTDs; however, supplementation in European or Australian countries is not required and has become a topic of controversy. Pregnant women are encouraged to maximize their dietary intake of folic acid; however, more than 1,000 µg daily affords no additional benefits and any adverse effects at this dosage have not yet been elucidated. The U. S. Department of Health and Human Services encourages dietary intake of folic acid through fortified dry cereals, supplements, or by eating fruits and vegetables high in folic acid. Folic acid is being examined in the cardiovascular arena with studies showing a promise of improved heart health, a decreased incidence of stroke, and a decrease in congenital heart defects.

SEE ALSO: Anemia; Neural Tube Defects; Vitamin and Mineral Supplements.

BIBLIOGRAPHY. Centers for Disease Control and Prevention, "The Basics about Folic Acid," www.cdc.gov (cited November 2005); Centers for Disease Control and Prevention, "Folic Acid Now," www.cdc.gov (cited November 2005); M. Tarek Elghetany and Katalin Banki, *Henry's Clinical Diagnosis and Management by Laboratory Methods: Erythrocytic Disorders* (Saunders, 2006); L.L.M. Lindsey, et al., "Use of Dietary Supplements Containing Folic Acid among Women of Childbearing Age," *Morbidity and Mortality Weekly Report* (v.54/38, 2005); National Women's Health Information Center, "Folic Acid—Frequently Asked Questions," www.womenshealth.gov (cited January 2005); Edward Reynolds, "Vitamin B12, Folic Acid, and the Nervous System," *Lancet* (v.5, 2006).

STEPHANIE F. INGRAM
UNIVERSITY OF SOUTH FLORIDA
COLLEGE OF MEDICINE

Fondation Jean Dausset (CEPH)

Founded in 1984 as the Centre d'Etude du Polymorphisme Humain (CEP), this foundation was renamed the Fondation Jean Dausset in 1993. Dausset, a world-renowned scientist, won the Nobel Prize in Physiology or Medicine in 1980. Since its inception the foundation has developed essential tools in the genetic and physical mapping of human chromosomes.

During the 1990s the foundation began concentrating on polyfactorial diseases, making a significant contribution to the understanding of the etiology of inflammatory bowel maladies. Through a positional cloning strategy the foundation succeeded in identifying three mutations in a new gene that increases the susceptibility to Crohn's disease.

The foundation is also involved with a large international consortium concentrating on research for susceptibility genes for breast and prostate cancer. In 1991, the Foundation, along with the French Muscular Dystrophy Association, created the Généthon, a nonprofit research institute, in order to provide tools to the scientific community for the localization and cloning of disease determining genes. The Fondation Jean Dausset is headquartered in Paris, France, and each year sponsors a number of meetings and seminars related to the organization's mission.

SEE ALSO: Breast Cancer; Gene Mapping; Prostate Cancer; Muscular Dystrophy.

BIBLIOGRAPHY. Association Française Contre les Myopathies (AFM), www.afm-france.org (cited October 2006); Fondation Jean Dausset (CEPH), www.cephb.fr (cited October 2006).

ERIN FITCH
INDEPENDENT SCHOLAR

Food Allergy

A food allergy, or hypersensitivity, is an exaggerate immunological response to a food that can cause symptoms from tingling lips to difficulty breathing and life-threatening anaphylaxis.

The prevalence of food allergies has been estimated to be around 1 to 3 percent in adults and 4 to 6 percent in children and rising, and more than 70 foods have been reported as causing food allergies. There is no current treatment for food allergies, and avoidance of the causative food is the only recommended prevention method. Access to care is crucial with food allergy; without it, the reaction can lead to inflammation of the airways, restricted breathing, and subsequent death.

Many food allergies begin in childhood. Children develop allergies in order of their exposure to the causative agent, so food allergies begin when food is introduced into the diet. Food allergy can develop from a combination of genetic factors and environmental exposures, as part of overall *atopy*, a genetic predilection toward overreactive immune responses against harmless environmental exposures. Many people outgrow their food allergies, although many of the most serious allergies are lifelong.

Food allergies are not the same as intolerance, which can cause abdominal cramping, but is not associated with an allergic response mediated by immunoglobulin E (IgE). The most common foods that trigger food allergies are eggs, fish, peanuts, soybeans, milk, tree nuts, gluten, and shellfish/crustaceans, and it is usually a protein in the food that acts as the allergen. Because foods that trigger allergy depend on exposure, food allergies vary across the world. In central Europe, allergy to celery is common, whereas east Asia has a substantial population with rice allergy.

As in any other allergic reaction, a person must be previously sensitized to the particular allergen, so that the immune system is able to identify and memorize a specific molecular "footprint" for each allergen. On encountering the allergen for the first time, IgE is produced. Once IgE has been synthesized, a second exposure to the allergen induces IgE to cause release of many inflammatory molecules. The signs and symptoms of an allergic food reaction can include tongue swelling, hives, difficulty breathing, vomiting, diarrhea, eczema, sudden decrease in blood pressure, loss of consciousness, and death.

Most symptoms are classified according to the organ system they affect. Gastrointestinal signs can include vomiting, pain, or diarrhea and can develop rapidly after consumption of the allergen. Oral allergy syndrome is a result of cross-sensitivity to foods that also cause allergic rhinitis in the individual; it manifests as itchy, swelling lips and tongue. Atopic dermatitis, or eczema, can be caused by food allergy, as can hives and angioedema, or deep tissue inflammation.

The most severe result of food allergy is anaphylaxis. The annual incidence of anaphylactic reactions is about 30 per 100,000 persons, and individuals with asthma, eczema, or hay fever are at greater relative risk of experiencing anaphylaxis. There are other causes of anaphylaxis besides food allergy, including medication allergy, insect stings, and latex, but foods are a common cause of anaphylaxis. Anaphylaxis is a systemic reaction that can affect several organ systems at the same time and can be life threatening without immediate treatment. An anaphylactic reaction may begin with a tingling or itching sensation in the mouth, and progress to hives, swelling of the mouth and throat area, difficulty breathing, vomiting, diarrhea, abdominal cramping, and loss of consciousness. The main treatment for an anaphylactic food response is injection with epinephrine or adrenaline. This can be self-administered with an EpiPen®, which is designed to inject a controlled amount of drug. The epinephrine constricts the swollen blood vessels and decreases inflammation, to decrease hives, tongue, throat and airway constriction, and to restore normal blood pressure.

In the case of those with milder symptoms, food allergies can be difficult to detect. The timing of a reaction can be delayed due to the digestive process, and a detailed food diary can help in detecting the timing of reactions, as well as the amount of food that triggers them, and the duration and severity of symptoms. An elimination diet, in which one particular food is eliminated in order to see if the existing reaction (eczema, hives, respiratory difficulty) resolves, is a good way to confirm suspected food allergens.

Other options for diagnosis, where allergists are present, include a skin prick test or oral challenge. In a skin prick test, small amounts of common allergens are scratched onto the skin and a red, itchy wheal will develop within minutes to indicate the specific allergens for that person. An oral challenge, which should only be undertaken under medical supervision, consists of feeding the suspected food and waiting for a reaction. In the case of anaphylactic reactions, oral challenge is not a good idea, especially in areas unequipped to treat severe allergic reactions.

Because there is no prevention method analogous to allergy shots and respiratory allergies for food allergies, those with food allergies are advised to avoid their triggering food(s) at all costs. If labels are present on foods, these should be read and screened against the allergy. If no labels are available, one should avoid the food or contact the manufacturer for more details of its contents. In a resource-poor environment, where food labels and available epinephrine are rare, food allergies can be especially deadly.

SEE ALSO: Allergy.

BIBLIOGRAPHY. Food Allergy and Anaphylaxis Network (FAAN), www.foodallergy.org; World Health Organization International Food Safety Authorities Network, "Food Allergies," www.who.int/entity/foodsafety/fs_management/No_03_allergy_June06_en.pdf (cited April 28, 2007).

ERIN FITCH
OREGON HEALTH AND SCIENCE UNIVERSITY

Food and Agriculture Organization of the United Nations (FAO)

Founded in 1945, the Food and Agriculture Organization of the United Nations (FAO) leads international efforts to defeat hunger throughout the world. Serving both developed and developing countries, the FAO acts as a neutral forum where all nations meet on an equal footing to negotiate agreements and debate policy. The organization also serves as a source of information related to world hunger and global agricultural issues. It helps developing and transitional countries modernize and make improvements in agriculture, forestry and fisheries to ensure optimum production with an emphasis on nutrition. Since its inception, the organization has focused special attention on rural areas, which are home to almost three-quarters of the world's poor and hungry. In general terms, the FAO's goals revolve around making sure that the world's population has regular access to enough quality to lead active, healthy lives. The organization is charged with raising levels of nutrition, improving agricultural production and contributing to the overall growth of the world economy. As part of its mission, the FAO serves as an ever-expanding information network, calling on the expertise of its staff, including agronomists, foresters, fish and livestock specialists, social scientists, nutritionists, economists and statisticians, to collect, analyze and impart data. The organization also lends its years of experience to member countries in devising agricultural policy, supporting, planning and drafting effective legislation, and creating national strategies to alleviate hunger in impoverished areas. With regard to practical application, the organization promotes and maintains thousands of field projects around the world and manages millions of dollars contributed in large part by industrialized nations, development banks and private sources. In crisis situations, the FAO works with the World Food Program and other humanitarian agencies to help protect the livelihoods of individuals living in rural areas. The FAO also sponsors a variety of publication and produces a number of annual reports in various areas related to food production, world hunger, and the status of FAO projects.

The FAO is governed by the Conference of Member Nations, which meets every two years to review the activities of the organization and approve the appropriate budgets. The conference elects a director general and governing council, which acts as a general governing body between Conference gatherings. The FAO is divided into eight departments: Administration and Finance; Agriculture; Biosecurity, Nutrition and Consumer Protection; Economics and Statistics; Fisheries; Forestry; General Affairs and Information; and Sustainable Development and Technical Cooperation.

The organization maintains an international headquarters in Rome as well as a number of regional, subregional, and country offices and employs more than 3,700 individuals. In the 1990s, the FAO underwent significant restructuring to cut costs and decentralize its operation. This effectively increased the organizations emphasis on food security and focus on developing and transition nations while it increased interaction with the private sector.

SEE ALSO: Food and Drug Administration (FDA); World Health Organization (WHO).

BIBLIOGRAPHY. *Ethics Update: World Hunger*, ethics. acusd.edu/Applied/WorldHunger/index.asp (cited September 2006); European Public Health Alliance, www. epha.org (cited September 2006); Food and Agriculture Organization of the United Nations, www.fao.org (cited September 2006); United Nations World Food Program www.wfp.org/english (cited September 2006); World Health Organization, www.who.int/en (cited September 2006).

BEN WYNNE, PH.D.
GAINESVILLE STATE COLLEGE

Food and Drug Administration (FDA)

The United States Food and Drug Administration (FDA) is responsible for guaranteeing the safety of food, drugs, cosmetics, biological products, and medical devices and in monitoring the labels on these products to make sure that manufacturers do not make false or misleading claims about their contents. FDA activities are divided into new product reviews, product use and risk monitoring, ensuring safe manufacturing and handling, enforcing FDA standards, and conducting relevant research. The history of the FDA began in 1862 when President Abraham Lincoln named Charles M. Wetherill to head the Chemical Division of the newly established Department of Agriculture. In 1901, the Bureau of Chemistry was established and was subsequently charged with implementing the provisions of the Federal Food and Drugs Act of 1906, which Congress had passed in response media and public crusading. The Food, Drug, and Insecticide Administration was founded in 1927 as a regulatory agency of the Bureau of Chemistry. By 1930, the agency had become known as the Food and Drug Administration.

Congress enacted the landmark Food, Drug, and Cosmetic Act in 1938, which still forms the statutory foundation of FDA activities. The Act was designed to ensure the safety of drugs, therapeutic devices, and cosmetics before they were marketed, establish food standards, and authorize the FDA to conduct factory inspections. In 1940, the FDA was transferred to the Department of Health, Education, and Welfare (HEW) and was incorporated into the Public Health Service branch of HEW in 1968. In 1980, the Department of Education assumed independent status, and HEW became the Department of Health and Human Services (HHS). Over time, the FDA was given responsibility for testing insulin and antibiotics, regulating chemical pesticides and food and color additives, establishing distinctions between prescription and over-the-counter (OTC) drugs, regulating drug efficacy, monitoring manufacturing processes, controlling prescription drug advertising, regulating biological therapeutic agents, and monitoring nutrition labeling.

In the 21st century, FDA priorities are focused on mitigating public health risks, improving the quality of information available to consumers, enhancing postmarketing safety, strengthening the ability of the agency to prepare for potential terrorist attacks, responding to any attacks that occur, and recruiting the best possible experts to carry out the agency's mission.

The FDA considers its main focus to be on protecting public health through ensuring that safe and effective products are not unnecessarily delayed in reaching the public, monitoring in-use products for safety, and supplying accurate, science-based information in the interests of public health. The FDA's most visible role from a public perspective is in verifying products, which include foods, medical and surgical devices, drugs, and consumer and medical products that emit radiation. Decisions are frequently made on a benefits-versus-risks basis, and the methods that the FDA uses to evaluate items are flexible according to the product under review.

Eighty percent of all food consumed by Americans is monitored by the FDA, including half of all seafood and more than a fifth of fruits and vegetables sold across the country. The FDA monitors four million food imports each year. Foods are checked for contaminants, and additives are examined for safety. Infant formulas, medical food, and dietary supplements come under the auspices of the FDA, but ensuring the safety of meat and poultry products is the responsibility of the United States Department of Agriculture (USDA). The FDA shares the responsibility for regulating water with the Environmental Protection Agency (EPA), with the FDA monitoring the safety and labeling of bottled water and the EPA monitoring and protecting all other water sources.

Drugs that are used for treatment and prevention of disease in both humans and animals and medical devices that range from tongue depressors and thermometers to pacemakers and dialysis machines must pass FDA tests that demonstrate safety and effectiveness. Biologics such as vaccines, blood products, and gene therapy are also vetted for safety and effectiveness. Products such as X-ray machines and microwave ovens are evaluated according to performance standards. Cosmetics and dietary supplements may reach the public without FDA approval. However, the agency may remove products that are deemed to be unsafe or fine manufacturers whose labels are discovered to be misleading or inaccurate.

The FDA employs around 9,000 workers, including biologists, chemists, physicians, biomedical engineers, pharmacologists, veterinarians, toxicologists, public health and communication specialists, administrators, and support personnel. Product reviews and regulatory policy are the responsibility of the Washington staff, and field employees are generally engaged in inspection, surveillance, laboratory research, and educating the public and industries about safety and effectiveness. The national headquarters of the FDA is located at 5600 Fishers Lane, Rockville, Maryland 20857. Information on the agency is available by telephone (1-301-443-6367) or over the internet (http://www.fda.gov/).

Part of the public health responsibility of the FDA is to provide consumers with informational resources. Consequently, FDA publications include *FDA Consumer*, which offers up-to-date health news and articles of interest on a bimonthly basis, and a plethora of brochures and fact sheets. These publications may be obtained from FDA offices, on the agency Web site, or by telephone. Periodic public service announcements and press releases also keep the public informed about ongoing issues of concern to consumers. The FDA History Office is responsible for maintaining administration history through records, data, and oral accounts. This office houses the FDA museum, which boasts a variety of exhibits ranging from a box of Pilsbury blueberry pancake mix that contained no blueberries to Lady Ample bust developers, which failed to deliver on their promise. Less whimsical exhibits include samples of thalidomide, which caused a myriad of deaths, injuries, and birth defects in the early 1960s and Lash Lure, which blinded users in the 1930s.

SEE ALSO: Food Contamination/Poisoning; Food Safety.

BIBLIOGRAPHY. Stephen J. Ceccoli, *Pill Politics: Drugs and the FDA* (Lynne Rienner, 2004); Fran Hawthorne, *Inside the FDA: The Business and Politics behind the Drugs We Take and the Food We Eat* (Wiley, 2005); Food and Drug Administration, http://www.fda.gov/; Jeanne Herzog, *Recurrent Criticisms, A History of Investigations of the FDA* (University of Rochester Medical Center, Center for the Study of Drug Development, 1977); Robert Higgs, *Hazardous to Our Health? FDA Regulation of Health Care Products* (Independent Institute, 1995); Sandra A. Hoffmann and Michael Taylor, eds., *Toward Safer Food: Perspectives on Risk* *and Priority Setting* (Resources for the Future, 2005); Stanley T. Omaye, *Food and Nutritional Toxicology* (CRC Press, 2004); Barbara Rasco and Gleyn E. Bledsoe, *Bioterrorism and Food Safety* (CRC Press, 2005).

Elizabeth R. Purdy, Ph.D.
Independent Scholar

Food Contamination/ Poisoning

Food contamination or poisoning covers any disease of an infectious or toxic nature caused by the consumption of food or water. It includes cases caused by chemical contamination as well as those caused by microbes and their toxins, or any other case where harm can be done by consuming unsafe food or water.

Despite the huge developments in food production, processing, distribution, and preparation, reflecting concerns with food safety, not all populations have access to safe food and water. Nowadays, this situation is still responsible for many cases of disease and a considerable number of deaths, particularly in developing countries. Although the exact numbers are difficult to calculate, the World Health Organization (WHO) estimates unsafe food causes approximately 1.5 billion annual cases of diarrhea in children, resulting in an estimated 2.1 million deaths from diarrhea worldwide, most of them caused by contaminated food and/or water.

According to the second United Nations (UN) World Water Development Report, almost one-fifth of the world population (1 billion people) does not have access to safe drinking water. This issue is a re-emerging public health problem as new foodborne disease threats occur, caused by a number of reasons. These include the current globalization as international travel and trade is flourishing, microbial adaptation, and changes in the food industry, as well as the changes in human demographics and lifestyle.

Contamination generally has a negative impact on the quality of food and may imply a risk to human health; therefore, close monitoring of this situation is vital. Surveillance of foodborne disease is a fundamental component of food safety systems, particularly in developed countries. Surveillance data can be used

for planning, implementing, and evaluating public health policies. These tasks can accomplish a further development of the health of consumers, while cooperating with the food industry, which has known massive developments during the last few years. The new food and water processing techniques need to be assessed for their safety. This has created very strict regulations worldwide, thus causing severe restrictions in international commerce and some tension between exporting and importing countries.

There are many aspects connected with food contamination, and those may include chemical, microbiological, and radiological contaminations. There are several sources of contamination by chemical hazards: environmental pollution of the air, water, and soil, such as the case with toxic metals and dioxins, or the intentional use of various chemicals, such as pesticides, animal drugs, and other agrochemicals.

Current policy has set acceptable levels of intake of certain compounds, thus ensuring food safety. Even so, there are several naturally occurring toxins, such as mycotoxins, marine biotoxins, cyanogenic glycosides, and toxins occurring in poisonous mushrooms, which periodically cause severe intoxications. Other chemicals frequently involved in food contamination are dioxins and polychlorinated biphenyls (PCBs). Dioxins are unwanted by-products of some industrial processes and waste incineration. On the other hand, metals such as lead and mercury can cause neurological damage in infants and children. Exposure to cadmium can also cause kidney damage, usually seen in the elderly. If preliminary toxicological evaluations and/or exposure estimates suggest that adverse health effects might be expected in the population, and the risk becomes sufficiently characterized, various management options may be considered, including the establishment of Codex Alimentarius standards.

Foodborne illness caused by microorganisms is considered a large and growing public health problem. Bacteria-related food poisoning is the most common, but fewer than 20 of the many thousands of different bacteria are actually the culprits. More than 90 percent of the cases of food poisoning each year are caused by *Staphylococcus aureus, Salmonella, Clostridium perfringens, Campylobacter, Listeria monocytogenes, Vibrio parahaemolyticus, Bacillus cereus,* and entero-pathogenic *Escherichia coli.* These bacteria are commonly found in many raw foods. Normally, a large number of food-poisoning bacteria must be present to cause illness. Therefore, illness can be prevented by controlling the initial number of bacteria present, preventing the small number from growing, destroying the bacteria by proper processing, and avoiding recontamination. With globalization and the thorough use of antibiotics, microorganisms are traveling faster and resulting in much more resistance, creating big problems in the control of these diseases.

Recent outbreaks of H5N1 avian influenza in poultry in Asia and, more recently, in Europe and Africa, have quickly raised awareness about new sources of infection and the risk to humans from various exposures. The vast majority of cases reported are connected with direct contact with infected poultry and airborne transmission. Although there is a possibility that the virus could also spread to humans through consumption of contaminated poultry products, so far, there is no scientific evidence that eating properly cooked food can be responsible for contamination of humans with avian influenza.

In the last years of the 20th century, bovine spongiform encephalopathy (BSE), more commonly known as mad cow disease, was making headlines on a daily basis. This fatal, neurodegenerative disease in cattle is caused by the accumulation of a misfolded cellular protein, and is also thought to be the cause of variant Creutzfeldt-Jakob disease (vCJD), a human brain-wasting disease. The misfolded protein accumulates in the central nervous system and is responsible for a rapidly progressive dementia and some patients manifest a cerebellar ataxia. The discovery of this new model of infection mechanism entitled Dr. Stanley Prusiner the 1997 Nobel Prize for Medicine.

Recent concerns have arisen concerning radioactivity, which has always been around and exists naturally in the atmosphere, soil, seas, and rivers. It is also created by human activity during energy production and military operations. Inevitably, some of this radiation contaminates food. Being invisible, tasteless, and not mentioned on food labels, it is frequently overlooked, but levels in food are strictly monitored and controlled.

Contamination from nuclear contamination from radionuclides is still a particularly present problem in Chernobyl, more than 20 years after the nuclear reactor exploded. Close monitoring of radioactivity in products coming from that region is usual and, for instance, in dairy products, special attention is being taken to ensure that the amount of radioactivity is compliant with government regulations.

In order to monitor the quality and safety of food and water, frequent analysis of different components, including elements (toxic and nutrient), pesticide residues, industrial chemicals, volatile organic compounds, and radionuclides, must be performed. These analyses are costly and often have economical sanctions should an abnormal value be found. This has led to strong opposition from the food industry and heavier restrictions on worldwide trade.

There have been several efforts to implement worldwide policies to prevent disease attributable to unsafe food or water. These policies cover the entire food chain from production to consumption and will make use of different types of expertise, including strengthening food safety systems, promoting good manufacturing practices, and educating retailers and consumers about appropriate food handling.

Education of consumers and training of food handlers in safe food handling is one of the most critical interventions in the prevention of foodborne illnesses. Taking this into consideration, the UN General Assembly has decided to designate March 22 as World Water Day. In 2007, the theme was "Coping with Water Scarcity," highlighting the significance of cooperation and importance of an integrated approach to water resource management of water at both international and local levels, as well as taking into account the need to provide easy and inexpensive solutions that can ensure sources of safe drinking water to all populations.

There were also some worldwide programs taking into account that most food-related illnesses can be avoided by some simple, inexpensive measures and common-sense hygiene.

The "Five Keys to Safer Food" campaign supported by WHO is one of the best examples, trying to set simple rules to improve food safety, such as keep clean; separate raw and cooked; cook thoroughly; keep food at safe temperatures; and use safe water and raw materials.

As with so many diseases, food poisoning is more likely to affect people with lowered resistance to disease. Therefore, people most at risk are children, pregnant women, and the elderly. Extra care should be taken when preparing food for these vulnerable groups to minimize the risks of their developing symptoms.

Clinical management of patients with acute symptoms of foodborne disease is generally the same regardless of cause (rest and rehydration). However, in more complicated cases, hospital care may be needed and prompt action must be taken to ensure the swift solution of these cases.

SEE ALSO: Drinking Water; Foodborne Diseases; Joint FAO/WHO Expert Committee on Food Additives (JECFA); Lead Poisoning; Mercury.

BIBLIOGRAPHY. Food Standards Agency, "Food Standards Agency," http://www.food.gov.uk (cited April 2007); International Atomic Energy Agency, "Mobile Radiation Unit Helps Fight Food Contamination," www-tc.iaea.org/tcweb/news_archive/Chernobyl/fightfood/default.asp (cited April 2007); World Health Organization, "Foodborne Emerging Diseases," www.who.int (cited January 2002).

RICARDO MEXIA, M.D.
INDEPENDENT SCHOLAR

Food Safety

Food safety is paramount in today's society as it is vital that individuals trust the food they are consuming, especially as it frequently has been produced quite far from them. A complete approach is essential, so addressing food safety issues along the entire food production chain from production to consumption is crucial. These methods provide efficient, science-based tools to improve food safety, thereby benefiting both public health and economic development.

Although there has been widespread improvement in food safety, the occurrence of foodborne disease remains a significant health issue in both developed and developing countries. Unsafe food has been a public health problem for centuries, addressed by governments and organizations all over the world, still, many food safety problems encountered today are not new.

Estimates show that each year 1.8 million people die as a result of diarrheal diseases and most of these cases can be attributed to contaminated food or water. Many of these foodborne diseases can be prevented through proper food preparation, using simple and effective techniques.

There are more than 200 known diseases transmitted through food, so close monitoring and deployment of food safety procedures is very important, enabling huge reductions in the burden of disease.

Food safety needs to focus on several aspects, including chemical safety, microbiological safety, and radiological safety.

Chemical safety deals with the contamination of food by chemical hazards Contamination may occur through environmental pollution of the air, water and soil, such as the case with toxic metals and dioxins, or through the intentional use of various chemicals, such as pesticides, animal drugs, and other agrochemicals.

When exposure to a chemical in food approach or exceed the acceptable level of intake, maximum levels for chemicals in food may be set, rendering some processing techniques inadequate for the food industry. This is a leading cause of trade problems internationally as it is a economically very competitive, and is broadening the gap between developing and developed countries.

On the other hand, foodborne illness caused by microorganisms is a large and growing public health problem. Most countries with systems for reporting cases of foodborne illness have documented significant increases over the past few decades in the incidence of diseases caused by microorganisms in food, including pathogens such as *Salmonella, Campylobacter jejuni* and enterohaemorrhagic *Escherichia coli*, and parasites such as cryptosporidium, cryptospora, trematodes. With globalization and the thorough use of antibiotics, microorganism are travelling faster and creating much more resistances, creating big problems in the control of these diseases.

Recent concerns have arisen concerning radioactivity, which has always been around and exists naturally in the atmosphere, soil, seas, and rivers. It's also created by human activity during energy production and military operations. Inevitably, some of this radiation contaminates food. Being invisible, tasteless, and not mentioned on food labels, it is frequently overlooked, but levels in food are strictly monitored and controlled.

The World Health Organization (WHO) has long been aware of the need to educate food handlers about their responsibilities for food safety. In 2001, after extensive consultation with food safety experts and risk communicators, WHO introduced the Five Keys to Safer Food concept, trying to reach a broader audience. The Five Keys to Safer Food poster incorporates all the messages of the Ten Golden Rules for Safe Food Preparation under simpler headings that are more easily remembered and also provides more details on the reasoning behind the suggested measures. The core messages of the Five Keys to Safer Food are: keep clean; separate raw and cooked; cook thoroughly; keep food at safe temperatures; and use safe water and raw materials.

Addressing the food industry, in 1963 the United Nations, through the Food and Agriculture Organization of the UN (FAO) and WHO, has created the Codex Alimentarius Commission to develop food standards, guidelines and related texts such as codes of practice under the Joint FAO/WHO Food Standards Program. The main purposes of this Program are protecting health of the consumers and ensuring fair trade practices in the food trade, and promoting coordination of all food standards work undertaken by international governmental and nongovernmental organizations.

The Codex Alimentarius, also known as the food code, has become the global reference point for consumers, food producers and processors, national food control agencies and the international food trade. The code has had an enormous impact on the thinking of food producers and processors as well as on the awareness of the end users—the consumers. Its influence extends to every continent, and its contribution to the protection of public health and fair practices in the food trade is immeasurable.

Simply stated, the Codex Alimentarius is a collection of standards, codes of practice, guidelines, and other recommendations. Some of these texts are very general, and some are very specific. Some deal with detailed requirements related to a food or group of foods; others deal with the operation and management of production processes or the operation of government regulatory systems for food safety and consumer protection. One of the techniques most widely spread to ensure food safety is HACCP (Hazard Analysis and Critical Control Point). It was initially developed for the U.S. Space Program and provided a new approach to the food safety requirements the astronauts needed. Instead of focusing on final product sampling and some items concerning manufacturing conditions, this technique focuses on preventing hazards that can cause foodborne illnesses.

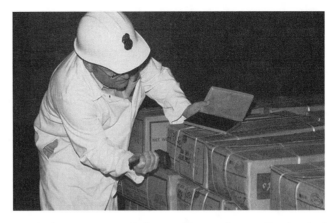

Food safety inspector marks boxes of imported meats. Two hundred known diseases are transmitted through food.

There are seven basic principles involved: (1) analyze hazards; (2) identify critical control points; (3) establish preventive measures with critical limits for each control point; (4) establish procedures to monitor the critical control points; (5) establish corrective actions to be taken when monitoring shows that a critical limit has not been met; (6) establish procedures to verify that the system is working properly; (7) establish effective recordkeeping to document the HACCP system.

In the context of global markets thriving and the growing need for international regulations concerning food safety, HACCP has been adopted by the Codex Alimentarius Commission as the international standard for food safety.

Nowadays, there is a new concern regarding food safety. Modern biotechnology has created a new field of development in the agriculture and food industries by introducing the use of genetically modified organisms (GMOs) in the food production chain. By artificially modifying the genetic characteristics of organisms such as plants, animals, and micro-organisms (bacteria, viruses, etc.), scientists have been able to give them a new property (a plant's resistance to a disease or insect, improvement of a food's quality or nutritional value, increased crop productivity, a plant's tolerance of a herbicide, etc.).

In the late 1990s, there was some dispute over the safety of GMO, originated food, mainly after research by a scientist in Scotland suggested that procedures routinely used in genetic engineering could make plants harmful. The massive controversy that followed, in the aftermath of the bovine spongiform encephalopathy

(BSE, commonly known as mad cow disease) scandal, was responsible for a "moratorium" on GMOs and enforcement of very strict regulations.

SEE ALSO: Center for Food Safety and Applied Nutrition (CFSAN); European Food Safety Authority (EFSA); Food and Agriculture Organization of the United Nations (FAO); Food Contamination/Poisoning; Foodborne Diseases.

BIBLIOGRAPHY. WHO Food Safety site, http://www.who.int/foodsafety/en/ (cited SJune 2007); John Pickrell "Instant Expert: GM Organisms" NewScientist.com September 2006 Codex Alimentarius, http://www.codexalimentarius.net/ (cited June 2007).

RICARDO MEXIA, M.D.
INDEPENDENT SCHOLAR

Foodborne Diseases

A significant health burden in the United States, foodborne diseases cause an estimated 76 million illnesses, 325,000 hospitalizations, and 5,000 deaths annually. Known pathogens, however, only account for a small portion of these illnesses, hospitalizations, and deaths; unknown agents account for the majority of foodborne diseases. Annually, $6 billion is spent on medical care and lost productivity due to foodborne diseases. Underreporting of foodborne illnesses continues to hinder the public health community's ability to accurately report the incidence, prevalence, and etiology of foodborne diseases. Prevention of foodborne diseases targets the safety of the food supply, manufacturing and processing of foods, and the transport of foods from the farm to the grocery store.

Foodborne diseases consist of viruses, bacteria, and protozoa. The most common causes of annual foodborne diseases are the following: Norwalk-like virus (23 million cases), *Campylobacter* (2.5 million), *Giardia lamblia* (2 million), *Salmonella* (1.4 million), *Shigella* (450,000), and *Cryptosporidium* (300,000). Surprisingly, *E. coli*, a common known cause of outbreaks in the United States, accounts for only 110,000 cases. Transmission of foodborne illnesses occurs through the fecal-oral route and ingestion and improper handling of contaminated foods.

Clinically, foodborne diseases can cause a variety of symptoms, including abdominal pain, diarrhea, nausea, and vomiting. Some diseases do not present with gastrointestinal symptoms, but can cause paralysis, headaches, or amnesia. The timing of symptom presentation after ingestion of a contaminated food can help to determine the offending pathogen. Some pathogens like *Staphylococcus aureus* have preformed toxins, and symptoms can occur within six to 12 hours of ingestion, while other pathogens like *E. coli* produce toxins within 24 hours once they are ingested.

When a foodborne illness is suspected, stool specimens may be helpful in isolating the offending pathogen; however, many patients may be diagnosed clinically and do not require confirmatory laboratory testing. Treatment of foodborne illnesses can consist of intravenous hydration if a patient is volume-depleted and/or antibiotic therapy. Increasingly, antibiotic resistance is becoming a problem in the treatment of these infections; thus, physicians must carefully weigh the risks and benefits of starting antibiotics in patients.

Currently, surveillance systems track the epidemiology of foodborne illnesses and outbreaks. The Centers for Disease Control and Prevention's FoodNet is an active surveillance program that covers over 44 million Americans. Yet, the underestimation of foodborne diseases occurs due to underreporting by health care professionals to the proper authorities and the low use of diagnostic studies. Additionally, not every patient with a foodborne illness will visit their primary care physician.

Prevention is an important tool to control foodborne illnesses and outbreaks. Proper hand washing and food handling can decrease the transmission of pathogens, particularly among immunocompromised persons, a susceptible population. Hepatitis A, an illness transmitted mostly through raw shellfish, can be prevented with a vaccine. Food safety must be ensured by enforcing regulations from the Food and Drug Administration and the Department of Agriculture.

SEE ALSO: Bacterial Infections; Botulism; Center for Disease Control and Prevention (CDC); Digestive Diseases (General); Drinking Water; E. Coli Infections; Food and Drug Administration (FDA); Food Contamination/Poisoning.

BIBLIOGRAPHY. Centers for Disease Control and Prevention. "Preliminary FoodNet data on the Incidence Of Infection With Pathogens Transmitted Commonly Through Food—10 States, United States, 2005," *MMWR Morbidity and Mortality Weekly Report* (2006); Richard Guerrant, et al., "Practice Guidelines for the Management of Infectious Diarrhea," *Clinical Infectious Diseases* (v.32, 2001); Morten Helms, Jacob Simonsen, Kare Molbak "Foodborne Bacterial Infection and Hospitalization: A Registry-based Study." *Clinical Infectious Diseases* (v.42, 2006); Paul Mead, et al., "Food-related Illness and Death in the United States," *Emerging Infectious Diseases* (v5, 1999); Robert Tauxe. "Emerging Foodborne Diseases: an Evolving Public Health Challenge," *Emerging Infectious Diseases* (v.3, 1997); UpTo-Date. "Differential Diagnosis of Microbial Foodborne Disease," www.uptodateonline.com (cited September 2006).

LINDSAY KIM, MPH
EMORY UNIVERSITY SCHOOL OF MEDICINE

Foot Health

Feet are the foundation of our bodies, and a disorder in the foot may alter the biomechanics of the balance between the feet and the rest of the body. Due to the complex structure of the feet, an otherwise small discomfort may become magnified once the effects of gravity take place on the feet due to the load they carry. Problems with the skin of the foot may lead to an altered gait, causing hip or back problems. Footwear can lead to problems as well, pushing on nails and altering the normal stresses that are applied to the bones of the feet. A person with altered sensation of the feet due to a metabolic condition such as diabetes mellitus may be unaware that they even have a foot problem, causing severe consequences. Through education and appreciation for the feet, one can prevent serious problems. Foot care may be provided by allopathic and osteopathic physicians (MDs and DOs), and also by doctors of podiatric medicine (podiatrists) whose practice is limited to the foot and ankle.

Each foot has 26 bones surrounded by a complex network of muscles, ligaments, tendons, blood vessels, nerves, subcutaneous tissue, and skin. The foot is specifically designed to ensure ultimate strength, flexibility, and functioning. Feet must withstand pressure from body weight, aid in locomotion, and allow for complex movements. This complicated structure, coupled with weight bearing, leaves many chances for malfunctioning. An estimated 75 percent of Americans have experienced a foot ailment, making it a common health concern. Although this includes many minor concerns, at times, foot disorders may be very serious, or a sign of systemic disease.

COMMON FOOT AILMENTS

Education about common foot ailments is necessary for proper foot health. Many conditions may begin small, but can develop into more serious disorders as well as a source of constant pain. Some minor disorders that can compromise the health of the foot are blisters, corns/calluses, warts, fungal infections (athlete's foot), ingrown toenails, bunions, hammer toes, and heel spurs.

Blisters arise in an area of skin exposed to extensive friction. A blister should not be popped but permitted to spontaneously rupture. It should be washed and covered by an adhesive bandage until the skin repairs itself, and the inciting rubbing force stopped. Corns/calluses are layers of dead skin that have encrusted onto each other. They form in places of repetitive microtrauma to provide protection to the foot. Plantar warts are caused by viruses in the human papillomavirus (HPV) family that have entered the skin, usually through a cut. The virus is commonly contracted from walking barefoot, especially in damp public areas, such as pools and showers. This is a noncancerous growth but should be treated to prevent pain and spread of the virus around the foot. Tinea pedis (athlete's foot) is a fungal skin infection, which results in dry skin, itching, inflammation, and at times, blisters. Onychomycosis is a fungal infection of the toenails, causing yellowing, thickened, and misshapen toenails. Fortunately, many of these minor ailments can be treated with over-the-counter remedies. However, if the problem gets worse, has changing symptoms, or is not responding to treatments, a physician should be consulted.

Ingrown toenails are nails that have grown into the skin, causing pain or infection. This typically results from improper nail cutting, trauma, or infection. Most ingrown toenails can be prevented if the toenails are clipped straight across, so that they are longer than the skin edge, which prevents the corners from digging into the skin. If the nail becomes infected, a relatively minor condition can become very serious and painful, and will need the care of a physician or podiatrist.

A bunion is a misalignment of the bones of the big toe, causing it to point toward the other toes, which alters the joint motion, and later, can cause inflammation and pain. A hammertoe is a bent, contracted toe, commonly seen on the second toe. It may result from ill-fitting shoes that may cramp the toes together into a fixed position, or from an imbalance of the muscles. Bunions and hammertoes can be treated with conservative treatment, such as changing shoes, orthotics, and antiinflammatory medications. However, in certain cases, a doctor must surgically realign the bones and debride the swollen tissue to reduce persistent pain.

Heel spurs are bony growths that develop on the underside of the calcaneus (heel) bone, leading to pain in the heel region, both standing and with ambulation. Heel pain and spurs can also result in plantar fasciitis, an inflammation of the fascia running along the bottom of the foot. To reduce the pain, one must treat the associated inflammation and avoid added pressure on the spur. Treat with local ice applications, antiinflammatory medications, and orthotic devices or shoe inserts to take pressure off the heel region. Rarely, but in extreme cases, is surgery performed to treat chronically inflamed spurs.

FOOT HEATH AND DIABETES

The feet can also be the first place to detect certain systemic disease, such as diabetes, gout, arthritis, anemia, kidney problems, and circulatory disorders. It is important to be aware of these signs and symptoms, because they can be indicators of systemic disease.

There are approximately 21 million people in the United States who have diabetes, a disease where the body does not produce or effectively use insulin, a hormone needed to convert sugar into energy. Diabetes causes blood sugar levels to be higher than normal and can have devastating effects on the blood vessels and nerves. When the blood vessels in feet become damaged, there is decreased blood and micronutrient supply to surrounding tissues leading to nerve damage. This results in a burning pain or loss of feelings in the surrounding areas, and is known as diabetic neuropathy. The combination of damaged vessels and nerves often causes diabetics to have trouble with their

feet. A loss of sensation in the feet makes it difficult to detect problems such as cuts, blisters, or ulcers. In addition, once a problem begins, the decreased blood flow from the damaged vessels will hamper healing due to lack of perfusion by oxygen and micronutrients that aid in tissue healing.

There are several key steps to maintaining adequate foot health in the diabetic patient. In addition to controlling blood sugar and adhering to other medical advice, a diabetic must also take precautions to protect and care for their feet. This includes a daily wash and inspection of their feet, trimming toenails, wearing proper footwear, and routine physician visits. If these precautions are not taken, a sore on the foot of a diabetic patient may go undetected and lead to a serious infection, which can ultimately lead to systemic infection or amputation of the gangrenous foot or limb. Although foot problems are a common complication of diabetes, with adequate blood sugar control and foot care, they are preventable.

WOMEN'S FOOT HEALTH

Overuse and improper foot care may disrupt the delicate balance between design and performance. High-heeled shoes are a perfect example of when a compromise in balance can cause a disorder. High-heeled shoes position the foot in a manner in which pressure is transferred to the ball of the foot, the Achilles tendon is shortened, and the toes are compressed together, all of which place unnatural stresses on the feet. Footwear is one of leading causes of foot problems in women. These positional changes may result in blisters, corns, hammertoes, bunions, as well as other medical conditions, such as osteoarthritis of the knee and low back pain. There are over-the-counter treatments for some of these foot ailments, but most of them are permanent and may require surgery to alleviate pain and restore function.

The best practice for avoiding these problems is to not wear high-heeled shoes. However, many women prefer the fashion of wearing high heels. The American Podiatric Medical Association recommends that women limit the time they wear heels and vary the heel height. It is also important that women find heels that properly fit the length and width of their feet. Finding the proper balance between fashion and comfort can have long-term effects on women's foot health.

There are a wide range of disorders that may alter the health of the foot. Although many are minor and can be treated with over-the-counter therapies, there are serious and systemic conditions that can also cause foot ailments. The best way to ensure proper foot health is to be aware of foot disorders and maintain a balance between the structure and function of the foot.

SEE ALSO: Endocrine Diseases (General); Fungal Infections Hip Injuries and Disorders; Leg Injuries and Disorders; Podiatrist; Ulcers; Virology.

BIBLIOGRAPHY. American Diabetes Association, "Diabetes Statistics," www.diabetes.org (cited October 2006); American Podiatric Medical Association, www.apma.org (cited October 2006); Mayo Clinic, "Foot Problems in Women: High Heels and Your Health," www.mayoclinic.com/health/foot-problems/WO00114 (cited October 2006).

Gautam J. Desai, D.O.
Ericka L. Scheller, MS II
Kansas City University of Medicine
and Biosciences

Foot Injuries and Disorders

As the weight-bearing portion of the body, injuries and disorders of the feet are common and can be quite disruptive to an individual's lifestyle. With 26 bones, 23 joints, and 20 muscles in each foot, compounded with athletic exercise plans and improperly fitting shoes, there is plenty of room for injuries and disorders in the human foot. Below are the most common foot injuries and disorders, their symptoms, and treatment options.

ACHILLES TENDONITIS

The Achilles tendon connects the calf muscle to the back of the leg. With overuse of the tendon, it can often become inflamed and stiff. Common in young athletes, Achilles tendonitis usually occurs after a runner's calf muscle becomes tighter and prevents normal functioning of the Achilles tendon. The Achilles tendon will often become strained and inflamed. Symptoms for acute inflammation of the Achilles tendon are pain of the tendon during exercise. Achilles pain will gradually increase with prolonged exercise but will be resolved with rest. As soon as pain is felt, excessive use of the tendon must stop. If usage continues despite pain, a partial rupture of the tendon may occur. Treatment of Achilles tendonitis includes antiinflammatory drugs two to three times a day. In addition, a heel pad should be used to take the strain off the tendon. Last, if pain does not subside, a sports rehabilitation professional should be seen.

ANKLE SPRAINS

Ankle sprains are one of the most common injuries of the lower extremities. They result from a tearing or stretching of ligaments that surround the ankle. Usually, this occurs when the ankle is forced into a position that is not normally encountered. The most frequent type of sprain occurs when the foot inverts and rolls, when weight is applied to the ankle on an uneven surface. Situations like this usually result in a sprain to the lateral portion of the ankle. Occasionally, patients report hearing a "snapping" sound which is then followed by swelling of the ankle. There are three categories of sprains: Grade I—stretch and/or minor tear of the ligament without laxity (loosening), Grade II—tear of ligament plus some laxity, and Grade III—complete tear of the affected ligament (very loose). The most important way to treat a sprain is to rest the ankle, treat it with ice, and compress and elevate the ankle. To prevent ankle sprains, one should avoid uneven terrain and wear shoes that are firmer which will provide more support.

ATHLETE'S FOOT

Athlete's foot is a skin infection in the foot caused by a fungus called Trichophyton. When the feet, or other areas of the body, stay moist, warm, and irritated, this fungus can thrive and infect the upper layer of the skin. The fungus usually infects between the toes or the arch of the foot. The foot is vulnerable to this fungus because shoes create a warm, dark, humid place for the fungus to grow. Symptoms of athlete's foot include dry skin, itching, burning, pain, swelling, and blisters. Athlete's foot usually arises in places where bare feet come in contact with moist surfaces, such as swimming pool locker rooms and showers. Preventative measures include avoid walking barefoot; use shower shoes; and reduce perspiration by using talcum powder, wear light and airy shoes, and wear socks that keep your feet dry, and change them frequently if you perspire heavily. Antifungal drugs are often prescribed to treat athlete's foot. A physician should be consulted if improvement is not seen after two weeks of improved self-care and hygiene.

HALLUX VALGUS: BUNIONS

A bunion is a bony growth on the side of the base of your big toe. Pressure from your shoe and motion at that joint can cause pain. Bunions gradually become worse until running and even walking are extremely painful. Arthritis of the great toe joint, diminished or altered range of motion, and discomfort with pressure applied to the bump or with motion of the joint may all accompany bunion development. Symptoms that occur at the site of the bunion include pain or soreness, redness and inflammation, a burning sensation, and some numbness. If the patient thinks the bunion is caused by overpronation, he or she should try an arch support or custom orthotic device, which will reduce overpronation and minimize the growth of the bunion. It is advised to also wear a pad over the bunion to reduce friction. Severely disabling bun-

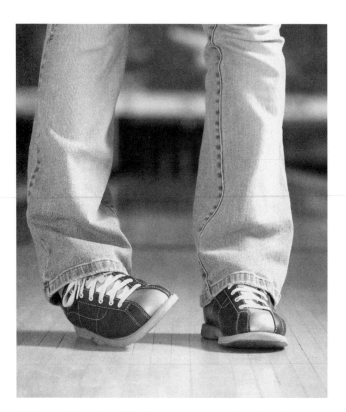

Injuries and disorders of the feet are common and can be quite disruptive to an individual's lifestyle.

ions eventually require surgery. Because bunions are progressive, they will usually get worse over time. However, some bunions progress more rapidly than others. Once your foot and ankle surgeon has evaluated your particular case, a treatment plan can be developed that is suited to your needs.

PLANTAR FASCIITIS

Plantar fascia is a fibrous sheath which helps in maintaining the arch on the bottom of the foot. This fascia is shaped like a bowstring, attached to the heel bone, and spreads out to the toes. Plantar fasciitis is inflammation of the insertion of the plantar fascia on the medial process of the calcaneal tuberosity. Symptoms include pain on the weight-bearing portion, pain on the first step in the morning that comes back later in the day. Tell-tale signs of plantar fasciitis include tenderness, tightness of plantar fascia, warmth of the affected area, and redness of the adjacent skin. Treatment includes stretching and strength-building exercises, weight control, oral antiinflammatory medications, steroid injections into the heel, physical therapy, plantar fascia night splints, and plaster or synthetic casts.

SEE ALSO: Foot Health.

BIBLIOGRAPHY. M.J. Breitenseher, "Injury of the Ankle Joint Ligaments," *Der Radiologe* (v.47, 2007); C. R. Daniel III and N. J. Jellinek, "The Pedal Fungus Reservoir," *Archives of Dermatology* (v.142 , 2006); R.A. Mann and M.J. Coughlin, "Hallux Valgus—Etiology, Anatomy, Treatment and Surgical Considerations," *Clinical Orthopedics and Related Research* (v.11/1, 1981); Frank Mayer, et al., "The Effects of Short Term Treatment Strategies over 4 Weeks in Achilles Tendinopathy," *British Journal of Sports Medicine* (January 2007); "Non-Surgical Way to Heal Severe Heel Pain. A New Twist on an Old Exercise Might Bring Relief from Chronic Plantar Fasciitis," *Health News* (November 2006).

MALA GURBANI, B.A.
UNIVERSITY OF SOUTHERN CALIFORNIA

Forensic Medicine

Forensic medicine refers to the application of medical facts to legal problems. It includes the medical examination of both the living and the dead in civil or criminal cases, along with the ethical and legal aspects of the behavior and practice of healthcare personnel. The terms *forensic medicine*, *forensic pathology*, and *legal medicine* are often used interchangeably to describe all aspects of forensic work, which nowadays involves the application of a broader range of sciences than those provided by medical knowledge alone.

The antecedents of forensic medicine go back several millennia. The Hippocratic Oath, the basis of medical ethics, dates from the 4th century B.C.E. In ancient Greece and Rome, physicians served as expert witnesses in medical matters, albeit in an ill-defined manner. In 13th-century China, Song Ci first documented how medicine and entomology could be used to solve criminal cases, and described how to distinguish drowning from strangulation. Forensic medicine further developed in 16th-century Europe as the legal system and the state of medical knowledge matured.

During this time, army and university physicians started to collect information on the manner and cause of death. Separate tracts appeared in late-18th-century Italy, France, Germany, and England on what was variously described as police, legal, or forensic medicine. Criminal investigations increasingly adopted forensic science during the 19th century and the first-known chemical confirmation of arsenic poisoning as a cause of death in a murder trial occurred in England in 1836. A number of European universities appointed chairs of Medical Jurisprudence, confirming the emergence of the field. The subject became obligatory for British medical students in 1833, but did not develop into a robust academic discipline.

Forensic pathology is the academic foundation for forensic medicine. It is predominantly made up of death investigation through autopsy and associated procedures, and develops justified explanations. Patient medical histories are obtained, witness statements reviewed, and laboratory tests conducted to recreate the events surrounding a sudden, unexpected death under suspicious circumstances. Crime scenes are investigated directly or indirectly, through testimonies and photographs that may be reproduced for the benefit of a court. An autopsy is performed if the cause of death is not determinable without dissection. Although religious groups may sometimes raise obstacles to conducting autopsies, such objections can often be mitigated through new technologies like laparoscopic examination and computed tomography (CT) scans.

Forensic medicine increasingly calls upon a broader range of sciences to answer legal questions related to crimes or civil actions. For example, a forensic anthropologist may be called to recover and identify skeletal human remains; a forensic toxicologist may be required to identify poisons or drugs and their effects on the human body; a forensic odontologist may be needed to identify a deceased person through dental examination; and a forensic entomologist may help establish the time or location of death through examining insects in, on, or around human remains, and to assess whether a body was moved after death. A forensic engineer may assess injury patterns to evaluate how an injury occurred or how and why a device or structure failed. Forensic psychologists and psychiatrists may be needed to help resolve equivocal suicides or to demonstrate mental illness and thereby incompetency to stand trial, a technique sometimes used in an insanity defense. The need for clinical forensic medicine to devote more attention to the care of living victims of crime or liability-related accidents has driven the development of forensic nursing. Although long established in England, Canada, and Australia, forensic nursing is relatively new in the United States and is just emerging in countries such as India, China, Turkey, Pakistan, Japan, and South Africa. The growing presence and credibility of forensic nursing has expanded the frontiers of forensic medicine.

Biological fluids and stains may be identified by toxicology testing of specimens. For example, blood may be obtained to measure alcohol levels and urine samples may be tested for opiates, diazepines, or cocaine. Small portions of internal organs may be removed for microscopic examination. Semen is the most commonly analyzed body fluid in criminal cases. In sexual assault cases, vaginal swabs may be obtained from the posterior vaginal fornix to show that ejaculation occurred by evaluating for known semen markers: acid phosphatase (AP), prostate specific antigen (PSA, also known as p30), or MHS-5 antigen. The AP test is the most common screener for seminal fluid, but AP can also be found in other biological samples such as saliva or fecal matter. The presence of semen must be confirmed by identifying spermatazoa microscopically or by detecting PSA. If more than 48 hours have elapsed since the incident, one or two endocervical swabs are also taken because sperm remains longer in this area. The sensitivity of some of these confirmatory tests has recently been considerably improved.

Advances in genetic analysis have been quickly integrated into forensic medicine. The DNA found in forensic samples, such as blood stains or hair samples, can be used to identify a suspect, an unknown person, or human body parts. DNA fingerprinting can be used to compare a person's genetic makeup with material evidence gathered at a crime scene. The pattern of DNA fragments seen after hybridization with specific probes gives the DNA fingerprint which, like an ordinary fingerprint, is specific to an individual. Y-chromosome STR typing is an important new forensic method for processing sexual assault samples.

There are no clear repeatable patterns of clinical forensic medicine practice when viewed on an international basis. In Britain, forensic pathologists rarely deal with living individuals, but general practitioners who work as police surgeons part time are often called upon to assess cases of substance abuse or sexual assault, injured prisoners, and those with preexisting morbidity to gauge their fitness for detention, release, transfer, or police interview. In the United States, forensic pathologists working as private practitioners are frequently involved in medical malpractice cases and vehicular injury litigations. Those working in the public sector are often called upon to date or evaluate wounds in assault cases, evaluate child abuse, and provide toxicological testimony. Also, there are no international standards of forensic medicine training, although international standards exist for fingerprint identification and bloodstain analysis, and recommendations exist for the harmonization of autopsy rules.

Despite the importance of independence and impartiality in forensic work, the medical care of detainees in police custody and the investigation of police complaints are variable. In some countries, there are disturbing omissions concerning causes of death in custody statistics. There has also been adverse publicity in high-profile cases involving miscarriages of justice. Unsound practices may occur because forensic science may become part of the culture of government prosecution and laboratories run by law enforcement personnel may sometimes have relatively lenient or inadequately managed quality assurance standards.

The practice of forensic medicine requires a stable legal system and adherence to ethical and human rights standards. In addition, by helping to identify and prosecute the perpetrators of human rights abuses, forensic medicine contributes to the protection of human rights in at least five ways. First, it may document injuries attributable to torture or ill-treatment. Second, it may establish the manner and cause of death and a victim's identity in cases where fatal abuse is alleged. Third, it facilitates investigation of mass graves and other war crimes. Fourth, it may identify unknown, deceased, or missing persons through DNA analysis or other means. Fifth, it sets standards for torture investigation and autopsies. Forensic specialists have been heavily involved in missions to countries beset by recent genocides such as the former Yugoslavia, Rwanda, Sierra Leone, and East Timor. They have also been increasingly engaged by human rights and nongovernmental organizations.

The word *forensics* has become common in the media, which has publicized the work of forensic practitioners. Perhaps the best-known crime detective is the fictional character Sherlock Holmes, believed to be based on a forensic surgeon and first introduced to the world in book form in 1887, when fingerprinting began to be applied in criminal investigations. At the start of the 21st century, a number of television crime detection dramas featured the forensic pathologist as the key person in solving murder cases, performing autopsies, examining DNA, and other bodily evidence using high-tech methods, and providing expert witness. This has stimulated general interest in forensic medicine.

SEE ALSO: DNA; Laboratory Tests; Pathology; Poisoning; Toxicology.

BIBLIOGRAPHY. Stuart H. James and Jon J. Nordby, eds., *Forensic Science: An Introduction to Scientific and Investigative Techniques* (Taylor & Francis, 2005); Jason Payne-James, Anthony Busuttil, and William Smock, eds., *Forensic Medicine: Clinical and Pathological Aspects* (Greenwich Medical Media, 2003); Richard Shepherd, *Simpson's Forensic Medicine* (Arnold, 2003).

ANDRZEJ KULCZYCKI, PH.D.
UNIVERSITY OF ALABAMA, BIRMINGHAM

Fractures

Bones are living tissue which serves to provide support and structure to the human body. Fractures as defined in the most basic meaning is the breaking of a bone. Under normal circumstances, bones are able to take a certain amount of force. However, if the force put upon the bone exceeds the limit that the bone can withstand, a fracture will result.

There are several clinical subtypes that fractures can be divided into. The first is a fragility fracture, which is a result of minor trauma. An example of this would be a fracture in an individual with osteoporosis whose bones are frail. Even a simple accident could result in a fracture. The second type of fracture is a pathological fracture, which is a result of a structurally abnormal bone. An example of this is a fracture in an individual who has a type of bone disease which makes their bones abnormally susceptible to fractures. The fractures in an individual with a pathological cause can result spontaneously or secondary to trauma. The third type of fracture is a high-energy fracture which is a result of serious trauma. An example of this would be an individual who falls off the roof and breaks a bone. This third type of trauma is equal to stress fractures; however, an example of stress fractures would be in an athlete who does repetitive minor trauma. The key to stress fractures and high-energy fractures is that they occur in people who have normal bones. Finally, if the fracture occurs in such a way that the bone pierces through the skin, it is called an "open" fracture.

The typical clinical presentation of a fracture would be acute pain followed by swelling. In most cases, the physician's differential diagnosis would be whether the bone is broken or there is a soft tissue injury. A fracture is fairly easy to diagnose. Signs of a fracture are pain, swelling, abnormal movement of the limb with the fracture, and deformity. Symptoms vary according to the area in which the bone is affected. A plain radiograph taken in two views is useful in confirming a suspected fracture. Although this will often confirm a suspected diagnosis, a higher type of imaging method may be used if a fracture is still not found after a plain radiograph and the symptoms are still highly suggestive of a fracture.

When treating a fracture, it is important to treat it according to the location of the fracture, as well as the type. The initial management of a fracture is to immobilize the area where the bone has been broken

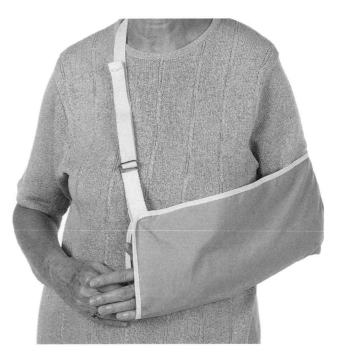

If the force put upon the bone exceeds the limit that the bone can withstand, a fracture will result.

so that additional damage can be prevented. Other things that can be done are elevation of the broken bone to reduce bleeding and swelling. According to the Academy of Orthopedics, the treatment of broken bones follows one rule: "The broken pieces must be put back into position and prevented from moving out of place until they are healed." After the healing process of the broken bone, rehabilitation is also important. Rehabilitation helps to avoid joint stiffness as well as muscle wasting around the affected bone.

The best way to avoid fractures is to do regular exercise and follow a diet high in calcium, both of which encourage bone strength.

SEE ALSO: Bone Health; Orthopedics; Orthopedist.

BIBLIOGRAPHY. American Academy of Orthopedics Surgeons, "Fractures: Types and Treatments," orthoinfo.aaos.org/brochurBroberg, K. Bertram, *Cracks and Fractures* (Academic Press, 1999), Ronald McRae, *Pocketbook of Orthopedics and Fractures,* (Churchill Livingstone, 2006).

Angela J. Garner
University of Missouri-Kansas City
School of Medicine

Framingham Heart Study

The Framingham Heart Study was a study of cardiovascular problems based in Framingham, Massachusetts. This town, officially the largest town in New England, was first established in 1650 and had an important place in the American War of Independence, as the birthplace of Crispus Attucks—the first African American killed in the war.

The study started in 1948 when 5,209 adults from Framingham were examined, and it continues to the present day with grandchildren of some of the original participants being tested. It was coordinated by the National Heart Institute (now the National Heart, Lung, and Blood Institute), which has worked with Boston University since 1971. It has also drawn people from hospitals and universities in the entire Greater Boston area. The original cohort of 5,209 men and women were between the ages of 30 and 62, an offspring cohort was added in 1971 in research conducted by Boston University, and the study of a third-generation cohort began in April 2002, allowing for a study of hereditary problems. By the middle of 2005, the study involved a survey of 4,095 people.

The idea of an intensive study of one community was partially that of Thomas Royle Dawber, who from 1949 until 1966, was the chief epidemiologist in the study, taking over after its early shaky start. Born in British Columbia, Canada, he attended Harvard Medical School and after 12 years in the U.S. Coast Guard, he started work near Boston and managed to keep the Framingham study going after it initially ran out of funds. He was methodical in his approach and ensured that medical professionals all around the world were aware of causes of coronary heart disease. Dawber and his colleagues published more than 100 papers including one study in the *Annals of Internal Medicine* in 1961 listing the major risk factors. These included aspects such as high blood pressure, high blood cholesterol, smoking, obesity, diabetes, and physical inactivity, most of which are now widely known. Dawber was nominated for the Nobel Prize on three occasions.

The Framingham study, because of its intensity and because of the long period of the surveys, has produced much of the knowledge of heart disease as well as on the effects of diet and exercise, and on the side effects from common medications such as aspirins. Often when diagnosing patients, medical professionals compare patients with those studied at Framingham. Some critics of the Framingham Heart Study claim that it overestimates the risk posed to people, with lower-risk groups, such as some communities in other countries, being far less prone to suffer from particular aspects of heart disease. Nevertheless, many medical professionals continue to use the data collected by the Framingham study, and another study has also been undertaken at Busselton, Western Australia, although the results from Framingham are more widely cited.

SEE ALSO: Cohort Study; Heart Diseases (General); Heart Diseases—Prevention; National Heart, Lung, and Blood Institute (NHLBI).

BIBLIOGRAPHY. Framingham Heart Study, www.framinghamheartstudy.org; Daniel Levy and Susan Brink, *A Change of Heart: How the People of Framingham, Massachusetts, Helped Unravel the Mysteries of Cardiovascular Disease* (Knopf, 2005).

JUSTIN CORFIELD
GEELONG GRAMMAR SCHOOL, AUSTRALIA

France

One of the most technically advanced nations in the world, France has a per capita income of $29,600 and ranks as the 27th richest nation. The United Nations Development Programme's (UNDP) Human Development Report ranks France 16th of 177 nations on overall quality-of-life issues. France has an enormous national budget, and the tax burden is heavy. The process of privatizing is ongoing, and the government continues to maintain control of several mega businesses, including Air France, France Telecom, Renault, and Thales.

Unemployment hovers at 10 percent and is heavily correlated with the poverty rate of 6.5 percent. France ranks 32.7 on the Gini inequality index, with the richest 10 percent of the population claiming 25.1 percent of resources and the poorest 10 percent holding on to only 2.8 percent. The population of 60,876,136 expe-

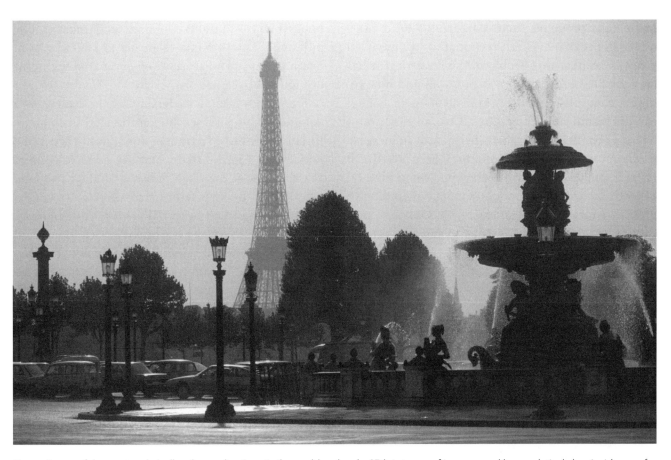

France is one of the most technically advanced nations in the world and ranks 27th in terms of income, and has a relatively low incidence of death from heart disease when compared with other industrialized nations.

riences a life expectancy of 79.73 years, with females outliving males an average of eight years. Virtually all of the relevant population is enrolled in primary and secondary school. Safe drinking water and improved sanitation are universally available.

France spends an average of 16 percent of the total budget on healthcare. Just over ten percent of the Gross Domestic Product (GDP) is used to finance healthcare programs, and $2,902 (international dollars) is allotted per capita. The French government accounts for 76.3 percent of all health spending, and 96.7 percent of that amount is earmarked for social security. The private sector provides 23.7 percent of total health spending with out-of-pocket expenses comprising 43.20 percent of private expenditures. There are 3.37 physicians, 7.24 nurses, 0.26 midwives, 0.68 dentists, and 1.06 pharmacists per 1,000 population in France.

Social security covers all employed individuals, but some groups such as railroad and mining employees and farmers are covered under special systems.

Nonworking heads of household, the unemployed who serve as adult care givers, and French citizens who live abroad may opt to be covered under the pension. In addition to elderly benefits, the system provides assistance, including a family allowance, to single parents. Social security is financed through employee and employer contributions and supplemented by the government. A separate program for sickness and maternity benefits is responsible for benefits to the disabled and survivors. Significantly ill persons may receive half of their salaries for up to a period of six months. If a condition is chronic, coverage is extended to three years. Pregnant women on maternity leave earn full salary for six weeks before and 18 weeks after giving birth. Adjustments are made for subsequent and multiple births. Adoptive parents receive the same benefits in the postpartum period as do other mothers.

Teen pregnancy is a major problem in France, and between 3,000 and 4,000 girls under the age of

16 become pregnant each year. From 700 to 1,000 of those pregnancies are terminated in any given year. To combat this problem, the government has launched a public awareness program and now requires compulsory education in all schools, colleges, and handicapped facilities. Overall birth rates began to climb in 2001, partly because of an increase in the number of multiple births. Three-fourths of French females report that they use some method of birth control, and French women currently give birth at a rate of 1.84 children each. Only one percent of births occur outside the presence of trained medical personnel, and 99 percent of women receive antenatal care. The maternal mortality rate of ten deaths per 100,000 live births has remained stable in recent years.

France has the 12th lowest infant mortality rate in the world at 4.21 deaths per 1,000 live births. Between 1990 and 2004, the government succeeded in cutting the infant mortality rate from seven to four deaths per 1,000 live births. During that same period, under-5 mortality was reduced from nine to five deaths per 1,000 live births. Despite general good health, 7 percent of French infants are underweight at birth. Infant immunizations are high in the areas of diphtheria, pertussis, and tetanus (DPT1) at 98 percent. Vaccinations for DPT3 and polio drop slightly (97 percent each), as do those for measles and *haemophilus influenzae* type B (86 percent each). Tuberculosis immunizations (85 percent) fall even further. The lowest rate of immunization is among children receiving hepatitis B vaccinations (28 percent).

HIV/AIDS is of concern to the French government due to an adult prevalence rate of 0.4 percent. Some 120,000 people are living with this disease, which has taken the lives of around 1,000 individuals. Other communicable diseases surface periodically in France. Leptospirosis and listeria were reported in 2000, and meningococcal disease generated concern in 2000 and 2001. In 2003 and 2004, France experienced outbreaks of influenza. In 2003, legionellosis and Severe acute respiratory syndrome (SARS) provided scares. Rabies appeared in 2004 and chikungunya in 2006.

Cancer is the leading cause of death in France among the general population, but circulatory diseases rank first among the elderly. Smoking is banned in restaurants, schools, and most public buildings. France has a relatively low incidence of death from heart disease when compared with other industrialized nations.

France has taken a leadership role in dealing with communicable diseases among the world's children. In fall 2006, the government announced that it had joined with Brazil, Britain, Norway, and Chile under the auspices of the Geneva-based Unitaid to target taxes imposed on air fares for funding treatment for children diagnosed with HIV/AIDS, tuberculosis, and malaria. The group is working with a foundation headed by former president Bill Clinton to obtain discounted drugs for affected children. Ultimately, the program hopes treat 200,000 people affected with AIDS, 150,000 children diagnosed with tuberculosis, and 28,000,000 infected with malaria.

SEE ALSO: European Public Health Association (EUPHA); Healthcare, Europe.

BIBLIOGRAPHY. Central Intelligence Agency, "France," World Factbook www.cia.gov/cia/publications/factbook/geos/fr.html; Commission on the Status of Women, France," www.un.org/womenwatch (cited August 2007); Spencer Di Scala, *Twentieth Century Europe: Politics, Society, Culture* (McGraw-Hill, 2004); Celia W. Dugger, "Five Nations to Tax Airfare to Raise Funds for AIDS Drugs," *New York Times*, (September 19, 2006); Sandra Halperin, *War and Social Change in Modern Europe: The Great Transformation Revisited* (Cambridge University Press, 2004); Martin A. Levin and Martin Shapiro, eds., *Transatlantic Policymaking in an Age of Austerity: Diversity and Drift* (Georgetown University Press, 2004); Jeremy Rifkin, *The European Dream: How Europe's Vision of the Future Is Quietly Eclipsing the American Dream* (Jeremy P. Tarcher/Penguin, 2004).

ELIZABETH R. PURDY, PH.D.
INDEPENDENT SCHOLAR

Fraternal Twins

Twins are two children who share the same pregnancy and are born during the same birthing process. Fraternal twins, or nonidentical twins, are twins who are the

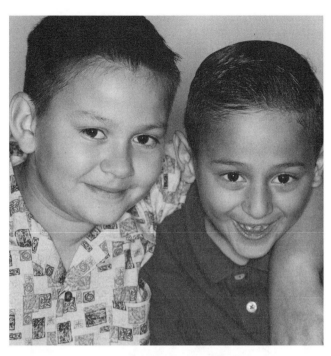

The rate of fraternal twins in the general population is estimated to be around two to 14 per 1,000 births.

products of two separate eggs fertilized by two separate sperm in contrast to identical twins who are formed from one sperm and one egg. Fraternal twins result in two independent zygotes that both implant in the uterus. Thus, fraternal twins are also known as dizygotic twins. In regards to genetics, fraternal twins are exactly like any other pair of siblings. They are extremely unlikely to have identical genes, can be the same or opposite gender, and can appear similar or different.

As with all twins, fraternal twins are more likely to be born prematurely due to the size restriction of the female uterus. Such premature newborns are susceptible to more complications that full-term newborns. With current medical technology and the capability to successfully care for premature babies, twins generally do as well. The rate of fraternal twins in the general population is estimated to around two to 14 per 1,000 births, but is higher among couples who undergo infertility treatments. Fraternal twins are rare because women usually release one ovum per menstrual cycle. However, those who are undergoing in vitro fertilization may be implanted with multiple embryos to increase the chances of at least one taking hold in the uterus and those taking drugs such as clomifene are intentionally stimulated to release multiple eggs from their ovaries.

Therefore, these women have a higher chance of having fraternal twins. In recent years, there has been an increase in the rate of fraternal twin births. Some attribute this to changing practices in society where some women are having children at later ages. Such older woman are more likely to need fertility treatment and thus are more inclined to give birth to multiple babies.

SEE ALSO: Pregnancy; Premature Babies.

BIBLIOGRAPHY. March of Dimes, "Quick References and Fact Sheets: Twins, Triplets, and Beyond," www.marchofdimes.com (cited October 2006).

E. JOHN LY, M.D.
BROWN UNIVERSITY MEDICAL SCHOOL

Fredrickson, Donald (1924–2002)

Donald Fredrickson was an American physiologist and leader in the field of biomedical research who made significant contributions to medicine over the course of four decades. He devised a system of classification of abnormalities in fat transport which was adopted by the World Health Organization (WHO). Fredrickson's classification became an international standard for identifying increased risks of coronary artery disease linked to the consumption of fats and cholesterol. He also discovered two genetic diseases caused by disorders in lipid metabolism. Throughout his career, Fredrickson proved an innovative researcher and an able administrator of the many prestigious institutions he chaired.

Donald Fredrickson was born in Cañon City, Colorado, on August 8, 1924. He attended the University of Michigan which awarded him a bachelor's degree in 1946 and a medical degree in 1949. Fredrickson enrolled for postgraduate studies at Harvard University Medical School and Massachusetts General Hospital and, during this period, he was largely supported by his Dutch wife Henriette Priscilla Dorothea Eekhoff. In 1953, Fredrickson started working for the National Institutes of Health (NIH) in Bethesda, Maryland, and was certified by the American Board of Internal Medicine in 1957. His successful combination of laboratory research with clinical practice allowed him to become director of the National Heart Institute (now National Heart, Lung, and Blood Institute) in 1966. During Fredrickson's two-year term as director, the South African surgeon Christiaan Barnard performed the first heart transplant in a person.

In 1974, Fredrickson was named the second president of the Institute of Medicine, a healthcare and medical research policy group established in Washington, D.C., by the National Academy of Sciences. A year later, Fredrickson returned to the NIH, becoming its director for the next six years. This was a difficult time to serve as director of the NIH as fears over genetic manipulation were spreading rapidly through the general public and economic stagnation prompted the federal government to reduce public funds for the Institutes. Fredrickson, however, was a painstaking mediator who was able to preserve the freedom of scientific inquiry and, at the same time, to placate public fears of genetic manipulation. He was also capable of assuring a steady influx of funds to the Institutes. In the mid-1970s, Fredrickson was appointed personal physician to King Hassan II of Morocco.

After he completed his tenure in 1981, Fredrickson spent two years as Scholar-in-Residence at the National Academy of Science and then became president, chief executive officer, and trustee of the Howard Hughes Medical Institute (HHMI). He died at his home in Bethesda on June 7, 2002.

SEE ALSO: Cholesterol.

BIBLIOGRAPHY. Donald S. Fredrickson, *Recombinant DNA Controversy: A Memoir: Science, Politics and the Public Interest, 1974–1981* (ASM Press, 2001); "Biographical Note," Web site of the United States National Library of Medicine, www.nlm.nih.gov/(cited June 2007).

LUCA PRONO
INDEPENDENT SCHOLAR

Fungal Infections

Fungi are eukaryotic (contain a true nucleus) organisms that lack chlorophyll and rely on preformed

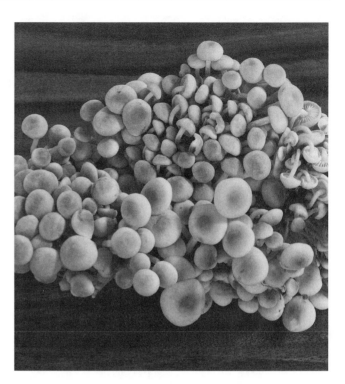

Of more than 100,000 fungal species, only several hundred cause infection and disease in humans.

organic matter as their energy source. Fungi may be grouped into two broad categories—yeasts and molds—based on their physical characteristics (single cells or hyphae) and mode of reproduction (budding or spore formation). Many species are dimorphic and may exist as yeast and as molds depending on the temperature or other characteristics of the physical environment. In general, fungi grow in damp, dark environments. The specific type of fungi present in a particular area depends on environmental conditions and available substrates. Of more than 100,000 fungal species, only several hundred cause infection and disease in humans. Fungi are found ubiquitously in the environment; however, despite this constant exposure, serious fungal diseases are rarely found in immunocompetent individuals.

Fungal infections, called mycoses (*myco* Latin for fungus), may be superficial, deep, or systemic, and may cause very mild to life-threatening disease.

The most common types of fungal infections are superficial skin infections caused by a variety of fungal species known as dermatophytes. While most fungal infections are not spread from person to person, superficial mycoses often are. The clinical conditions, tinea pedis, tinea manis, tinea corporis, and tinea capitis, affect the feet (athlete's foot), hands, body, and head, respectively. These infections are most often an itchy nuisance which can usually be easily controlled with topical medications. Pytiriasis versicolor is a fungal skin infection most often found around puberty and causes hyper- or hypopigmentation of the skin. Onychomycosis is a fungal infection of the finger or toe nails which can be chronic and difficult to treat. Piedra is a fungal colonization of the hair shaft in which the color and steadfastness of the fungal nodules depends on the species of fungus. A species of yeast called candida albicans is responsible for superficial infections of mucous membranes such as the vagina or mouth and are known commonly as yeast infections. Candida species can also cause skin infections in warm, moist areas, particularly in babies (diaper rash) or in adults in intertriginous areas or folds of fat in the breasts or abdomen.

In people with HIV/AIDS, on chemotherapy, or with other immunocompromising conditions, superficial mycoses can progress to serious life-threatening conditions. For example, candidal infections can spread from the oral cavity to the esophagus, causing candidal esophagitis which can be very painful and prevent already-ill people from eating or drinking. Fungal infections of the eyes, though superficial, can be very serious. Mycotic keratitis (fungal infection of the cornea of the eye) can take many forms, and is associated with contact lens use, eye surgery, and immunosuppressive illnesses.

Fungal infections that infect deeper skin tissues include sporothrix schenckii, a dimorphic fungi classically contracted from a piercing from a rose bush. Sporotricosis manifests as pain and redness that tracks up lymphatic vessels in the arm or leg and treated with oral antifungal medications. Mycetoma or madura foot is a fungal infection of an extremity, usually the foot, which invades and destroys skin and subcutaneous tissue. It can spread to deeper tissues such as bone and tendon, and cause very serious disability.

Systemic fungal diseases are those that enter through a break in the skin, the lungs, or mucous membranes and progress to infect other parts of the body. These are much more serious infections that are usually only found in specific geographical regions where the fungi are found in the environment. For example, paracocidiomycosis is a fungal infection found only in Latin America. Spores of the fungus are inhaled and immediately invade the body, but the infection may remain dormant for many years. When it manifests, patients, usually men, present with painful ulcers in the mouth, nose, and throat. Paracoccidiomycosis is very difficult to treat and may progress or present as a lung infection resembling tuberculosis.

Histoplasmosis is a systemic fungal infection found throughout the world and usually affects the lungs, but may involve any body organ. It has become much more common since the HIV epidemic and, depending on the individual, it may cause anything from flu-like illness to death. The histoplasma fungus is most often found in soil enriched by bat or bird droppings and is, therefore, classically found in spelunkers. It may also be acquired occupationally by those working in mines, excavation sites, or other activities that may disrupt and aerosolize spores.

Cryptococcosis is caused by an encapsulated yeast, which like histoplasmosis, is inhaled, and is also common in AIDS sufferers. One of its most severe manifestations is cryptococal meningitis which is a fungal infection of the membranes surrounding the brain, often leading to death. Blastomycosis is a fungal disease which is found in southeastern and south-central United States and Canada. This fungi is found near streams or in areas with moist soil where its spores are inhaled by people working or recreating in these areas. The spores then enter the lungs and develop into yeast which causes an asymptomatic infection in over 50 percent of people. In others, it can cause acute lung infection resembling a bacterial pneumonia, or chronic lung infections that may mimic lung cancer on X-ray. Blastomycosis, like other systemic mycoses may also affect other body systems, particularly bones, and the genitourinary tract.

Antifungal medications exploit the fact that fungal cells use ergosterol in their cell walls whereas human cells use cholesterol. Medications from the azole group (ketoconazole, clotrimatzole, etc.) inhibit the synthesis of ergosterol, whereas polyene antimycotics (amphotericin) disrupt the ergosterol cell wall, killing the cells. Newer echinocandins (mycafungin) inhibit the synthesis of glucan, another cell wall component.

Fungal infections may be simple or difficult to treat using these agents, with the success of treatment often depending as much on the host as on the medication or the fungus itself. Serious fungal infections in the developed world became more common during the height of the AIDS epidemic, but since the advent of highly active antiretroviral therapy (HAART), they have become less frequent. Fungal infections are still a cause of significant morbidity and mortality in the developing world, particularly in those with high HIV prevalence.

SEE ALSO: Molds.

BIBLIOGRAPHY. Eugene Braunwald, et al., eds., *Harrison's Principles of Internal Medicine*, 15th ed. (McGraw-Hill, 2001); Tony Hart, *Microterrors: The Complete Guide to Bacterial, Viral and Fungal Infections That Threaten Our Health* (Firefly Books, 2004).

BARRY PAKES, M.D., M.P.H.
UNIVERSITY OF TORONTO

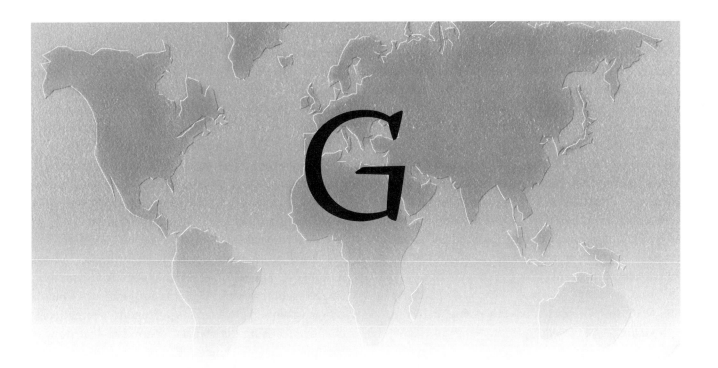

Gabon

Gabon, known officially as the Gabonese Republic, is located in western Africa, with a coast on the Gulf of Guinea. The country was part of colonial French Equatorial Africa from 1910 to 1960. Per capita income in Gabon is four times that of other sub-Saharan nations, largely because of the rich offshore oil deposits that form most of its exports. Despite being home to 40 distinct ethnic groups, Gabon is mostly free from internal strife. In 2007, Omar Bongo became the longest-serving African president and celebrated his 40th year in power.

The population is 1,455,000, growing at 2.04 percent annually. The birth rate is 35.96 per 1,000 and the death rate is 12.45 per 1,000. More people are migration out of Gabon than into it, with a migration rate of minus 3.15 migrants per 1,000. Median age is 18.6 years. Life expectancy is currently 52.85 years for males and 55.17 years for females. Gross national income is U.S. $5010, high for the region. However, it is not equally distributed, and many Gabonese live in poverty. About 60 percent of the population relies on agriculture.

Gabon has had several small but highly publicized outbreaks of the Ebola virus in recent years. Still, the main killers of the Gabonese are more routine communicable diseases, such as malaria, which is endemic, and typhoid. Only 88 percent of the population has access to clean drinking water and 37 percent use sanitary waste facilities. Gastrointestinal and parasitic infections are common.

HIV/AIDS affects 7.9 percent of the adult population, with 60,000 Gabonese infected with the virus and 4,700 having already died. Gabon is among the 13 nations participating in the Joint United Nations Programme on HIV/AIDS (UNAIDS) Accelerating Access Initiative to buy drugs for reduced rates from suppliers, although currently only 23 percent of those infected are on antiretorviral drug therapy. Less than 1 percent of at-risk pregnant women are receiving drugs to reduce mother-to-child transmissions.

Girls in Gabon marry young, sometimes as early as 10 or 12 years of age. The fertility rate is 4.71 children per woman. Contraception is avaliable to 33 percent of women. Abortion is legal in only a few situations, so many women rely on illegal abortions, often suffering major complications as a result. Ninety-four percent of pregnant women receive some prenatal care. Eight-six percent have the help of trained assistance during childbirth. The maternal mortality rate is 420 deaths per 100,000 live births.

Infant and child mortality rates have held steady since 1990. Sixty of every 1,000 infants die before the age of 1; 91 of every 1,000 children die between their first and fifth birthdays. Immunization rates are low, and children are most vulnerable to malaria and other communicable diseases. Malnutrition is not a serious issue in Gabon, although 12 percent of children are underweight and 21 percent show signs of stunted growth.

Gabon spends more on healthcare per capita than most of its neighbors, at U.S. $181. There are 27 hospitals and 660 clinics spread across the country, although access to care is uneven. There is a medical school at Université Omar Bongo. Three institutions, the Université Omar Bongo, the Albert Schweitzer Hospital, and the International Center for Medical Research, conduct research into malaria, AIDS, and other regional health concerns.

SEE ALSO: Joint United Nations Programme on HIV/AIDS (UNAIDS).

BIBLIOGRAPHY. Central Intelligence Agency, World Factbook, "Gabon," www.cia.gov/library/publications/the-world-factbook (cited June 15, 2007); IPS: Inter Press Service, "HEALTH-GABON: Abortions Mostly Illegal, But in Demand," ipsnews.net (cited June 15, 2007); Researchafrica.rti.org: Sub-Saharan Africa-Gabon," researchafrica.rti.org (cited June 15, 2007); UNAIDS: The Joint United Nations Programme on HIV/AIDS, "Gabon", www.unaids.org/en (cited June 15, 2007); UNICEF, "UNICEF-At a glance: Gabon-Statistics," www.unicef.org/infobycountry (cited June 15, 2007).

HEATHER MICHON
INDEPENDENT SCHOLAR

Gage, Phineas (1823–60)

Phineas Gage was a railroad foreman who endured a traumatic brain injury resulting in significant changes in his mental capacities. Over 160 years since his accident, Gage continues to play a significant role in defining the function of the brain in emotion and personality.

On September 13, 1848, near Cavendish, Vermont, working with the Rutland and Burlington Railroad, a 25-year-old man, Phineas Gage, was clearing rocks to level the ground. The task involved placing an explosive charge deep into the rock by drilling a hole. The hole was then filled with gunpowder and a fuse was set. Sand was added on top of the explosive material to prevent contact. A tamping rod was then used to pack the explosives deep into the rock. Unfortunately, on that fateful afternoon, Gage was distracted and he tamped down the powder without the addition of the sand. As his three-foot-long iron tamping rod, with a diameter of 1.25 inches, struck against the side of the rock, it ignited the gunpowder, shooting the rod completely through Gage's head, landing almost 30 yards behind him. The 13.5 pound rod inserted into Gage's skull just below his left cheekbone exiting from the top of his skull.

Extraordinarily, Gage survived the accident. He sustained no motor or speech impairments and his memory remained intact. Within a matter of months, Gage regained his physical strength and was able to return to work. However, his personality dramatically changed, causing his colleagues to state that he was "no longer Gage." A once-efficient, focused, and well-balanced man with a strong work ethic, Gage had become restless, disrespectful, and unreliable, unable to execute plans. He eventually died in 1860, nearly 12 years after his tragic injury, of epileptic seizures. Gage's skull and the iron tamping rod are on permanent exhibition at Harvard Medical School's Warren Anatomical Museum in Cambridge, Massachusetts.

The exact location and extent of injury to Gage's brain continues to hold controversy, as it is uncertain if the lesion involved only the left or both frontal lobes. His ensuing personality change was the first clinical case to suggest the role of the frontal lobes in emotion and socially appropriate behavior.

SEE ALSO: Brain Diseases; Phrenology.

BIBLIOGRAPHY. John Fleischman, *Phineas Gage: A Gruesome but True Story about Brain Science* (Houghton Mifflin, 2004); Malcolm Macmillan, *An Odd Kind of Fame: Stories of Phineas Gage* (MIT Press, 2000).

SHANNON GEARHART, M.D.
INDIANA UNIVERSITY SCHOOL OF MEDICINE

Gallbladder and Bile Duct Diseases

The production of bile is important for digestion and aids in the absorption of dietary fat. Bile is a heterogeneous mixture formed in the liver as an isotonic fluid and secreted into the bile duct. Bile is stored in the gallbladder, and food stimulates the release and secretion of the bile. Once released, bile flows into the duodenum and mixes with the food incoming content. Bile functions: (1) to aid absorption by making dietary cholesterol, fats, and fat-soluble vitamin soluble; (2) induce water secretion in the colon; and (3) excrete bilirubin, degradation products from worn-out red blood cells. The formation of calculi (gallstones) occurs in the gallbladder and can lead to acute and chronic inflammation of the gallbladder. The passage of the stone into the common hepatic duct obstructs the flow of secretion from the liver and pancreas and leads to serious and lethal complications.

BILE PRODUCTION

Bile is an isotonic fluid whose electrolyte composition resembles that of blood plasma. It is produced by the liver and contains bile acids, bilirubin, cholesterol, phospholipids, and electrolytes. Soluble bile acids, the major solute components of bile (80 percent), are synthesized from water-insoluble cholesterols. The primary bile acids are cholic acid and chenodeoxycholic acid (CDCA). They are formed by conjugating glycine or taurine into cholesterol molecules.

BILE SECRETION

Bile formed in the hepatic lobules are secreted into a network of bile ducts that eventually forms the right and the left hepatic ducts. The two hepatic ducts then converge to form the common hepatic duct. Off of the common hepatic duct is the gallbladder which is connected via the cystic duct. The cystic duct and the common hepatic duct join together to form the common bile duct, which enters the duodenum through the ampulla of Vater. Joining the ampulla are pancreatic ducts, through which exocrine pancreatic secretions are made. The sphincter of Oddi surrounds the common bile duct and the pancreatic duct.

During fasting state, bile is secreted by the liver and about 50 percent of the secreted bile flows into the gallbladder via the cystic duct and is stored there. The remaining secretion flows into the common bile duct and is trapped in the duct due to the constriction of the sphincter of Oddi. The bile secretion that is stored in the gallbladder is highly concentrated because up to 90 percent of the water in the secretion are absorbed in the

gallbladder. When an individual eats and food enters the duodenum, a series of hormonal and neuronal processes are activated that causes the contraction of the gallbladder and the relaxation of the sphincter of Oddi.

CHOLELITHIASIS

Cholelithiasis is the formation or the presence of calculi in the gallbladder. Gallstone is the most frequent cause of clinical disorders relating to extrahepatic biliary tracts. In the United States, it is estimated that at least 20 million individuals have gallstones and the incidence of cholelithiasis is 1 million per year. More than 500,000 cholescystectomies are performed each year. Gallstones are divided into two major types: cholesterol stones and pigment stones. The predominant composition of cholesterol stones is cholesterol monohydrate, while pigment stones primarily are composed of calcium bilirubinate.

Cholesterol gallstones formation is primarily due to the supersaturation of cholesterol in the bile. Other causes include the nucleation of cholesterol monohydrate and hypomotility of the gallbladder leading to delayed emptying. Pigment gallstone formation is primarily due to the presence of increased amounts of unconjugated and insoluble bilirubin in the bile, which then precipitates to form stones. Risk factors that predispose individuals to gallstone formation are 1.) obesity, 2.) rapid weight loss (low caloric intake), 3.) female sex hormones (i.e., pregnancy, contraceptives), 4.) age, 5.) gallbladder hypomotility, 6.) high fat diet, 7.) cystic fibrosis, and 8.) alcoholic cirrhosis. Treatment of cholelithiasis include surgical removal of gallbladder, medical dissolution of gallstones via medication, and stone fragmentation via the administration of extracorporeal shock wave.

CHOLECYSTITIS

Cholecystitis is the inflammation of gallbladder. Cholecystitis can be categorized as acute or chronic. Acute cholecystitis, inflammation of the gallbladder wall occurring as a response to cystic duct obstruction by a gallstone, is the most common cause of cholelithiasis. Symptoms of acute cholecystitis are recurrent worsening colicky pain in the right upper quadrant, often radiating into the right lower scapula, nausea, and vomiting.

An enlarged and palpable gallbladder is present in about half of individuals with acute cholecystitis.

During deep inspiration, pain increases and there is sudden stop of breathing (Murphy's sign). The attack of acute cholecystitis typically resolves within a week. The triad sign of right upper quadrant pain, fever, and leukocytosis are highly suggestive of acute cholecystitis. Treatment and management include rehydration via intravenous fluids and electrolytes and parenteral antibiotics are given to prevent infection. Cholecystectomy will cure acute cholecystitis.

In chronic cholecystitis, there are pathological findings of fibrotic, thick-walled, and contracted gallbladder. The mucosa may be ulcerated and scarred and stones or sludge often obstruct the lumen. It is thought that chronic cholecystitis results from the persistent bouts of acute cholecystitis and/or the mechanical irritation of the gallbladder wall from gallstones. The treatment and management of chronic cholecystitis is the same as that of acute cholecystitis.

CHOLEDOCHOLITHIASIS

Choledocholithiasis is the formation or the presence of the stones in the common bile duct. The passage of stones into the common bile duct occurs in about 15 percent of cholelithiasis patients. The incidence of stone in the common bile duct increases with age and it is estimated that up to 25 percent of elderly cholelithiasis patients have stones in the common duct. Stones in the common bile duct is the most common cause of extrahepatic obstructive jaundice and it can lead to serious or lethal infection (cholangitis), pancreatitis, or chronic liver disease. The obstruction of the biliary tree is a major source of bacteremia and systemic infection as gram-negative bacteria quickly colonize the area. Endoscopic and/or surgical interventions are required to decompress the area.

SEE ALSO: Bacterial Infection; Liver Diseases (General).

BIBLIOGRAPHY. Thomas E. Andreoli, et al., "Disorders of the Gallbladder and the Biliary Tract," *Cecil Essentials of Medicine* (Saunders, 2003); "Gallbladder Disease," *Medline Plus*, www.nlm.nih.gov/medlineplus (cited March 2007); Marshall Kaplan, "Medical Progress: Primary Biliary Cirrhosis," *New England Journal of Medicine* (v.335, 1996).

JAMES S. YEH
BOSTON UNIVERSITY SCHOOL OF MEDICINE

Gallbladder Cancer

The gallbladder is an organ located beneath the liver which participates in the digestion of food, specifically in the breakdown of fats, which are catalyzed by the liquid stored in the gallbladder known as bile. Cancerous cells can infest the tissue of the gallbladder, although this is a rare condition, which is slightly more common in women than in men. Hard clusters of material can form in the gallbladder (gall stones) and these can be painful and require surgery. The entire gallbladder can be removed if required without causing any particular problems to the patient. It is often during this procedure that any cancer of the organ is detected, because there are no characteristic symptoms of gallbladder cancer and the organ itself is quite difficult to access or to inspect. Some symptoms that can be caused, for example, jaundice, fever, weight loss, loss of appetite, and others, may arise from a number of different causes and, indeed, diagnosis is likely to attribute the symptoms to one of the more common conditions. People with a history of passing gallstones may have a slightly higher susceptibility to gallbladder cancer, but the underlying cause of the cancer is not fully known.

Gallbladder cancer is best treated, as in the case of most cancers, if the disease is detected at an early stage and, particularly, before the cancer spreads or metastasizes. The extent to which the cancer has spread before it is detected will determine the nature of the treatment chosen. Surgery is possible if the disease remains localized in the gallbladder, which may be excised in a cholecystectomy, which might also involve removing part of the nearby liver. An alternative is to bypass the bile ducts where the passage has been blocked by cancerous cells. Some other surgical procedures may be effective depending on the spread of the disease. A catheter may be used to reroute the bile in some cases. It is also possible that surgery can be used to relieve painful or distressing symptoms caused by the buildup of cancerous masses in the body. If the cancer can be resected (excised) by surgery, then patients may have an 80 percent chance of survival; if this cannot be managed either because of the extent or the configuration of the spread, then survival chances can fall to 5 percent in some cases. Of course, advice from medical practitioners should be sought for a particular diagnosis and because of the possibility of the introduction of effective new techniques. It is also possible for the cancer to recur even when excised. Tests for recurrence are difficult to conduct effectively for similar reasons to those that make initial detection problematic.

Surgery may be used in addition to either or both of chemotherapy and radiotherapy. External-beam radiation therapy may be used to attack the cancerous cells, but given the location of the gall bladder, this is once again often practically difficult to implement. Some drugs may act to make the relevant cells more sensitive to the radiotherapy and these are generally injected intravenously. As the cancer spreads, it may lead to general ill health and weakness which make the patient less resistant to the side effects of any such treatment and its sometimes debilitating effects. Drugs that have been used with some success include Mitomycin c and 5-FU, although these are associated with side effects, while capecitabine, a drug that is administered orally, shows promise in attacking gallbladder cancer. However, this drug is also associated with many side effects which will require careful management. Attention to general health issues such as diet and nutrition, exercise, and a positive psychological approach can in some cases assist in enabling the body to resist these effects. Specific remedies at this stage may include assistance with sleeping to overcome sleep disorders and nausea, frequent small meals to combat reduced size of the stomach, diuretics to reduce swelling, and often quite high dosages of pain-relief medications. Pain-relief drugs may require careful management because these are metabolized in the liver and the patient may suffer from an imperfectly working liver as a result of the cancer.

SEE ALSO: Cancer (General); Cancer Alternative Therapy; Cancer Chemotherapy; Cancer Radiation Therapy; Cancer—Coping with Cancer.

BIBLIOGRAPHY. E. J. Boerma, "Towards an Oncological Resection of Gall Bladder Cancer," *European Journal of Surgical Oncology* (v.20/5, 1994); Alan P. Venook and Sabrina Selim, "Cancer of the Gall Bladder," http://www.cancersupportivecare.com/gallbladder.html (cited June 2007).

JOHN WALSH
SHINAWATRA UNIVERSITY

Galton, Sir Francis (1822–1911)

Francis Galton was born in Birmingham, England, in 1822. He is best known for coining the term *eugenics*, from the Greek for "well born," in 1883. Galton was heavily influenced by his cousin Charles Darwin's book *On the Origin of Species* (1859) and his position as a member of the British elite. He began doing quantitative research on heredity in the 1860s to demonstrate how it worked and how it might be used to manipulate the *germ plasm*, or what might today be called the gene pool, to improve society. Ruth Schwartz Cohen has argued that Galton redefined "heredity," thus eventually helping the progress of genetics as a field. Galton developed the field of biometrics, the statistical study of hereditary patterns on a population level. Galton's student Karl Pearson (1857–1936) continued his research program.

Heredity was of ongoing interest to 19th-century intellectuals and laypeople, both of whom thought that children inherited traits and tendencies their parents acquired along with heritable physical characteristics. The idea that social and biological decline should be reduced through responsible marriage and moral behavior was on the minds of especially the upper class, who attributed rising crime and disease rates in urban areas to increasing numbers of degenerate people. Galton's research did not demonstrate a radical break with previous attitudes about heredity and its relationship to civilization, but rather it attempted to redefine heredity and locate the solution to societal problems in science.

He thought that stockbreeding techniques should be applied to humans. Galton's contributions to eugenics lay primarily in his late-19th–century publications about the relationship between social class and the inheritance of ability and his development of biostatistics (also called biometry) as a discipline. While known primarily as an advocate of eugenic reform and for his statistical studies of heredity, Galton was also an active member of the Royal Geographical Society, an explorer, meteorologist, anthropometrist, and leading researcher on the statistical study of evolution. He was knighted in 1909 and died in 1911.

SEE ALSO: Darwin, Charles; Genetics; Phrenology.

BIBLIOGRAPHY. Daniel J. Kevles, *In the Name of Eugenics: Genetics and the Uses of Human Heredity* (Harvard University Press, 1985); Ruth Schwartz Cohen, *Sir Francis Galton and the Study of Heredity in the Nineteenth Century* (Garland, 1985); Francis Galton, *Hereditary Genius* (Macmillan, 1869); Francis Galton, *Inquiries into Human Faculty and Its Development* (J. M. Dent, 1883).

CHRISTINE L. MANGANARO
UNIVERSITY OF MINNESOTA

Gambia

Gambia is located in western Africa, completely surrounded by Senegal except for a 80 kilometers (50 miles) long coast on the Atlantic Ocean. Only 48 kilometers (30 miles) across at its widest point, Gambia follows the track of the River Gambia for 740 kilometers (460 miles). The country is overwhelmingly rural, with only 20 percent of Gambians living in urban areas. Poverty is widespread, with much of the population working as subsistence farmers; the chief export crop is the groundnut (or peanut).

The population is 1,688,000, growing at 2.78 percent annually. The birth rate is 38.86 per 1,000 population and the death rate is 11.99 per 1,000 population. Median age is just 17.8 years, with 49 percent of Gambians under the age of 18. Life expectancy is 52.68 years for males and 56.46 years for females. Only a quarter of the population lives in urban areas, and 75 percent are involved in agriculture, either for subsistence or trade. Gross national income is just $290 a year, with 59 percent of Gambians getting by on $1 a day or less.

Gambians are threatened by any number of communicable diseases, including malaria, dengue, Crimean-Congo hemorrhagic fever, yellow fever, schistosomiasis, trypanosomiasis, meningococcal meningitis, tuberculosis, acute respiratory disease, and others. Sanitation rates are low, with 82 percent of the population able to access clean water and 53 percent using adequate sanitary facilities.

HIV/AIDS certainly exists in The Gambia, but there is little information on its spread or impact. The Joint United Nations Programme on HIV/AIDS (UNAIDS) does not list an adult prevalence rate for the country, although some groups put the rate at 1.2 percent. A national coordinating committee was instituted in 2001.

While communicable diseases are the most urgent threat to the health of Gambians, they are not the only ones. Diabetes is an emergent problem noted by the Secretary of State for Health and Social Welfare in mid-2007. There are an estimated 29,600 Gambians suffering from diabetes today, with about 500 deaths in the first part of 2007. The number of cases are expected to climb to 53,600 by 2025.

Female genital mutilation (FGM) is another issue for Gambians. Gambia has one of the highest rates of FGM in the world, with estimates of between 60 and 90 percent of women in the county having gone through some form of the procedure. Rates seem to vary by ethnic group, with reports that 100 percent of Mandinga and Serehule women (about 50 percent of the total population) undergo FGM, along with 93 percent of Fula women (18 percent of the population). Excision is common,with some cases of infibulation. There is also a regional technique called "sealing," about which little is known. There is an active campaign both nationally and internationally to end FGM.

The fertility rate for Gambian women is 5.21 children. Only 18 percent use contraceptives. Although 91 percent receive at least some prenatal care, only 55 percent give birth with the help of trained attendants. The maternal mortality rate is 540 deaths per 100,000 births.

Infant and child mortality rates have stayed steady since 1990, with 97 deaths per 1,000 for infants younger than one and 137 deaths per 1,000 for those between the ages of 1 and 5 years. Immunization rates are 88 percent for most vaccine-preventable childhood diseases. Seventeen percent of children under 5 are underweight, and 19 percent show signs of stunting.

Gambia spends around U.S. $5 per capita on healthcare. There are three major hospitals and a number of community-level health centers. The University of Gambia maintains a medical school, and along with the Medical Research Council Laboratories, conducts research into a number of regional diseases, including HIV. Gambia has suffered from a "brain drain" of medical personnel in recent years, as young professionals leave the country in search of better opportunities elsewhere. There are 3.5 doctors and 12.5 nurses per 100,000 population.

SEE ALSO: Dengue; Female Circumcision; Malaria.

BIBLIOGRAPHY. "allAfrica.com: Gambia: 2025—53,600 at Diabetes Risk". allAfrica.com, allafrica.com (cited June 2007); CIA World Factbook, "Gambia" . www.cia.gov/library/publications/the-world-factbook, (cited June 2007); "Female Genital Mutilation: Gabon, Gambia, Germany, Ghana," .ipu.org/wmn-e/fgm-prov-g.htm (cited June 2007); UNICEF. "UNICEF—At a Glance: Gambia—Statistics". www.unicef.org/infobycountry (cited June 2007). World Health Organization; "WHO|A Guide to Statistical Information at WHO," www.who.int/whosis/en/ (cited June 2007); World Health Organization, "WHO Global InfoBase," www.who.int/infobase/report (cited June 2007).

HEATHER K. MICHON
INDEPENDENT SCHOLAR

Gastroenterologist

A gastroenterologist is a physician who specializes in the diagnosis, treatment, and management of disorders of the digestive system. The digestive or gastrointestinal (GI) system includes the esophagus, stomach, small intestine, colon, and rectum, which are the organs through which food passes in the body. It also includes the liver, gallbladder, and pancreas, which are organs directly related to the digestion, absorption, and removal of nutrients and waste. Therefore, a gastroenterologist is trained to deal with a broad range of disorders such as gastroesophageal reflux disease (heartburn), peptic ulcer disease (PUD), gallbladder and bilary tract disease, hepatitis, pancreatitis, inflammatory bowel diseases (IBD), celiac disease, and colon polyps or cancer.

Both pediatric and adult gastroenterologists generally receive five to six years of training after graduating from medical school. In the United States, pediatric gastroenterologists complete their initial residency in pediatrics and then a fellowship (further specialized training) in pediatric gastroenterology while adult gastroenterologists complete their initial residency in internal medicine and then a fellowship in gastroenterology.

One of the diagnostic and therapeutic tools that gastroenterologists frequently use is endoscopy. It is a specialized skill in which gastroenterologist receive extensive training and involves the use of a flexible, lighted tube with a built in camera in order to directly visualize parts of the upper gastrointestinal system (esophagus, stomach, duodenum) or the lower gastrointestinal system (rectum, sigmoid colon, colon). Endoscopy can be utilized for diagnosis of gastrointestinal disorders by visualization or biopsy for such things as peptic ulcers or colon cancer. It can also be used for therapeutic procedures such as dilatation for disorders of narrowing of the GI tract such as achalasia, hemostasis (to control bleeding) for a bleeding ulcer, or the removal of colon polyps.

SEE ALSO: Acid Reflux; Colonic Disease (General); Esophageal Disorders; Gastroenterology; Gastrointestinal Bleeding.

BIBLIOGRAPHY. American College of Gastroenterology, "What Is a Gastroenterologist?" www.acg.gi.org (cited October 2006); Tom MacDonald, *Immunology for Gastroenterologists* (Remedica, 2003).

E. JOHN LY, M.D.
BROWN UNIVERSITY MEDICAL SCHOOL

Gastroenterology

Gastroenterology is the branch of medicine that focuses on the structure, function, and diseases of the digestive system. The gastrointestinal tract breaks down food as it is digested to provide energy for the human body to function. During the digestive process, food and liquids travel from the mouth to the anus where elimination takes place. The digestive function is a complex process involving the esophagus, the stomach, the small and large intestines, the liver, the pancreas, and the gallbladder. If any part of this digestive process fails, it can lead to a host of gastric conditions that range from minor discomfort to potentially fatal malignancies.

The first signs of gastric problems may be discoloration or ulcers in the cheeks, hard and soft palates, and tongue. Gastric conditions include dyspepsia, gastric reflux, bowel-related conditions, malabsorption syndromes, ulcerative colitis, Crohn's disease, hepatitis, and malignancies of the gastric tract. Tools used in diagnosis include blood tests, gastroscopy, X-rays, and measurements of esophageal acidity and neuromuscular dysfunction. Treatments vary according to the condition and may include drugs, antacids or alginates, weight loss, elevation of the head when sleeping, and the elimination of smoking, alcohol, caffeinated beverages, fruit juices, and fatty and spicy foods. Surgery is used in more serious cases and may be followed by radiation and chemotherapy in the case of gastric cancers.

DYSPEPSIA

Gastric upsets are particularly common in Western countries because of nutritional and lifestyles. Approximately 10 percent of all visits to general practitioners involve gastric conditions, and 40 percent of the adult population in Western nations experience at least one serious gastrointestinal attack each year. Ninety percent of all gastric cases diagnosed by healthcare professionals are identified as dyspepsia, which is an umbrella term for gastric conditions. Dyspepsia includes indigestion, reflux (heartburn), gastritis, and duodenal and gastric ulcers. It is impossible to estimate how many people self-medicate and never seek professional help for dyspepsia. Dyspepsia can be caused by eating too quickly or eating on the move so that food is not digested properly. Stress may also be a factor in gastric disorders. Particular medications such as aspirin, nonsteroidal antiinflammatory drugs (NSAIDs), antacids containing magnesium, antibiotics, dioxin in large amounts, proton-pump inhibitors, and thiazide diuretics may also lead to dyspepsia.

Diagnosis is based on observation and patient reports of abdominal discomfort accompanied by belching, bloating, flatulence, feelings of fullness, and heartburn. It may be necessary to rule out peptic ulcers. Pain associated with common forms of dyspepsia tends to be aching or uncomfortable. Sharp and stabbing pains or pain that radiates to other body parts may be indicative of more serious conditions. Symptoms that call for professional consultation include persistent vomiting with or without blood and unintentional rapid weight loss. Discomfort alleviated by pain suggests peptic ulcers, while pain relieved by food is indicative of a duodenal ulcer.

GASTRIC REFLUX

If the muscles at the lower end of the esophagus fail to close after contents are emptied into the stomach, gastric reflux may occur, causing partially digested food to back up. The result is heartburn, belching, and other gastric distress. The condition could also be indicative of a hiatal hernia. Virtually all human beings experience gastric reflux at some point in their lives. Infants are particularly prone to the condition. Between the ages of birth and three months, one-half of all infants suffer gastric reflux that causes them to "spit up" undigested milk or food. Between 4 and 6 months, two-thirds of all infants experience gastric reflux at least once a day. Incidences decline after eight months as the infant's digestive system matures. In some cases, reflux may require hospitalization. Warning signs include malnutrition due to inadequate caloric intake or loss of calories through continual regurgitation, and pain, inflammation, or bleeding in the esophageal tract. Gastric reflux may also affect the airways, leading to constant hoarseness, laryngitis, cough, apnea, exacerbation of asthma, or pneumonia.

Treatment for gastric reflux varies from lifestyle and nutritional changes to drugs and surgery. Elevating the head may reduce gastric attacks when sleeping. Smaller and more frequent feedings may also reduce attacks in infants. Older children and adults should avoid caffeinated beverages, peppermint, chocolate, onions, fatty and spicy foods, citrus fruits, and tomato-based products. Smoking and alcohol are contraindicated for anyone experiencing gastric attacks. Weight loss may reduce the frequency of attacks in adults and children who are obese.

CONDITIONS OF THE BOWEL

All individuals suffer from bowel conditions at some point in their lives. Approximately one-fourth of the Western population suffers from irritable bowel syndrome (IBS), which is most common in individuals under the age of 45. IBS is accompanied by common symptoms of dyspepsia, lower abdominal pain, and altered bowel habits. Diarrhea, which is the most common bowel complaint, may be either viral or bacterial. It is characterized by increased frequency or passage of soft and watery stools. Diarrhea may be acute (lasting more than seven days), persistent (lasting more than 14 days), or chronic (lasting more than a month). Acute diarrhea is generally accompanied by the rapid onset of nausea and may be accompanied by nausea, vomiting, and abdominal cramping or tenderness. Patients with viral diarrhea may have a cough or cold that disappears within two to four days. In developing countries, diarrhea frequently results from giardiasis, a protozeal infection of the small intestine that is contracted from drinking contaminated water. This condition may also be contracted by tourists who travel to these countries. Giardiasis is characterized by watery and foul-smelling diarrhea, bloating, flatulence, and epigastric pain. Antibiotics are required to treat the condition.

If diarrhea persists in individuals over the age of 50 or following travels in tropical and subtropical climates, professional help should be sought. Other trigger points include duration of more than two to three days in infants, blood or mucus in stool, rectal bleeding, and severe abdominal pain. Of itself, diarrhea is rarely life threatening, but in developing countries, acute infectious diarrhea is a leading cause of death. Persistent diarrhea may lead to dehydration, and death may care if patients are not rehydrated. Infants are particularly vulnerable to dehydration. In Western countries, liquids designed to restore fluid and electrolytes are widely available. In developing countries, access to such products is more limited. Infant mortality rates have dropped in many developing countries in response to the involvement of the World Health Organization (WHO) and United Nations Children's Fund (UNICEF) in promoting rehydration with solutions containing sodium, potassium, chloride, bicarbonate, and glucose.

It is estimated that most of the world's children under the age of 5 will experience an attack of diarrhea caused by a rotavirus. Each year, more than 600,000 children die from the effects of the virus, and some 2,000,000 are hospitalized. In 1998, the Food and Drug Administration (FDA) approved a rotavirus vaccine that has reduced the incidences of associated dehydration by half in the United States. In 2003, a number of international organizations and the Centers for Disease Control and Prevention (CDC) joined together to reduce rotavirus-related child mortality in developing countries.

Another common bowel complaint is constipation, which is characterized by a reduction in normal bowel habits. Although it may occur at any age, constipation is most common in the elderly. From 25 to 40 percent of sufferers are over the age of 65. Constipation can be caused by medications, IBS, pregnancy-related problems, difficulties encountered during potty training, depression, and colorectal cancer. If constipation is accompanied by weight gain, lethargy, coarse hair, and dry skin, it may be an indication of hyperthyroidism.

Common treatment for constipation includes laxatives, stool softeners, and fiber. Bloody stools, constipation that endures for more than seven days, and depression call for professional consultation.

Hemorrhoids (piles) may also affect bowel habits. Around 80 percent of the population experiences this condition at some time, and incidences are common among pregnant women and the elderly. Hemorrhoids are characterized by rectal bleeding, pain, and itching. Over-the-counter medications are generally effective, but more serious cases call for professional consultation.

Both ulcerative colitis and Crohn's disease are IBD, which are characterized by chronic inflammation and ulcers in the lining of the rectum and colon. With Crohn's disease, inflammation occurs deeper within the walls of the intestine and may spread to the small intestines, mouth, esophagus, and stomach. Ulcerative colitis occurs among all age groups but is most common among individuals between the ages of 15 and 30. There is a strong genetic link with both diseases. The most frequently recognized symptoms are diarrhea and the presence of bloody stools.

OTHER CONDITIONS

Gallstones are another common cause of gastric problems and are asymptomatic in 60 percent of all cases. Since the late 20th century, most gallbladder surgeries are laparoscopic, which is less invasive than traditional abdominal surgery, and reduces postoperative effects and recovery time. Individuals who imbibe large amounts of alcohol frequently suffer from liver disease, particularly from potentially fatal cirrhosis of the liver.

Hepatitis, which is an inflammation of the liver, is found in three forms. The mildest form is hepatitis A, which may be contracted by contact with infected food, objects, or stool. Because of its mildness, it may go undiagnosed. Hepatitis B is uncommon in the general population because of blood screening tests. However, it continues to occur among drug abusers who use unsterilized needles, and it may be transmitted through sexual contact or from mother-to-child during birth. Because it is viral in nature, it may lead to chronic liver disease or liver cancer. Hepatitis C is spread in ways similar to A and B, and is a chronic problem in kidney dialysis centers. The majority of patients with hepatitis C never completely recover, and many develop diseases of the liver. Since 1992, blood screening has significantly reduced incidences of hepatitis C in the United States. Symptoms of all three types of hepatitis include a generally feeling of malaise, fever, aching muscles, loss of appetite, nausea, vomiting, diarrhea, and jaundice.

Some individuals may experience malabsorption syndromes such as lactose intolerance in which individuals are unable to properly digest dairy products. This condition, which is frequently diagnosed in infants, is characterized by loose bowel movements, fever, vomiting, and failure to grow at acceptable levels. A much rarer malabsorption condition is known as coliac disease, which renders sufferers unable to properly digest grain products. In its most often diagnosed in early infancy when cereal products are introduced into the diet and between the fourth and fifth decades or life. A gluten-free diet is mandatory for individuals diagnosed with coliac disease.

Only 2 percent of cases referred to gastric specialists by internists involve malignancies. The most common malignancies of the gastrointestinal tract are colorectal cancer, pancreatic cancer, and gastric carcinoma. In the earliest stages, these conditions may not be evident. Professional help is sought only when individuals begin to have difficulty swallowing or experience unintentional weight loss. Other warning signs of possible malignancies include bloody, dark, or tarry stools, persistent changes in bowel habits, debilitating pain that persistently causes sufferers to awaken at night, and persistent vomiting with or without blood. Colorectal cancer, which has a strong genetic factor, may be accompanied by persistent diarrhea and a feeling that the bowel has not been fully emptied.

SEE ALSO: Acid Reflux; Alcohol Consumption; Caffeine; Cancer (General); Celiac Disease; Colonic Disease; Colorectal Cancer; Diarrhea; Esophageal Disorders; Gastroesophageal Reflux/Hiatal Hernia; Liver Diseases; Pancreatic Diseases; Ulcers.

BIBLIOGRAPHY. "CDC Advance Data Number 212: Prevalence of Major Digestive Disorders and Bowel Symptoms," (March 25, 1992); "CDC Advance Data Number 322: National Ambulatory Medical Care Survey, 1999 Summary," (July 17, 2001); Donald K. Cherry, et al., "Casebook: Abdominal Pain," *The Practitioner* (May 31, 2006); Michael Fried, et al, "Global Guidelines: Is Gastroenterology Leading the Way?" *The Lancet* (December 9, 2006); Paul Hungin and Greg Rubin, *Gastroenterology in Primary Care* (Blackwell Science, 2000); Felicia LeClere, et al., "Key Developments in Gastroenterology," *The Practitioner* (May 5, 2004); Carolos H. Lifschitz, editor, *Pediatric Gastroenterology and Nutrition in Clinical Practice* (Marcel and Dekker, 2002); Paul Rutter, *Community Pharmacy: Symptoms, Diagnosis, and Treatment* (Churchill Livingstone, 2004); Jenny du Toit, "Assessing Patients for Risk of Colorectal Cancer in Primary Care," *The Practitioner*, (December 31, 2006).

ELIZABETH R. PURDY, PH.D.
INDEPENDENT SCHOLAR

Gastroesophageal Reflux/ Hiatal Hernia

Up to 40 percent of people in Western countries are estimated to regularly experience heartburn, the most characterisitic symptom of gastroesophageal reflux disease (GERD). GERD is a digestive disorder that affects the lower esophageal sphincter (LES)—the muscle connecting the esophagus with the stomach. The LES has no anatomic landmarks, but its presence is identified by a rise in pressure over gastric baseline pressure. In normal digestion, the LES opens to allow food to pass into the stomach and closes to prevent food and acidic stomach juices from flowing back into the esophagus. The LES also relaxes when the stomach is distended with gas allowing it to vent (a belch). With GERD, however, the sphincter relaxes between swallows resulting in chronic regurgitation of acid into the lower esophagus.

The inner lining of the stomach resists corrosion by acid because of specialized cells that secrete large amounts of protective mucous. The esophagus lacks this protective barrier and constant acid backwash irritates its inner lining resulting in inflammation called esophagitis. Esophagitis may lead to ulceration, narrowing of the esophagus (stricture), or cellular changes called metaplasia that are associated with an increased risk of esophageal cancer.

In most cases, GERD can be relieved through diet, lifestyle changes, and over-the-counter medications. However, if the symptoms persist or worsen, patients should seek medical advice and may require more potent medications or surgery.

SIGNS AND SYMPTOMS

Persistant heartburn, also called acid indigestion, is the most common symptom of GERD. It is a burning pain that starts in the center of the chest, and sometimes spreads upward to the neck and throat. It may be associated with a sour or bitter taste in the mouth. The pain of heartburn can last as long as two hours and is usually worse after eating. Lying down or bending over can precipitate heartburn or make it worse.

Some patients with GERD do not report heartburn and rather suffer from a variety of symptoms that ranges from a bitter taste in the mouth or regurgitation of food or sour liquid to a persistant dry cough, hoarsness especially in the morning, wheezing, and asthma. These are called atypical symptoms and are the primary complaints in 20 percent of patients with GERD.

CAUSES AND RISK FACTORS

The exact etiology of GERD is not known. Several risk factors weaken or relax the LES making reflux possible. Fatty and fried foods, chocolate, garlic, caffeine, spicy and acid foods, and mint flavorings relax the LES sphincter. Similarly, alcohol and cigarettes as well as certain medications such as nitrates and calcium channel blockers weaken the LES and increase the likelihood of reflux. Eating large meals or eating right before bedtime can also contribute to GERD. Certain medical conditons such as obesity and pregnancy are strongly associated with reflux disease.

A hiatal hernia occurs when part of the stomach protrudes through the diaphragm into the lower chest. The diaphragm is the respiration muscle that seperates the chest from the abdominal cavity. Recent studies show that the opening in the diaphragm acts as an additional sphincter around the lower end of the esophagus. Studies also show that hiatal hernia results in retention of acid and other contents above this opening. These substances can reflux easily into the esophagus.

TREATMENT

The first step in treatment consists of lifestyle and dietary changes. Head elevation during sleep, weight loss, avoiding certain foods, as well as cutting down on alcohol consumption and cigarette smoking help reduce the symptoms of GERD. Antacids neutralize acid in the esophagus and stomach and provide temporary or partial relief.

When GERD symptoms persist, medications such as histamine-2 receptor blockers (H2-blockers) and proton pump inhibitors (PPIs) are used to decrease stomach acid production. H2-blockers inhibit the histamine-induced acid production. PPIs block the protein that secrete acid into the stomach. They are more effective and more expensive than H2-blockers. Patients with GERD have an excellent response to PPIs.

If symptoms continue for more than six weeks despite medical therapy, patients are further evaluated to document the extent and degree of tissue damage at the lower esophagus. Upper endoscopy is the standard procedure to evaluate esophagitis. A tissue biopsy can be obtained to check for cellular metaplasia, a condition called Barrett's esophagus. Esophageal pH monitoring is the best study to document acid reflux, but is unnecessary in most patients with GERD. Esophageal manometric studies assess esophageal motility and determine the LES pressure. They are particularly useful in patients considered for antireflux surgery.

A small number of patients with GERD may need antireflux surgery because of severe reflux and poor response to medical treatment. Fundoplication is a surgical procedure that increases pressure in the lower esophagus. It is performed laparoscopically with a low complication rate and good to excellent relief of symptoms.

SEE ALSO: Acid Reflux.

BIBLIOGRAPHY. F. Charles Brunicardi, *Schwartz's Principle of Surgery*, 8th ed. (McGraw-Hill, 2005); John L. Cameron, *Current Surgical Therapy*, 8th ed. (Mosby, 2004).

ELIAS DARIDO
INDEPENDENT SCHOLAR

Gastrointestinal Bleeding

Gastrointestinal (GI) bleeding arising from lesions in the alimentary canal can be attributed to a variety of pathological and rarely even physiologically normal conditions such as simple tearing, vomiting, or excessive coughing. The entire digestive tract, consisting of the esophagus, stomach, small intestine, large intestine (colon), rectum, and anus, may be susceptible to damage, with certain gut segments showing greater frequency of insult in certain diseases. Although the location of injury may be ascertained through diagnostic exam and laboratory testing, conclusive determination of the specific bleeding site usually requires endoscopy. This is also used as treatment and to resolve complications.

UPPER GI INFLAMMATION/ULCER

The mucosal lining of the esophagus, stomach, and duodenum is especially susceptible to inflammation from infection, radiation therapy, damage caused by ingested materials such as alcohol and oral medications, and exposure to stomach acid and digestive enzymes. Initially, simple abrasion and erosion of the mucosal lining may be followed by a more severe lesion, which penetrates deeper layers of the gut wall, exposing blood vessels and underlying tissue. Repeated insult and resulting compensatory replacement of lining cells can also lead to the development of cancers also capable of damaging the luminal covering.

The most common etiology of an inflamed esophagus is gastroesophageal reflux disease, characterized by heartburn and abnormal acid reflux due to a dysfunctional lower esophageal sphincter. In the stomach and duodenum, peptic ulcers are caused by overproduction of hydrochloric acid by parietal cells in gastric glands due to hormonal or parasympathetic nervous stimulation. A majority of cases are also strongly associated with bacterial infections of *Helicobacter pylori* which invade gastric pits and cause autodigestion of the stomach wall by gastric enzymes.

ANATOMICAL MALFORMATIONS/ AGE-RELATED WEAKENING

Various anatomical malformations may also contribute to the etiology of gastrointestinal bleeding. On its course to the stomach, the esophagus passes from the chest cavity to the abdomen through a hole in the muscular diaphragm called the esophageal hiatus. In enlarged or age-related weakened openings, the upper cardiac part of the stomach herniates through the diaphragm into the chest cavity, increasing regurgitation and likelihood of bleeding characteristic of

acid reflux. In very rare cases, torsion and volvulus or twisting of the gut may cause mechanical stress induced bleeding.

DIVERTICULITIS

Diverticulitis a condition associated with diet, constipation, and obesity, involves small outward herniation of the gut lining through small, natural, peripheral openings created by perforating intestinal nutrient arteries. Thin outpouches, of gut wall, are highly susceptible to perforation from fecal blockage, resulting in intestinal bleeding and other complications

LOWER GI INFLAMMATION

Inflammatory bowel disease is a broad category of conditions including ulcerative colitis, Crohn's disease, and postinflectional colitis. Inflammation that arises from infection, genetic influence, immune abnormalities, stress, food allergy, or idiopathic causes may be significant enough to cause ulcerations and bleeding in the lower bowel. In Crohn's disease, these lesions are deeper, discontinuous, and may occur along the entire digestive tract.

VARICES/HEMORRHOIDS/POLYPS

Veins draining deoxygenated blood from the gut tube carry newly absorbed nutrients first to the liver through portal circulation before draining into the inferior vena cava and heart for pulmonary circulation. Portal hypertension is a condition resulting in impeded blood flow to the liver, causing enlargement, thinning, and increased blood pooling and pressure in portal veins that drain the gut.

The result is varicose veins, which jut out from underlying connective tissue layers into the gut lumen, becoming vulnerable to abrasion. In the esophagus and anus, which experience the greatest physical stress due to food boli and hardened stools, respectively, these exposed veins are particularly susceptible to rupture and bleeding. In a similar condition, hemorrhoids occur when anorectal veins are similarly swollen and inflamed due to strained bowel movements, not hypertension.

Colon polyps are benign overgrowths in the gut lining, which also protrude into the lumen. The mechanism of injury related to bleeding is the same as that of varicies and hemorrhoids. Polyps, if left untreated, may form malignant cancers with similar bleeding pattern.

DIAGNOSIS AND TREATMENT

Bleeding that originates from the upper gut results in vomiting red blood, and stools with blood that is either black, occult, or red. Black tarry stool, also called melena, is the result of blood that has undergone bacterial breakdown by the naturally occurring intestinal flora to produce dark colored hematin. If the bleeding is slow, sometimes the invisible occult blood in the stool is detectable only by chemical tests. In bleeding that occurs more distally, near the anus, frank blood in the stool takes on a brighter red hue. The pain associated with GI bleeding may be nonexistent, poorly circumscribed, or highly localized depending on the location and severity. In general, blood tests and stool sample tests are used in the first step of diagnostic procedure to derive an etiology for the bleeding. Sometimes, the lesions are caused by bacterial or other parasitic pathogens, which are detected by these tests and resolved with antibiotics. If the cause of the bleeding is still unclear, however, endoscopy is the next step, which allows visual localization and biopsy sampling of inflamed tissues for ulcerative and precancerous cells. Endoscopic procedures, such as banding, can also be used to resolve bleeding, in cases of varicies and hemorrhoids. Other diagnostic methods include manometry, pH monitoring, and barium swallow X-rays.

SEE ALSO: Anemia; Colorectal Cancer.

BIBLIOGRAPHY. Christine A. Iacobuzio-Donahue and Elizabeth A. Montgomery, *Gastrointestinal and Liver Pathology: A Volume in the Foundations in Diagnostic Pathology Series,* (Churchill Livingstone, 2005); NIH/NIDDK National Digestive Diseases Information Clearinghouse, "Digestive Diseases," digestive.niddk.nih.gov (cited April 2007); Patient Centered Guides, "Colon and Rectal Cancer," www.oreilly.com/medical/colon/news/crc0101.gif (cited December 2005); U.S. National Library of Medicine Medline Plus, "Gastrointestinal Bleeding," www.nlm.nih.gov/medlineplus/ency/article/003133.htm (cited December 2005).

Chanukya R. Dasari
Angela Garner, M.D.
University of Missouri–Kansas City

Gaucher's Disease

Gaucher's disease (GD) is a rare genetic disease that was first described by French physician Philippe Gaucher in 1882. Despite being the most common lysosomal storage disease, it afflicts fewer than 10,000 worldwide. Caused by one of over 200 inheritable defects in the gene coding for ß glucocerebrosidase, it is also the most common genetic disease in Jews. ß glucocerebrosidase is an enzyme responsible for breakdown of glycolipids within the cell.

FORMS OF DISEASE

Three forms of GD have been reported. The form of disease determines the person's symptoms and their severity. According to data from the Gaucher Registry, type 1 accounts for 94 percent of cases. Fortunately, these symptoms often manifest later in life and are less severe than the other forms. That is why type 1 GD is called the adult form. People with type 1 GD may have enlargement of the liver and spleen with the potential for subsequent destruction, reduced platelet count, anemia, reduced white blood cell count, and lung disease. The clinical course is variable and can range from barely detectable to wheelchair confinement at an early age.

Forms 2 and 3 are much less common. They are not linked to the Jewish population. In addition to the symptoms suffered in type 1, GD patients with types 2 or 3 suffer neurologic squeal. Type 2, also called the infantile form, is fatal within the first three years of life. Type 3 GD, also called the juvenile form, progresses more slowly. However, it still results in neurologic problems, such as seizures and poor coordination.

DIAGNOSIS

The best way to diagnose GD is with a genetic test. A doctor will send someone for this test if he or she is suspicious of GD. Some scenarios that may raise this suspicion are family history of GD, enlarged liver, enlarged spleen, or low platelet count.

GENETIC SCREENING

Screening for type 1 GD is available. It is typically performed as part of a Jewish genetic screening panel, a battery of screening tests performed when a Jewish couple begins to plan for a family. This has brought up a number of ethical concerns. Will the knowledge of a couple's carrier status impact the decision to move forward with a family?

This carves out a niche for genetic counseling as more individuals are being screened. GD is inherited in an autosomal recessive pattern. If two parents are carriers for the same genetic mutation, the child has a 25 percent chance of having the disease. If one parent has the disease and the other does not, the child will be a carrier for GD.

TREATMENT

Imiglucerase (Cerezyme®, Genzyme) replaces the deficient ß glucocerbrosidase. It is used only in type 1 GD. Approximately 3,500 patients around the world are on this course of treatment. Enzyme replacement therapy is extremely costly, ranging from $250,000 to $600,000 annually, depending on the patient's body mass. Again, ethical issues arise. How much is society willing to pay in order to extend life? What social obligations, if any, does the pharmaceutical industry have? Very severe cases of GD may require splenectomy if the spleen has been damaged. This is done much less frequently since the approval of Imiglucerase.

SEE ALSO: Genetic Disorders; Genetic Testing/Counseling; Rare Diseases.

BIBLIOGRAPHY. G. Anand, "Uncertain Miracle: A Biotech Drug Extends a Life, but at What Price?" *Wall Street Journal* (November 16, 2005); Cerezyme Home Page, www.cerezyme.com/home; J. Charrow, et al., "The Gaucher Registry: Demographics and Disease Characteristics of 1698 Patients with Gaucher Disease," *Archives of Internal Medicine* (v.160, 2000); National Gaucher Foundation, www.gaucherdisease.org/; National Organization for Rare Disorders, Inc., www.rarediseases.org.

Ross E. Breitbart, M.S.
Philadelphia College of Osteopathic Medicine

Gay Gene

Plato may have offered the first explanation of homosexuality as an inborn trait in the *Symposium*, written in the 5th century B.C.E.: he suggests that all humans originally were paired, and homosexuals are the separated halves of male-male pairs. Two pioneers of the modern study of sexuality, Karl Heinrich Ulrichs (1825–95) and Magnus Hirschfeld (1868–1935) also believed that homosexuality was an innate characteristic. Interest in discovery of a biological explanation for homosexuality remains strong in some quarters, and beginning in the mid-1990s, several scientists have announced discovery of results which would suggest a biological basis for homosexuality, although none of these claims have held up to sustained scrutiny.

In 1991, Simon LeVay published results from a series of autopsies which found that the hypothalamus was smaller in homosexual men than in heterosexual men. This study has been criticized on many grounds, including the fact that the homosexual men in the study died from AIDS, which is known to affect the brain; in addition, other studies have failed to replicate his results. In 1993, Dean Hamer claimed that his studies of self-identified homosexual men and their family members suggested the presence of a "gay gene," in this case a set of markers on the X chromosome, which was highly prevalent although not universal among the gay men in his sample. Hamer's results received a great deal of publicity at the time, although interest has lessened as subsequent studies have failed to replicate his results and the design of his original research has been criticized.

Most modern theorists believe that sexuality is a complex human behavior which cannot be reduced to a simple biological or genetic explanation. Another question whether the discovery of such an explanation would be good for the gay community. Some believe that establishing homosexuality as an inborn characteristic would lead to greater acceptance and stronger legal protections against discrimination such as that afforded to people based on their race or gender. Others argue that it could lead to further discrimination, including termination of pregnancies if a fetus was found to be carrying the "gay gene", or early behavioral interventions on boys carrying that gene.

SEE ALSO: Homosexuality; Genetics.

BIBLIOGRAPHY. Council for Responsible Genetics, "Do Genes Determine Our Sexuality?" www.gene-watch.org/educational/genes_and_sexuality.pdf (cited May 2007); Dean H. Hamer, et al., "A Linkage between DNA Markers on the X Chromosome and Male Sexual Orientation," *Science* (July 13,

1993), Simon LeVay, "A Difference in Hypothalamic Structure Between Heterosexual and Homosexual Men," *Science* (August 30, 1991).

Sarah Boslaugh
BJC HealthCare

Gel Electrophoresis

Gel electrophoresis, sometimes called cataphoresis, is a group of techniques used by scientists and medical researchers who separate molecules based on the physical characteristics of these molecules on the basis of their shapes, size, or isoelectyric point. Although there is no prescribed use for gel electrophoresis, the techniques are usually undertaken to partially purify molecules before they are used for a number of procedures including DNA sequencing, polymerase chain reaction (PCR) cloning, mass spectrometry, or immunoblotting. The term *gel* refers to the matrix used to separate the molecules, which in many instances, is a crosslinked polymer where the composition and porous ability is chosen on the weight and the composition of the target molecules being isolated. The main method of electrophoresis involves the movement of electrically charged particles in a fluid, after they are put under the influence of an electric field. If, however, the liquid instead of the particles are set into motion through use of a fixed diaphragm or through other techniques, the phenomenon is given the name electroosmosis.

Although some electrophoresis techniques date from the 19th century, much of the development took part in the 20th century, with the Swedish chemist Arne Tiselius first using electrophoresis as an analytic technique in about 1930 when he was an assistant to the Sverdberg at the University of Uppsala. Tiselius was able to separate proteins in suspension on the basis of the protein's electrical charge, thus developing the main technique still used in electrophoresis. He was awarded a doctorate for his research in 1930, and 18 years later, he won the Nobel Prize for Chemistry.

Much of the current interest in electrophoresis is in human genetics with the technique being used to identify hundreds of variants of hemoglobin. The annual journal *Advances in Electrophoresis* reviews the literature being published in the field.

SEE ALSO: DNA; Polymerase Chain Reaction (PCR).

BIBLIOGRAPHY. Anthony T. Andrews, *Electrophoresis: Theory, Techniques, and Biochemical and Clinical Applications*, 2nd ed. (Oxford University Press, 1986); Milan Bier, ed., *Electrophoresis: Theory, Methods and Applications* (Academic Press, 1959–67); Barry L. Karger, Lloyd R. Snyder, and Csaba Horváth, *An Introduction to Separation Science* (Wiley, 1973).

Justin Corfield
Geelong Grammar School, Australia

Gene Array Analysis

Gene array analysis is a method to simultaneously evaluate the expression of many genes. It can be used for sequence identification such as mutation analysis as well. Gene arrays are solid surfaces, such as a microscope slide, on which a number of nucleotide sequences belonging to a gene have been placed at defined locations by spotting or by direct synthesis. The aim of using this technology is to recognize the existence and abundance of labeled nucleic acids in a biologic sample, which is hybridized to the nucleotide sequences on the gene array. This technology is a very young one and is growing very fast. One of the most important features of gene arrays is the amount of quantitative data they can provide. The major challenge for using this technology is the methods that can be used for dealing with such a huge amount of data. These data can be interpreted in different ways. Bioinformatics is capable of helping to interpret the data provided by gene arrays by using mathematics, statistics, and computer science technology. In other words, gene array analysis is the analysis of data provided by gene arrays to obtain the correct interpretations and significant results.

The nucleic acids attached to the array or the labeled nucleic acid of the sample are called target, while the labeled nucleic acids compromising the sample are called probes. The amount of probe hybridized to each target spot provides information about specific nucleic acid composition of the sample. A gene array experiment has the advantage of getting the information on thousands of targets in a single experiment.

There are different kinds of gene arrays including nylon membrane arrays, glass slide arrays, and affymetrix's gene chips.

There are several terms that are used to refer to gene arrays including biochip, DNA chip, GeneChip® (Affymetrix, Inc.), DNA array, microarray, and macroarray. In general, biochip, DNA chip, or GeneChip refers to gene arrays on glass slides. Microarray and macroarray indicate the spot size or the number of spots on the slide.

Gene arrays are powerful tools to compare complex sample RNA populations. For example, using array analysis, the expression profiles of normal and tumor tissues, treated and untreated cell cultures, developmental stages of an organism or tissue, and different tissues can be compared. A typical gene array experiment involves the following:

1. Isolating RNA from the samples to be compared;
2. Converting the RNA samples to labeled cDNA via reverse transcription;
3. Hybridizing the labeled cDNA to identical membrane or glass slide arrays;
4. Removing the unhybridized cDNA;
5. Detecting and quantization the hybridized cDNA; and
6. Comparing the quantitative data from the various samples.

For validating the differences in expression of special genomic sequences, another method of analysis, such as RT-PCR, Northern analysis, or nuclease protection assays, is used. These procedures can be used for relative or absolute quantization of specific data recognized by gene array analysis. The most challenging part of a gene array experiment is the data analysis, which is performed with the help of computer and bioinformatics. Just one gene array experiment can offer thousands of data points. Then, making sense of the provided data is of great importance.

For dealing with this challenge, the novel field of gene array bioinformatics has become available. The computational analysis of a gene array consists of several steps: image processing, normalization, and measuring and quantifying the gene array variability. During these steps, the data resulting from a gene array experiment can be interpreted. Gene array analysis by bioinformatics methods can help to find which genes are differentially expressed in one set of samples relative to another. It can be applied to determine the relationships between genes or samples measured. It will also provide the possibility to classify samples based on gene expression measurement.

SEE ALSO: Gene Pool; Genes and Gene Therapy; Genetics; Genomic Library.

BIBLIOGRAPHY. Ambion, "The Basics: What Is a Gene Array?" http://www.ambion.com/techlib/basics/arrays/index.html (cited July 2007); Dov Stekel, *Microarray Bioinformatics* (Cambridge University Press, 2003).

IMAN TAVASSOLY
MAZANDARAN UNIVERSITY OF MEDICAL SCIENCES, IRAN
OMID TAVASSOLY
TARBIAT MODARES UNIVERSITY

Gene Mapping

Gene mapping describes identifying the location of specific genes on chromosomes. It is a key step in understanding genetic diseases. The goal of gene mapping is to understand and treat genes that cause genetic disease.

The Human Genome Project (HGP) was essentially completed in 2003. It was a 13-year project sponsored by the United States Department of Energy and the National Institutes of Health. Major contributions were made by China, France, Germany, Japan and Great Britain as well as others. Its goal was to build detailed guides to the type and location of all genes on chromosomes.

Every human being has 46 chromosomes. Twenty-three are inherited from the mother and 23 from the father of the child. The X and Y chromosomes make the essential difference between male and female. If the chromosomes that determine the sexual inheritance are both X then the child will be a female. If one is an X and the other is a Y the child will be a male. The other chromosomes contain the genes that regulate the growth and functioning of all of the cells in the human body.

The creation of a genetic map plotting the locations of genes on DNA strains of the respective chromosomes is the goal of gene mapping. A genome is the total set of genes on chromosomes. The genome may be that of a human (human genome) or a chicken or pig (chicken genome and pig genome). When researchers begin the process of gene mapping there is nothing on the map. As the genome is investigated the chromosomes are identified and the respective genes are also identified and their location plotted on their respective chromosomes. The end product is a complete map reporting the location of all the respective genome's genes and the DNA sequencing of the bases of each gene.

Genetic markers are fragments of DNA that identify differences in strains. The genetic markers are unique sequence-dependent patterns or DNA. The ordering of the different bases in genes is made by observing recombinant frequencies. The makers are somewhat like finger prints because of their unique characteristics.

It was estimated that there were between 50,000 and 100,000 genes in humans. However, the number of genes turned out to be much smaller. The number of genes is only between 20,000 and 25,000. The additional goal of determining the sequences of the three billion chemical base pairs that make up human DNA was also a goal.

There are two ways to do gene mapping—genetic mapping and physical mapping. Gene mapping identifies the order of genes along each chromosome. Genetic mapping analyzes the locus of genes on chromosomes. The locus of a gene (loci of genes) on a chromosome can allow it to be linked to another gene, in which case the two genes are "linked." If genes are not linked to each other although linked to the chromosome then they are separated by an independent assortment.

Alleles are the sequences of chemical units that compose the genetic sequence of the gene. The loci may be the genetic inheritance of both the father and the mother of the human whose genetics are being mapped.

The genes may have different loci, but during DNA crossover there may be a recombination of loci so that the order of the genes on the chromosomes is changed. The closer two genes are the less likely recombination is to occur. This failure to recombine is due to the fact that recombination frequency is more likely to occur when there is a chiasma between the two loci.

If two DNA molecules are homologous and they combine the new combination is called DNA crossover. During meiosis if two homologous pairs of sister chromatids align side by side then DNA crossover is likely to occur.

The point at which two homologs connect is the chiasma. This is where the two homologs exchange DNA segments. The exchange is from the chiasma to the end of the chromosomes. If during the DNA exchange the sequences of chemicals on the DNA do not match exactly on the chromatid then the exchange will be an unequal crossover. The effect is to mis-code the genetic sequence.

Physical gene mapping techniques are more precise than those used in gene mapping. The methods seek to establish the distances of genes on the chromosome and their distance from each other. Physical gene mapping include somatic cell hybridization and fluorescent in situ hybridization (FISH).

Both the gene mapping and the physical mapping methods use genetic markers. These are specific physical or molecular features that differ among individual people. These markers are also transmitted genetically to succeeding generations.

Physical mapping seeks to understand the process of DNA replication. When DNA replicates it creates a group of clones, but it does not have to replicate all of the DNA. With a map the clones are used to map the workings of the whole genome. The clones allow for the visualization of stretches of DNA in operation.

Once mapping is completed genes can be investigated for a number of features. The most common is to identify the location of genetic disorders on genes. Then the investigation seeks to find ways to overcome the gene deficiency. There are many diseases that are genetically based. These include achondroplasia, agammaglobulinemia, albinoism, ankylosis, cellac disease (celiac sprue), Huntington's Chorea, Christmas disease (hemophilia B), cystic fibrosis, Downs syndrome, dwarfism, Ehlers-Danlos syndrome, epilepsy, Friedreich's ataxia, Gaucher's disease, hemolytic disease of the new born, hemophilia, Hirschsprung's disease (megacolon), Klinefeiter's syndrome, myotonia congentia, osteogenesis imperfecta, phenylketonuria, polycystic kidney, sickle cell anemia, Tay-Sachs disease (gangliosidosis), Thalassemia (hemolytic anemia), Turner's syndrome (gonadal dysgenesis), Von Recklinghausen's disease (neurofibromatosis), Wilson's disease, and many others.

The process of identify the genetic locations responsible for genetically based diseases is also a form of gene mapping. It requires development of a very fine map of the base sequences on the gene responsible for the disease. It can also be used to investigate the origin and the manifestation of genetic disease in large families. For these data it is also possible to project the demographics of the disease in the general population.

There are numerous benefits that will be harvested in the short run from gene mapping. Among these are contributions to molecular medicine, environmental applications, advances in anthropology and especially in bioarchaeology which seeks to trace the linage of people, forensic DNA and the precise identification of criminals, and advances in agriculture, livestock breeding and other bioprocesses.

Advances in genome science now being applied to all plants and animals are making biology the great science of the 21st century. It has created a biotech industry that producing billions of dollars in goods and services in the near future.

SEE ALSO: Genetic Code; Genetic Testing/Counseling; Genetics.

BIBLIOGRAPHY. Minou Bina, ed., *Gene Mapping, Discovery, and Expression: Methods and Protocols* (Springer-Verlag, 2006); T.A.A. Brown, *Genomes 3 3E* (Taylor & Francis, 2006); Ian Dunham, ed., *Genome Mapping and Sequencing* (Horizon Scientific Press, 2003); Lawrence B. Schook and Haris A. Lewin, eds., *Gene-Mapping Techniques and Applications* (Marcel Dekker, 2001); Matt Ridley, *Genome: The Autobiography of a Species in 23 Chapters* (HarperCollins, 2006); David Siegmund and Benjamin Yakir, *The Statistics of Gene Mapping* (Springer-Verlag, 2007).

ANDREW J. WASKEY
DALTON STATE COLLEGE

Gene Pool

In a population of sexually reproducing organisms, a gene pool is the sum of that population's genetic material at a given time. In terms more specific to a particular genetic locus on a chromosome, it is the sum of the alleles in a population at that locus.

As is currently posited by the "Out of Africa" hypothesis, the species of homo sapiens, and its gene pool, began as a relatively small group of individuals (roughly in the hundreds) in east Africa. Over some tens of thousands of years, some groups left Africa and increasingly populated the rest of the world. This hypothesis finds wide agreement by modern evolutionary theorists. At the end of the 20th century, it has also found strong confirmation from the molecular genetic and chromosomal studies of population origins that have mapped the specific route taken by different human subgroups or races throughout evolutionary time.

Evolution is the change in composition of a population's gene pool. This can occur by a variety of mechanisms, including mutations, natural selection, and genetic drift. As populations left Africa, each faced different environments, different novel diseases, diets, and climates. To the extent that this was the case, over time, the surviving composition of each subpopulation's gene pool was altered to be attuned to the needs of its specific environment. Two well-studied examples are illustrative of this point.

As a population moved away from the equator where the average amount of sunlight (and also the risk of skin cancer) is less, over time pigments in the skin were selected to allow more translucency per sunlight exposure. This allowed a more efficient manifestation of the endogenous synthesis of vitamin D, an absolutely critical vitamin for proper human bone development and therefore proper childbirth. Second, as Europeans domesticated new animals and increasingly relied on such animals for sustenance, they had to evolve the enzymes necessary to digest specific novel nutrients (lactose). It is interesting to note that most of the world is lactose intolerant because the gene for the enzyme to digest lactose originated in Europeans. As populations change or evolve in response to different environments, their gene pools are changing their composition and character.

Evolutionary "fitness" is defined not from the perspective of the human person but from the unconscious perspective of the gene: it is the ability to pass on one's genes, the ability to reproduce. Because populations often face difficult and rapid changes in their environments (e.g., famine, plagues, ice ages as in Eurasia 20,000 years ago, social selection, etc.), the advantages gained in fitness by the adaptive specificity of a gene pool must be balanced by the risks posed to evolutionary fitness by too narrow of a genetic profile. A large and diverse gene pool allows a greater chance for future adaptation to an ever-uncertain environment.

SEE ALSO: Allele; DNA; Genetic Code.

BIBLIOGRAPHY. Richard Dawkins, *The Selfish Gene* (Oxford University Press, 1976); Jared Diamond, *Guns, Germs and Steel* (Norton, 1999); Richard Leakey, *The Origins of Humankind* (HarperCollins, 1996); Nicholas Wade, *Before the Dawn: Recovering the Lost History of Our Ancestors* (Penguin, 2006).

OMAR SULTAN HAQUE
HARVARD UNIVERSITY

Gene Silencing

Gene silencing is a process in which a gene is switched off. It is different from gene mutation. In fact, in gene silencing the mechanisms regulating gene expression are changed so that the gene will not be expressed and, in other words, the gene expression is down-regulated or the gene is turned off. It is believed that innate gene silencing has been a tool for protecting the genomes of organisms from infectious DNA elements such as viruses during the evolution. In other words, gene silencing has been an innate cellular immune surveillance system. Gene silencing has been proposed as a method for gene therapy in different diseases.

Because genes are regulated by transcriptional and posttranscriptional mechanisms, gene silencing can be a transcriptional or posttranscriptional procedure. Gene silencing at the transcriptional level is made by creating an environment with modified histone proteins. In this environment, gene cannot be expressed because of changes in transcriptional agents. For gene silencing at the posttranscriptional level, the messenger ribonucleic acid (mRNA), which is the transcriptional result of that gene, must be destroyed to stop translational process.

There are different methods for gene silencing at the transcriptional and posttranscriptional levels. Using oligodeoxynucleotides is a way for performing gene silencing as a therapeutic tool. Synthetic oligodeoxynucleotides are used for gene-specific expression interruption. Introduction of gene-specific oligodeoxynucleotides with their binding to target gene or mRNA inhibits transcription or translation of that specific gene. This strategy is called antisense strategy. Another strategy, which is called antigenene strategy, is based on avoidance of interaction between transcription factor and a target gene which will result in inactivation of that gene.

The most famous gene silencing method is RNA interference (RNAi) which has brought hopes for gene therapy of many diseases. The discovery of RNAi has been one of the transforming events in biomedical sciences. This novel technology can result in gene silencing or even omitting functions of specific sequences from the genome. RNAi technology involves introduction of double-stranded RNA result in inhibition of gene expression at the posttranscriptional level. In order to target mRNA for destruction and perform a posttranscriptional gene silencing, short interference RNA (siRNA) or silencing RNA is used. siRNA is a short oligonucleotide of about 19 to 23 nucleotides with a high specificity for target genes which are supposed to be turned off. There are many ongoing trials to test the capability of RNAi for curing several diseases such as cancers and AIDS.

Although gene silencing is an ancient immune cellular system, man-made gene silencing technology is a state-of-the-art approach for meddling with specific gene expression with applications in treatment of many important diseases.

SEE ALSO: DNA; Gene Pool; Genetic Code; Genes and Gene Therapy; Genomic Library.

BIBLIOGRAPHY. Roman Gardlik, et al., "Vectors and Delivery Systems in Gene Therapy," *Journal of Medical Sciences Monitor* (v.11/4, 2005); Gregory J. Hannon and John J. Rossi, "Unlocking the Potential of Human Genome with RNA Interference," *Nature* (v.431, 2004); Wei Lv, Chao Zhang, and Jia Hao, "RNAi Technology: A Revolutionary Tool for the Colorectal Cancer Therapeutics," *World Journal of Gastroenterology* (v.12/29, 2006).

IMAN TAVASSOLY
MAZANDARAN UNIVERSITY OF MEDICAL SCIENCES, IRAN
OMID TAVASSOLY
TARBIAT MODARES UNIVERSITY

Gene Transfer

Gene transfer is the process of transferring genetic material from one cell to another by mechanical or surgical means. This process can help overcome the problems inherent in finding or manufacturing viruses which might be used to transfer the material and offers a genuine opportunity to redress some of the issues concerning genetic disease. Vertical gene transfer involves moving genetic material from a cell to its successor, while horizontal or lateral gene transfer involves the transfer of material among cells which do not have such a relationship.

Scientific understanding of the role and nature of genes in single-celled organisms was more or less complete by the end of the 1960s. Since then, researchers have been working on expanding understanding to higher organisms. Although many advances have been made, the complexity of genetic interactions and bodily functions means that there have also been many failures and even deaths resulting from clinical trials. Inserting genetic material via virus has proved to be more difficult than anticipated because the human body has spent millennia fighting to resist viruses and the legacy of this conflict is multifactorial and difficult to document exactly. Clearly, those researchers who could discover breakthroughs and convert this knowledge into marketable treatments for pharmaceutical companies would find their careers transformed into glittering success and this, together with the need to obtain research grants, can produce pressure on scientists to work with maximum speed and at the limit of understanding.

It is clear that bacteria contain genetic material that may have been spliced together from quite unrelated or at least diverse organisms. The altered genetic material has led to quite distinct changes in the ecological niche which the bacteria has subsequently occupied. To some extent, these changes are understood and can be manipulated to create distinctive forms of bacterial life. If the same processes can be more properly understood in more complex life forms and the changes that would be brought about therefore predicted, then it would be possible to modify living creatures, including people, in whatever ways might be desired. It is obvious that this would have major benefits in that it could assist people suffering from genetically inherited diseases and conditions. However, a number of social and ethical issues need to be resolved to determine wheth-

er the same technology would be deemed acceptable to root out other genetic conditions which some may consider undesirable—obesity, perhaps, or unattractive features. It is clear that even if this technology became sufficiently well established as to make it available on an open market, prohibitive costs are likely to rule it out from all but the most wealthy members of the most wealthy societies, at least for the foreseeable future. This brings about additional equity issues that should be considered.

SEE ALSO: Gene Pool; Genetic Code; Genes and Gene Therapy; Genomic Library.

BIBLIOGRAPHY. Horace Freeland Judson, "The Glimmering Promise of Gene Therapy," *Technology Review* (v.109/5, 2006); Harold Ochman, Jeffrey G. Lawrence, and Eduardo A. Groisman, "Lateral Gene Transfer and the Nature of Bacterial Innovation," *Nature* (v.405, 2000).

JOHN WALSH
SHINAWATRA UNIVERSITY

Generic Drug

Generic drugs, sometimes known colloquially as generics, are drugs that are bioequivalent to a brand-name drug with respect to the pharmacokinetic and pharmacodynamic properties. However, because of the registration of brand-name drugs, generic drugs tend to be sold at a much lower price, enabling health service providers and customers to make substantial savings. Generic drugs and medicines have to have exactly the same active ingredient as the brand-name versions and must meet identical pharmacopeial requirements for preparation. They also must be of exactly the same strength and use the same method of administration, safety, efficacy, and intended use.

The sole reason for the use of generic drugs is to allow drugs to be made at a much cheaper price or to make drugs available that are not elsewhere for whatever reason. The reason why they are cheaper is that the company making the generic drug has generally not been involved in the extremely expensive research and development of drugs, the costs associated with obtaining regulatory approval in various countries,

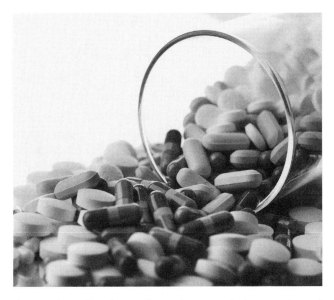

Generic drugs allow drugs to be made at a much cheaper price and make drugs available that are not elsewhere.

Although generic drugs are said to be identical as brand-name drugs, in terms of having the same medical properties, some people have found adverse reactions to changing from medication with brand-name drugs to generic drugs. In some countries such as Australia, patients are allowed to ask for brand-name drugs or request that pharmacists substitute it with a generic drug to alleviate any of these problems, both actual and perceived.

SEE ALSO: Pharmacist; Pharmacologist; Pharmacology; Pharmacopeia/Pharmacopoeia; Pharmacy.

BIBLIOGRAPHY. M. Laurence Lieberman, *The Essential Guide to Generic Drugs* (HarperCollins, 1986); Donald L. Sullivan, *The Consumer's Guide to Generic Drugs* (Berkley Publishing Group, 1996).

JUSTIN CORFIELD
GEELONG GRAMMAR SCHOOL, AUSTRALIA

and also the cost of marketing these drugs, and making medical professionals around the world aware of their existence and use. As a result, makers of generic drugs do not have to go through the lengthy process of developing drugs and spending resources on drugs which are later found to be unsuitable. Furthermore, they do not need to undertake clinical trials—the test for a generic drug is solely that it has exactly the bio-equivalent makeup as the original.

The making of generic drugs is legal in three circumstances. The first and major use is when the original patent for the brand-name drug as expired or there has never been a patent issued. The second instance is when the generic company certifies that the original brand-name drug patents are invalid, unenforceable, or will not be infringed. Generic drugs are also made when the patent for the brand-name drug is not enforceable in the country where the generic drugs is being manufactured and sold. To preempt the expiry of patents, many drug companies producing brand-name drugs produce their own generic product or license their own product to be made by generic companies. In a few cases, some countries have also allowed their own manufacturers to produce generic drugs to treat major diseases when the health service of that country has not been able to fund the cost of brand-name drugs. This has happened recently in Brazil and Thailand.

Genes and Gene Therapy

Genes are chemical compounds that act as genetic codes. They instruct cells to make proteins.

Each gene is a collection of DNA (deoxyribonucleic acid) in sequence. DNA molecules are long double-helix molecules resembling a spiral staircase. The steps in the spiral staircase were fixed at conception when the individual inherited 46 chromosomes from two parents (23 from each). The steps consist of pairs of four types of chemicals. Each is a molecule called a base (nucleotide). The four types are adenine (A), thymine (T), guanine (G), and cytosine (C).

The genetic code of each individual is written in triplicate so that the combination of A with G or G with C or T creates sequences such as AAA, or AGT or GCT. The genetic codes are so arranged that they instruct the manufacturing of one of twenty amino acids. For example, the sequence GCT is the code for the manufacture of amino acid lysine.

Each gene codes for the manufacture of one protein. This means that each gene is a stretch of DNA in a coded sequence. The sizes of genes vary. The size depends upon the size of the molecule that it is coded to manufacture.

Obvious inherited characteristics are hair, skin, or eye coloring. These inherited characteristics are the product of the genes acquired at conception. Some traits are regulated by more than one gene.

Each gene contains a set of nucleic acid molecules that comprise a set. The segment contains the coded information needed to produce a functional RNA (ribonucleic acid). The gene uses the coded information in an orderly manner. The code includes information in the segments that acts as rules directing the manufacturing of another molecular product. The gene also has in is program regions that carry instructions on how to function.

The genetic makeup of an individual is a genotype. The genotype contains information for the physical development of the body. Phenotype is the name for the manner in which the genotype is expressed (phenotype expression). The interaction of the genes with each other and with the environment (e.g., food available, minerals in water, and other environmental factors) guides the physical development of the individual.Genes are the units of genetic inheritance. Often more than one gene is involved in the expression of the genetically determined characteristics of an individual. For some reason genes normally contain noncoding regions.

GENES AND DNA

The genes in cells are composed of a long strand of DNA. A promoter region controls the activity of the gene. The code also controls gene products that are used by the body. The code contains a sequence or a set of instruction for engaging in the process of transcription. The transcription process creates an RNA copy of the gene's code. The RNA then directs the synthesis of proteins using the code. Gene expression is the gene using its code to manufacture gene products that are either a protein or an RNA copy.

During RNA transcription the DNA molecule splits open along its length. One strand of the DNA molecule will be inactive. The strand becomes a template that is used to form an RNA molecule. The bases of the RNA are arranged in the same sequence as are the bases of the inactive strand of DNA with one difference. The RNA contains uracil (U) instead of thymine (T).

In the next step of replication, the RNA copy becomes the messenger RNA (mRNA). The mRNA RNA acts as a template for protein synthesis. An RNA polymerase II in the nucleus of the cell uses protein coding to a precursor RNA which contains the intron sequence that will be removed by splicing. It separates from the DNA and travels into the cytoplasm of the cell. In the cytoplasm it combines with a ribosome. The ribosomes are the cells manufacturing centers for making proteins. The mRNA in the next step instructs the ribosome to construct an amino acid which will be used to make a protein. The amino acids are free-floating chemicals in the cytoplasm. A transfer RNA (tRNA) brings them into what becomes a growing chain of proteins. The molecule chain will be folded into the exact shape needed because it is influenced through close by chaperon molecules.

When cells divide DNA replicates itself. The DNA helix unravels. Step by step, a new molecule of DNA is formed. The replication leads to the formation of a new cell which then divides into two new cells. During DNA helix replication, it is possible for a mutation to occur. If the mistake is severe enough, the cell will die. Most mutations are trivial and will not have any significant consequence. However, some changes can introduce changes that may be detrimental or beneficial in some cases.

When mutations that are deleterious mistakes occur these may affect only the individual. However, if the mistake affects the germline cells that are involved with reproduction then there can be genetic consequences that contribute to the expression of genetic disorders in the offspring. Humans have cells that are eukaryotic organisms, that is, most of the cells of the body contain chromosomes which contain the genes needed to do the chemical reactions which transfer energy, build tissue, reproduce and other activities of life. There are in the genes of eukaryotic organism noncoded regions (introns). When RNA transcription is taking place these are spliced away by the RNA messenger by regions called exons. The result is that a single gene can used different exons to produce differing splicings that then produce different proteins.

GENE THERAPY TECHNOLOGY

The Human Genome Project, completed in 2003, put the number of genes in the human genome at 20,000 to 25,000. The exact number is close to 20,500. The number was a surprise because earlier estimates had imagined a much larger number. The number of base pairs residing in the DNA double helix is estimated to be nearly three billion pairs.

Gene therapy is a new technology which seeks to change the function of some genes in individuals in order to cure or prevent certain diseases. At the present time gene therapy is still experimental in most of its forms.

The goal of gene therapy is to replace or repair defective genes that cause disease. In the case of some diseases such as immune deficiency diseases sample cells of the immune system are taken from the patient. The cells may be in the patient's blood or bone marrow. The normal gene is inserted into the cells form the patient. The replacement cells are then grown in a laboratory. When there is a sufficient supply they are reintroduced into the patient. In other forms of gene therapy the cells are fixed within the cell inside of the patient.

Some diseases such as diabetes, hemophilia, and cystic fibrosis are caused by defects in the genetic code inherited from the parents of an individual. The therapy seeks to replace the defective genes with a healthy genetic code. The modified genetic code will then replicate itself in the cells of the individual being treated. However, it will not prevent the transmission of the defective gene(s) to offspring. Gene therapy has the potential to counteract a health gene. In diabetics this would mean that the cells of the islets in the pancreas that are no longer producing insulin would be replaced with genes that would then instruct the pancreas to manufacture insulin. The health benefits if successful would be enormous. The focus of gene therapy is upon the most fundamental level of biochemistry. For example the gene which causes type 2 diabetes mellitus has been identified. Research into the transference of genetic material into the chromosome that carries the gene is being conducted which if successful would restore some or all of the individual's ability to manufacture insulin.

Somatic gene therapy is research into gene therapy has been limited so far to targeting specific cells in the body. These are called somatic cells. When somatic gene therapy is successful it alters the genetic code or makeup of the individual. The changes in characteristics however, will not be transmitted to succeeding generations.

Germline gene therapy seeks to produce changes in the individual's genetic code that would alter genes and also make them transmissible to succeeding generations. So far, they have not been successfully developed.

A major challenge for gene therapy is to develop methods for delivering the genetic material that will be the new genetic code. Genetic code is the genetic information that is present as a biochemical language. A genetic code is present in all living things including humans, animals, plants, bacteria, fungi and viruses. The genetic code is used by the DNA molecule to instruct cells to do specific functions. Or in the case of noncellular organism such as viruses the code instruction the interactions that replicate the virus usually to the detriment or death of the cell in which it is living.

Using viruses to deliver the gene therapy is one strategy that is being explored. The virus will have been effectively neutralized as a harmful agent. It will then have been spliced so that the genetic code that will be the gene that is therapeutic is added to the virus. The part of the virus' genetic code that is harmful will be spliced off rendering it harmless. The virus will when implanted in the body invade the specific cell tissue it normally effects but will instead add the genetic material that will give beneficial instructions to the cells of the tissue.

The deliver systems of viruses make them strategically interesting vectors. Research is currently in progress to develop viral vectors for genetic therapy.

Another strategy is the use of chemicals that act as vehicles to deliver the needed genes as chemical messengers. The chemical vehicle or chemical "vector" delivers the genetic material to the target cells. The chemical vector reacts with the target cells so that the gene therapy can become a part of the target cells.

The first experiments with gene therapy were aimed at two genetic diseases. These were the inherited forms of immune deficiency in children and a genetic disorder that causes very high levels of serum cholesterol in both children and adults. The American Society of Gene Therapy (a nonprofit medical and science organization) has reported that X-linked immunodeficiency has been treated successfully with foamy viruses as vector in gene therapy.

X-linked severe immunodeficiency (SXCID) is a rare genetic disorder which results from defects in the immune hormone receptor (common gamma chain). It is found on the surface of lymphocytes and immune blood cells. Patients with SXCID usually develop fatal infections in infancy unless they undergo a bone marrow transplant. However, in a percentage of cases the bone marrow transplant is ineffective. The new therapy holds considerable promise children suffering from SXCID.

In the early 1990s gene therapy was attempted on patients with severe combined immune deficiency (SCID). The first two patients chosen for gene therapy were chosen because bone marrow transplants had indicated that replacing the defective gene was possible. In addition, studies with mice had indicated that enzyme replacement therapy was a model that gene therapy could follow. However, most of the first 3,000 patients with a variety of immune diseases were not helped significantly. Since 2000, advances in understanding the human genome and advances in understanding the immune system have aided the effectiveness of bone marrow transplants. However, they have not provided a permanent gene therapy cure for SCID victims.

Researchers have been able to develop a gene therapy in mice for the immune deficiency disease agammaglobulinemia which is X-linked (XLA). The disorder affects only males. The researchers were able to identify the specific defective gene, and were able to replace it with a therapeutic gene. Research has not yet advanced enough to be applicable to humans.

Stem cell transplantation is being used to treat individuals with T cell defects. The defect interferes with the victim's body's ability to ward off disease. The immune system is defective because of the genetically inherited defect. The use of stem cell is taken from the umbilical cord upon the birth of a normal infant. The blood containing the stem cells is transplanted into the immune deficient recipient. The procedure has met with some success.

Two forms of SCID have been proven as successful treatments side effects have kept them from active use in the United States. The use of gene therapy is also only for genetically caused illnesses. In the future, it might be possible to use gene therapy for a wider range of diseases.

Early experiments with gene therapy were also conducted upon cystic fibrosis (CF) patients. CF is caused by a defective gene which interferes with the balance of salt/water balance in the lungs. The CF gene is designed to manufacture a protein that will regulate the flow of salt and water in and out of the cells of the lungs. Instead, in CF patients the protein is dysfunctional. It causes the air passages to accumulate thick, sticky mucus. The mucus is an inviting environment for bacteria. Infections that occur damage the airways and the lungs.

The gene therapy used to treat CF is targeted at the mucus linings of the lungs of the patient. The vectors used at first were viruses that are known to cause respiratory infections. While there was some risk of respiratory infection this was an inviting choice of vectors.

Current research on animals using a non-viral vector has been successful in reducing the DNA molecule as a compacted molecule to the point where it can penetrate the cell wall membrane. This allows the therapeutic DNA molecule to enter into the cell nucleus. The goal is to deliver a gene which will manufacture enough protein to counteract the CF protein deficiency that causes breathing problems. The gene transfer method if successful will open a new way to treat many forms of genetic disorders.

Gene therapy has been used to treat single cell disorders such as hemophilia, muscular dystrophy and sickle cell anemia. These therapies are still very experimental. Other applications of gene therapy include cancer treatments, heart disease and some infectious diseases. Gene therapy has also been investigated for infectious diseases such as AIDS.

SEE ALSO: Gene Mapping; Gene Pool; Genetic Testing/Counseling.

BIBLIOGRAPHY. Roman Espejo, *Gene Therapy* (Thompson Gale, 2004); Linda George, *Gene Therapy* (Thompson Gale, 2006); Anthony J. F. Griffiths, et al., *Introduction to Genetic Analysis* (W. H. Freeman Company, 2007); Leland Hartwell, Michael L. Goldberg, and LeRoy Hood, *Genetics: From Genes to Genomes* (McGraw-Hill, 2000); Benjamin Lewin, *Genes IX* (Jones & Bartlett, 2007); Jeffrey R. Morgan, ed, *Gene Therapy Protocols* (Springer-Verlag, 2001); Clay Farris Naff, *Gene Therapy* (Thompson Gale, 2004); Michael A. Palladino and Mary Colavito, *Gene Therapy* (Benjamin Cummings, 2006); Sandy B. Primrose, Giuseppe Bertola, Bob Old and Richard Twyman, *Principles of Gene Manipulation* (Blackwell Publishers, 2005); Matt Ridley, *Genome: the Autobiography of a Species in 23 Chapters* (HarperCollins, 2006); Gabor M. Rubanyi and S. Yla-Herttuala, eds., *Human Gene Therapy* (Springer-Verlag, 2003).

ANDREW J. WASKEY
DALTON STATE COLLEGE

Genetic Brain Disorders

Genetic brain disorders are defined as disease states that affect the differentiation and function of the neuroectoderm and its derivatives via defective genes. The Human Genome Project has suggested that there may be approximately 30,000 genes. In a particular disease, there may be one or more defective genes that contribute to the particular brain disorder. The defect may be a gain of function or loss of function. The inheritance of these defective genes may be autosomal dominant, autosomal recessive, sex-linked recessive, or mitochondrial. Many of these brain disorders not only affect the brain, but also affect many other organ systems. Hereditary genetic disorders involving the central nervous system may have a wide variety of clinical presentations, including that of developmental delay, neurological or developmental regression, varying levels of consciousness, multisystem involvement, and focal neurologic deficits.

INBORN ERRORS OF METABOLISM

The study of genetic brain disorders was largely established when Archibald Garrod published *Inborn Errors of Metabolism* in 1923. Inborn errors of metabolism are uncommon individually, but occur quite frequently when taken as a whole. Collectively, there is approximately 1 in 1,400 to 1 in 5,000 disorders per live birth. The incidence among different racial and ethnic groups varies among the diseases. They are often due to defective genes that regulate enzymes or transport proteins. These diseases can be divided into the following categories: carbohydrate metabolism, amino acid metabolism, organic acidemias, lysosomal storage diseases, fatty acid metabolism, and mitochondrial disorders. Most of these disorders are of autosomal recessive inheritance. The presentation of the disease can vary even within each specific disease type, ranging from differing ages of onset to variable levels of clinical severity.

Various types of inherited disorders will result in differing mental deficits. For example, the psychoses and hallucinations may be due to any of the following disorders: lysosomal defects (Sanfilippo and Hunter diseases, GM2 gangliosidosis, neuronal ceroid lipofuscinosis, Krabbe disease), purine metabolism defects (Lesch-Nyhan syndrome), peroximsomal defects (adrenoleukodystrophy), Wilson's disease, acute intermittent porphyria, and homocystinuria. Developmental delay may also result from metabolic defects such as lysosomal defects, disorders of amino acids, organic acids, carbohydrates, copper metabolism (Menke's disease, Wilson's disease), and peroxisomes (adrenoleukodystrophy, Zellweger syndrome). Seizures and ataxias can manifest secondary to metabolic diseases.

It is important to diagnose and treat patients with inborn errors of metabolism because a delay in either may lead to long-term neurologic impairment. Patients should also be referred to appropriate counseling, as there exist many profession and peer support groups for individuals with these disorders. Genetic counseling should also be offered to evaluate recurrence risks, familial screening, and prognosis.

HEREDITARY MOVEMENT DISORDERS

Hereditary movement disorders may include neurologic deficits such as ataxia, dystonia, and chorea. Ataxia is the inability to maintain posture or smooth movement. Dystonias are defined as diseases that cause an abnormal muscle tone, while choreas are diseases associated with involuntary spastic movements. The differences in disorders are largely due to the gene and location of the gene deficits. The spinocerebellar pathways are involved in the majority of hereditary ataxia syndromes. These disorders can be associated with three different types of mutations.

One set of diseases is due to nucleotide triplet repeat expansions. A common nucleotide expansion is that of the nucleotides cytosine; adenine and guanine are repeated which results in a polyglutamine tail as in the spinocerebellar ataxias and Huntington's disease. Huntington's disease is characterized by chorea, dementia, and psychiatric symptoms. Other hereditary ataxias include dentatorubral-pallidoluysian atrophy (DRPLA, also known as Haw River syndrome or Naito-Oyanagi disease), Friedreich's ataxia, adrenoleukodystrophy, and Refsum disease.

Movement disorders may also be due to defects in the mitochondrial DNA. Mitochondrial disorders are due to defects in either the nuclear- or mitochondrial-encoded mitochondrial proteins. These defects are passed to subsequent generations via nonmendelian inheritance. Specific examples of mitochondrial diseases include Friedreich's ataxia, mitochondrial myopathy, encephalopathy, lactic acidosis, stroke syndrome (MELAS), ataxia with selective vitamin E deficiency (AVED), and X-linked ataxia with sideroblastic anemia.

Finally, diseases may be due to defects in DNA repair. In particular, ataxia telangiectasia mutated protein, aprataxin, and senataxin are proteins involved in DNA repair that can be altered to cause movement disorders. Specific examples of these mutations include ataxia telangiectasia, ataxia with oculomotor apraxia types 1 and 2, and spinocerebellar ataxia with sensory neuropathy (SCAN1).

MUSCULAR DYSTROPHIES

Duchenne muscular dystrophy (DMD) is an X-linked autosomal recessive disorder that presents in early childhood. The disease is caused by a mutation in the dystrophin gene on the X chromosome. It is a rapidly progressive disease that is associated with muscle weakness, mental retardation, and cardiomyopathy. It often leads to patients being wheelchair-bound before they reach their teenage years and often results in death by the second to third decade of life.

MOTOR NEURON DISORDERS

Motor neurons are the cells that control voluntary muscle activity. Diseased motor neurons cause difficulty with voluntary movement. Many of these diseases are hereditary in nature and are associated with neurologic symptoms. For instance, Kearns-Sayre syndrome (KSS) is a maternally inherited disorder causing progressive ophthalmoplegia, atypical pigmentary retinal degeneration, heart block, ataxia, and dementia. Myoclonus is another symptom of motor neuron disease and can be associated with brain disease as in myoclonus epilepsy with ragged red fibers (MERRF). These patients also inherit the disease maternally and demonstrate myoclonus, ataxia, seizures, dementia, and hearing loss. MELAS syndrome is also associated with motor neuron disease, as described above.

EPILEPSY

Epilepsy is a seizure disorder defined as the occurrence of two or more unprovoked seizures. Seizures are caused by the abnormal hypersynchronous firing of neurons in the brain. Seminal works by Fritsch, Hitzig, Ferrier, and Caton in the 1870s initiated the development of the epilepsy field. Seizures have many etiologies, some which have genetic components. Progressive myoclonus epilepsy (Unverricht-Lundborg type) is one form of inherited epilepsy. It is an autosomal

recessive disorder characterized by epilepsy, ataxia, and myoclonus. Tuberous sclerosis complex is another inherited epilepsy disorder. It has autosomal dominant inheritance and is associated with hamartomas in the skin, lung, heart, kidney, and brain.

SEE ALSO: Huntington's Disease; Metabolic Disorders; Wilson's Disease.

BIBLIOGRAPHY. T. N. Feraro, D. J. Dlugos, and R. J. Buono, "Role of Genetics in the Diagnosis and Treatment of Epilepsy," *Expert Reviews of Neurotherapeutics* (v.6/12, 2006); G.F. Hoffman, W.L. Nyhan, and J. Zschocke, *Inherited Metabolic Diseases* (Lippincott Williams & Wilkins, 2002); C.R. Scrivner, et al., eds., *The Metabolic and Molecular Bases of Inherited Disease*, 7th ed. (McGraw-Hill, 1995).

Darrin J. Lee
University of California, Irvine

Genetic Code

The genetic code governs the production of protein synthesis in the cell by mapping DNA (deoxyribonucleic acid) sequences to proteins that are utilized for various cellular functions. The process of protein synthesis does vary between prokaryotes (single-cell organisms; i.e., cyanobacteria, *E. coli*) and eukaryotes (multicellular organisms; i.e., animal, plant); however, both cell types are characterized by the processes of transcription and translation that are mediated by the genetic code.

In the eukaryotic cell, chromosomes are located within the nucleus of the cell. These chromosomes contain DNA that are composed of sequence(s) of the basic unit of genetic information—the gene. Governed by noncoding and coding sequences, the gene plays an integral role in the encoding of proteins. The essential component of the gene is the segment or portion that is necessary for transcription to produce the RNA (ribonucleic acid) transcript, being the mRNA (messenger RNA), to serve as a carrier of genetic information from DNA to the ribosomes for the production of proteins.

Translation guides amino acid (protein building blocks) production by the sequence of nucleotide triplets, called codons, that stem from the RNA transcript. The RNA transcript is produced in the cell's nucleus and during this process three other types of RNA molecules are manufactured: tRNA (transfer RNA), rRNA (ribosomal RNA), and snRNA (small nuclear RNA). With the exception of snRNA, all RNA molecules eventually leave the nucleus via the nuclear pores and are involved in the process of translation that occurs mainly outside the nucleus. The snRNA are components of spliceosomes, which aid in removing introns (noncoding sequence) from the genetic sequence of DNA. The snRNAs interact with other subunit nuclear proteins to form these spliceosomes. The tRNA molecules are composed of 70 to 90 nucleotides that fold and are representative of another triplet nucleotide sequence, called the anticodons, that base pairs with complementary codons of the mRNA molecule on the ribosome for translation and the production of amino acids and the polypeptide chain —resulting in the synthesis of proteins. Thus, the "coding" defined by the triplet base pairing of codons and anticodons is instrumental for the production of a particular amino acid and subsequent protein.

SEE ALSO: Chromosome; DNA; DNA Repair; Genetics; Gene Mapping; Gene Pool; Gene Silencing; Gene Transfer; Genes and Gene Therapy; Genetic Disorders; Genetic Transformation; Genetics; Genome; Genomic Imprinting; Genomic Library; Genomics; Genotype; Watson, James.

BIBLIOGRAPHY. Jeremy M. Berg, John L. Tymoczko, and Lubert Stryer, *Biochemistry*, 5th ed. (W.H. Freeman, 2002); Harvey Lodish, et al., *Molecular Cell Biology*, 5th ed. (W.H. Freeman, 2003); Tom Strachan and Andrew Read, *Human Molecular Genetics*, 3rd ed. (Garland Science/Taylor & Francis Group, 2003).

Dino Samartzis, DSc, MSc, Dip. EBHC
Harvard University and Erasmus University

Genetic Disorders

Genetic disorders are medical conditions that are caused by errors in the replication of genetic code. Genetic diseases may be evident at birth, while others will only be manifested later in life. Some involve inconveniences, while others are life threatening or fatal.

There are many diseases caused by genetic abnormalities. They create deformity, disease or a tendency to develop certain diseases. Genetic disorders include achondroplasia, agammaglobulinemia, albinoism, ankylosis, cellac disease (celiac sprue), Huntington's Chorea, Christmas disease (hemophilia B), cystic fibrosis, Downs syndrome, dwarfism, Ehlers-Danlos syndrome, epilepsy, Friedreich's ataxia, Gaucher's disease, hemolytic disease of the new born, hemophilia, Hirschsprung's disease (megacolon), Klinefeiter's syndrome, myotonia congentia, osteogenesis imperfecta, phenylketonuria, polycystic kidney, sickle cell anemia, Tay-Sachs disease (gangliosidosis), Thalassemia (hemolytic anemia), Turner's syndrome (gonadal dysgenesis) Von Recklinghausen's disease (neurofibromatosis, Wilson's disease, and many others.

Some genetic disorders such as myopia, color blindness or inherited blepharitis (*Seborrheic blepharitis*) have mild symptoms. Other genetic diseases such as cystic fibrosis (CF) have severe symptoms. In some cases of inherited diseases such as Huntington's Chorea, death is an inevitable result. Prion diseases (spongiform encephalopathies) such as fatal familial insomnia (FFI) are genetic disorders that are also fatal.

Some genetic disorders arise from a single gene. For this to occur, it is necessary for the single-gene disorder to be carried on a dominant gene. The dominant gene can express the disorder from a single gene. In the case of a recessive gene, two copies of the gene are needed for it to be expressed. The abnormality is expressed as the production of too little or too much of a particular protein.

Genetic diseases may be rare disorders or they may be common. They can be the result of a mistake in the genetic coding of a single gene, or they may involve the whole chromosome. The mistakes may be the result of a reproduction in the mitochondria (self-reproducing) part of cells, or the mistake(s) may be due to chemical or radiation exposure. Radiation exposure included both atomic radiation and natural sunlight.

Skin cancer is the most common type of cancer in United States, South Africa, and Australia. Fair-skinned people, who are exposed to strong sunlight, especially in childhood, are likely to develop some form of skin cancer after the age of 65. They ultraviolet radiation (UV) exposure damages the skin and creates mistakes in the genetic reproduction. Artificial sources of UV light such as tanning beds are also sources of skin cancer.

Abnormalities in genes are common. They are more common in recessive genes than in dominant genes. All human beings carry abnormal genes. On average, each person has from six to eight abnormal recessive genes. Normally these genes are inoperative or do not cause a problem. Only if there is an inheritance from both parents of the same abnormal gene is there a problem. It is the presence of two copies of the abnormal gene that creates genetic disorders.

In the human population at large, there is only a small likelihood that a person will have two copies of an abnormal recessive gene. However, in cases of children born to parents who are close relatives is the risk high. In groups of people such as Orthodox Jews in come communities, and Amish and Mennonites who have intermarried for some generations, the risks are much higher. Abnormal genes that create genetic disorders may be inherited. However, they may also be the result of some spontaneous action that caused a mutation in the genetic code of the gene. The spontaneous mutation may be the result of several causes or of no identifiable cause. In cases where the mutation does not affect the reproductive cells the mutation will simply die out with the individual. However, if the mutation is included in the reproductive cells then the mutation will be transmitted to offspring.

Gene mutation that produces an abnormal gene may or may not be a "bad" event. The mutation is a matter of interpretation. For example, sickle cell anemia is an inherited blood disease found among people with African, Mediterranean, and Middle Eastern heritage. It is caused by the inheritance of two copies of the abnormal gene. Sickle cell anemia affects the hemoglobin (protein in red blood cells) of the red blood cells. These carry oxygen to all parts of the body.

People with sickle cell anemia have inherited two copies of the abnormal gene. It causes their red blood cells to change shape from a flexible disk-shaped cell into one that is less flexible and is shape like an old-time farm sickle (crescent moon shaped). The sickle shaped hemoglobin cells eventually clog blood vessels and prevent oxygen from reaching all parts of the body. The sickle cells are fragile and break down easily creating fatigue. People with a single sickle cell gene have the sickle cell trait. It does not cause the disease, but it does afford protection from malaria.

Some genetic disorders can occur at conception which may be so severe that the fetus does not survive or the infant if carried to full term does not survive. These mutations are rare, but the mutation dies with the individual. The mutation, as tragic as is the loss of the individual to family and friends, is not transmitted to the next generation. Mutations that affect radically the immune system are also in this category of severe mutations.

Sometime mutations can give an advantage. It may be that a mutation improves the ability to survive in the local environment including the diseases prevalent in the environment. The effect is to increase the survival potential of succeeding generations. For example, people who have genes that produced an immune system that was able to withstand and to recover from a severe influenza strain while many others dies will transmit genes that are better for succeeding generations.

If one parent has an abnormal gene and the other does not, then each child has a 50 percent chance of inheriting the abnormal gene. However, if one parent (rare occurrence) has two copies of the abnormal gene, then all of the children will inherit the abnormality. If only one parent has the abnormality and a child is born without the abnormal gene, then it will not transmit it to any offspring. For those who inherit the gene in a single copy, the odds are again set at 50 percent for the offspring (grandchildren) inheriting the gene assuming that the child mate does not have the same abnormal gene. In the modern world, medical advances have led to the survival and the reproduction of many people with inherited genetic disorders. Juvenile diabetes was until recent times fatal in childhood. Other hereditary disorders also prevented the individual from living long enough to reproduce and to thus transmit the disorder to their offspring. The net effect is that natural selection has been modified by human interference. It means that there is an increase in the number of individuals in the "gene pool" who have significant genetic defects. So the number of people born with genetic disorders can be expected to rise.

SEE ALSO: Genes and Gene Therapy; Genetic Brain Disorders; Genetic Testing/Couseling.

BIBLIOGRAPHY. Suzanne B. Cassidy, *Management of Genetic Syndromes* (Wiley, 2004); Muin J. Khoury, Julian Little and Wylie Burke, *Human Genome Epidemiology:*

A Scientific Foundation for Using Genetic Information to Improve Health and Prevent Disease (Oxford University Press, 2003); Robert L. Nussbaum, et al., *Thompson & Thompson Genetics in Medicine* (Elsevier Science, 2004); Joel L. Spitz, *Genodermatoses: A Full Color Clinical Guide to Genetic Skin Disorders* (Lippincott Williams & Wilkins, 2004); Helga V. Toriello, Robert J. Gorlin and William Reardon, eds., *Hereditary Hearing Loss and Its Syndromes* (Oxford University Press, 2004).

ANDREW J. WASKEY
DALTON STATE COLLEGE

Genetic Testing and Counseling

Genetic testing is the use of biochemical and cytological techniques to determine the carrier and disease status of an individual with regard to any number of genetic or chromosomal states which may manifest themselves in disease states. Genetic counseling is the provision of information and assistance to individuals (consultands) who are, or may be, affected by a disease of genetic origin. Consultands may themselves be suffering from a disease, may be a relative (usually a parent) of such an individual, or may have questions about their own carrier status (typically for purposes of reproductive planning). Advice given in genetic counseling includes calculation and interpretation of pretest and posttest probabilities (both for development of disease and of disease appearance in offspring) as well as provision of information and advice on follow-up actions individuals might take given their newfound knowledge.

COMMON GENETIC TESTS

Because genetic testing is neither universal nor inexpensive, genetic testing methods vary widely by geography and available resources. As a broad distinction, genetic testing may be divided into cytological and molecular techniques. The principle cytological method in genetic testing is the karyotype. Karyotyping examines the gross appearance of all 46 chromosomes. While not able to detect point mutations, this method can detect abnormalities caused by unequal crossing over or nondisjunction. The latter are a class of abnormalities caused when meiosis is abnormal and subsequent fertilization leads to cells with either more or less than two of a particular chromosome. Syndromes caused by nondisjunction which can be detected by karyotyping include Down syndrome and Turner's syndrome.

Among molecular techniques, the most accurate is gene sequencing where various methods are used to determine the exact base sequence of a relevant locus. While sequencing allows precise determination of genotype, it is not always appropriate. Because sequencing is not cheap, it is not feasible to sequence an entire genome. Instead, counselors and/or physicians work with consultands to determine the region of DNA that should be sequenced. More commonly, when many different loci are of interest, tests are done that determine the presence or absence of specific alleles known to cause or cosegregate with disease. Such testing methods, unlike sequencing, cannot confirm the presence of a wildtype allele, only the absence of specified mutant alleles.

KEY PRINCIPLES AND EVENTS

Generally, patients are not told what decisions to make regarding the various testing and management options. Instead, they are given information and support and empowered to make their own decisions. This is known as the principle of nondirective counseling and has been widely adopted as standard practice, particularly in North America and western Europe. It should also be

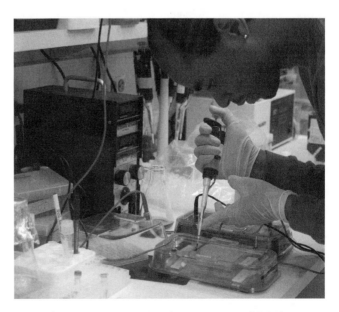

National Human Genome Research Institute researcher Milton English, Ph.D., using a pipette to load DNA into a gel.

emphasized that although the activities of counseling are commonly described in relation to genetic testing, counseling requires the ability to identify and address complex psychosocial issues associated with both the disorder of interest and the family of the consultand.

The events in genetic counseling case management can be broadly classified into four chronological phases: collection of information, assessment, counseling, and follow-up. Genetic counselors collect information on family history and medical history as well as work with consultands to determine which further tests to order. In assessment, this information is combined with a physical examination to validate or establish a diagnosis. The counseling phase can only begin when this information has been established either definitively or in a probabilistic manner. The nature and consequences of the diagnosis are explained with emphasis not just on the consultand, but on the consequences for relatives. In the case of potential parents, the risk to current and future children is also explored. Decisions about case management and referrals to other health professionals are also made in this phase. Finally, responsible genetic counseling entails follow-up for psychosocial support and to help assess and incorporate emergent information into improved case management.

SEE ALSO: American Society of Human Genetics (ASHG); Down Syndrome; Turner's Syndrome.

BIBLIOGRAPHY. D.L. Baker, J.L. Schuette, and W.R. Uhlmann, *A Guide to Genetic Counseling* (Wiley, 1998); R.J.M. Gardner and G.R. Sutherland, *Chromosome Abnormalities and Genetic Counseling*, 2nd ed. (Oxford University Press, 1996); R.L. Nussbaum, et al., *Thompson & Thompson: Genetics in Medicine*, 6th ed., revised reprint (Saunders, 2004).

BIMAL P. CHAUDHARI
BOSTON UNIVERSITY

Genetic Transformation

Transformation is the consequence of the introduction and incorporation of foreign genetic material, such as DNA or RNA, into a cell that brings about alteration of the genetic makeup. It was first discovered in 1928 by Dr. Frederick Griffith, and subsequently in 1944, Drs. Oswald T. Avery, Colin M. MacLeod, and Maclyn McCarty demonstrated that the gene transfer in bacteria *Streptococcus pneumoniae* was through DNA. Nowadays, genes from unrelated species can be combined in laboratories using molecular biology techniques which facilitate production of therapeutics such as insulin.

In single-cell organisms such as bacteria, genetic transformation can be achieved in laboratory setting using strains such as *Escherichia coli*. Foreign genetic materials can be transferred to these bacteria either naturally or artificially. Some species of bacteria routinely take up foreign genetic materials from their surrounding environment that is thought be used as a source of nucleotides. It has been suggested that this uptake of foreign genetic information might have been developed through evolution to allow the organisms to gain ability to adapt to their environment. The second way to accomplish genetic transformation in organisms is via artificial methods utilizing either thermal (heat shock) or electrical (electroporation) means. Both methods involve making the cell walls permeable for the entry of genetic material, such as DNA, into the cells.

In multicell organisms, such as plants, genetic transformation can also be achieved using particle bombardment or biolistics, which involves coating small gold or tungsten particles with DNA and then shooting them into plant cells. This process randomly incorporates DNA of interest into the plant genome.

In addition, foreign DNA can be introduced into mammalian cells DNA via transfection (heat shock or liposome-based methods), microinjection (injection of DNA directly into the cells using tiny needles), or viral transduction (delivery of genetic material packaged in virus to target host cells). Mammalian cells can sometimes be rendered tumorigenic when viral genes, such as oncogenes, transform normal cells into those with abnormal cellular appearance and properties regulating growth, proliferation, or differentiation.

SEE ALSO: Avery, Oswald Theodore; Cancer; Gene Transfer; Genetics.

BIBLIOGRAPHY. Bruce Alberts, et al., eds., *Molecular Biology of the Cell*, 4th ed. (Garland, 2002); J.F. Jackson and H.F.

Linskens, eds., *Genetic Transformation of Plants* (Springer-Verlag, 2003).

STEPHEN CHEN
UNIVERSITY OF TORONTO

Genetics

Genetics is the branch of biology that studies heredity. The passing of biological information from parents to offspring occurs through the combination of genes that are unique to each individual person, animal or plant that reproduces through living cells. As a field of study, it is concerned with the origin of individual characteristics and the way that these are transmitted to offspring. Genetics has developed over the centuries from the view of Aristotle and others that the species are fixed. One ancient idea being that inside of the seed of a man was another tiny little man. Inside of his seed was another tiny little man and so on through the generations.

Charles Darwin's ideas on evolution sparked controversy in part over how it was possible for species to develop into different animals from "lesser" species. The prevailing view in his time was that of Jean-Baptiste Lamarck (1744–1829) who had viewed heredity as proceeding according to natural laws, in particular through "acquired characteristics." His theory which was also accepted by Darwin and by others until the discovery of the ideas of Gregor Johann Mendel (1822–84) was recognized at the beginning of the 20th century.

A particularly notorious result of the Lamarckian understanding of Darwinism occurred from its adoption into social and political ideas. Herbert Spencer adopted the idea of evolution directed by the acquired characteristics of human beings to his socioeconomic theory. Followers like William Graham Sumner brought his ideas to America where they were used with a moral component added to justify the capitalism of the Robber Barons and others in the late 19th century. The Supreme Court also incorporated the idea into its rulings. The effect of Social Darwinism was to say that the successful (the rich) are the evolutionarily advanced and the poor are those that should be left to die because society will be better for it. Other political theories also adopted this view. The rediscovery in 1900 of a paper published by Gregor Mendel, an Augustinian monk from Moravia set modern genetics on the path of genes as the bearers of inheritance.

Mendel's work as a gardener revealed to him that pea plants inherited traits. The traits came from the parents to the offspring. Having practiced gardening in his youth between 1850 and 1863 he grew and test over 29,000 pea plants (*Pisum sativum*). He observed that all traits were not inherited by the offspring, just some of the traits of each parent. He was able to show the genetic inheritance of the pea strains. One in four of the pea plants had pure bred recessive alleles. Two out of four were hybrids and one out of four was the dominant purebred type. He show that the inheritance of traits followed laws. These laws have since become known as Mendel's Laws of Inheritance. He published his theory ("Experiments on Plant Hybridization") in an obscure journal in 1866 (*Proceedings of the Natural History Society of Brunn*) in Brunn, Moravia (now Brno, Moravia). His theory was ignored until 1900 when the importance of his work was recognized. His paper was republished in a journal with an international readership.

The development of statistics in the 20th century along with the gene theory enable a modern evolutionary synthesis to occur that when combined with the revealing of the structure of DNA and the mapping of the human genome has made it possible to understand the specific genetics of an individual and to trace the genetic heritage of people and animals to distant ancestors.

Genetic information is located in the base sequences in the genes that are attached onto the DNA double helix. The constitute codes are read as gene expressions when the cells decode the information in order to manufacture proteins that cells need to function. In order to synthesize a protein a complementary RNA molecule is produced. Its sequence orders a specific amino acid sequence of the protein.

The codes of the amino acids are 64-base triplets called codons. The codons encode the 20 possible amino acids. Most of the amino acids have more than one codon. The codons are synonyms if they encode the same amino acid. The "wobble" position is on the third base which can vary so that there are initiation codons and three stop codons.

Humans who have identical copies of a particular gene are described as being homozygous. Those with two different copies of a gene are described as heterozygous. As genes are copied they undergo mutations. Variant genes are called alleles. In describing alleles life scientists use the convention that dominant variant genes are designated with a capital letter, while recessive variants are designated with a lower case letter.

In the Mendelian genetic theory each inherited trait is a phenotype. All of the phenotypes are the result of specific genes or combinations of genes. In other words genes define the unique characteristics of individuals. All of the phenotypes are the sum of the genotype which constitutes the individual human or creature.

If the phenotypes produce hybrids then one phenotype will probably dominate another. Purebred lines of genes are strains of species that have been bred as exactly the same for generations. For example, breeds of dogs or cattle or grape vines are selectively bred for characteristics that aid agriculture or other needs. The breeding seeks to maintain the same phenotype so that, for example, a Concord grape or a Scottish Terrier is the same from generation to generation.

Crossbreeding of pure-breed types (homozygous) line will have different inherited characteristics. They will have offspring that will all have the same phenotype. The technical term for this cross-breeding is the F1 generation. The second generation (F2) will show the original phenotypes in a ratio of 3:1. The dominant phenotype will be the majority of the prodigy.

Purebred lines are organisms that have been inbred for many generations. Stock breeders breed cats, dogs, cattle, sheep, or other kinds of animals for a variety of purposes. There are strains of laboratory animals such as mice, rats, flies, and other animals or plants are used for experimentation with virtually fixed genomes that permit replication of experiments in any laboratory in the world.

DOMINANCE

Dominance within species arises between differences in the phenotype for one inherited characteristic. Hybrids produced from two different phenotypes produce offspring with only one phenotype. For example, experiments with short-winged fruit flies and long winged fruit flies have shown that when bred they produce only long-winged offspring.

Mendel's studies of pea plants showed that the offspring inherited several phenotypes. Focusing in on only the color of the petals, he crossed plants with

white petals with plants with violet petals. The offspring of the first generation F1 (first filial) all inherited violet petal flowers. This demonstrated that the violet color was dominant to the white petal color. He then allowed the F1 generation of offspring to self fertilize. The resulting F2 (second filial) offspring has both violet and white petal flowers. However, the colors were in a ratio of 3:1 (monohybrid ration) in which the violet color was three and the white color was one. Other experiments with crossbreeding show the same off spring ratio which led Mendel to conclude that the inherited trait was biological which today are called genes.

The monohybrid ratio is the basis for all pattern of inheritance in organism higher than peas. The 3:1 phenotype ration will be a 1:1 ration if an F1 individual is crossed with a homozygous recessive parent. The crossing will produce gametes with either a dominant or a recessive gene. A testcross is produced from a recessive parent crossed with the phenotype to determine if it is heterozygous. This ratio is important because in families with genetic diseases such as Huntington's disease the dominant allele is rare. As a result, the individual with the allele will not likely be homozygous.

Instances of partial or incomplete dominance also occur. For example snapdragon with white petals is crossed with a red petal parent the result will be a pink flower rather than the dominant ratio (F1). The next generation (F2) will produce red, white, and pink petal flowers.

Co-dominance occurs with crossbreeding as well. It is a departure from standard Mendelian order. When two alleles of a gene product are two distinct and detectable then they product is the results of co-dominance. Human MN blood typing is a commonly cited example of this phenomenon. This blood type is distinct from the common A, B, O, AB typing. The antigen formed by responses to antibodies that are found on the red blood cells identifies this type. The MN blood groups have two types of antigens. These two types are produced by the inherited alleles. People who are genetically heterozygotes inheritance produces both antigens and are classed as MN.

When co-dominance occurs, both alleles contribute equally to the phenotype. In contrast, in cases of incomplete dominance, the two alleles contribute unequally to the phenotype. When Mendel studies the genetic characteristics of the succeeding generations of peas he developed a concept of genetic inheritance based upon only two different alleles. When his work was rediscovered, life scientists soon found that nature was much richer than Mendel's theory had proposed. Indeed, there are cases of genes with three, four, and occasionally more alleles.

To investigate two alleles is a challenge, but the process becomes very complicated when more than two alleles have to be considered. In the case of the color of rabbit fur, the gene for color has four alleles.

The ratio produced is similar to incomplete dominance. There is a difference in that both alleles are dominant. This characteristic is found in blood groups that are inherited. In humans, the MN blood group is controlled by a single gene.

Dominance, co-dominance, and incomplete dominance affect human health. Some of the alleles carried on the genes of some humans affect their viability. In many cases the homozygous recessive does not survive. However, the heterozygotes may have a normal lifespan. If there is a phenotype that is observable such as yellow coats in mice, then the consequences can be observed. Yellow coats are dominant to black coats in mice. However, when two yellow-coated mice breed their offspring die in utero. This particular allele is lethal. There is a nuance that is significant in this instance. In yellow coated mice the allele that produces a yellow coat is dominant. However, in terms of viability, it is recessive. This is an important principle that occurs in many other alleles.

In the developmental genes, many that are mutations produce changes if one is present, but if two copies of the same allele are present, the outcome is lethal. In humans, Tay-Sach's disease, Huntington's disease and sickle cell anemia are diseases that manifest this genetic characteristic.

In some cases, semi-lethal genes are present. If a homozygote is present in a crossbreeding but is present in only reduced numbers, it is an alternation of the 3:1 ratio established by Mendel. Because many genes have a large number of alleles, there are also possibilities of variants that are not fatal.

The ideas developed by Mendel were developed in the first part of the 20th century. While the procedures have not been altered much since then, understanding DNA and the mapping of the human genome has created a huge number of polymorphic markers that enable useful genetic analysis.

Polymorphism in DNA sequences when identified allows alterations in DNA sequences to be understood. DNA polymorphisms are grouped into different classes and can be used in forensic genetics. They can also be used of other purposes as well.

GENETIC CODING

The genetic code is universal. It applies to all organisms which use the same codons for the same amino acids. However, as ever in nature exceptions can be found. Genes are measures of the response of each individual to the environment. Genes are inherited from parents usually without any genetic accidents. However, in rare cases mutations occur. These are variations in the copying the genetic sequence(s) which serves as a code. The "mistake" mars the expected genetic outcome. Some mutations are nonconsequential. Others are beneficial. Others are harmful or even fatal.

Genetic defects can occur spontaneously, be chemically induced, or caused by excessive exposure to radiation. The vast numbers of individuals that are born without any genetic defects is an improbably high number.

Medical genetics is field of study that deals with genetic defects which cause diseases through heredity. Diabetes and hemophilia are two such inherited diseases. Genetic diseases are a diverse group of genetic disorders. They are caused by one or more genes. Among the disorders are neurofibromatosis, hemoglobinopathies, thalassemias, Charcot-Marie Tooth Disease, multifactorial disease, and other disease. To identify genetic diseases, genetic screening is used. Its use however, is surrounded with ethical issues.

Recent research has indicated that cancer is genetically related. However, it also seems to be the case that there are DNA repair genes and tumor suppressor genes as well which use an in-activator gene. Because altered patterns of RNA are often found in tumors, it is currently thought that mutations in the introns or exon splice sites are responsible. Genes that have been identified as cancer causing are termed *oncogenes*.

Other areas of genetic research or applications of genetic knowledge include gene therapy with the introduction into cells copies of the necessary genetic code that will end or reawaken the appropriate genetic code.

The biotechnology industry is also the product of modern genetic research. Plants and animals have been the subject of extensive research and now development from genetic engineering. A major goal is the production of biologically useful proteins. Recombinant DNA is used to produce natural proteins. In addition, cloned genes are to produce proteins with modified amino acid sequences. Transgenic is the creation of useful plants and animals with altered genomes by the transfer of new genes. Cloning may be the ultimate act of genetic development. However, genetic work is filled with ethical issues arising from a respect for life.

SEE ALSO: Genetic Code; Genetic Disorders; Genetic Testing and Counseling.

BIBLIOGRAPHY. Helen V. Firth, Judith G. Hall, and Jane A Hurst. eds., *Oxford Desk Reference Clinical Genetics* (Oxford University Press, 2005); Leland Hartwell, et al., *Genetics: From Genes to Genomes* (McGraw-Hill, 2000); Bruce R.R. Korf, *Human Genetics: A Problem-Based Approach* (Blackwell Science, 2006); Robert L. Nussbaum, Roderick R. McInnes, and Huntington F. Willard, *Thompson & Thompson Genetics in Medicine* (Elsevier Health Sciences, 2007); Eberhard Passarge, *Color Atlas of Genetics* (Thieme Medical Publishers, Incorporated, 2006); Matt Ridley, *Francis Cricket: Discoverer of the Genetic Code* (HarperCollins, 2006); D. Peter Snustad, and Michael J. Simmons, *Principles of Genetics* (Wiley, 2005); Tom Strachan, and Andrew P. Read, *Human Molecular Genetics* (Taylor & Francis, 2003); Peter Turnpenny, and Sian Ellard, *Emery's Elements of Medical Genetics* (Elsevier Health Sciences, 2007); Spencer Wells, *The Journey of Man: A Genetic Odyssey* (Random House, 2004); Spencer Wells, *Deep Ancestry: Inside the Genographic Project* (National Geographic Society, 2006).

ANDREW J. WASKEY
DALTON STATE COLLEGE

Genital Herpes

Genital herpes is a sexually transmitted infection caused by the herpes simplex virus type 1 (HSV-1) and type 2 (HSV-2). Although most individuals are asymptomatic, following a two-week incubation period, patients will present with painful blisters surrounding the genitals and rectum. HSV-1 also commonly causes sores around or in the lips and mouth; these sores are known as cold sores. HSV-2 can also cause oral sores,

although these are not as common. The genital blisters will break, forming ulcers that can take up to four weeks to heal. Subsequent outbreaks, especially in those infected with HSV-2, can occur in the following months or even years, although outbreaks tend to decrease in frequency and severity over time. Other symptoms might include swollen glands in the genital region, painful urination, vaginal discharge, fever, or headache. Genital herpes infections usually do not cause serious long-term health problems.

Genital herpes is transmitted by contact with an infected sore, typically via sexual contact. Unlike some other sexually transmitted diseases, using condoms does not provide complete protection against transmission, as the condom may not cover the entire area. Using condoms, however, will cut down on transmission rates even if they are not 100 percent effective. Although close skin-to-skin contact can transmit these viruses, they are not transmitted via toilet seats, towels, or other forms of casual contact. Women seem to be slightly more susceptible to infection than men. Pregnant women can also pass genital herpes to their babies, who can subsequently have serious eye, skin, or brain problems, although the risk of transmission is low, especially if the woman is diagnosed and treated prior to delivery.

Although there is no cure or vaccine for genital herpes, antiviral drugs can decrease the risk of viral transmission as well as reduce the severity and frequency of herpes outbreaks. These drugs include acyclovir, famciclovir, and valacyclovir. The drug valtrex can also reduce the likelihood that an infected person will pass the disease on to a noninfected sexual partner. Reducing the frequency and severity of herpes outbreaks is especially important in patients who are also at risk of HIV infection, as coinfection with an actively ulcerating sexually transmitted infection such as herpes greatly increases the chances of HIV transmission.

Partly because transmission can occur even when a patient is not actively infectious or even aware of the infection, genital herpes is quite common in most populations. In the United States, approximately 25 to 30 percent of the adult population carries the HSV-1 or HSV-2 viruses, and incidence rates have been rising over time. Prevalence rates in other countries can range from 2 to 74 percent, and are generally much higher than those of other sexually transmitted diseases such as syphilis or gonorrhea. Although data are often scarce, many studies show that prevalence of herpes in countries outside the United States has also been increasing steadily since the 1970s, especially in Africa and countries of the former Soviet Union.

Promoting many of the measures that prevent HIV transmission will also help decrease herpes transmission, including condom use (although, as noted above, condoms are not as effective in preventing herpes as they are in preventing HIV), reducing the number of sex partners, and effectively treating active infections. Because herpes is an important cofactor of HIV infection, treating herpes infections is an important way to help cut HIV transmission rates.

SEE ALSO: National Center for HIV, STD, and TB prevention (NCHSTP); Sexually Transmitted Diseases.

BIBLIOGRAPHY. *Genital Herpes—A Medical Dictionary, Bibliography, and Annotated Research Guide to Internet References* (ICON Health Publications, 2004); Hunter Handsfield, *Genital Herpes* (McGraw-Hill, 2001) Lawrence R. Stanberry, *Understanding Herpes: Revised Second Edition* (University Press of Mississippi, 2006)

Annie Dude
University of Chicago

Genomic Imprinting

Genomic imprinting is an important process that occurs in some genes in the human genome wherein a gene is differentially expressed depending on whether it has been received from one's mother or one's father. Such "parent of origin" effects are only known to occur in sexually reproducing placental mammals. Imprinting is one of a number of patterns of inheritance that do not obey the traditional biallelic Mendelian rules of inheritance, which assume indifference about the parental origin of an allele. Traits are, therefore, able to be passed down maternal or paternal lines.

IMPRINTING MECHANISMS

One mechanism by which a given imprinted gene in an individual is differentially expressed is that one of the gene's parental alleles is silenced throughout the embryonic development of the individual by an alternation in parental DNA made during parental gametogenesis. The other parental allele is, therefore, allowed expression during embryonic development. An epigenetic mechanism by which this occurs is DNA methylation (the labeling of a $-CH_3$ group to specific regions of DNA) at imprinting control regions (ICRs). Intracellular DNA reading mechanisms exist after fertilization to check that the correct parental allele has been allowed differential expression.

IMPRINTING AND FETAL DEVELOPMENT

Imprinting has been able to explain a number of predicaments of life in utero as experienced by mother, father, as well as offspring. A number of imprinted genes are related to the manner in which the developing human must extract resources from its environment. As experimental work has confirmed predictions made by Robert Trivers's theory of parental investment, unfortunately, mother and father have different interests in how resources are extracted. Fathers and mothers have asymmetrical parental investment in each given child. This arises from the fact that mothers can only have one child every nine months for approximately 20 years, whereas a father could conceivably impregnate a different woman every day from puberty until death.

Systematic knockout studies of key imprinted genes, especially as performed on mice, have provided support for the hypothesis that imprinted genes that allow expression of paternally inherited alleles tend to drive more extraction of nutrients from the mother during gestation and after birth to produce a larger child. In contrast, imprinted genes that allow expression of maternally inherited alleles will tend to drive mechanisms to prevent the disproportionate utilization of resources by the fetus. A commonly cited example of this differential resource transfer is the paternally expressed Igf2, which enhances fetal growth and placental nutrient transport capacity, and the maternally expressed Igf2 receptor, which degrades excessive Igf2.

Many of the effects of imprinted genes occur at the placenta, a crucial site for resource and nutrient transfer. For example, an overgrown placenta (hydatidiform mole) results when maternal imprints are missing. Additionally, in Silver-Russell syndrome, a maternal uniparetal disomy, one finds growth restriction. Similar effects are found in other cases of disordered imprinting, as in preeclampsia, which also demonstrates growth restriction in utero. These diseases can only be understood within the context of imprinting as a common mechanism of parental conflict and manipulation of the phenotypic outcome of children.

IMPRINTING AND COGNITION AND BEHAVIOR AFTER BIRTH

Although only approximately 100 human genes are presently known to be subject to parent of origin effects, these prove to have tremendous implications for the development and eventual adult attributes of the human, including its cognitive and behavioral attributes. Imprinting effects, like other genetic expression patterns, need not be only all or none, but also may manifest as earlier age of onset effects or changes in severity.

In Turner's syndrome, a parent of origin effect exists in social and intellectual functioning. The phenotypic female (XO) could have received her only X chromosome from her father (Xp) or her mother (Xm). Xp Turner's women—who received a paternally derived X (the same as every non-Turner's woman)—were shown through surveys to display greater attributes of social intelligence. These data were confirmed by higher performance on tests of verbal IQ and social inhibition when compared to Xm Turner's women. Xm Turner's women—who receive a maternally derived X (which non-Turner's males always receive from their mothers)—performed better than Xp Turner's women on measures of visuospatial function.

Other prominent cognitive and behavioral manifestations of the effects of imprinting are seen in a number of neuropsychological disorders, including autism and schizophrenia, and can help explain such varied phenomenon as motor tic complexity in Tourette syndrome when relevant imprinted genes are maternally inherited (and greater verbal tic complexity when paternally inherited).

SEE ALSO: DNA; Gene Silencing; Turner's Syndrome.

BIBLIOGRAPHY. D.P. Barlow, "Gametic Imprinting in Mammals," *Science* (v.270, 1995); M. Constância, G. Kelsey, and W. Reik, "Resourceful Imprinting," *Nature* (v.432, 2004); A.R. Isles and L.S. Wilkinson, "Imprinted Genes, Cognition and Behavior," *Trends in Cognitive Sciences* (v.4, 2000); R.L. Trivers, "Parental Investment and Sexual Selection," in B. Campbell, ed., *Sexual Selection and the Descent of Man, 1871–1971* (Aldine, 1972).

OMAR SULTAN HAQUE
HARVARD UNIVERSITY

Genomic Library

A genomic library is a collection of genes or DNA sequences created using molecular cloning. These libraries are constructed using clones of bacteria or yeast that contain vectors into which fragments of partially digested DNA have been inserted. These bacteria and yeast are subsequently grown in culture and when these microorganisms replicate their genome, they also replicate the vector genome contained within them, that is, they replicate DNA fragments that had been inserted in vectors producing clones of the original DNA.

This collection of clones, in theory, contains all sequences found in the original source, including the sequence of interest. This sequence of interest is identified using screening methods that are very complex and capable of finding the original clone among 10 million starting clones. Genomic libraries can be constructed using various hosts like plasmids (insert size up to 15 kb), bacteriophage lambdas (insert size up to 20 kb), cosmids (insert size up to 45 kb), YACs and (insert size up to 2,000 kb), and many more. Some important ones are as follows:

CONSTRUCTING GENOMIC LIBRARIES USING PLASMIDS:

This is the process of cloning human DNA fragments by inserting them between two *Eco*RI digested sites of a plasmid cloning vector. After the human DNA fragments are inserted into the plasmid, the plasmids in turn are inserted into bacterial cells. In the end, these host bacterial cells contain their own chromosomal DNA together with plasmid DNA. As these bacteria replicate their chromosomes, they also replicate with them the plasmid cloning vectors. Plasmids are very convenient to work with because they contain one origin of replication, one of more selectable markers (such as a gene that confers resistance to antibiotics), and one or more restriction sites that can be cut and used for ligation of foreign DNA molecules.

CONSTRUCTING GENOMIC LIBRARIES USING BACTERIOPHAGE VECTORS:

The human genome is partially digested with a restriction enzyme like *Sau*3A in a specific way so that some of the sites are cleaved and others are not. By this way, random cleavage of the sites occurs and a collection of overhanging fragments of length suitable for cloning can be obtained, which are then ligated into bacteriophage lambda "arms" prepared so that the *Sau*3A ends of human DNA fragments can be ligated into the vector. The recombinant lambda chromosomes are then packaged into the infectious bacteriophage, and then the library, containing 1 million or more fragments of genomic DNA, can be stored for the future isolation of many genes. A collection of several hundred thousand phages would represent the entire DNA from the human genome.

CONSTRUCTING GENOMIC LIBRARIES WITH YEAST ARTIFICIAL CHROMOSOMES (YACS):

Large fragments of human DNA (over 500 kb) are generated by partial *Eco*RI digestion of human genomic DNA. Individual vector arms contain telomeres at one end and *Eco*RI compatible overhangs on at the other end. Individual vectors also carry a different selectable marker, and one arm also contains a centromere and selectable markers at each end and a yeast chromosome at the other end. The YACs are transferred into yeast, and the selectable markers are used to select only those yeasts that contain a properly constructed YAC.

ADVANTAGES OF MOLECULAR CLONING

The main task of modern medical genetics is to understand genetic disease in terms of mutations, and to find highly efficient methods of diagnosis and treatment. Medical geneticists, however, are faced by two difficulties when trying to find the basis of genetic disease. The first difficulty is obtaining enough amount of DNA to work with because cells generally have only two copies of a gene and some genes are only transcribed in specific tissues providing very little RNA to work with. The second difficulty is obtaining a purified form of the specific sequence of interest from all other sequences of DNA and mRNA present in the cell. To solve these two problems, scientists have come up with various techniques, one of them being molecular cloning. Molecular cloning allows us to obtain large sequences of purified DNA that were, otherwise, impossible to obtain.

SEE ALSO: Clone; Genetic Disorders; Genetic Testing/ Counseling; Genetics.

BIBLIOGRAPHY. Robert L. Nussbaum, Roderick R. McInnes, and Huntington F. Willard, *Genetics in Medicine,* 6th, ed., (Thompson & Thompson, 2001); Susan L. Speaker, Elizabeth Hanson, and M. Susan Lindee, *Guide to the Human Genome Project: Technologies, People, and Information* (Chemical Heritage Foundation, 2005).

RAHUL GLADWIN, M.D.
UNIVERSITY OF HEALTH SCIENCES ANTIGUA

Genotype

A genotype is the specific genetic constitution or makeup (genome) of an individual in terms of its DNA. The DNA through the genotype determines the hereditary potentials and also the limitations of an individual person (or indeed that of any organism) from its embryonic formation through to adulthood. For organisms that reproduce sexually, the inherited genotype contains the entire complex set of genes from both parents. This means that after sexual reproduction, it is certain that each individual will have a unique genotype, except for identical twins, triplets, and so forth, who are derived from the same fertilized egg. This contrasts with the phenotype of an individual which involves the physical appearance and constitution of an organism.

For medical research, the genotype is crucial in working out ways of treating diseases in general, separated from the person suffering from the disorder. This has been particularly important in the treatment of cancer, with oncologists and their research teams anxious to work on the fundamental causes of cancer and try to eliminate hereditary factors that might otherwise influence their work. Much of the original research and the development of ideas on genotypes was carried out by the Danish botanist and geneticist Wilhelm Ludvig

Johannsen. He conducted many experiments in plant heredity and these tended to support the mutation theory of the Dutch botanist Hugo de Vries, which argues in favor of gradual change through heredity rather than Charles Darwin's concept of natural selection. Johannsen coined the term *genotype*, based on *genus*, and also the term *phenotype*.

Although research in genotypes has aided much medical research, one of the emerging problems with the increased popularity of genotype research has occasionally led to some people, who have no real understanding of medicine, to become fatalistic and feel that particular disorders from which they suffer are part of their inherited genotype and ignoring environmental and other factors.

SEE ALSO: Phenotype.

BIBLIOGRAPHY. Steve E. Humphris and Sue Malcolm, *From Genotype to Phenotype* (Bios Scientific Publishers, 1994); Majit S. Kang and Hugh G. Gauch, Jr., *Genotype-by-Environment Interaction* (CRC Press, 1996); Amy Suzanne Richards, *The Effects of Genotype and Environment on the Chemical Composition and the Influence of Oxidative Stability of Brassica napus and Brassica Juncea Oils*, PhD thesis, University of Melbourne, 2006.

JUSTIN CORFIELD
GEELONG GRAMMAR SCHOOL, AUSTRALIA

Georgia

This Republic in the Caucasus was a part of the Russian Empire until 1922 when it became a constituent part of the Soviet Union. It became an independent nation in 1991. It has a population of 4,694,000 (2004) and has 436 doctors and 474 nurses per 100,000 people.

While Georgia was a part of the Soviet Union, healthcare was extensive and coordinated from Moscow, the capital, which established the basic policies for the whole country, although these were implemented by the health ministries of the constituent republics. There were also regional and local health authorities which provided healthcare. The main problem faced by Georgia was that the Soviet Union wanted to set national standards of health care, along with quotas for patient visits, and the provision of treatment and hospital beds with not much consideration for the regional differences in the need for healthcare. Georgia also became a place to where many people from elsewhere in the Soviet Union went to for health cures in spa resorts. Many of these were restricted to people who worked in state enterprises throughout the Soviet Union, with access being regarded as a privilege.

Traditionally much healthcare was provided in the home, with people being treated by family members, and elderly people remaining at home rather than going to hospitals, as institutional nursing care was often poor. The system, which operated in Tbilisi, the capital of Georgia, and to a lesser extent in the rest of the country, saw emergency first aid provided by ambulance teams that were often well equipped by regional standards, although their equipment lagged considerably to that used in western Europe. As regular hospitals did not have emergency rooms, there were special emergency hospitals which dealt with people treated by ambulance teams. In remote parts of Georgia, the system was often haphazard because of the problems with communications and roads.

When the Soviet Union was dissolved, the responsibility for looking after the health services of Georgia fell to the Ministry of Health. At that time, the healthcare of the population of Georgia had been exceedingly good. With Georgia having the highest number of doctors per capita, 59.2 doctors per 100,000 people, it also had more dentists per capita than any of the Soviet republics. Tuberculosis diagnoses, at 28.9 cases per 100,000 people, was the third lowest of any of the republics in the Soviet Union, and cancer, at 140.9 diagnoses per 100,000 people in 1990, was the lowest. However, there were problems with hospital bed availability which was low, and the rate of infant mortality was also high.

By this time, the healthcare system had become underfunded, and the decline in living conditions also led to the increased prevalence of some diseases. There were also more frequent problems of ill-health environmental hazards. These include some problems from nuclear waste left over from Soviet-era sites. A Georgian commission inquiry into radiation burns suffered by 11 soldiers in February 1997, concluded in November 1997 that there were 352 contaminated sites in the country. By contrast with the plight of the majority of the people in the country, the elite in Georgia continued to experience good healthcare having access to the best medical facilities.

Alcoholism and problems relating to it had always been a major factor in Georgia, and from the 1990s, there was a massive increase in drug use, but it remains low by international standards, with alcohol abuse being much more serious. The first cases of the HIV/AIDS were reported in 1993 with the Republic AIDS and Immunodeficiency Center in Tbilisi reporting the detection of sixteen cases, five from foreigners who were then deported. The number of cases has increased during the late 1990s, but is still much lower than many other countries in the world. There is now compulsory medical insurance for everybody, and there have been large increases in the amount of money spent on healthcare from the mid-1990s. The political infighting, and also the civil war and large numbers of refugees have led to more demand on medical facilities.

There are three medical associations in Georgia, with the Georgian Bio-Medico-Technical Society and the Georgian Society of Patho-Anatomists both being affiliated to the Georgian Academy of Sciences, and the Georgian Neuroscience Association founded in Tbilisi in 1996. There is also a Research Institute of Oncology in Tbilisi. The main center for medical training in the country remains the Tbilisi State Medical University, which was founded in 1918. It publishes the *Georgian Medical News* each month and *Georgian Medical Research* annually. It has 780 teachers and 4,000 students and maintains a library of about 520,000 volumes. Within it are located schools of general medicine, pediatrics, stomatology, health administration and management, pharmacy, medical biology, and nursing.

SEE ALSO: AIDS; Alcholism.

BIBLIOGRAPHY. W. Horsley Gantt, *Russian Medicine* (P.B. Hoeber, 1937); Galina Vasilevna Zarechnak, *Academy of Medical Sciences of the U.S.S.R.: History and organization 1944–1959* (U.S. Department of Health, Education and Welfare, 1960).

JUSTIN CORFIELD
GEELONG GRAMMAR SCHOOL, AUSTRALIA

Geriatrics

Geriatrics is the medical specialty concerned with elderly people and the field of human aging. Due to the important and worldwide population aging, geriatrics became an important specialty in medical care and in public health planning. Geriatrics deals with the human aging process and its implications, as well as with the prevention, diagnosis, and treatment of health problems in elderly people.

During human aging, people undergo transformations that change the likelihood of becoming ill, because the functional reserve of one person—the capacity of functioning of each human organ or system surpassing the needs of everyday life—decays in this process. Importantly, however, in the absence of health challenges (e.g., diseases), human aging does not impose restrictions to everyday life.

Since aging is a progressive phenomenon, this likelihood of illness tends to increase with age. As both susceptivity and reaction capacity for diseases change with age, so too do the clinical manifestations of many common diseases. A myocardial infarction may arise without pain in an older person, making the clinical picture very different from what medical doctors might generally expect.

Another specificity of geriatrics is the so-called comorbidity; because the effects of bad habits (e.g., bad nutrition, smoking, sedentarism, alcohol and abuse of other substances) tend to accumulate with time and the same is true for chronic diseases, it is common for an elderly person to have different diseases at one time. Comorbidities and bad health habits may increase the decay of functional reserve, making an individual more frail than he or she should be at a given age. This is called pathological aging, the phenomenon responsible for making people's health status different from each other's. A geriatrician, therefore, has to be able to give preventive care for anyone concerned with keeping good health, to care for multiple chronic diseases in an elderly person, or even to give palliative care for those dying. That makes geriatrics a very broad field.

Some conditions are common in the elderly and they are studied carefully within geriatrics. They include cognition-affecting diseases (notably Alzheimer's disease), depression and delirium (a mental disorder arising from clinical diseases), urinary symptoms and diseases (such as urinary incontinence or prostate diseases), malnutrition, immobility, and falls.

While caring for comorbid conditions, geriatrics concentrates on maintaining the functional status of patients, because this is what allows the engagement of daily living activities or prevents a person from doing so rather than the number or importance of the diseases per se. In this sense, rehabilitation (e.g., with physical or occupational therapy) after a loss of health status or adaptations in the environment (e.g., the substitution of a ladder for a slope allowing the passage of wheelchairs) may help a patient recover functional status even when the medical condition responsible for the loss is irreversible.

Polypharmacy is another common situation in geriatric care. Having more than one chronic condition, for example, diabetes, hypertension, and high low-density lipoprotein (LDL) cholesterol levels, may imply the need for simultaneous treatments, frequently with the use of multiple drugs, increasing the chances of adverse or antagonistic drug effects. The simultaneous use of different drugs may also be a burden in the patient's metabolism, because the metabolic reserve also diminishes with age. Finally, changes in the metabolism and body composition result in several pharmacological behaviors different of those observed in young adults. A common condition is related to the duration and intensity of a drug effect: lipid-soluble drugs tend to have longer-lasting effects in the elderly and water-soluble drugs tend to have more intense effects due to the fat increasing with aging at the same time that the proportion of water decreases.

Because of the particularities of pharmacology in the elderly and the likelihood of comorbid conditions, elderly people are at great risk of iatrogenics, defined as a medical intervention causing loss for the patient or the lack of a medical intervention that would have done good for the person. It is important to stress, nonetheless, that iatrogenics does not always mean a mistake, because the care of the elderly may be so challenging that giving standard care for a frail elderly may be the cause of iatrogenics. Finally, in this complex scenario, there are situations when a calculated iatrogenics may be essential to achieve a necessary result; the use of toxic antibiotics to cure an infection being one case in point.

Another important aspect in geriatrics is the need to establish treatment priorities, because caring for one disease may prevent the treatment of another condition or simply a patient may be so frail that the challenges of multiple drugs may result in worse consequences than carefully neglecting one mild disease. Priorities also must be established during terminal illness and palliative care, when relieving and avoid treatment-induced suffering is often more important than using all medical resources available in the quest for a cure that may not be achievable.

Geriatrics also studies the field of death and dying. To die with dignity and with the least suffering, surrounded by loved ones is achievable in most cases, mainly when consensus between the patient, family, caregivers, and the healthcare team is present. Geriatric care professionals seek this while making its knowledge available to those in need of it, respecting the will of the patient, who is the center and aim of care. In cases when the patient has no competence to decide, being unconscious or cognitively impaired, advance directives given in the past by the patient or by a person in care of the patient may inform the healthcare team of the amount of therapeutic maneuvers to perform in a terminal condition, for example. Some countries require that advance directives or the power of attorney for healthcare decisions be given by a document signed by the patient prior to the incapacity.

Although geriatrics, as a medical specialty, seeks to provide clinicians with the best training and knowledge to care for the elderly, it recognizes that there is no health-related profession or its specialty capable of giving good care in most complex cases, such as frail elders or those with multiple health-affecting conditions or situations. Such cases demand a broader, multidisciplinary team, ideally composed of different health professionals with background in elderly care.

Geriatrics itself is a multidisciplinary field that recognizes the different axes involved in the health of the elderly: not only does medical condition influence health and functioning, but environmental factors, psychological status, social conditions and opportunities, and financial matters all influence the health of an older person as well.

Geriatrics is a science that studies such fields as the medical therapy and palliative care for the elderly, but it emphasizes the need for health promotion and disease prevention as the only way to achieve long-lasting good health, a way far cheaper than the use of the most advanced therapeutic solutions.

SEE ALSO: Centenarians; Death and Dying; Pharmacology.

BIBLIOGRAPHY. W. Jacob-Filho and T. Monaco, eds., "Aging: Concepts and Misconcepts," in *Diagnóstico e Tratamento* (Manole, 2006); C. S. Landefeld, *Current Geriatric Diagnosis and Treatment* (McGraw-Hill Medical, 2004).

THIAGO MONACO, M.D., PH.D.
UNIVERSITY OF SÃO PAULO MEDICAL SCHOOL, BRAZIL

Germany

Despite the economic upheaval that Germany has experienced since reunification in 1990, the country ranks as the 24th richest nation in the world, with a per capita income of $30,100. The German economy is the largest in Europe, but growth has continued to slow in recent years. No official poverty rates are reported, but unemployment is high (11.7 percent). Income inequality also exists, and Germany ranks 28.3 percent on the Gini index of inequality. The poorest 10 percent of the population claims only 3.6 percent of resources as compared to 25.1 percent for the richest 10 percent. Direction of social funding to residents of the East German area has caused a great deal of dissatisfaction among some West Germans, and the rapidly aging population has added additional strain to the budget. However, the overall standard of living remains high, and the United Nations Development Programme's (UNDP) Human Development Report ranks Germany 21st of 177 countries on overall quality-of-life issues.

Health insurance in Germany can be either compulsory or voluntary, and approximately 90 percent of all Germans are covered by the compulsory state health insurance plan. Social security is compulsory, and it covers workers, students, trainees, the elderly, and dependents of various groups. Benefits include medical coverage, long-term care insurance, pensions, unemployment stipends, and worker compensation insurance. Employees below a set wage standard pay half the required contribution, and the other half is picked up by the employer. Individuals who earn higher wages contribute established percentages toward insurance coverage, generally about four percent if they choose to join the program. If they desire, salaried employees may choose a private insurance provider.

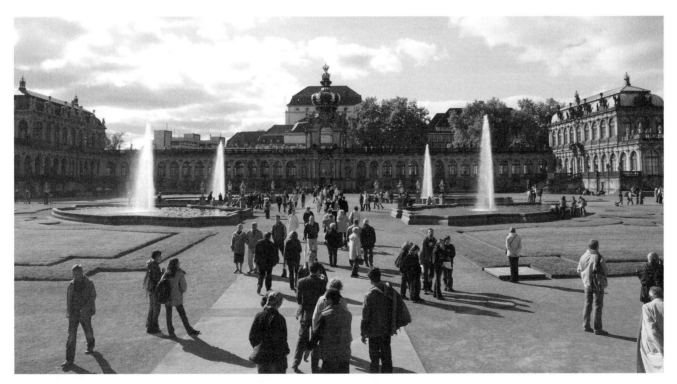

The UNDP Human Development Report ranks Germany 21st of 177 countries on overall quality-of-life issues. Germany has the second largest population in Europe (82,422,299), and people there enjoy a life expectancy of 78.8 years.

The government expends a good deal of money on healthcare in Germany, averaging 19 percent of the total budget. Just over 11 percent of the Gross Domestic Product (GDP) is used to fund healthcare, and $3,100 (international dollars) is allotted per capita. Most health spending in Germany originates with the government (78.2 percent), and social security spending accounts for 87.4 percent of all government health costs. The private sector is responsible for generating 21.8 percent of health expenditures, and nearly half (47.9 percent) of that amount involves out-of-pocket expenses. There are 3.37 physicians, 9.72 nurses, 0.10 midwives, 0.78 dentists, and 0.58 pharmacists per 1,000/ population in Germany. In March 2006, the German healthcare system experienced a medical crisis when physicians at all university clinics decided to strike over administrative demands that they work additional hours without a pay increase. After three months of negotiations, employers agreed to increase pay from eight to 18 percent and guaranteed bonuses to specialists who took on additional duties.

Germany has the second largest population in Europe (82,422,299), and the people enjoy a life expectancy of 78.8 years. Females outlive males an average of six years. Access to safe drinking water and improved sanitation is universal. The population is highly literate (99 percent), and virtually all children are enrolled in primary and secondary schools. Germany has the 25th lowest fertility rate among the nations of the world. Three-fourths of German women use some form of birth control, and births occur at a rate of 1.39 children per female. All births are attended by trained personnel, and the adjusted maternal mortality rate for German women is eight deaths per 100,000 live births. Women's health is a major concern, and programs have been initiated to target such areas as breast cancer screening, reproductive health, drug addiction, and domestic violence.

While East Germans have equal access to healthcare, some problems of assimilation continue to exist. At the time of reunification, major health indicators in the east were generally lower than those in the west. After reunification, East Germany's health system was abandoned in favor of the West German system. Over time, differences began to narrow but did not disappear. Life expectancy, for instance, remains lower in the east than in the west. Incidences of alcoholism and obesity have increased, posing greater health threats to East Germans than to West Germans.

At 4.12 deaths per 1,000 live births, Germany has the 11th lowest infant mortality rate in the world. Between 1990 and 2004, the infant mortality fell from seven to four deaths per 1,000 live births, and the mortality rate for children under the age of 5 dropped from nine to five deaths per 1,000 live births. Seven percent of all infants are underweight at birth. Most German infants receive the necessary vaccinations, and diphtheria, pertussis, and tetanus (DPT1) is reported at a rate of 98 percent. The number of infants receiving DPT3 is one percent lower than the rate for DPT1. Immunization rates fall still lower for other vaccinations: polio (94 percent), measles (92 percent), *Haemophilus influenzae* type B (90 percent), and hepatitis B (81 percent).

Air pollution resulting from coal-burning facilities poses a health threat in urban areas of Germany, and the proper disposal of hazardous waste is a national issue. The HIV/AIDS virus has also caused concern because Germany has a 0.1 percent adult prevalence rate. Around 43,000 people are living with the disease, which has proved fatal to some 1,000 people. Germany has also had problems with a number of communicable diseases in recent years, including some that were imported from developing countries. Lassa fever, for example, was imported into Germany in 2000 and 2006. That same year, incidences of meningococcal disease were reported. In 2003, Germany was involved in an outbreak of severe acute respiratory syndrome (SARS), and influenza appeared in January 2004.

About one-half of all deaths in Germany are a result of circulatory diseases. Cancer is another leading cause of death, partly because about a third of the population smokes. The government is particularly concerned about rising rates of smoking among women and young people. Consequently, in December 2006, the German government retreated from its traditional position on smoking and announced that it was following the lead of other European nations that had already placed limitations on smoking in restaurants, discos, schools, and some public buildings. Germany, unlike Britain, France, Ireland, and Italy, chose not to restrict smoking in pubs and bars.

SEE ALSO: European Association for Cancer Research (EACR); Healthcare, Europe.

BIBLIOGRAPHY. Central Intelligence Agency, "Germany," *World Factbook*, www.cia.gov/cia/; Jochen Clasen,

Reforming European Welfare States: Germany and the United Kingdom (Oxford, 2005); Commission on the Status of Women, Germany," www.un.org/women-watch/; Spencer Di Scala, *Twentieth Century Europe: Politics, Society, Culture* (McGraw-Hill, 2004); Sandra Halperin, *War and Social Change in Modern Europe: The Great Transformation Revisited* (Cambridge University Press, 2004); Wade Jacoby, *Imitation and Politics: Redesigning Modern Germany* (Cornell University Press, 2000); Mark Landler, "Germany to Restrict Smoking, Joining Other Nations in Europe," *New York Times*, (December 3, 2006); Martin A. Levin and Martin Shapiro, eds., *Transatlantic Policymaking in an Age of Austerity: Diversity and Drift* (Georgetown University Press, 2004); Jeremy Rifkin, *The European Dream: How Europe's Vision of the Future Is Quietly Eclipsing the American Dream* (Jeremy P. Tarcher/Penguin, 2004).

ELIZABETH R. PURDY, PH.D.
INDEPENDENT SCHOLAR

Germline Mutation

Germline mutation is an alteration of genetic matter which occurs after the time of conception and affects germ cells (eggs and sperm). A principal consequence of affecting germ cells is that such mutations may be passed to offspring.

Another key consideration is that a germline mutation will likely have few, if any, consequences for the individual with the mutation. Instead, the consequences accrue the offspring. Mutations of this sort are critical in understanding Alfred G. Knudson's two-hit hypothesis of heritable cancers as well as the spontaneous appearance of phenotypes associated with dominant inheritance in otherwise normal families.

Retinoblastoma is the paradigmatic model of the role of germline mutations in cancer caused by the loss of tumor-suppressor function. Retinoblastoma appears in two forms: heritable and sporadic, with heritable cancers accounting for 40 percent of the disease. In this form, a child inherits one wildtype allele and one mutant allele at the retinoblastoma locus. This first mutation is Knudson's first hit. Cells heterozygous at the retinoblastoma locus show a normal phenotype until a somatic mutation occurs at the wildtype retinoblastoma locus (Knudson's second hit). Because this mutation eliminates the only remaining DNA sequence to code for the working tumor suppressor, the resulting cell is without this tumor suppressor's capabilities and is likely to accumulate other somatic mutations at an increased rate and progress to a tumor.

In contrast, the 60 percent of sporadic cancers of this type require two somatic mutations of the retinoblastoma gene, an unlikely event in an otherwise normal cell. Because of these two different mechanisms of tumorigenesis, cancers of this type present differently in the heritable and sporadic modes. Because the underlying somatic mutation in the heritable form is much more likely, heritable cancers of this type occur simultaneously in multiple locations from multiple progenitor cells. Even if all such tumors are excised and the cancer goes into remission, relapse is likely throughout life. In contrast, sporadic cancers of this type occur singly, from a single progenitor cell and are unlikely to recur if cured.

There are two ways a dominant mutation can affect a child born to two parents who do not carry the mutation: somatic mutation early in embryogenesis giving rise to a mosaic dominated by the mutant phenotype or germline mutation in one of the parents. The former is exceedingly rare. However, for certain conditions such as osteogenesis imperfecta, certain hemophilias and Duchene's muscular dystrophy, germline mutation may increase the risk of recurrence by several orders of magnitude (to as high as 15 percent). Consideration of the role of mosaicism in atypical inheritance is now considered standard practice in genetic testing and counseling.

SEE ALSO: Cancer (General); Osteogenesis Imperfecta; Somatic Mutation.

BIBLIOGRAPHY. Justin C. St. John and Gerald P. Schatten, eds., *Mitochondrion in the Germline and Early Development* (Elsevier Science & Technology Books, 2007); R.L. Nussbaum, et al., *Thompson & Thompson: Genetics in Medicine,* 6th ed., revised reprint (Saunders, 2004).

BIMAL P. CHAUDHARI
BOSTON UNIVERSITY

Gerontology

Gerontology is the interdisciplinary study of aging and all that it encompasses, and gerontological studies have become increasingly significant as life expectancy expands around the globe. The word *gerontology* is derived from the Greek and literally means "old man." The term was coined by Nobel Prize-winning Russian immunologist Elie Metchnikoff (1845–1916) who worked at the world-renowned Pasteur Institute. In *The Nature of Man* (1903) and *The Prolongation of Life: Optimistic Studies* (1907), Metchnikoff argued that creativity was essential to longevity. He believed that aging was a process of cellular involution in which deteriorating cells countermanded cell growth of earlier life stages. This process could be halted, he believed, by the promotion of intestinal health. Geriatrics, which is related to gerontology, is concerned with the physical aspects of aging. The term was coined by Austrian American physician Ignatz Nascher (1863–1944) in 1908.

The field of gerontology was greatly advanced in 1992 with the publication of *Senescence: The Last Half of Life* by G. Stanley Hall (1844–1924), a pioneer in the fields of both psychology and education. Hall contended that aging should not signal an end to creativity and vitality. In 1939, professional handbooks become the major source of information for gerontologists, particularly in the United States, with the publication of American physician Edmund V. Cowdry's (1888-1975) *Problems of Aging*. After World War II, the study of gerontology further expanded as researchers began applying social science to the study of aging. In 1944, the American Social Science Research Council established a committee on aging, leading to Otto Pollack's (1887–1972) landmark publication of *Social Adjustment in Old Age* in 1948. The Gerontological Society was founded in 1945 and began publishing the *Journal of Gerontology* the following year.

In 1953, Robert J. Havighurst (1900–91) and Ruth Albrecht (1910-?) published *Older People* in which they took other gerontologists to task for not addressing the lack of social equality for the elderly by examining such areas as housing, healthcare, and social security. Some four decades later, Betty Friedan (1921–2006), the mother of the Second Wave of the women's movement, continued to fault gerontologists for their part in making the elderly invisible, accusing them of dismissing the possibility that the elderly could continue to grow and change as they aged.

APPLICATIONS OF GERONTOLOGY

Duke University conducted one of the first longitudinal (1955–80) studies that examined the impact of gender, ethnicity, and social status on aging. Two decades later, the Midtown Manhattan longitudinal Study and a National Center for Health Statistics study painted a discouraging picture of aging women. The report maintained that beginning in their 20s, women progressively deteriorated, with the most significant impairment occurring after the age of 40. In response to the women's movement, researchers began paying greater attention to women's physical and psychological health. Consequently, later studies indicated that women's health had significantly improved, while little change had occurred in men' health.

In 2007, American women had a life expectancy at birth of 80.97 years. Following a global trend, life expectancy for males was lower at 75.15 years. In most of the world, individuals are living longer in response to improved healthcare and technology, healthier lifestyles, and widespread access to safe food, clean water, and improved sanitation. All developed nations are currently faced with an aging population that demands a significant portion of available resources. In 2007, 12.6 percent of the American population was over the age of 65. By 2030, estimates place that number at a fifth of the population in response to the aging of baby boomers. One-fourth of those aged Americans will be people of color. At the international level, it is estimated that the world's population of those over the age of 60 will reach the two billion mark by 2030.

In the United States, as in the rest of the world, the quality of life for the aged is heavily dependent on economic status and access to healthcare. Because of unequal wages, women and African Americans are more financially vulnerable that white males. Social Security, which provides 44 percent of income for elderly Americans, accounts for 88 percent of income for elderly African Americans. White males are more likely than other elders to have employment pensions and private retirement accounts, resulting in unequal distributions of elderly income. In 2004, for instance, the Social Security median income for American males over 65 was $12,583, but only $8,799 for women. When other sources were factored in, the median income for males increased to $20, 800 and to $12,000 for females.

Without government aid through such programs as Social Security, Medicare, and Medicaid, elderly Americans would be even more vulnerable. This fact is evidenced by the decline in the poverty level for individuals over the age of 65, which dropped from 24.6 in 1970 to 9.8 in 2004. Despite the fact that the United States spends more on elderly healthcare than other developed nations, the care of aging Americans is considered poor when compared to those nations with government-sponsored programs that provide financial assistance to the elderly without requiring them to "poor themselves down" in order to qualify for residential long-term care. As a result of gaps in American healthcare coverage, two-thirds of elderly Americans are forced to purchase private insurance to supplement Medicare benefits.

By the 1980s, gerontologists were focusing on societal and political solutions to the problems of aging and promoting what they called the "new longevity." By the end of the century, the trend had shifted from relegating the aged to nursing homes to allowing the more affluent elderly to continue living as normally as possible in their own homes or in retirement communities. Since memory function declines as individuals age, gerontologists supported the use of physical and mental exercise to stimulate brain activity; and senior citizen centers offered a variety of programs to aid in continued growth and development.

Providing solutions to aging has become a billion dollar market in much of the developed world, offering everything from cosmetics to drugs to surgery to halt or offset the aging process. Some gerontologists have criticized the overuse of such methods. On the other hand, the use of nutritional supplements in fighting disease has been readily embraced by both mainstream gerontologists and practitioners of alternative medicine. Studies have indicated that elderly individuals who experience vitamin B-7 and B-12 deficiencies may exhibit signs of dementia. Vitamin D is believed to aid in preventing bone fractures, while calcium is promoted as having the capability to enhance nerve function, promote blood clotting and muscle contraction, and provide some defense against colon cancer. Vitamin E is considered to protect against all cancers. Some gerontologists suggest that products such as those containing caffeine and sugar may have greater negative impacts on the aged.

By the latter half of the 20th century, the global population of individuals over the age of 60 had nearly trebled. Global life expectancy increased from 46 years in 1950 to 66 years in 2000. Life expectancy in developing nations has increased by approximately 50 percent as fertility rates have decreased. Consequently, the aged make up larger proportions of populations. In response, the United Nations World Assemblies held two international conferences on aging. The first, held in Vienna in 1992, focused on aging in developed nations. The second conference in Madrid in 2002 examined aging in the developing world, which is home to more than one-half of the global population over the age of 60.

By 2050, it is estimated that 85 percent of the aged will live in developing nations, with the largest gains taking place China, Brazil, Nigeria, Indonesia, Colombia, Kenya, and Thailand. Among developed nations, the largest gains are expected to occur in Japan, Switzerland, Italy, and Germany. The only nations that are not expected to mirror this trend to some degree are those in sub-Sahara Africa where poverty and HIV/AIDS continue to exact a heavy toll on life expectancy. In 2002, the International Association of Gerontology sponsored the Valencia Forum, joining with the United Nations Office on Aging to develop a research agenda for the world's aging population. A number of variables such as sex, genetics, lifestyles, economic status, and access to healthcare, housing, and the environment are now regularly examined to develop gerontological theories and solutions to the problems of aging.

SEE ALSO: Administration on Aging; Alzheimer's Disease; Geriatrics; Medicaid; Medicare; Women's Health.

BIBLIOGRAPHY. M. Clemmitt, "Caring for the Elderly," *CQ Researcher* (v.16, 2006); Margaret Cruikshank, *Learning to Be Old: Gender, Culture, and Aging* (Rowman & Littlefield, 2003); Betty Friedan, *The Fountain of Age* (Simon & Schuster, 1993); Robert J. Havighurst, and Ruth Albrecht, *Older People* (Arno, 1953); Malcolm L. Johnson, ed., *The Cambridge Handbook of Aging* (Cambridge University Press, 2005); Stephen Katz, *Aging: Life Course, Life Style, and Senior Worlds* (Broadview, 2005); Donald H. Kausler, et al., *The Essential Guide to Aging in the Twenty-First Century:*

Mind, Body, and Behavior (University of Missouri Press, 2007); *The Merck Manual of Geriatrics* (Merck Research Laboratories, 2000); Debra J. Sheets, et al., eds., *Enduring Questions in Gerontology* (Springer, 2006).

ELIZABETH R. PURDY, PH.D.
INDEPENDENT SCHOLAR

Ghana

Ghana is located in western Africa on the Gulf of Guinea, between Togo and Côte d'Ivoire. Formerly a British crown colony called the Gold Coast, in 1957, Ghana became the first sub-Saharan nation to emerge from colonial rule. Now 50 years old, Ghana has suffered through a long string of political coups and the creation of a new constitution. Its economy, while better than its neighbors, is still heavily dependent on international aid, and about 60 percent of the workforce relies on subsistence agriculture. The population is 22,931,000, growing at 1.972 percent annually. The birth rate is 29.85 per 1,000 population and the death rate is 9.55 per 1,000. Median age is 20.2 years. Life expectancy is 58.31 years for males and 59.95 years for females. Forty-eight percent of Ghanians live in urban areas. The gross national income is $450 a year, with 45 percent of the population living on $1 a day or less.

With only 75 percent of the population able to access safe drinking water and 18 percent with sanitary waste facilities, Ghana suffers from a high rate of waterborne and parasitic infections, including diarrhea, typhoid fever, Guinea worm disease, and schistosomiasis.

Malaria and tuberculosis remain the biggest threat to Ghanian health. Recent years have seen a decline in malaria deaths, but it is still among the biggest killer of children under 5, and only three percent of Ghanians sleep under insecticide-treated nets. Tuberculosis (TB) cases have increased dramatically over the span of a decade. In 1995, there were 2,195 TB cases within the country. Today, there are 30,000 new cases a year, and 15,000 fatalities. Many cases are found to be multidrug resistant.

As in most country, the rise in TB cases has mirrored a rise in HIV/AIDS infections. The adult prevalence rate is 2.3 percent, with an estimated 320,000 cases, including 180,000 women. Ghana has a strong strategic plan and has secured international funding for programs, but the Ministry of Health notes that most patients have trouble affording even subsidized drugs. Only seven percent of patients are on antiretroviral therapy; 1.3 percent of pregnant women receive treatment to prevent mother-to-child tranmission.

The Ministry of Health says that the noncommunicable disease burden of Ghanians are "largely unknown." A major hospital found that hypertension was the third leading cause of mortality in their facility, after malaria and diarrhea. Antitobacco programs and diabetes awareness campaigns have met with limited success. Most medical facilities are poorly equipped to handle noncommunicable illnesses.

One in nine Ghanian children die before their fifth birthday. Malaria is the leading cause, although it has declined over the past five years. Immunization rates have increased, and are most apparent in the substantial reduction in measles cases, from 13,500 in 2001 down to just 487 in 2005. Malnutrition rates are "unacceptably high" according to the Ministry of Health. Fifty-seven percent of children work, and 28 percent marry before the age of 18.

The total fertility rate is 3.89 children per women. A quarter of Ghanian women use contraceptives. Less than half have a trained attendant to assist during childbirth. The maternal mortality rate is thus high, estimated at 540 deaths per 100,000 live births.

Medical services in Ghana are clustered along the coast, with limited services in the northern tier of the country. At least 40 percent of medical care comes from faith-based non-governmental organizations. Ghana suffers from a "brain drain" of trained staff: a 2002 report found that 30 percent of the physicians and nurses educated within the country between 1993–2002 left the country for better opportunities abroad.

SEE ALSO: Healthcare, Africa; Malaria; Tuberculosis.

BIBLIOGRAPHY. "Ghana" *CIA World Factbook*, www.cia.gov/library/publications/the-world-factbook/geos/gh.html (cited June 2007); UNAIDS: The Joint United Nations Programme on HIV/AIDS, "Ghana," www.unaids.org (cited June 2007); Ministry of Health, Republic of Ghana

"Pause, Get It Right, Move On: Review of Ghana Health Sector 2005 Programme of Work". Ministry of Health, Republic of Ghana. www.moh-ghana.org/moh/docs/Report2005.pdf (accessed June 2007); "UNICEF—At a glance: Ghana—Statistics". UNICEF. www.unicef.org/infobycountry (accessed June 2007).

HEATHER K. MICHON
INDEPENDENT SCHOLAR

Giardia Infections

Despite the controversy about the taxonomy of the species in the genus *Giardia*, this protozoan (*G. intestinalis/lamblia/duodenalis*) produces an important disease in the proximal portion of the small intestine, which could be asymptomatic, produce an acute self-limited diarrhea, and diverse intestinal symptoms such as chronic diarrhea, abdominal pain, cramps and tenderness, and weight loss, among others. Normally, there is no extraintestinal infections, but sometimes could produce a reactive arthritis (in recent years different studies revealed a clear relationship between giardiasis and inflammatory processes and allergy, possibly because infection by this protozoon enhances sensitization toward food antigens, due to increased antigen penetration through damaged intestinal mucosa). In severe *Giardia* infections, significant lesions of duodenal and jejunal mucose cells also are seen. Although many aspects of the infection are currently known, the mechanisms of pathogenicity and the major host defenses against *Giardia* infection are not well characterized.

This infection could lead to intestinal malabsorption that may be severe, and when it occurs in children, it could be associated with growth and development retardation. This pathogen has a considerable prevalence either in institutional and community settings.

This parasite, described in 1859 by Lambl, is a flagellated eukaryote organism (which belongs to the subphylum *Mastigophora*) with a relatively simple life cycle which includes trophozoites (vegetative stage) and cysts (infective stage). Humans can carry both forms, as can animals, and today, giardiasis is considered a zoonosis.

Diagnosis of *Giardia* infections is made by examining stools of suspected individuals or animals (including direct and stained observations as well as cultures of the organism); however, sometimes this is not enough and other diagnostic techniques should be used (immunological and molecular tests), even to the extent of studying the duodenal contents. *Giardia* can also be diagnosed when organisms are seen in intestinal biopsy specimens and/or at endoscopic evaluations.

The choice treatment for this infection is tinidazole or nitazoxanide. Alternative treatments may include metronidazole and paromomycin. In refractory patients, metronidazole and quinacrine may be used.

As with most infectious and parasitic diseases, prevention is the most important issue. In the case of giardiasis, safe water access is one of the primary priorities that should be considered, because cysts could be viable for a long time in water contaminated by human and animal feces. Additionally, as giardiasis is common in children, health education, especially in primary schools, is useful in preventing this infection.

Recently, the importance of this pathogen for travelers to zones with high prevalence of this parasitosis has been highlighted.

Finally, molecular tools that are now available will be useful in better understanding the frequency of zoonotic transmission as well as in developing more effective approaches to controlling giardiasis.

SEE ALSO: Gastroenterology; Infectious Diseases (General); Immunology; Parasitic Diseases; Pathology.

BIBLIOGRAPHY. Antonio Atias, *Medical Parasitology* (Mediterraneo, 2005); Paul Beaver, Rodney Jung, and Eddie Cupp, *Clinical Parasitology* (Lea & Febiger, 1984); Gordon Cook and Alimuddin Zulma, *Manson's Tropical Diseases* (Saunders, 2003); Becerri Flores and Romero Cabello, *Medical Parasitology* (McGraw-Hill, 2004); David Heymann, *Control of Communicable Diseases in Man* (APHA/PAHO/WHO, 2004); Pan American Health Organization, *Zoonoses and Communicable Diseases Common to Man and Animals: Parasitoses* (Pan American Health Organization, 2003).

ALFONSO J. RODRIGUEZ-MORALES, M.D., M.Sc.
UNIVERSIDAD DE LOS ANDES, VENEZUELA
CARLOS FRANCO-PAREDES, M.D., M.P.H.
EMORY UNIVERSITY

Gibbon, John H., Jr. (1903–73)

John H. Gibbon, Jr., was an American cardiovascular surgeon who successfully developed the first artificial machine to bypass the patient's heart and lungs during an operation. With his invention, Gibbon paved the way for modern open-heart surgery.

Gibbon was born in Philadelphia on September 29, 1903, into a family of medical doctors from four generations. He received his A.B. from Princeton University in 1923 and his M.D. from Jefferson Medical College of Philadelphia in 1927. He completed his internship at Pennsylvania Hospital in 1929. He then obtained a research fellowship at Harvard in the early 1930s and later became a Harrison Fellow of Surgical Research at the University of Pennsylvania. It was during these years that Gibbon worked to develop an artificial mechanism that could take over the functions of the human heart and lungs during an operation.

He was convinced that such a machine would allow better heart surgery techniques. His initial experiments in the field were met with skepticism by the medical establishment, but Gibbon continued his research independently. He first experimented on animals, keeping a cat alive for almost half an hour in 1935. During World War II, Gibbon suspended his experiments to serve in the China-Burma-India theater. After the war, Gibbon joined the faculty of Jefferson Medical College and became director of the Department of Surgery in 1946, a position he maintained until 1967. While at Jefferson, he resumed his experiments on animals, beginning a new series on dogs in the early 1950s.

On May 6, 1953, Gibbon first used his heart-lung machine in an operation on a human being. The 18-year-old Cecilia Bavolek underwent an operation for the repair of an atrial septal defect and was completely supported for 26 minutes by the machine. The development of the heart-lung machine catapulted Gibbon to international fame. Thanks to successive modifications and improvements, the machine can now be used for open-heart surgery and for heart transplant. While the name of Gibbon has become synonymous with the device he invented, he was also the editor of the *Annals of Surgery* and author of *Surgery of the Chest*. He received honorary degrees from the Universities of Princeton, Buffalo, and Pennsylvania, and

Dickinson College. For his invention, Gibbon received awards from the Gairdner Foundation, the International Society of Surgery, the Pennsylvania Medical Society, and the American Heart Association. Gibbon retired from Jefferson Medical College in 1967 and died on February 5, 1973.

SEE ALSO: Heart Bypass Surgery; Heart Diseases.

BIBLIOGRAPHY. Harris B. Shumacker, Jr., *Dream of the Heart: The Life of John H. Gibbon, Jr. M.D.: Father of the Heart-Lung Machine* (Daniel & Daniel, 1999); "Biographical Note," Web site of the United States National Library of Medicine, www.nlm.nih.gov/hmd/manuscripts/ead/gibbon.html (cited July 2007).

LUCA PRONO
INDEPENDENT SCHOLAR

Glaucoma

Glaucoma is a disease characterized by elevated intraocular pressure, optic nerve damage, and subsequent impaired vision. Glaucoma is one of the leading causes of adult blindness in the United States and worldwide. Risk factors include increased age, African-American race, and family history in a first-degree relative. The main types of glaucoma include primary open angle glaucoma, angle closure glaucoma, and congenital glaucoma. Primary open angle glaucoma is the most common form of glaucoma and occurs in 0.5 to 2.1 percent of the population over the age of 40. It is caused by a resistance to flow of aqueous humor. Aqueous humor is produced in the ciliary body and drained by the trabecular meshwork. Dysfunction of the trabecular meshwork leads to a disruption in the normal flow of aqueous humor. This results in an increase in the pressure of the eye and damage to the optic nerve. The increased pressure causes a decrease in the blood supply to the nerve and thus damage to the nerve. Over time, due to the damage to the nerve, patients will gradually lose peripheral vision. In advanced cases, the vision loss can lead to absolute blindness.

Angle closure glaucoma results from the peripheral iris, or colored part of the eye, blocking the trabecular meshwork. The angle closure leads to a rise of the in-

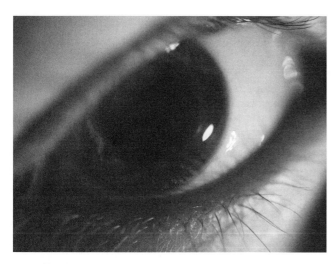

Glaucoma is one of the leading causes of adult blindness in the United States and worldwide.

traocular pressure from its normal level (10 to 21 mm Hg) to 30 mm Hg or more. This results in an increase in aqueous fluid inside the eye causing damage to the optic nerve. Prodromal symptoms occur as transitory attacks during which time patients may experience symptoms of decreased vision, eye pain, halos around lights, headache, nausea, and vomiting.

Another important type of glaucoma is congenital or infantile glaucoma. Congenital glaucoma has an incidence of 1 in 10,000 births with an increased incidence in males. The exact cause is unknown but appears related to a maldevelopment of the aqueous humor drainage system. Signs and symptoms include enlarged cornea (buphthalmos), photophobia, and tearing. Prompt surgical intervention offers the best method of controlling the intraocular pressure and long-term preservation of vision.

For the adult patient, the first signs of glaucoma include gradual loss of peripheral vision. Patients with angle closure glaucoma may present with pain and colored halos, but with primary open-angle glaucoma, patients may be asymptomatic until late in the disease. Glaucoma screening involves a complete ophthalmic history and examination, including evaluation of intraocular pressures, optic nerve, visual fields, and gonioscopy (evaluation of the drainage system of the eye). Intraocular pressure in most individuals ranges between 10 and 21 mmHg, with an average of approximately 16 mmHg. Patients with pressures above 21 are suspicious for glaucoma. Intraocular pressures can fluctuate throughout the day, so pressure levels cannot be the only screening tool for glaucoma.

During examination, the optic nerve is also observed. The optic nerve is examined by comparing the cup to disk ratio. A central depression exists in the optic nerve called the cup. An increase in the size of the cup relative to the rest of the nerve signifies glaucomatous damage. Physical examination should also include gonioscopy. Gonioscopy consists of a special lens placed on the eye that allows visualization of the trabecular meshwork, peripheral iris, cornea, and presence of angle closure. For patients with glaucoma, management includes intraocular pressure checks every three to six months, visual field examination every six to 12 months, gonioscopy and optic nerve evaluation yearly.

Treatment for glaucoma includes the use of medications, laser, and surgery. Although glaucoma cannot be completely attributed to increased intraocular pressure, most therapy is directed toward decreasing the pressure. Decreasing the pressure in the eye can decrease the risk of visual impairment dramatically. Medications include several types of eye drops directed at decreasing pressure. Several of the medications have mechanisms of action similar to medications taken for other systemic conditions. Patients with glaucoma should inform their ophthalmologist about other medications they are taking. Laser therapy involves laser treatment of the trabecular meshwork.

It is thought that a cascade of biological events that involves renewal of trabecular meshwork cells and accelerated turnover of the extracellular matrix, or tissues between the trabecular cells, enhances outflow through the trabecular meshwork following laser treatment. With angle closure glaucoma, laser therapy creates an opening in the iris, allowing for another route of aqueous fluid to be removed from the eye. Surgical treatment consists of a trabeculectomy or tube shunt placement that allows an alternate route of filtration of excess aqueous fluid out of the eye. Through the methods of medications, laser treatment, and surgery, intraocular pressure is reduced and optic nerve damage is offset. Appropriate and early diagnosis and treatment can prevent significant loss of vision in glaucoma patients. Continued efforts to improve early screening and prompt treatment for glaucoma patients are underway.

SEE ALSO: Eye Care; Eye Diseases (General); Ophthalmologist.

BIBLIOGRAPHY. G. Cioffi, and E. Van Buskirk, "Glaucoma Basics & Frequently Asked Questions," *American Glaucoma Society*, www.glaucomaweb.org (cited October 2006); Peter Kaiser, Neil Friedman, and Roberto Pineda. *The Massachusetts Eye and Ear Infirmary Illustrated Manual of Ophthalmology* (Saunders, 2004); Jack J Kanski, *Clinical Ophthalmology* (Butterworth-Heinemann, 2000); Derek Y. Kunimoto, Kunal D. Kanitkar and Mary S. Makar. *The Wills Eye Manual* (Lippincott Williams & Wilkins, 2004).

KOMAL BHARAT DESAI, M.D.
JACQUELYN STURM, M.S.
INDEPENDENT SCHOLARS

Global Health Council

The Global Health Council (GHC) was established in 1972 as the National Council of International Health. This established Council is a U.S.-based, nonprofit membership organization that is dedicated to saving lives and improving the health of people worldwide by working collaboratively to identify world health problems and reporting them to the international and domestic communities. GHC membership is extensive and includes government agencies, international healthcare professionals and organizations, nongovernmental organizations, corporations, and academic institutions. The mission of the GHC is "to ensure that all that who strive for improvement and equity in global health have the information and resources they need to succeed." In line with the Council's mission, the organization strives to serve as a voice to inform and educate those who wish to improve global health.

KEY ISSUES

The GHC has identified the following five key issues that are critical to improving global health:

- Women's health
- Child health
- Human immunodeficiency virus (HIV)/AIDS
- Infectious diseases
- Emerging threats

The GHC asserts that addressing all of the issues and key points involves coordinated global efforts to help eliminate the barriers to good health. The efforts necessary to effect change and to address the barriers are complicated and require many resources. The GHC seeks to make multifaceted approaches to fostering change easier by encouraging partnerships among key organizations/peoples. The GHC acknowledges that the common barriers to good global health include poverty, limited education, limited access to healthcare and family planning, limited employment, limited maternal and reproductive health, and violence (gender based and war). The GHC also works to identify potential emerging public health threats.

WHAT THE GHC DOES

The GHC works to ensure that all those who want to assist in achieving better global health have the resources to reach this goal. The Council's membership ensures that it can inform and educate all peoples/organizations who want to work toward improving global health, as well as educating key leaders, policy makers, the media, and concerned citizens.

The GHC also works to encourage investment in the betterment of global health and development of effective methods to improving health. The Council furthers its mission by mobilizing grassroots efforts (such as the International AIDS Candlelight Memorial and Take Action); advocating for increased resources and policy changes to achieve better health; generating media focused on the key issues; disseminating information (through publications including *HealthLink*, *AIDSLink*, and technical reports); conducting an annual conference to share knowledge and discuss the key issues; and working to identify evidence-based recommendations through their research and analysis department.

DEPARTMENTS

The GHC consists of the following departments:

- Research and analysis
- Government relations
- Policy analysis and communications
- Public outreach
- Administration

These departments work together to push forward the GHC mission statement. The GHC offers technical support in the form of training courses, consultation services, and networking. Additional publications include monthly newsletters, monthly job newsletters, and other reports that focus on the identified key ar-

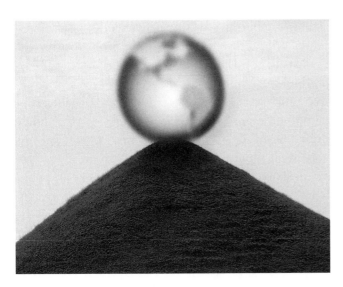

The Global Health Council is a U.S.-based, nonprofit membership organization that is dedicated to saving lives.

eas. The GHC seeks to develop a sustainable future which includes better global health and believes that illness has wide implications that affect all peoples.

SEE ALSO: Disease Prevention; International Center for Equal Healthcare Access; International Council of AIDS Service Organizations.

BIBLIOGRAPHY. Global Health Council, www.global-health.org/; Jay A. Levy, Claude Jasmin, and Gabriel Bez, eds., *Cancer, Aids and Quality of Life: Proceedings of the Second International Conference of the International Council for Global Health Progress* (Kluwer Academic Publishers, 1997).

SUDHA RAMINANI, M.S.
THE FENWAY INSTITUTE

Global Health Ethics

The Institute of Medicine refers to global health as "health problems, issues, and concerns that transcend national boundaries, may be influenced by circumstances or experiences in other countries, and are best addressed by cooperative actions and solutions." The notion of global health presumes a common bond between all of humanity, a common fate, and to some extent, a common interest in preventing death and alleviating suffering. For many, this common interest defines the ethics of global health; for others, global health ethics is a more complex and varied field.

The domain of global health ethics involves both philosophically justifying common interests and deciding how to expend resources to best achieve them. Even though there are clear values inherent in the concept of global health, there is no one ethical framework that guides the field of global health, just as there is no one strict definition of what global health really is.

Some of the most difficult questions in global health include the following:

1. What do we, as individuals or as countries, owe to each other in terms of medical aid?

2. How do we apportion scarce resources locally, nationally, and globally? How is it possible that some people have access to tertiary intensive care while others die from affordable vaccine-preventable diseases?

3. Do we have more of an obligation to prevent disease or to treat it? Must we focus on preventing human immunodeficiency virus (HIV) transmission or devote resources to treating those already infected?

4. What principles should be used in responding to global health threats such as pandemic influenza and bioterrorism?

5. How much should cultural preferences determine priorities? Are there moral absolutes in healthcare resource allocation?

6. Should we focus on ensuring equity and equality over maximizing potentially unequal health outcomes?

Ethics can refer both to the systematic study of moral concepts and theories, or to a set of rules, principles, values, and ideals that guide a discipline or group of people. The study of ethics is generally divided into the areas of meta-ethics, normative ethics, and applied ethics. Meta-ethics refers to the study of foundational issues such as the nature and sources for ethical principles. The two broad schools of thought in meta-ethics are relativism which understands ethical values as a subjective creation of societies and cultures, and realism which posits that a moral truth based on natural law or divine inspiration objectively exists. Normative ethical theories are approaches to determining what one ought to do—the rightness or wrongness of principles, beliefs, or actions. Theories of normative ethics generally fall into three groups.

Virtue ethics focuses on the ethical "actor" or "agent" and deals with qualities or virtues that are desirable. Aristotelian virtue ethics are the prototype of this way of thinking. Deontological ethics, pioneered by Immanuel Kant, emphasize moral duties as the most important element in judging ethical behavior. This approach focuses on certain moral principles that must guide actions, regardless of their consequences. For example, a strict follower of this view might say that it is immoral to lie even if it saves a human life. Teleological or consequence-based theories emphasize outcomes or ends, rather than duties or means. Consequentialist arguments are those most often used in public health and may seem straightforward, but they must resolve the complex task of specifying which outcomes are morally relevant and how they can be maximized.

Applied ethics seeks to develop and apply ethical theory to real practical dilemmas. Medical ethics, research ethics, and public health ethics are all areas of applied ethics that may be relevant to problems of global health. Medical ethics usually refers to the ethical principles governing the relationship between healthcare professionals and patients. While medical ethics may extend beyond this narrow definition, it is this small area of medical ethics that has been most extensively studied and taught. Research ethics also received a great deal of attention in the decades following the horrors of Nazi experimentation on human subjects. As a result, there is an extensive, multifaceted regulatory framework that governs medical experimentation and protects research subjects.

Public health ethics is a relatively new field that seeks to understand how to apply ethical principles to broader health issues, and balance the needs of individuals and communities. Public health ethics focus more on health promotion and disease prevention in populations than on clinical healthcare in individuals. Frameworks for public health ethics are derived from ethical theory but borrow from the related fields of political and legal theory for justification or implementation. Because promoting global health is necessarily a multidisciplinary and complex endeavor, many ethical paradigms may apply. The approach of public health ethics is probably the most relevant and appropriate to use in addressing global health dilemmas and in defining global health ethics.

Some public health ethics frameworks describe potential approaches to public health problems through the lens of political theory. They describe the underlying philosophy and rationale of subjective and objective utilitarians, libertarians and liberal egalitarians, communitarians, and others, and the corresponding public health decisions that can be derived from the consistent application of one of these approaches. Others describe and try to resolve the tensions in public health practice and focus on key areas such as confinement and the limits of liberty, paternalism and the limits of autonomy, and surveillance and the limits of privacy. Still others outline principles and processes that should apply and guide public and global health activities. These include substantive principles such as duty of care, equity, individual liberty, privacy, proportionality, protection of the public from harm, reciprocity, solidarity, stewardship, and trust. Relevant procedural principles include openness and transparency, accountability, inclusiveness, reasonableness, and responsiveness.

Global health ethics is a critically important, complex, and currently ill-defined field. While it may seem obvious that improving global health and minimizing health disparities are ethical imperatives in global health, the setting of priorities and defining effective and appropriate means of achieving these goals are neither intuitive nor straightforward. The various approaches and frameworks of global health ethics can begin to solve these dilemmas and aid in developing an implementable global health agenda.

SEE ALSO: Global Health Council; Institute of Medicine (IOM).

BIBLIOGRAPHY. Howard Frumkin, *Environmental Health: From Global to Local* (Wiley, 2005); Global Health Council, www.globalhealth.org/ (cited July 2007).

BARRY PAKES, M.D., M.P.H.
UNIVERSITY OF TORONTO

Glomerular Diseases

Glomerular diseases are a group of disorders that directly affect the main filtering unit of the kidney, which is called the glomerulus. The glomeruli are groups of blood vessels in the body that clear extra fluid and waste substances from the body. The glomeruli are attached to a series of small tubes (tubules), which also contribute the filtration process by controlling sodium and water concentrations in the body. Glomerular diseases damage the glomeruli and cause leaking of protein and other cells. This leakage disturbs the fragile environment of the kidney and without this balance; it is harder for the body to rid of wastes and extra fluid.

There are two main groups of glomerular diseases: nephrotic syndromes and nephritic syndromes. Both of these syndromes affect the glomerulus in different ways and show different symptoms. Nephrotic syndrome has a more insidious onset and commonly occurs in association with systemic diseases that affecting multiple organs in the body. This includes illnesses like diabetes mellitus, systemic lupus erythematous, or amyloidosis. Nephritic syndrome has a quicker onset and occurs in association with infections of single organ systems. An example of this is a bacterium in untreated strep throat, which can damage the kidneys or a virus like chicken pox.

Proteinuria, protein in the urine, is the hallmark finding of glomerular disease. Normally, the glomerular wall sorts blood proteins based on the size and charge and blocks proteins that are too large or charged from entering the urinary tubules. With glomerular damage this sorting ability is hindered, so large and charged proteins are allowed into the urine. Proteinuria is present in both nephrotic and nephritic syndrome so to differentiate the amount of 3.5 grams/deciliter is the cutoff, above this level is considered nephrotic and below it is nephritic. Nephrotic syndrome also shows low levels or blood protein, which manifests as swelling in face and extremities that occurs gradually over time. Another sign of nephrotic syndrome is high levels of blood cholesterol and triglycerides, which can show as fatty casts in the urine.

Hematuria, blood in the urine, is a common finding in nephritic syndromes. Hematuria can be defined as gross, or visible to the naked eye, or microscopic, only seen by high-power microscopy. In nephrotic syndrome, hematuria is due to disturbance and damage to glomerular cells caused by inflammation. The presence of blood in the urine can also been seen by the presence of bloody casts in a urinary specimen. Other symptoms of nephritic syndrome include generalized aches and pains in joints and muscles, swelling in extremities and face, lethargy, blurry vision, and fatigue or malaise.

MANAGEMENT OF GLOMERULAR DISEASES

The first step in the management of glomerular disease is treatment of the underlying condition. In nephrotic syndrome, it is important to control the systemic inflammation in order to preserve remaining kidney structure and function. In nephritic syndrome, the underlying bacterial, viral or immune infection must be treated with proper medication. By doing this, the infections are stopped from spreading even further. The next step in management is administration of diuretics and antihypertensives to facilitate ridding of the excess fluid and control of blood pressure. Another management step is to replace any vitamins and electrolytes that are lost with glomerular damage. It is also important to take measures to decrease blood cholesterol and monitor for risk of thrombotic events.

SEE ALSO: Kidney Failure and Dialysis; Nephrology.

BIBLIOGRAPHY. Abul Abbas, et al., *Robbins and Cotran: Pathologic Basis of Disease* 7th ed., (Elsevier Saunders, 1999); Mark Beers, Thomas Jones, and Robert Porter, *Merck Manual of Diagnosis and Therapy* 18th ed., Section 17, (Merck & Co. Inc, 1995-2006); Arthur Schneider and Phillip Szanto, *Pathology BRS* 2nd ed. (Lippincott, Williams & Wilkins, 2001).

ANGELA GARNER, M.D.
UNIVERSITY OF MISSOURI–KANSAS CITY

Goiter

Goiter leads to a swelling in the front of the neck, just below the Adam's apple or larynx, owing to an enlarged thyroid gland. This often results in the normal thyroid gland weighing 20 to 30 grams (0.75 ounces), turning into a goitrous gland which can swell to 1 kilogram (more than 2 pounds). The main cause of goiter is an iodine deficiency, and this is often called endemic goiter. It is curable by consumption of food heavily supplemented with iodine, in the form of iodate or iodide, and this remains largely a problem in poor countries. However, there are some other causes such as congenital hypothyroidism, thyroiditis, Hashimoto's thyroiditis, Graves-Basedow disease, and other relatively uncommon disorders. Goiter can also occur when the thyroid gland has the normally functioning tissue but enlarges for reasons that are currently unknown. All these disorders causing goiter tend to result in the thyroid gland not being able to secrete sufficient amounts of the thyroid hormone, and hence the gland grows larger to try to make more to compensate for this.

Goiter was common in parts of the English Midlands where there was an iodine deficiency in the soil. This led it to be called, colloquially, the "Derbyshire Neck." For the same reason, goiter used to be found in the area around the Great Lakes, Midwest, and the Intermountain regions of the United States. It is also common in Tasmania. The man who realized that goiter should be treated with iodine was Jean-Baptiste-André Dumas, a professor at the University of Paris. Anton Freiherr von Eiselberg recognized that tetany cramps often resulted after a goiter operation. Nowadays, it is mainly found in India, Pakistan, central Asia, and central Africa. Peter Pitt, a doctor working in Nepal, spent many years curing people suffering from goiter in the Himalayan kingdom. Part of the reason for its prevalence there, it has been suggested, is because of the increased use of rock salt and/or sea salt which has not been fortified with iodine. People with goiter appear in many stories. In *Little Dorrit* by British writer Charles Dickens, there is a person "sunning his big goitre [sic]." Goiter also tends to be popular in novels set in imperial Rome.

SEE ALSO: Thyroid Diseases.

BIBLIOGRAPHY. R.I.S. Bayliss, *Thyroid Disease: The Facts* (Oxford University Press, 1998); Leslie J. DeGroot, *The Thyroid and Its Diseases* (Wiley, 1984); Franz Merke, *History and Iconography of Endemic Goitre and Cretinism* (MTP Press, 1984); Peter Pitt, *Surgeon in Nepal* (John Murray, 1970).

JUSTIN CORFIELD
GEELONG GRAMMAR SCHOOL, AUSTRALIA

Gonorrhea

Gonorrhea is a very contagious sexually transmitted disease (STD). It is one of the most common venereal diseases in the world. It can be successfully treated with antibiotics, but without prompt treatment, sterility may occur. In addition, it may also cause congenital blindness.

The gonorrhea bacterium (*Neisseria gonorrhoeae*) is the cause of the disease. It causes inflammation of the mucous membranes of the urogential tract. They may also affect the membranes of the throat, the conjunctiva, and the rectum. These infections are most likely if the infected person has engaged in oral or anal sex.

Gonorrhea infections of the throat (*gonoccal pharyngitis*) can cause a sore throat, but often the infection is asymptomatic. Diagnosis can be made with a throat culture. In cases of rectal gonorrhea (*gonococcal proctitis*), symptoms may include anal discharge, pain on defecating, and rectal bleeding.

The gonorrhea bacterium usually infects the *columnar epithelium* of the urethra and the *endocervix*. Symptoms of gonorrhea in men are a thick yellow-green discharge from the penis. The symptomatic discharge can occur as early as two days after infection but usually no later than 14 days after infection. Most case present symptoms within two to five days after infection. In addition, the urethra will also be inflamed which will cause significant pain in urinating. Urination will be slow and difficult. In a small number of males, no symptoms are presented; however, they become carriers who can infect their sexual partners.

In women, the cervix is usually the first place infected. Symptoms of gonorrhea are often absent which will allow infection of new partner(s) in future sexual encounters. In some females, symptoms do develop. These are usually slowly presented as vaginal discharge, painful urination, frequent urination, or pain in the lower abdomen.

Infection with gonorrhea may occur in the throat or rectum. Symptoms are asymptomatic. Discovery of the disease occurs only with coincidental medical tests.

Diagnosis of gonorrhea for males is made with a Gram's stain test of the urethral discharge. The diagnosis is reliable in men. It can be performed in a physician's office with a sample of the patient's discharge. However, the test is not as reliable in women because gonorrhea bacteria can be confused with other naturally occurring organisms in the vagina or uterus. Definitive diagnosis in women is made with a culture. New testing techniques examine the genes of the bacteria from a urine or cervical swab. This test is somewhat more accurate than the culture method.

Treatment for gonorrhea with antibiotics is usually successful. However, successful treatment will not protect against reinfection through subsequent sexual contacts. Resistant strains of the gonorrhea bacteria since the 1970s have rendered penicillin and tetracycline ineffective. The problem of resistance is a continuing problem that threatens vast numbers of people globally. The Centers for Disease Control and Prevention declared gonorrhea bacterium a "super bug" in 2007.

Antibiotics now used to treat gonorrhea include fluoroquinolones, spectinomycin, amoxycillin, ampicillin, and others. If the patient is pregnant, fluoroquinolones cannot be used.

There are no known home cures for gonorrhea. Treatment has to be made by a physician. In addition all sexual partners must be identified to its further spread.

Treatment for gonorrhea in an age of HIV/AIDS is very important because in increases the risk of contracting or transmitting HIV/AIDS. The weakening of the mucosal surface by the gonorrhea infection increases the opportunity for the AIDS virus to successfully invade the body.

The use of a condom provides limited protection. If not treated and allowed to become chronic gonorrhea, it can spread from the mucous membranes into deeper tissues. The bladder, prostrate gland, and the epididymis may all become infected. Scarring of the urethra can occur, which will make urination slow and difficult. Sterility can occur in males and in females as well.

In females, chronic infection with gonorrhea can lead to infection of the uterus, the fallopian tubes, and ovaries leading to eventual sterility. At child birth, a woman infected with gonorrhea can transmit the disease to her newborn baby as it passes through the birth canal. Treatment of all newborn's eyes is standard in modern hospitals as a prophylactic measure. In women, chronic gonorrhea can enter the blood stream. Fever, infections of the joints, tendons, liver, skin, and rarely the heart or brain can occur in severe cases.

SEE ALSO: Sexually Transmitted Diseases.

BIBLIOGRAPHY. Linda Kollar, *Gonorrhea* (Chelsea House Publishers, 2005); *Gonorrhea—a Medical Dictionary, Bibliography, and Annotated Research Guide to Internet References* (ICON Health Publications, 2004); Amy L. Sutton, *Sexually Transmitted Diseases SourceBook: Basic Consumer Health Information about Chlamydial Infections, Gonorrhea, Hepatitis, Herpes, HIV/AIDS, Human Papillomavirus, Pubic Lice, Scabies, Trichomoniasis, Vaginal Infections, and Others* (Omnigraphics, 2006).

Andrew J. Waskey
Dalton State College

Gout and Pseudogout

Gout and pseudogout are painful inflammatory disorders caused by the deposition of crystals in the joints. They are the two most common crystal-induced arthropathies. Gout results from high blood levels of uric acid which leads to a buildup of monosodium urate monohydrate crystals in joint tissue. Gout actually encompasses a variety of clinical presentations including hyperuricemia (elevated levels of uric acid in the blood), acute gouty arthritis (attacks of acute inflammatory arthritis due to the collection of monosodium urate monohydrate crystals in joint fluid), tophi (accumulations of monosodium urate monohydrate crystals within and around a joint and its surrounding soft tissues), gouty nephropathy (impairment of the kidneys due to crystal deposition), and uric acid urolithiasis (also known as urinary tract stones). Pseudogout is caused by the accumulation of calcium pyrophosphate crystals in the cartilage and joint fluid.

EPIDEMIOLOGY

Gout has become more prevalent over the last 30 years, not only in the United States, but also abroad. British and American studies have estimated gout to affect 2.6 to 8.4 per 1,000 adults. More than 2 million people in the United States live with this disease. Gout is nine times more common in men than in women. The 1995 National Health Interview Survey (American study) reported 8.5 per 1,000 adults have gout, and 5 percent of all arthritis cases are gouty arthritis. The onset of gout is most common in the fifth decade of life (ages 40–49). The disease is most prevalent in the elderly population; this is supported by a rate of 24 per 1,000 men and 16 per 1,000 women aged 65–74 years. These rates are increased from those published in 1986: 13.6 per 1,000 men and 6.4 per 1,000 women. It is the most common cause of inflammatory arthritis in men over 30 years of age. This condition is rarely seen in male children and teenagers as well as premenopausal women. Increased systemic estrogen during the reproductive years is likely to be the reason for lower rates of gout in women. Estrogen acts to increase elimination of uric acid from the body via the kidneys. There is also a racial predilection for gout: it is more common among Pacific Islanders. In the United States, it is twice as prevalent in African-American males than it is in Caucasian males.

Gout is twice as prevalent as pseudogout. The conditions are similar in that incidence increases with age: calcium pyrophosphate crystals are found in approximately 3 percent of adults in their 60s; however radiologic surveys show evidence of chondrocalcinosis (calcium deposits in the joints) in 50 percent of people in their 90s. Studies have differed on whether the disease is predominant in men versus women.

PATHOGENESIS

Gout is due to hyperuricemia, or high levels of uric acid in the bloodstream. Uric acid is produced when purines are metabolized by liver enzymes (such as uricase). Purines are a part of all normal tissue. They may be endogenously produced as a by-product of normal cell turnover or they may come from the diet (seafood, liver, beans, gravy, sweet breads, anchovies, beer, wine). Typically, the body is able to regulate the amount of uric acid by balancing production with excretion. If the body produces too much uric acid or if an insufficient amount is excreted from the body, uric acid builds up in the blood and precipitates as monosodium urate crystals. Most people with gout tend to be underexcretors of uric acid. This may be due to kidney or digestive system malfunction.

Pseudogout is due to the buildup of calcium pyrophosphate crystals. The crystals are produced by nucleoside triphosphate pyrophosphohydrolase (NTPPPH), an enzyme found within the cartilage of joints with preexisting osteoarthritis.

Active gout and pseudogout represent an inflammatory host response to monosodium urate and calcium pyrophosphate crystals, respectively. The crystals are perceived as foreign bodies, and so they are enveloped by white blood cells (the body's natural defense system). White blood cells, specifically neutrophils, attempt to destroy the crystals, but the crystals trigger lysis of these cells. This causes a release of enzymes which damage local tissues, produce pain, and cause joint swelling (arthritis).

THE STAGES OF GOUT

Gout can progress through four stages: asymptomatic hyperuricemia, acute gouty arthritis, intercritical gout, and chronic tophaceous gout.

Asymptomatic hyperuricemia is often a precursor to gout. This first stage is not yet considered gout, because some patients with high uric acid levels do not go on to develop crystal deposits or symptoms. They simply have high bloodstream levels of uric acid. However, many patients with hyperuricemia will go on to have deposition of crystals in the joint space and surrounding tissue prior to the onset of their first gouty arthritis episode.

Acute gouty arthritis is characterized by a sudden onset of intense pain and swelling in a joint. It is the most common early presentation of gout. The attack usually occurs at night, and it may be triggered by stressful events, alcohol or drug ingestion, or a concurrent illness. The most common site to be affected is the metatarsophalangeal joint of the first toe. This site will eventually be involved during the overall course of illness in 75 percent of gout patients. The ankle, foot, and knee are other common sites of initial involvement. The affected joint(s) will be warm, tender, and red. A diffuse redness is usually evident surrounding the joint as well. An early attack may include chills, fever, pressure or tightness in the joint, and gnawing pain. Acute gouty arthritis episodes typically last three to 10 days, after which, a patient is often asymptomatic. The patient may be symptom-free for months to years. Subsequent attacks may occur more frequently, last longer, and involve multiple joints.

Intercritical gout describes the asymptomatic periods between gout attacks. Despite the absence of symptoms, crystal deposition is still present. Therefore, a patient can still be diagnosed with gout during this time. Intercritical gout intervals can last months or years, but the majority of patients will have a second attack within two years.

Chronic tophaceous gout usually develops over a period of approximately 10 years. This advanced stage involves multiple joints; the pain persists without interruption and tophi are evident. Tophi (singular: tophus) are subcutaneous crystal deposits that can accelerate joint degeneration and lead to disability and deformity. They are often large, painless, and irregular; they contain white tophaceous material. If a tophus exists close to the skin surface, the chalky material can be removed by aspiration. Tophi may also ulcerate through the skin, and the white chalk or paste will exude from that opening. Tophi most frequently occur in the synovium (joint lining), subchondral bone, olecranon bursa, infrapatellar and Achilles tendons, extensor surface of the forearms, overlying joints, and on the helix of the ear. Chronic crystal deposition and inflammation cause erosion of the cartilage and underlying bone. Deformation is a potential complication of these processes. Other complications seen with advanced chronic gout include kidney damage (uric acid deposits can cause renal failure), urinary stones, hypertension, and albuminuria (abnormal presence of protein in urine; indicative of kidney disease). Diabetes mellitus, atherosclerosis of the heart and brain, and hypertrigliceridemia (high cholesterol) are more common among gout patients.

PRESENTATION OF PSEUDOGOUT

Pseudogout, as the name implies, has a very similar presentation to gout. Patients experience sudden joint pain that begins without warning. Pseudogout may affect one or multiple joints simultaneously; the affected joint(s) are red, swollen, warm, and stiff. Unlike gout which most commonly affects the first toe, pseudogout is most likely to attack the knees. Other common sites include the wrist, ankle, shoulder, elbow, and fingers. Attacks of pseudogout typically resolve spontaneously without treatment, although they may continue for weeks. Recurrences may occur quickly after an earlier attack.

CAUSES OF GOUT AND PSEUDOGOUT

The main predisposing factors for gout are a family history of the condition, obesity, alcohol abuse, a high purine diet, and high cholesterol.

In describing the causes of gout, patients may be broadly classified as overproducers or underexcretors of uric acid. The majority of patients (90 percent) are underexcretors; their kidneys excrete less uric acid than is necessary to maintain balance in the body. Underexcretion may be due to a genetic issue (primary hyperuricemia) or may be attributed to other factors, such as impaired renal function, ketoacidosis, lactic acidosis, dehydration, diuretics, hypertension, hyperparathyroidism, medications, and the effects of lead exposure. Overproducers of uric acid may have a variety of acquired and genetic disorders, and these are typically associated with high rates of cell turnover. Examples include hemolytic anemias, anemias associated with ineffective red blood cell production, psoriasis, myeloproliferative diseases (i.e., chronic myelogenous leukemia, polycythemia vera, essential thrombocythemia), and lymphoproliferative diseases (i.e., Hodgkin's lymphoma, non-Hodgkin's lymphoma). Uric acid overproduction may also be due to excessive dietary purine intake, glycogen storage diseases, severe muscle exertion, alcohol abuse, or fructose intolerance.

Cases of pseudogout are classified as familial, associated with metabolic diseases or trauma (including joint surgery), or sporadic. Any kind of insult to the joint can trigger the release of the calcium crystals, inducing a painful inflammatory response. Research suggests that genetics play a role, as many patients with pseudogout have a family history of the disease. Although the exact cause of pseudogout is unknown, several risk factors have been determined for this condition: hypothyroidism, hemochromatosis (excessive iron storage in the body), hyperparathyroidism, stroke, heart attack, and hypercalcemia. Attacks of pseudogout may be precipitated by injury, stress, surgery, severe dieting, alcohol abuse, and use of thiazide diuretics.

LABORATORY AND RADIOLOGIC FINDINGS

The diagnosis of gout and pseudogout is unequivocally made by taking fluid from the inflamed joint through a needle (joint aspiration) and examining the joint fluid with polarized light microscopy. A smear of joint fluid from a gout patient will show strongly negatively birefringent, needle-shaped uric acid crystals. A sample of fluid from a pseudogout patient will show positively birefringent calcium pyrophosphate crystals.

X-rays can also be useful in diagnosing these two diseases. Typical radiographic features of gout are soft tissue swelling around the affected joint, subcutaneous and periarticular masses adjacent to eroded bone, overall retention of bone density and joint spaces, asymmetric distribution of erosions, and a thin overhanging edge of displaced bone at erosion sites. Septic changes and chondrocalcinosis (calcification of the cartilage) may also be present. The main radiographic feature of pseudogout is chondrocalcinosis. Calcified deposits are most likely to be seen at the lateral and medial meniscus of the knee, the acetabular labrum of the hip, the symphysis pubis of the pelvis, the articular disc of the wrist, and the annulus fibrosus of the intervertebral discs of the spine.

In addition to joint fluid analysis and X-rays, a thorough history and physical examination is critical to making the diagnosis. Information regarding the use of medications, alcohol abuse, and environmental exposures (such as lead) may suggest the presence of gout or pseudogout. Routine laboratory tests may also be done to detect comorbid conditions or associated diseases, such as chronic renal disease, sickle cell disease, polycythemia vera, leukemia, and Hodgkin's disease.

TREATMENTS

The first-line therapies for both gout and pseudogout are nonsteroidal antiinflammatory drugs (NSAIDs). NSAIDs decrease joint swelling and are effective for pain relief. Occasionally, additional medication is needed for pain; examples include codeine and meperidine. Colchicine is an alternative to NSAIDs for treatment of acute attacks. It can be administered orally every hour until symptoms are relieved or can be given intravenously to relieve inflammation and pain. Joint pain typically begins to wane after 12 hours and is completely relieved in 36 to 48 hours. It was once the treatment of choice for gout; however its use has been curtailed due to side effects of severe abdominal pain and diarrhea. Occasionally, colchicine has caused bone marrow damage. Since other effective treatments with fewer side effects are currently available, use of colchicine has fallen out of favor. Corticosteroids, such as prednisone, are another treatment option for acute attacks. These medications can be given orally (systemic steroids) or be prepared as a suspension which is injected into the joint (intra-articular steroids). Corticosteroids are often given to elderly patients with impaired renal function that cannot take NSAIDs.

Besides addressing acute attacks, treatment should also be aimed at preventing recurrences. Prevention of attacks does not prevent or heal joint damage which has already been done, but it will limit its progression. Lifestyle modifications should be encouraged, including avoiding alcoholic beverages, limiting the intake of purine-rich foods, stopping medications that increase blood levels of uric acid, and losing weight. Long-term prophylaxis may be accomplished with allopurinol. This medication should be started one month after an acute attack. Allopurinol blocks the production of uric acid in the body; it is a valuable option for patients with severe hyperuricemia. Side effects include nausea, hypersensitive skin rash, immunocompromise, and liver damage. Uricosuric drugs, such as probenecid and sulfinpyrazone, are also used for prophylaxis. These drugs promote excretion of uric acid in the urine. Patients who are given this therapy should have good kidney function in order to be able to tolerate the increase in renal workload. Last, colchicine and NSAIDs may be taken daily to prevent attacks.

Treatment of pseudogout parallels the recommendations for gout. NSAIDs and corticosteroids can be given to decrease inflammation and pain. NSAIDs are the most commonly prescribed treatment. Joint aspiration can be done in order to remove fluid, and thus crystals from the area, to relieve pressure, pain, and stiffness from the joint. In severe chronic cases, surgery is a possibility. Calcified or otherwise damaged cartilage can be removed from the joint and bone can be repaired. Joint replacement is the most intense therapeutic option. Currently, there is no effective prevention for pseudogout attacks. Muscle strengthening and stretching are recommended to improve joint stability (thereby reducing injury which may trigger pseudogout episodes) and mobility over the long term.

SEE ALSO: Arthritis; Calcium; Rheumatoid Arthritis.

BIBLIOGRAPHY. Daniel J. McCarty, "Calcium Pyrophosphate Dihydrate Crystal Deposition Disease," *Primer on the Rheumatic Diseases* (Arthritis Foundation, 1993); Lawrence M. Ryan and Daniel J. McCarty, "Arthritis Associated with Calcium-Containing Crystals," *Internal Medicine,* Ed. Jay H. Stein (Mosby, 1998); Guillermo A. Tate, and H. Ralph Schumacher, Jr., "Gout: Clinical and Laboratory Features," in *Primer on the Rheumatic Diseases* (Arthritis Foundation, 1993); Robert Terkeltaub, and Jay H. Stein, eds., "Gout and Hyperuricemia," *Internal Medicine,* (Mosby, 1998); Robert Terkeltaub, and H. Ralph Schumacher, Jr., eds., "Gout: Epidemiology, Pathology, and Pathogenesis," in *Primer on the Rheumatic Diseases* (Arthritis Foundation, 1993).

Stacy A. Frye, M.D.
Michigan State University

Greece

With a per capita income of $22,300, Greece is the 45th richest nation in the world. The population has easy access to healthcare. The Greek economy is basically strong and is currently growing at a rate of 3.7 percent. However, unemployment (9.9 percent) and inflation (3.5 percent) are both higher than average for members of the European Union. Around 12 percent of the workforce is involved in the agricultural sector, and almost three-fourths are involved in services. Because of its ancient heritage and temperate climate, Greece draws visitors from all over the world, and tourism provides 15 percent of the Gross Domestic Product (GDP). The government does not issue an official poverty report, but some of the poorest residents are immigrants who are concentrated in menial jobs. Income disparities do exist, and Greece ranks 35.1 on the Gini index of inequality. The poorest 10 percent are able to claim only three percent of resources while the richest 10 percent hold 28.3 percent. The standard of living is reasonably high, and the United Nations Development Programme's (UNDP) Human Development Report ranks Greece 24th of 177 countries on overall quality-of-life issues.

Much of the responsibility for healthcare in Greece is concentrated in the private sector, which accounts for 48.7 percent of health costs. Some 95.40 percent of private resources involve out-of-pocket expenses. On the average, seven percent of the total government budget is allocated to healthcare. Approximately 10 percent of the GDP is directed toward healthcare, and the government allocates $1,997 (international dollars) to health-related programs. The government is responsible for over half (51.3 percent) of all health expenditures, and 32 percent of funding is earmarked for Social Security. All regular employees and some self-employed workers are covered under the social insurance plan. The program is financed through a combination of employee contributions (6.67 to 8.86 percent of wages), employer benefits (13.33 to 14.73 percent of payroll), and government supplements (10 percent). Reforms to the existing pension system are under way. Workers receive cash benefits for illness and maternity leave. Both mothers and fathers are eligible for a one-year leave for the birth of a child, and leave time is expanded for the birth of additional children. Parents with children in public schools receive a family allowance, distributed at the beginning of each school year, for all children 16 and under. There are 4.38 physicians, 3.86 nurses, 0.18 midwives, 1.13 dentists, and 0.82 pharmacists per 1,000 population in Greece.

In order to improve access to healthcare, the government instituted the Integration Action Plan and charged the Ministry of Health and Social Care with establishing 50 socio-medical centers and two mobile units. The services of a doctor, a nurse, a social worker, a physical trainer, and a special health promoter are available at each center. Patients who need further treatment are directed to area hospitals. Help for families in crisis is provided by the National Center of Immediate Social Assistance, which provides care and support for neglected children, victims of domestic violence, and the elderly who live alone.

Life expectancy is the 25th highest in world, and the Greek population of 10,688,058 people can expect to live an average of 79.24 years. Females outlive males by about five years. While the vast majority of all Greeks over 15 are able to read and write, there is a slight disparity between male (98.6 percent) and female (96.5 percent) literacy rates. Most children attend primary school regularly, but only 87 percent of females and 85 percent of males regularly attend secondary school. Greek women give birth at a rate of 1.34 children each. The adjusted maternal mortality rate is nine deaths per 1,000 live births. Birth control has become a government concern, and information on family planning, abortion, and sexually transmitted diseases is widely distributed Family Planning Centers are set up in many hospitals, operating under the auspices of the Foundation for Social Insurance.

Infant mortality is currently reported at 5.43 deaths per 1,000 live births. Between 1990 and 2004, infant and under-5 mortality were more than halved, dropping from ten to four and from 11 to five deaths per 1,000 live births, respectively. Eight percent of all infants are underweight at birth. While 96 percent of infants are immunized against diphtheria, pertussis, and tetanus (DPT1), all other immunization rates are in the high 80s: 88 percent of infants are immunized against DPT3, tuberculosis, measles, hepatitis B, and *Haemophilus influenzae* type B (Hib3) and 87 percent against polio.

Earthquakes may present a safety hazard in Greece, and industrialization has led to air and water pollution that threaten general health. HIV/AIDS also causes some concern in Greece. With a 0.2 percent adult prevalence rate, some 9,100 Greeks are living with HIV/AIDS. The disease has caused the deaths of around 100 people. An outbreak of severe acute respiratory syndrome (SARS) created a public scare in spring 2002. Human trafficking poses a constant to threat the general well-being of the population, and both children and adults are victims of forced labor and sexual exploitation.

Greece has the highest rate of smokers in Europe and one of the highest rates in the world. According to recent studies, 51 of men and 39 percent of women smoke. While the governments in several other European nations have imposed major restrictions on public smoking, cultural dictates make the government of Greece reluctant to do so. A new law prohibiting smoking in the workplace is generally ignored. Tobacco products do carry warnings, but opinion polls indicate that most Greeks consider them as annoyances rather than deterrents. Antismoking efforts have been greatly hindered by the presence of a strong tobacco lobby.

SEE ALSO: European Public Health Association (EUPHA); Smoking; World Health Organization (WHO).

BIBLIOGRAPHY. Central Intelligence Agency, "Greece," *World Factbook*, www.cia.gov/cia/publications (cited July 2007); Commission on the Status of Women, "Greece," www.un.org/womenwatch (cited July 2007); Spencer Di Scala, *Twentieth Century Europe: Politics, Society, Culture* (McGraw-Hill, 2004; Sandra Halperin, *War and Social Change in Modern Europe: The Great Transformation Revisited* (Cambridge University Press, 2004); Martin A. Levin and Martin Shapiro, eds., *Transatlantic Policymaking in an Age of Austerity: Diversity and Drift* (Georgetown University Press, 2004); Jeremy Rifkin, *The European Dream: How Europe's Vision of the Future Is Quietly Eclipsing the American Dream* (Jeremy P. Tarcher/Penguin, 2004); Social Security Administration, "Greece" www.ssa. gov (cited July 2007); UNICEF, "Greece" www.unicef.org/infobycountry/greece_statistics.html; C.I. Vardavas and A. Kafatos, "Greece's Tobacco Policy: Another Myth?" *The Lancet*, (May 6, 2006); World Bank, "Greece Data Profile," /devdata.worldbank.org (cited July 2007).

ELIZABETH R. PURDY, PH.D.
INDEPENDENT SCHOLAR

Grenada

Grenada is a small island at the southern end of the Grenadines, a short archipelago at the boundary of the Caribbean Ocean and the North Atlantic. At just 344 square kilometers, it is one of the smallest independent nations in the western hemisphere. Few Americans had heard of Grenada before October 1983, when hundreds of U.S. troops invaded the island to oppose Cuban troops building an airstrip. Operation Urgent Fury lasted just a few days and took the lives of 19 U.S. servicemen and 100 Cubans and Grenadians. The Cubans retreated, and the Grenadians welcomed the United States as liberators.

Since the 1980s, Grenada has been a peaceful place, with an economy based on tourism, offshore finance, agricultural exports, and manufacturing. The total population is 89,700, and the growth rate is only 0.26 percent. Grenada has a birth rate of 22.08 per 1,000 people and a death rate of 6.88 per 1,000 people, but its migration rate is minus 12.59 per 1,000.

Sixty-two percent of Grenadians work in the service industry, 24 percent in agriculture, and 14 percent in industry. Unemployment is 12.5 percent. Per capita income is $4,060, although a third of Grenadians live below the poverty level. Grenada lies at the edge of the Atlantic hurricane belt, with little to protect it from tropical systems. In 2004, Hurricane Ivan swept the island, taking no lives but destroying or damaging 90 percent of the residential housing. The economy is still recovering from the blow.

Life expectancy at birth is 63.06 years for males and 66.68 years for females; healthy life expectancy is 58.4 years for men and 60 years for women. Infant mortality is just 14 deaths per 1,000 live births, and almost every child survives childhood. Immunization for the major diseases of childhood is almost universal. Between 1990 and 2004, there was only one reported death in childbirth. All Grenadian women have a trained attendant monitoring their deliveries, and 98 percent receive prenatal care.

The local diet is based on cereal grains, yams, cassava and other root vegetables, shrimp, and fish. Nutmeg, mace, cinnamon, cloves, citrus fruits, and bananas are major export crops. The government has launched a campaign to "grow what you eat and eat what you grow" to encourage both a healthy diet and a reduced dependence on expensive, imported foods.

With the exception of a few isolated cases of dengue fever, Grenadians are not plagued with major infectious diseases. Between 95 to 97 percent of citizens use safe drinking water and sanitary facilities. The HIV/AIDS rate is low, with 139 cases diagnosed between 1996 and 2001. Workplace accidents are common. Cardiovascular disease and cancers are the most common causes of death.

The government allocates $212 per capita for medical care. There is one general hospital in St. George's and two rural hospitals in the countryside. The Ministry of Health plans to establish several local "polyclinics" to better serve people for basic health needs.

For the past 30 years, doctors have been a chief export for Grenada, thanks to the St. George's University (SGU) School of Medicine. Since its establishment in 1977, SGU has used its low tuition and tropical locale to attract medical students from around the globe. Today, there are 5,000 SGU-trained physicians practicing in 35 countries and all 50 U.S. states.

SEE ALSO: Healthcare, South America.

BIBLIOGRAPHY. Pan American Health Organization, "Grenada," http://www.paho.org/English/SHA/prflgre.htm (cited June 2007); World Health Organization, "Grenada," http://www.who.int/countries/grd/en/ (cited June 2007).

HEATHER K. MICHON
INDEPENDENT SCHOLAR

Growth Disorders

Child growth is internationally recognized as an important public health indicator for monitoring nutritional status and health in populations. Growth is influenced by many factors such as heredity, genetic or congenital, illness and medications, nutrition, hormones, and psychosocial environment. Measurements of growth—height and weight—are a very inexpensive service that should be offered by all healthcare providers rendering care to children.

The internationally recommended way to assess malnutrition at population level is to take body or anthropometric measurements (e.g., weight and height). Based on combinations of these body measurements, anthropometric indices are constructed. These indices are essential for the interpretation of body measurements as, for example, weight alone has no meaning unless it is related to an individual's age or height. In children, the three most commonly used anthropometric indices are weight for height, height forage, and weight for age. These indices can be expressed in terms of z-scores, percentiles, or percentage of median, which enable comparison of a child or a group of children with a reference population.

A normal growth pattern does not guarantee overall health; however, children with abnormal growth patterns frequently have nutritional complications of specific clinical disorders (e.g., cystic fibrosis, inflammatory bowel disease) or poor socioeconomic conditions. A child who is two standard deviations (SDs) or more below the mean height for children of that sex and chronologic age (and ideally of the same racial ethnic group) is said to have short stature. A single measurement of height is much less important in assessing growth than is the pattern of growth over a period of time; the key finding is slowed growth that progressively deviates from a previously defined growth channel (or percentile).

Children who suffer from growth retardation as a result of poor diets and/or recurrent infections tend to have more frequent episodes of severe diarrhea and are more susceptible to several infectious diseases, such as malaria, meningitis, and pneumonia. In addition, there is strong evidence that impaired growth is associated with delayed mental development, poor school performance, and reduced intellectual capacity.

CAUSES OF POOR GROWTH

Children are a reflection of their parents' growth patterns and height. Parents who were late bloomers and experienced slow growth and late pubertal development may see the same pattern in their children. The final height these children achieve is usually normal. Parents who have short stature usually have children whose adult height potential is in the shorter range. Conversely, tall parents usually have tall children. As a general rule, a child's potential adult height ranges between the average of the parents' heights toward that of the parent who is the same sex as the child.

Congenital (those present at birth) causes for growth failure include intrauterine growth retardation, skeletal abnormalities, and chromosome changes. Intrauterine growth retardation may result from maternal infections, smoking, or alcohol/drug use while pregnant. Skeletal causes, such as short-limbed dwarfism, result from abnormal production of new bone and cartilage. These children usually have unusual trunk/limb proportions. Chromosome variations causing short stature can include Turner's syndrome in girls and Down syndrome.

Conditions that are considered chronic can reduce growth because they interfere with the body's ability to use nutrients properly. Diseases that involve the kidneys, digestive tract, heart, or lungs are examples of such conditions that may influence growth. Some medications that are used in large doses or for long periods of time may affect growth. Nutritional problems can influence growth in two ways. More commonly, the problem is a poor diet with inadequate nutrients, not enough calories, or the wrong food groups. Second, diseases that interfere with the absorption of food from the bowel will prevent the body from using those nutrients for growth. In these cases, symptoms may include nausea, vomiting, excessive gas, diarrhea or constipation, poor weight gain, or being underweight for height. After diagnosis, these problems usually improve with a special diet and or medications. With proper correction of these disorders, growth will also improve.

Children in situations where home life is disrupted or unhappy or where there is a lack of love, of consistency, or of emotional support, experience severe stress. This stress can precipitate growth failure. Growth resumes when the problems are relieved and the stress is gone. Growth failure caused by endocrine disorders is uncommon, but is often easily remediable. Thyroid function should always be evaluated, because growth failure may be the first or even the only manifestation of hypothyroidism. The evaluation should include measurements of both serum thyrotropin (TSH) and thyroxine; both primary and central hypothyroidism can cause growth failure, and measurement of serum TSH alone will not detect central hypothyroidism.

Cushing's syndrome is rare in children except when due to the toxicity of glucocorticoid therapy. It is initially a clinical diagnosis that is suggested by the clinical findings and then confirmed by biochemical and imaging tests. A corticotrophin (ACTH)-secreting pituitary adenoma (Cushing's disease) is by far the most common cause. The two major findings are weight gain (90 percent) and growth retardation (83 percent); bone age tends to be normal at diagnosis in most patients. If growth hormone deficiency is congenital and complete, the diagnosis is relatively easy to confirm. Affected children present with severe growth failure, delayed bone age, and very low serum concentrations of growth hormone, IGF-I, and its major binding protein, IGF-binding protein-3. Provocative testing of growth hormone secretion with insulin-induced hypoglycemia, as may be performed in adults with suspected growth hormone deficiency, is not recommended in children.

The rare children with growth hormone insensitivity have high serum growth hormone concentrations but low serum IGF-I and IGF binding-protein-3 concentrations. In its complete form, this condition is called Laron-type dwarfism (complete growth hormone insensitivity).

CAUSES OF EXCESSIVE OR RAPID GROWTH

Children who are above the 95 percentile in height or are growing unusually fast for their age may need to be evaluated by their physician. Although tall stature is almost as common as is short stature, few children or their families seek medical attention, presumably because tall stature is socially acceptable and often advantageous. Nevertheless, it is critical to be able to identify situations in which tall stature or an accelerated growth rate provides a clue to an underlying disorder. Determining the heights of the biological parents is of critical importance because their height reflects the genetic component for growth and development of the child. When dysmorphic features are found, special effort should be made to rule out the disorders and syndromes that are associated with excessive growth. Causes of rapid growth that may be abnormal include excessive growth hormone production, some congenital growth hormone production, some congenital genetic conditions, or early puberty. Signals of these problems may include unusual body proportions, breast growth, enlargement of the genitals, and axillary and pubic hair growth.

Central (or true) precocious puberty refers to the early occurrence of normal puberty. Precocious puberty has been defined as sexual development in girls before the age of 8 years and in boys before the age of 9 years; however, current data for girls, particularly black girls, indicate that the age of onset of normal puberty is younger. The hallmarks of precocious puberty are accelerated growth and advanced bone age, plus breast development in girls and penile enlargement and sexual hair growth in boys. The pattern of secretion of pituitary gonadotropins and gonadal sex steroids is normal but early.

Pseudoprecocious puberty refers to sexual precocity due to adrenal or gonadal disorders or rarely tumor production of human chorionic gonadotropin. The clinical manifestations are similar to those of central precocious puberty, except that the sexual development may be that of the opposite sex, for example, androgen effects in girls with congenital adrenal hyperplasia. Any cause of sexual precocity (including exogenous) can awaken the hypothalamic-pituitary axis for normal pubertal development and "induce" central puberty as well.

Excessive growth hormone secretion causes gigantism in growing children and acromegaly after fusion of the epiphyseal growth plates, usually in adults. Although rare in children, the possibility of gigantism should be considered when the height exceeds +3 to +4 SDs.

Pituitary growth hormone-secreting tumors usually are eosinophilic or chromophobe adenomas. Their cause is unknown, although many result from somatic mutations that generate activated G proteins with reduced guanosine triphosphatase (GTPase) activity. Growth hormone-secreting tumors also have been reported in patients with multiple endocrine neoplasia type 1, neurofibromatosis, or tuberous sclerosis.

Hyperthyroidism caused by endogenous overproduction or overtreatment with exogenous thyroxine may lead to increased growth, advanced bone age, and, in early life, craniosynostosis. The tall stature and transient increase in linear growth usually do not require intervention, and the growth rate normalizes with treatment of the hyperthyroidism.

Permanent hypogonadism, that is, permanent deficiency of testosterone in males or of estrogen in females, results in delayed skeletal maturation, a prolonged period of growth, tall stature, and eunuchoid proportions, with long legs and low upper-lower segment ratio. As an example, several patients with estrogen deficiency resulting from aromatase deficiency or estrogen resistance caused by a mutation of the estrogen receptor gene who were tall have been described.

Familial glucocorticoid deficiency is a rare autosomal recessive disorder characterized by hypoglycemia, seizures, increased skin pigmentation, and in some cases tall stature or advanced bone age. Biochemical findings include extremely high serum corticotrophin (ACTH) concentrations together with low or undetectable serum cortisol concentrations that do not respond to exogenous ACTH stimulation. Type 1 familial glucocorticoid deficiency is caused by mutations in the ACTH receptor gene, whereas some other defect is responsible for type 2 familial glucocorticoid deficiency.

Excessive production of adrenal androgens probably is responsible for the tall stature. Another suggestion is that the high serum ACTH concentrations could activate melanocyte-stimulating hormone receptors in cartilaginous growth plates and that the increase in height is caused by the unopposed anabolic action of growth hormone.

Primary cortisol resistance is a rare cause of hypercortisolism but may cause excessive growth because of the effects of the increased ACTH levels on adrenal androgen production. Because this is gonadotropin-independent precocity, the size of the testis is relatively small compared to the degree of growth and virilization. The bone age is advanced and many quite tall boys do not become excessively tall adults.

Congenital total lipodystrophy is a rare autosomal recessive disorder. The main clinical features, in addition to overgrowth and acromegaloid changes, are generalized absence of subcutaneous fat, muscular hypertrophy, hyperpigmentation, enlargement of the penis or clitoris, advanced bone age, insulin resistance, hyperinsulinemia, hyperlipidemia, and nonketotic hyperglycemia. Large doses of insulin are given to avoid decompensation, but normoglycemia may not be attainable. Adult height in these patients tends to be normal or tall.

Klinefelter syndrome is caused by an abnormality in chromosome number in which two or more X chromosomes are present in phenotype males. The most common abnormal karyotype is 47 XXY. Prepubertal boys often are tall for their age, with relatively long legs, and they may have learning disabilities, mainly in expressive language. Small testes and gynecomastia are the most common features on physical examination. Serum luteinizing hormone and follicle-stimulating concentrations are high in patients with Klinefelter syndrome. Usually, serum testosterone concentrations are in the low normal adult range. Testosterone treatment can be initiated during the pubertal years to facilitate development of secondary sexual characteristics and minimize the psychological complications of hypogonadism. This approach also may diminish adult height.

Marfan syndrome is an autosomal dominant abnormality of connective tissue characterized by tall stature, long thin fingers (arachnodactyly), hyperextension of joints, and superior lens subluxation. Pectus excavatum, scoliosis, aortic or mitral regurgitation, and aortic root dilatation may be present. Female and male patients with this syndrome may attain excessively tall height, and treatment with estrogen in women and testosterone in men may be indicated, especially if any orthopedic problem is present.

Homocystinuria is an inherited inborn error of methionine metabolism, caused by a deficiency of the enzyme cystathionine synthetase. Some of the clinical features are similar to those of Marfan syndrome, with subluxation of the lens being the most consistent finding. In addition, 50 percent of patients have mental retardation, life-threatening thromboembolic phenomena may occur at any age, and early onset of osteoporosis is seen.

Neurofibromatosis type 1 is an autosomal dominant disorder that comprises approximately 90 percent of all cases of neurofibromatosis. It is caused by an abnormality of neural crest differentiation and migration during the early stages of embryogenesis. Short stature is common, but some patients are excessively tall. Thus, neurofibromatosis should be considered in patients with overgrowth.

For many years, the World Health Organization (WHO) Department of Nutrition has been using anthropometric data to monitor trends in child malnutrition. A major difficulty has been the nonuniformity of survey analyses and presentation of their results. Although numerous nutritional surveys have been conducted since the 1970s, many of them have used distinct definitions of malnutrition (i.e., different anthropometric indices, reporting systems, cutoff points, and reference values), thus making comparison of results between studies difficult.

This lack of comparable data prompted the beginning of WHO's systematic collection and standardization of information on the nutritional status of the world's under-5 population. The WHO Global Database on Child Growth and Malnutrition was initiated in 1986 to compile, standardize, and disseminate results of nutritional surveys performed worldwide. The specific objectives of this database are to characterize nutritional status; enable international comparisons of nutritional data; identify populations in need; help evaluate nutritional and health interventions; monitor secular trends in child growth; and raise political awareness of nutritional problems. A distinct feature of the database is the systematic analysis of raw data sets in a standard format to produce comparable results.

SEE ALSO: Endocrine Diseases (General); Klinefelter's Syndrome; Marfan Syndrome; Tanner Stages.

BIBLIOGRAPHY. C.E. Brain and M.O. Savage, "Growth and Puberty in Chronic Inflammatory Bowel Disease," *Baillière's Clinical Gastroenterology* (v.8, 1994); P. Chatelain, "Trends in the Diagnosis and Treatment of Short Stature as Revealed by KIGS," in M.B. Ranke and P. Wilton, eds., *Growth Hormone Therapy in KIGS: 10 Years' Experience* (Johann Ambrosius Barth Verlag, 1999); A. Grimberg, J.K. Kutikov, and A.J. Cucchiara, "Sex Differences in Patients Referred for Evaluation of Poor Growth," *Journal of Pediatrics* (v.146, 2005); S.L. Kaplan and M.M. Grumbach, "Pathophysiology and Treatment of Sexual Precocity," *Journal of Clinical Endocrinology and Metabolism* (v.71, 1990); A.D. Rogol and E.L. Lawton, "Body Measurements," in J.A. Lohr, ed., *Pediatric Outpatient Procedures* (J. B. Lippincott, 1991); J.M. Tanner, H. Goldstein, and R.H. Whitehouse, "Standards for Children's Heights at Ages 2 to 9 Years Allowing for Height of Parents," *Archives of Disease in Childhood* (v.45, 1970).

BARKHA GURBAN, B.A.
UNIVERSITY OF CALIFORNIA, LOS ANGELES

Guatemala

Guatemala girdles the width of Central America, wedged between Mexico and Belize on the north and Honduras and El Salvador on the south. Most of the coastline is on the Pacific Ocean, but there is access to the Atlantic on the Gulf of Honduras. Guatemala is a beautiful country, with a volcanic mountain range and lush tropical lowlands and an ancient indigenous culture. Still, life there is difficult, with 75 percent of the people living below the poverty line. The country has a population of about 12.3 million (2006 estimate), growing at 2.27 percent annually. The birth rate is 29.88 per 1,000 people, the death rate 5.2 per 1,000 people, and the migration rate is minus 1.94 migrants per 1,000 people. The urbanization rate is 46 percent, with more and more people moving into the cities in search of work.

The economy is driven mainly by agricultural exports, particularly coffee, bananas, and sugar. Fifty percent of the workforce is involved in agriculture. Per capita income is $4,080, but uneven distribution of land and wealth means that poverty is widespread. Sixteen percent of Guatemalans live on $1 a day or less.

There are two Guatemalas when it comes to both wealth and health. Sixty percent of the population is of Amerindian-Spanish descent, known as mestizo or ladino. The rest of the people are indigenous, with 23 Mayan groups alone. Indigenous people tend to live in the mountains, far from adequate healthcare or decent food sources. For Guatemalans overall, life expectancy at birth is 67.65 years for males and 71.18 years for females, with healthy life expectancy averaging 54.9 years for men and 59.9 years for women. However, the life expectancy for indigenous people is, on average, 17 years shorter. Maternal mortality is 89 deaths per 100,000 live births nationally, but in the indigenous region of Alta Verapaz, it is 192 deaths per 100,000 live births.

Guatemala's location and geography make it vulnerable to a number of natural disasters affecting health and safety. Active volcanoes in the mountains lead to frequent damaging earthquakes. Tropical storm systems routinely cross the country. In October 2005, Hurricane Stan made a direct hit on the Yucatán Peninsula; flooding and mudslides caused the deaths of an estimated 2,000 to 3,000 people in Guatemala alone.

Ninety-five percent of Guatemalans have access to clean drinking water and 61 percent have sanitary

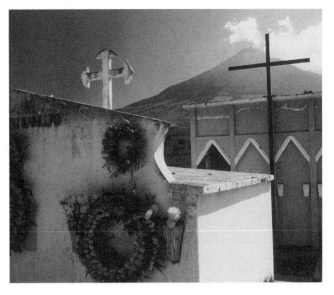

Life in Guatemala is difficult; 75 percent of the people are living below the poverty line.

facilities, although, again, these rates are much different in indigenous areas. Major infectious diseases are largely under control, with only sporadic outbreaks of cholera, leptospirosis, and meningitis in recent years. Pneumonia and acute diarrhea are still common.

The average Guatemalan is more likely to be affected by cardiovascular disease, cancer, or diabetes. In the cities, death by accident, suicide, or violent crime is common. Guatemala is a major transit point for cocaine and heroin, and in 2004, the country reawakened its dormant opium industry.

Domestic violence and random violence against women is common in urban areas. More than 2,300 young women have been found raped, mutilated, and murdered since 2001. These crimes, like most homicides in Guatemala, go unsolved.

The HIV/AIDS rate has remained fairly low, with 1.1 percent of the population estimated to be infected as of 2003. About 78,000 Guatemalans are living with the virus, and 5,800 people have already died of it.

The government spends $112 per person annually on healthcare. The constitution recognizes health as a fundamental human right, and healthcare is supposed to be free for those without means. In recent years, the government has worked to improve healthcare among the Mayan, Garifuna, and Xinka people, although this investment has not yet paid off. In 2000, there were 43 hospitals and 1,309 mixed healthcare posts, maternity centers, general clinics, emergency centers, and mental health centers spread throughout the country. The World Health Organization estimated that there are 9,965 physicians and 44,986 nurses to serve the population.

SEE ALSO: Healthcare, South America.

BIBLIOGRAPHY. Walter Randolph Adams and John Palmer Hawkins, *Health Care in Maya Guatemala: Confronting Medical Pluralism in a Developing Country* (University of Oklahoma Press, 2007); Gerard M. La Forgia, ed., *Health System Innovations in Central America: Lessons and Impact of New Approaches* (World Bank Publications, 2005).

HEATHER K. MICHON
INDEPENDENT SCHOLAR

Guillain-Barré Syndrome

In 1859, Jean Landry first described what is likely now called Guillain-Barré syndrome or acute inflammatory demyelinating polyradiculoneuropathy (AIDP). William Osler later elaborated on this description in 1892. In 1916, Georges Guillain, Jean Alexandre Barré, and Andre Strohl refined the definition and clinical picture of Guillain-Barré syndrome by analyzing the cerebrospinal fluid of these patients. With this information, one could then distinguish Guillain-Barré syndrome from anterior horn cell disease processes.

Guillain-Barré syndrome is an autoimmune-mediated disease that involves demyelination of peripheral nerves and associated inflammatory cells or an axonal degeneration with or without demyelination and inflammation. It most commonly causes muscle weakness or paralysis and is thought to be due to an irregular immune response often preceded by an infection, such as Epstein-Barr virus (EBV), cytomegalovirus (CMV), hepatitis, varicella, *Mycoplasma pneumoniae*, or *Campylobacter jejuni*. Specifically, the mechanism of action involves the destruction of peripheral nerve fibers via T-cell lymphocytes and macrophages.

When Guillain-Barré syndrome was first described, it was believed to be a single disorder, but now the syndrome has been associated with many variants. The National Institute of Neurological Disorders and Stroke (NINDS) developed the criteria for the diagnosis of Guillain-Barré syndrome. At a minimum, the individual must have progressive weakness of at least two limbs as well as areflexia. The most common form of Guillain-Barré syndrome in Europe and the United States is the acute inflammatory demyelinating polyradiculoneuropathy (AIDP). Other less common variants include the Miller-Fisher syndrome, acute motor axonal neuropathy (AMAN), and acute sensorimotor axonal neuropathy (AMSAN).These other variants occur more commonly in regions of the world such as China, Japan, and Mexico.

This syndrome afflicts approximately 2 in 100,000 individuals and is not associated with any particular race or geographical distribution. However, adult men have a slightly greater risk of having Guillain-Barré syndrome than adult women. After the age of 40, the risk for acquiring Guillain-Barré syndrome increases until the age of 80. The most recent epidemic of Guillain-Barré syndrome in the late 20th century occurred in northern China (AMAN variant) and had been attributed to *C. jejuni* infection.

Typically, the afflicted individual has progressive motor weakness and areflexia starting in the proximal legs. The progression of Guillain-Barré syndrome is variable, ranging from hours to weeks. Often, they will complain of balance problems, paresthesias, and ascending weakness from the lower extremities to the upper extremities. The extent of weakness ranges from mild weakness to complete paralysis. Lower extremity weakness may manifest as foot drop. One of the most severe complications of this disease is respiratory compromise, resulting from weakness of the respiratory muscles.

Dysautonomia is a common comorbidity that may manifest itself as arrhythmias, urinary retention, decubitus ulcers, constipation, gastritis, or ileus. The individual may also suffer from mood or anxiety problems. The disease process usually occurs within two to four weeks of an illness or immunization. In addition to weakness, the disease may manifest as pain, leading to misdiagnosis, particularly in children. Guillain-Barré syndrome may not present with weakness as the primary symptom. In fact, the Miller-Fisher variant is defined by the presence of ophthalmoplegia, ataxia, and areflexia.

Once Guillain-Barré syndrome is suspected based upon physical findings and a clinical history, a lumbar puncture should be completed to look for demyelination without active infection. A magnetic resonance imaging (MRI) of the spine may help to confirm the diagnosis generally two weeks after the first onset of ascending weakness. The lumbosacral MRI will show enhancement of the cauda equina nerve roots. Abnormal electrodiagnostic studies may be useful within the first two weeks as well. Glycolipid antibody analysis is also useful because different forms of Guillain-Barré syndrome express different antibodies. For example, GQ1b antibodies are present in the Miller-Fisher variant, while GD1b has been linked to pure sensory GB syndrome.

Current treatment is focused on immunomodulation. Initially, intravenous immunoglobulin (IVIG) is given to the patient. While an individual may benefit from short-term IVIG treatments, there is no definitive evidence that IVIG is beneficial in the long term. Another potential treatment is plasmapharesis. Recent studies have suggested that plasmapheresis may decrease the severity and duration of the disease. This treatment may have complications, including autonomic instability, hypercalcemia, or bleeding. Steroids have also been used in the past but are no longer considered efficacious. Physical activity is encouraged in these patients, although patients should be monitored for autonomic symptoms. If respiratory distress is noted, intubation may be required.

Studies have shown that recovery usually occurs within six months to one year, although children generally have more favorable outcomes. Deaths are rare with this disease, especially if the disease is treated early on its course. Mortality rates are usually quoted at less than 5 percent. After Guillain-Barré syndrome has been treated, it has been known to recur in approximately 5 percent of cases. A total of 5 to 10 percent of the entire patient population is left with permanent disability.

SEE ALSO: Autoimmune Diseases (General).

BIBLIOGRAPHY. A. K. Asbury and D. R. Cornblath, "Assessment of Current Diagnostic Criteria for Guillain-Barré Syndrome," *Annals of Neurology* (v.27/Suppl, 1990); J. W. Griffin, et al., "Guillain-Barré Syndrome in Northern China. The Spectrum of Neuropathological Changes in Clinically Defined Cases," *Brain* (v.118/Pt 3, 1995); R. A. Hughes and R. H. Rees, "Clinical and Epidemiological Features of Guillain-Barré Syndrome," *Journal of Infectious Diseases* (v.176, 1997); J. R. Jones, "Childhood Guillain-Barré Syndrome: Clinical Presentation, Diagnosis and Therapy," *Journal of Child Neurology* (v.11, 1996); A. H. Ropper, "The Guillain-Barré Syndrome," *New England Journal of Medicine* (v.326, 1992).

Darrin J. Lee
University of California, Irvine

Guinea

Guinea is located in western Africa, with a coastline on the Atlantic Ocean. It is sometimes referred to as Guinea-Conakry to differentiate it from the neighboring country of Guinea-Bissau. A former French colony, Guinea won its independence in 1958. Although it managed to avoid being drawn into the civil strife that rocked Sierra Leone and Liberia on its southern borders, political and economic discontent was leading toward demonstrations and general strikes in 2006 and early 2007, and some international observers believe Guinea could soon fall into chaos.

Guinea's population now stands at 9,948,000 and is growing at a rate of 2.62 percent annually. (These population figures do not include several large refugee groups living in camps along the borders.) The birth rate is 41.53 per 1,000 and the death rate is 15.33 per 1,000. Median age is 17.7 years. Life expectancy is 48.5 years for males and 50.84 years for females. Despite ample natural resources, Guinea's economy is still characterized as "underdeveloped." Gross national income is a mere $370 per capita.

Malaria is the primary cause of morbidity in Guinea. Lassa fever, a viral hemmorhagic disease transmitted through animal waste, is endemic in Guinea; 80 percent of those infected are asymptomatic, but the fatality rate is high for those who become symptomatic. Acute respiratory infections are common, especially in the overcrowded refugee camps. Guinea also suffers from a high burden of yellow fever in some region, along with schistosomiasis, meningococcal meningitis, measles, and cholera. Sanitation is minimal within the country, with about half the population able to find clean water, and only 18 percent using adequate waste facilities.

Estimates on the HIV/AIDS epidemic vary, but the Joint Programme of the United Nations on HIV/AIDS (UNAIDS) puts the adult prevalence rate at 1.5 percent. This translates to around 85,000 cases, of which 53,000 are women and 7,000 are children under age 15. At present, only 0.4 percent of pregnant women are receiving drugs to help prevent mother-to-child tranmission of the virus, despite the fact that in some areas, 6.5 percent of pregnant women are infected. Health officials have but Guinea on the fast track for improvements in their treatment and educational programs.

Child mortality rates have dropped from 1990 levels, but remains high at 98 deaths per 1,000 for infants younger than 1, and 150 deaths per 1,000 for children aged 1–5. AIDS and other diseases have left an orphan population estimated at 370,000. Per capita government expenditures on health were around U.S. $13 in 2001. Medical facilities are spread around the country, often forcing the sick or injured to walk for many miles before finding healthcare. There are few ambulances to transport the seriously ill to district or general hospitals. Facilities around the country are in poor physical condition, and often lack safe water. The large refugee population has strained resources to the breaking point in some regions. Understaffing is also a problem, with 0.9 physicians and 4.7 nurses and midwives per 10,000 population.

SEE ALSO: Cholera; Healthcare, Africa; Malaria.

BIBLIOGRAPHY. The Johns Hopkins University Center for Communications Programs, "Guinea, Country Overview," www.jhuccp.org/africa/guinea/index.shtml (cited July 2007); World Health Organization, "Guinea," www.who.int/countries/gin/en/ (cited July 2007).

HEATHER K. MICHON
INDEPENDENT SCHOLAR

Guinea-Bissau

Guinea-Bissau is a small country on the Atlantic coast of Africa, between Senegal and Guinea. Formerly called Portuguese Guinea, it won independence in 1974 and took its name to differentiate itself from its southern neighbor, itself a former French colony. Guinea-Bissau is one of the world's 10 poorest countries. Political turmoil in the late 1990s sparked a brief civil war that in turn caused severe disruptions in the country's agricultural and fishing industries.

The population is 1,473,000 and growing at 2.05 percent annually. The birth rate is 36.81 per 1,000 population, and the death rate is 16.29 per 1,000. Median age is 19 years. Life expectancy is 45.37 years for males and 49.04 years for females. Gross national income is $180 per capita. Only 36 percent of the population lives in urban areas; 62 percent of Guineans work in agriculture.

Vectorborne and waterborne diseases are common through Guinea-Bissau. Malaria is likely the chief killer. There is also a high risk of yellow fever, cholera, meningococcal meningitis, schistosomiasis, typhoid, hepatitis A, and diarrhea. Less than 60 percent of the population have access to clean water, and only 35 percent have sanitary waste disposal. Little is known about the dimension of the AIDS epidemic in Guinea-Bissau. In 2003, the adult prevalence rate was estimated at 10 percent, with 17,000 people believed to be infected as of 2001.

Guinea-Bissau has abysmal rates for infant and child mortality, with 124 of every 1,000 infants dying between birth and age 1, and 200 deaths per 1,000 for children aged 1–5. In 2005, the United Nations Children's Fund (UNICEF) estimated the total number of deaths at 16,000 children 5 and younger. A quarter of Guinean children are underweight, 30 percent show signs of stunting, and 10 percent are defined as wasting. Immunization rates run at around 80 percent. Fifty-five percent of children go to work during the school-age years.

The health profile for women is similarly grim. The total fertility rate is 4.79 children per women. Only 8 percent of women use birth control. Just 62 percent have prenatal care, and 35 percent have a trained attendant during childbirth. Consequently, Guinea-Bissau has one of the highest maternal mortality rates in the world, with 1,100 women per 100,000 dying in childbirth.

The medical system in Guinea-Bissau barely functions. Facilities are understaffed, and staff often goes for long periods without pay. There are 188 physicians, 912 nurses, and 160 midwives working within the country; per capita expenditures on healthcare by the government amounts to $8.70. Hospitals often lack electricity and running water. What equipment exists is often antiquated, and most facilities lack the most basic drugs and medical supplies. The necessity for up-front payment for care puts it out of the reach of many Guineans.

SEE ALSO: Cholera; Healthcare, Africa; Malaria.

BIBLIOGRAPHY. "A Guide to Statistical Information at WHO". www.who.int/whosis/en/index.html (cited June 2007); "Guinea-Bissau: Health Service Far From Well". www.plusnews.org (cited June 2007); United Nations Children's Fund, "At a Glance: Guinea-Bissau—Statistics". www.unicef.org (cited June 2007).

HEATHER K. MICHON
INDEPENDENT SCHOLAR

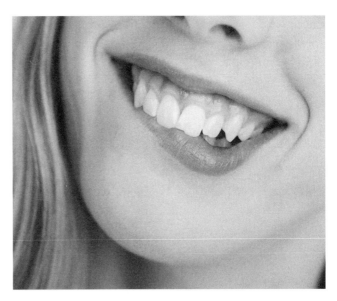

Gum disease is an inflammation of oral tissues caused by bacteria collecting around the base of the teeth.

Gum Disease

Gum disease, also called periodontitis or peridontal disease, is an inflammation of oral tissues caused by bacteria collecting around the base of the teeth. Prolonged inflammation destroys bone and connective fibers and can lead to tooth loss and a host of other health problems. Gum disease affects people throughout the world without regard to region, class, or development.

According to the American Academy of Periodontology, there are several types of gum disease. *Gingivitis* is the mildest form, causing the gums to become red and swollen but causing little discomfort. It is the easiest form of gum disease to reverse. *Agressive periodontitis* is the next stage, where inflammation has caused loss of tooth attachment and bone loss. *Chronic (or severe) periodontitis* is the most frequently diagnosed form of gum disease, especially among adults. Bacteria and inflammation causes the formation of pockets around the base of the teeth, or the recession of the gums, along with loss of tooth attachment. *Necrotizing periodontal disease* is generally seen in those with diseases such as HIV/AIDS or other systemic diseases, or in cases of severe malnutrition. It causes the loss of gingiva and the formation of lesions on gum tissue.

While periodontitis has long been viewed as arising from a lack of oral hygiene, there are in fact several other risk factors for the development of the disease. New research indicates that tobacco use may be the most significant risk factor in both periodontitis and oral cancers. Genetics may also play a large role, with around 30 percent of the population predisposed to gum problems. In women, hormonal changes around puberty and during pregnancy may spur the development of inflammation. Lifestyle issues like stress, poor nutrition, and the use of some medications are known to reduce the ability of the body to fight off infections. Bruxism, or the involuntary clenching or grinding of the teeth, causes a variety of gum problems, including recession.

The ultimate result of untreated, advanced periodontitis is tooth loss, but researchers are now finding that even mild cases of gum disease has an impact far beyond the mouth. Periodontitis is believed to increase the risk of cardiovascular disease, perhaps as a reaction to the presence of bacteria in the bloodstream. It also may increase the risk of certain respiratory diseases. Pregnant women with periodontitis are seven times as likely to give birth prematurely. Some studies indicate that periodontitis can raise the risk of developing diabetes, or it can develop as a result of having diabetes.

Most of the global population has some form of gum inflammation, with severe periodontitis affecting five to 15 percent worldwide. The World Health Organization has identified oral health as a major part of overall health and quality of life, and has launched a Global Oral Health Programme designed to raise awareness of the issue. Among their goals is increasing availability of dental care in disadvantaged regions and reducing the global consumption of tobacco products.

SEE ALSO: American Dental Association (ADA); Child Dental Health; Dental Health.

BIBLIOGRAPHY. American Academy of Periodontology "Frequently Asked Questions About Gum Disease and General Health," www.perio.org (cited July 2007); "What Is the Burden of Oral Disease?" World Health Organization. www.who.int (cited July 2007); World Health Organization, "World Oral Health Report 2003," www.who.int (cited July 2007).

HEATHER K. MICHON
INDEPENDENT SCHOLAR

Guyana

Guyana is located on the eastern coast of South America, bordered by Venezuela, Surinam, and Brazil. It is a small country with a long and complicated history. For two centuries, Guyana was a Dutch colony, but in 1815, it became a British possession; it did not gain independence until 1966. During these years of British rule, there was an influx of immigrants from India. So this small South American country has English as its primary language, and the majority of the population is of East Indian descent. Thirty percent of Guyanese are practicing Hindus.

Guyana is about the size of Idaho and has an estimated population of 767,000. The population growth rate only 0.25 percent a year, with 18.28 births per 1,000 people and 8.28 deaths per 1,000 people. The migration rate is deeply in the negative column at minus 7.49 migrants per 1,000 people.

Eighty percent of Guyana is covered by tropical rainforest. Most of the population lives in urbanized coastal areas. The climate is hot and humid, with some relief coming from the northeast trade winds. Winter is the rainy season, and flash flooding is common. In recent years, the government has opened the rainforest to Malaysian logging interests and palm oil producers, which environmentalists warn could devastate local ecosystems.

However, with per capita income for most Guyanese at $990 annually, the government has little choice but to woo foreign investors. The national economy has long depended on agricultural imports such as sugar, rice, molasses, and shrimp, along with gold and bauxite mining, but it is not profitable enough to improve the daily lives of the citizens.

The Guyanese manage to get by on very little. Their average caloric intake is 2,450 per day, which is actually above the recommended averages. Staple foods are peas, rice, bread, and starchy vegetables such as plantain, cassava, and breadfruit. The calories are more than adequate, but malnutrition is still a problem, as this diet lacks key vitamins and protein.

Life expectancy at birth is 63.21 for males and 68.65 for females; healthy life expectancy is 53.1 for men and 57.2 for women. Infant mortality is 32 deaths per 1,000 live births and 64 children in 1,000 die between the ages of 1 to 5 years. Maternal mortality is 170 deaths per 100,000 live births. Eighty-six percent of births are monitored by a trained attendant. About 37 percent of women have access to birth control.

Like most of Latin America, there is a high rate of parasitic infections. About 83 percent of the population has access to clean drinking water and 70 percent can access sanitary facilities. Malaria, typhoid fever, and filariasis are common. Measles remains a problem. Immunization rates for children average about 90 percent for all major childhood diseases, and the country maintains an active malaria-eradication program. Communicable diseases are closely monitored, and the country has not suffered a major epidemic in several years.

The HIV/AIDS rate is 2.5 percent, with an estimated 11,000 Guyanese living with the virus. More than 1,100 have died so far. Tuberculosis rates are also high.

The Ministry of Health has launched an AIDS awareness program and has 14 treatment sites scattered throughout the country. Many AIDS patients are now receiving life-extending drug treatments, but it remains a struggle for the government to provide the recommended three-drug cocktail. In 2006, Health Minister Leslie Ramsammy announced that the government could not yet afford the new one-pill daily protocol, at a cost of $1,000 per patient per month.

Basic healthcare is available throughout most of Guyana, with four regional hospitals, 22 district hospitals, 70 health centers, 32 health posts, and one psychiatric hospital. Ambulance service to more advanced care at the regional hospitals is spotty. There are 366 doctors and 1,738 nurses, leaving facilities frequently understaffed.

SEE ALSO: Healthcare, South America.

BIBLIOGRAPHY. Pan American Health Organization (PAHO) and World Health Organization (WHO), "Health Sector Analysis: Guyana," www.lachealthsys.org (cited July 2007); World Health Organization, "Guyana," http://www.who.int/countries/guy/en/ (cited July 2007).

HEATHER K. MICHON
INDEPENDENT SCHOLAR

Gynecologist

A gynecologist is a medical doctor who specializes in the health and diseases of women's reproductive organs. While medical training is broad and exposes a future physician to a wide array of medical problems and treatments, gynecologists have chosen to pursue a four-year residency in obstetrics and gynecology in order to train in the specialty of women's reproductive health. Unlike most medical specialties, the practice of gynecology represents a blend of both medical and surgical skills making the gynecologist both a physician and a surgeon. They typically see female patients of all ages and are equipped to deal with a wide variety of reproductive health and basic medical issues.

A gynecologist is an important caregiver in the context of global health because of the relevance of elevated maternal mortality rates, increasing prevalence of AIDS and other sexually transmitted infections among women, lack of screening for cervical cancer, and gender-based violence in the developing world.

While all patients who visit gynecologists are female, their ages can range from the prepubescent to the elderly. Young females are often medically treated by a pediatrician or family physician into their teenage years, and most females generally begin to see a gynecologist around age 18 or once they have become sexually active. However, there is plenty of variation within this scheme. Many women begin to see gynecologists at age 18 for a Pap smear. The Pap smear is a screening test for cervical cancer and current guidelines indicate that women should begin to receive Pap smears at age 18 or the onset of sexual activity. Once initiated into the care of the gynecologist, most women continue to see one throughout their reproductive years, through menopause, and into the postmenopausal years when different types of problems can occur.

Women seeking care from gynecologists require services ranging from prescriptions for oral contraceptive pills, to Pap smears, to assessment and treatment of abnormal vaginal bleeding, to lower abdominal or pelvic pain, to sexually transmitted infections, to urinary incontinence, to vulvar, vaginal, cervical, endometrial, or ovarian cancer. Gynecologists also need to tend to the mental and social health needs of their patients by screening them for depression, substance abuse, or gender-based violence. In addition, many women utilize their gynecologist as their primary health provider which means that these physicians are also evaluating their patient's general medical health.

A woman's reproductive tract includes her ovaries, fallopian tubes, uterus, cervix, vagina, vulva, and breasts. It is worth noting that most breast surgery (for biopsy or excision of cancerous tissue) is done by gen-

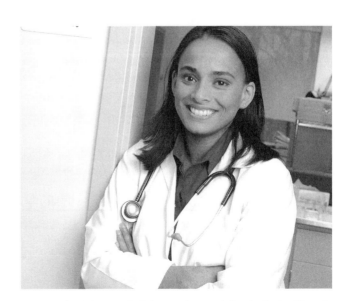

A gynecologist is a medical doctor who specializes in the health and diseases of women's reproductive organs.

eral surgeons who specialize in surgery of the breast. However, there are a growing number of gynecologists, often gynecologic oncologists, who pursue fellowship training in breast surgery and are qualified to offer this service to their patients. The remaining reproductive organs located in the pelvis are the main focus of the gynecologist. There are a wide range of diseases or other problems that can affect these organs.

Training to become a gynecologist is a lengthy process. First, she/he must complete four years of medical school and then complete four years of residency in obstetrics and gynecology. All residency programs that prepare medical school graduates to practice in this field train residents in both obstetrics and gynecology. It is up to the individual physician to chose whether she/he goes on to practice both obstetrics and gynecology or focus solely on gynecology upon completion of the program.

Many obstetricians/gynecologists go on to pursue fellowship training. This means that they choose to further specialize in one area of gynecology and spend an additional one to three years honing their skills. Examples of fellowships that gynecologists pursue include gynecologic oncology, urogynecology, reproductive endocrinology and infertility, and family planning. There are other fellowships that pertain more directly to the practice of obstetrics such as maternal-fetal medicine.

SEE ALSO: Gynecology; Obstetrician/Gynecologist; Obstetrics.

BIBLIOGRAPHY. P. R. Bennett and G. E. Moore, *Molecular Biology for Obstetricians and Gynecologists* (Blackwell, 1991); Duane E. Townsend, *Maverick of Medicine Speaks to Women: A World-Renowned Gynecologist's Solutions for a Better World in Women's Health Care* (Woodland Publishing, 2003).

MEGAN K. GUFFEY, M.D., M.P.H.
INDEPENDENT SCHOLAR

Gynecology

Gynecology (alternately, gynaecology) is the branch of medicine that deals with the female reproductive organs. It is closely related to the field of obstetrics, which is involved with the care of women and fetuses during pregnancy. OB/GYN is a common medical specialty. Gynecological problems are rare in pre-adolescence except in cases of birth defects or conditions precipitated by sexual abuse. The onset of menstruation, which generally occurs around the age of 12, marks the beginning of puberty. Even in cases where physical abnormalities are present, they may not surface before puberty. Dysmenorrhea (painful menstruation), for instance, may be either primary or secondary to pelvic disease. Around 50 percent of all women of childbearing age experience dysmenorrhea to some extent, but it is severe in only one in 10. Incidences of the disorder tend to decline after the age of 24 and may disappear earlier in women who become pregnant. In some women, amenorrhea, the absence of menstruation, is experienced without a clear physical cause. In most cases, it is associated with autoimmune or infectious diseases or cancer treatments. It may also occur in female athletes and in females with eating disorders.

It is estimated that 95 percent of all premenopausal women experience Premenstrual Syndrome (PMS), occurring seven to 10 days before the beginning of the menstrual cycle. Symptoms tend to disappear once bleeding starts. Experiences with PMS vary greatly. Common symptoms include facial acne, breast swelling and tenderness, fatigue, insomnia, gastrointestinal problems, bloating, constipation, diarrhea, headache, backache, appetite variations, joint or muscle pain, and concentration and memory difficulties. Caused by fluctuating hormone levels, the classic symptom of PMS is wide mood swings involving tension, irritability, crying jags, anxiety, or depression. While there is no specific treatment for PMS, pain medication, vitamin B6, oil of evening primrose, and serotonin inhibitors offer relief to some women.

In some cultures and religions, the most pressing gynecological problem is female genital mutilation (FGM), also known as female circumcision. The purported purposes of altering a girl's external sexual organs are to prolong virginity and enhance marriageability. Performed in Africa, the Middle East, and in Muslim areas of Indonesia and Malaysia without anesthesia, FGM poses major health risks for females. Because the procedure is also performed among immigrant populations in Western countries, many nations have passed laws to make the practice illegal.

However, physicians are encouraged to show compassion in dealing with women who have undergone FGM. In 1995, the landmark Beijing Conference on women's rights condemned the practice as a violation of human rights.

Throughout the world, sexually transmitted diseases (STDs) continue to present major difficulties for the medical community, society, and governments. Health clinics are established to screen for STDs and to provide treatment and follow-up. Once diagnosed, all sexual partners of infected persons must be notified in order to prevent individual health problems and the spreading of the disease. Even women who have had sex with only one partner may be vulnerable to infection if that partner has practiced unsafe sex or had sex with multiple partners. The human papillomavirus (HPV) is the most prevalent of all STDs, and around 70 strains of the virus have so far been identified. In many developing nations, HIV/AIDS has become the most pressing gynecological problem for both women and for the children they deliver because of the risk of mother-to-child transmissions during the birthing process.

GYNECOLOGICAL DISORDERS

Infections may occur in all parts of the reproductive system for a variety of reasons. Visits to gynecologists are often made in response to unexplained pelvic pain. One of the most common sources of pelvic pain is fibroids, noncancerous growths that take root in the smooth muscle layer of the uterus. Fibroids occur in from 30 to 50 percent of all women over the age of 30. They tend to occur earlier in African Americans. While fibroids may be asymptomatic, they are often associated with menstrual abnormalities and changes in menstrual patterns.

Behaviors linked to the formation of fibroids include being physically inactive and consumption of alcohol and caffeine. Some physicians believe that taking vitamin B6 and eating more fiber may reduce the risk. Adenomyosis, a disorder in which endometrium tissues grow outside the walls of the uterus, is also common, occurring at a rate of 10 to 90 percent of all women over the age of 50. Both fibroids and adenomyosis may improve after menopause as estrogen levels decrease. As a general rule, germ cell tumors are most common in younger women, and epithelial growths are associated with older women. Half of all tumors found in older women are benign.

Postmenopausal women, particularly those over the age of 60, may experience a prolapsed uterus, a condition in which the uterus partially descends into the vagina in response to the weakening of pelvic floor muscles. A prolapsed uterus may also result from a difficult labor, having a large baby, multiple pregnancies, obesity, chronic constipation, fibroids, or pelvic tumors. Symptoms include heaviness or pressure in the vagina, incontinence, backaches, painful or difficult intercourse, and constipation. Mild cases may be treated with hormone therapy and lifestyle changes. Kegel exercises that involve tightening the vaginal and uterine muscles may also offer some relief. In the most severe cases, surgical repositioning of the uterus is necessary.

Early in pregnancy, women who experience severe abdominal pain on one side, spotting, vaginal bleeding, nausea, vomiting, fainting and dizziness may be experiencing an ectopic or tubal pregnancy in which a fertilized egg has implanted outside the uterus, usually in the fallopian tubes. If not treated promptly, the condition may lead to rupture, hemorrhage, and infection. Nine percent of all pregnancy-related deaths in the United States are a result of ectopic pregnancies. Risk for ectopic pregnancies include pelvic inflammatory disease or endometriosis, being over the age of 30, a history of ectopic pregnancies, smoking, and past surgeries of the abdomen or fallopian tubes. Endometriosis involves the depositing of tissues that normally line the womb outside the uterus. The condition occurs in three to seven percent of all women, but it may be more prevalent because of underreporting. Endometriosis normally peaks between the ages of 30 and 45 years. Symptoms include pain, menstrual disturbance, and infertility, and treatment may include medication or surgery.

Gestational trophoblastic tumors, also referred to as "molar pregnancies," involve the growth of moles that occur after abnormal fertilization. They may be either benign or cancerous. Researchers have not been able to establish a clear link between race and these cancers, but they are more common in some Asian countries, leading to the assumption that they may be related to diet. These tumors are 10 times more common in women over the age of 45. Warning signs include uterine bleeding, severe nausea, and vomiting. In general, such pregnancies resolve after uterine evacuation. In 10 to 20 percent of all case, moles transform into malignancies; but there is a cure rate of 90 to 95 percent.

GYNECOLOGICAL CANCERS

The most common cancers in women are breast, cervical, uterus, and ovary. Breast cancer is the second leading cause of death in the United States. Endometrial cancer is the most common gynecological cancer found in American women. Out of 37,000 cases diagnosed each year, the cancer is fatal in 3,000 to 4,000 women. It may strike at any age, but three-fourths of endometrial cancers occur after the age of 50. Warning signs are postmenopausal bleeding, and estrogen and obesity are established links. The condition known as polycystic ovarian syndrome (PCOS) involves a functional derangement of the hypothalamo-pituitary ovarian axis. PCOS may be genetic. Risk factors include obesity, abnormal menstrual disorders, hirsutism, acne, and infertility. Women with PCOS have three times the risk of developing endometrial cancer and are at increased risk for developing diabetes, hypertension, and cardiovascular disease. Growths in the vulva may be either benign or malignant, but vulva cancer is generally considered curable. The cancer is most common in women between the ages of 60 and 79; fewer than 15 percent occur in women under 40. Risk factors include a past history of the human papillomavirus or cancer and smoking.

Eighty percent of cervical cancers are squamous in origin and were once assumed to have an ethnic risk factor. Incidences are rising among young white women and declining among black women. Accepted risk factors include a past history of HPV, smoking, alcohol abuse, early onset of sexual activity, marriage or conception at an early age, and multiple sex partners. Many women with these risk factors will not get cervical cancer, while women who have had only one sexual partner may contract the disease. Warning signs include bleeding or spotting after intercourse and bloody discharge. In the early stages, pain is rarely a factor. Cervical cancer is treated with surgery and radiation. Early in the 21st century, a vaccine to protect girls against cervical cancer was released. Despite the move for universal vaccinate of the relevant age group, the vaccine remains controversial. Ovarian neoplasms may result from normal changes to existing malignancies. Risk factors for ovarian cancer include early menstruation, late menopause, and never having had children. Symptoms of ovarian cancer are acute pelvic pain and hemorrhage. Women who have used oral contraceptives are at a reduced risk for ovarian cancer, as are those who have had early pregnancies or several children.

In the past, dilation and curettage (D&C) in which the lining of the uterus was scraped was used as both a diagnostic and surgical tool. However, new and less invasive technologies such as laparoscopy have become more common. The most common gynecological procedure performed is the hysterectomy, which involves surgical removal of the uterus. In 40 percent of all cases, one or both ovaries are removed, in part to remove the risk of developing ovarian cancer. Estimates suggest that without ovarian removal, one in every 700 women who undergo hysterectomies would have later developed ovarian cancer. After hysterectomies are performed, women abruptly enter menopause, a cessation of the menses that signals the end of fertility.

Women who undergo menopause, before the age of 40 are said to experience premature ovarian failure. Before the scare over the link between breast cancer and hormone replacement therapy (HRT), estrogen and progesterone therapies were routinely prescribed for women after hysterectomies. The new findings have caused many women to look for alternative therapies. Early detection of gynecological cancers through self-examinations, mammograms, and Pap smears is a key factor in survival rates. Preventive care is similar to that of other cancers and involves controlling hypertension and cholesterol, not smoking, healthy eating habits, being physically active, using birth control, practicing safe sex, and managing stress.

CONTRACEPTION AND INFERTILITY

Most women of childbearing age are sexually active, and studies show that approximately one-half of all American women between the ages of 15 and 19 have had sexual intercourse. Large numbers of sexually active women do not use any form of birth control to prevent unwanted pregnancies or the transmission of STDs. Teenage pregnancies are a major problem in many countries throughout the world, and they present major health risks because they pose greater health risks to both mother and child and place onerous burdens on social service systems.

Humans have practiced birth control throughout much of history. The most common method, which was used in biblical times, was coitus interuptus in which the male withdraws from the female before climax to prevent the release of sperm. Natural forms of birth control, including the rhythm method, which estimates fertility by charting menstrual cycles, are still in use today. Since the women's movement of the 1960s, research into contraception has produced a variety of birth control technologies, including spermacides, condoms, diaphragms, intrauterine devices, and the highly effective birth control pill.

Common surgical contraception methods include tubal ligations in females and vasectomies in males. In both cases, the intent is to prevent the female's eggs from being fertilized by sperm. In many societies, abortion remains the most controversial method of birth control. It is generally controlled by strict guidelines that serves the dual purpose of protecting the health of the mother and serving the interest of those who object to abortion on either religious or moral grounds. Abortions that occur spontaneously are called miscarriages, and those performed for health reasons are considered therapeutic.

Approximately one in six couples are said to be infertile, but only 42 percent of infertile women seek professional help. The classification of infertility is made only after a couple fails to conceive after a year of unprotected intercourse. In about 40 percent of all cases, the male is either the sole or a contributing cause of infertility. In females, the most common causes of infertility are abnormalities or diseases of the fallopian tubes, ovulation disorders, cervical abnormalities, uterine failure, chronic infections, debilitating diseases, severe nutritional deficiencies, and advancing age. Modern medicine has provided a plethora of alternatives to traditional pregnancies that include artificial insemination from a partner or donor's sperm, in vitro fertilization, fertility drugs, embryo transfer from a donor, and surrogacy.

SEE ALSO: Abortions; Adolescent Health; AIDS; Birth Defects; Breast Cancer; Diabetes; Gastroenterology; Hormones; Hypertension; In vitro; Infectious Diseases (General); Infertility; Menopause; Obesity; Obstetrician/Gynecologist; Obstetrics; Preventive Care; Pregnancy; Sexually Transmitted Diseases (STDs); Women's Health (General).

BIBLIOGRAPHY. Phyllis L. Carr, et al., *The Medical Care of Women* (Saunders, 1995); Allen H. DeCherney, and Martin L. Pernoll, eds., *Current Obstetric and Gynecologic Diagnosis and Treatment* (Appleton and Lange, 1994); Valerie Edge, and Mindi Miller, *Women's Health Care* (Mosby, 1994); Stephen S. Entman, and Charles B. Rush, eds., *Office Gynecology* (W.B. Saunders, 1995); Neville F. Hacker, and J. George Moore, eds., *Essentials of Obstetrics and Gynecology* (Saunders, 1998); Norman E. Himes, *Medical History of Contraception* (Schocken Books, 1970); John H. Mattox, eds, *Obstetrics and Gynecology* (Mosby, 1998); David McKay and Jane Norman, *Gynaecology Illustrated* (Churchill Livingstone, 2000); Angus McLauren, *A History of Contraceptives: From Antiquity to the Present Day* (Basil Blackwell, 1991); Ann McPherson, ed., *Women's Problems in General Practice* (Oxford University Press, 1993); Manuel Penalver, et al., eds., *Gynecologic Oncology* (Saunders, 2001).

ELIZABETH R. PURDY, PH.D.
INDEPENDENT SCHOLAR

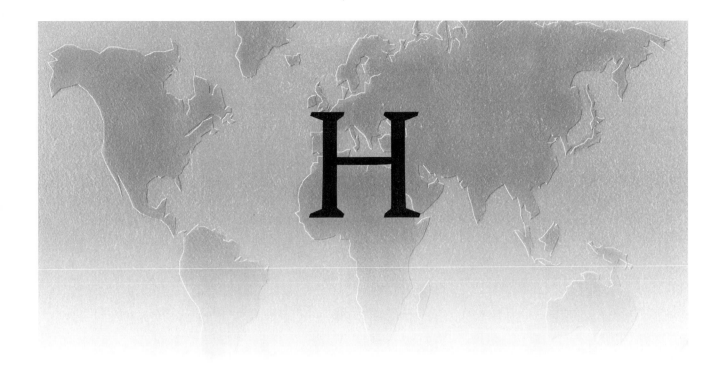

Hair Diseases and Hair Loss

Hair grows from hair follicles located in the layer of skin called dermis, lying immediately below the surface layer. The dermis all over the body contains hair follicles except for lips, palms of hands, and soles of feet. Hair color originates from a pigment called melanin, which also gives skin its color. Hair grows in cycles of growth consisting of a long growing phase followed by a short resting phase. Human hair growth is regulated by hormones like testosterone and dihydrotestosterone, which are present in both the sexes. These hormones influence hair growth in the underarms and pubic area. Beard hair grows due to stimulation from dihydrotestosterone. Hair disorders include hair loss, excessive hairiness (hirsutism), and ingrown beard hair. These disorders may be caused by physical causes or abnormal hormone secretion. Hair diseases may not be life threatening, but may be a cosmetics issue. Some common diseases are below:

Alopecia Areata. This autoimmune disease results in patches of hair loss over the head. These patches may remain for years or may go away. This disease is caused when the immune system attacks hair follicles causing hair loss.

Folliculitis. Folliculitis is a bacterial infection of hair follicles caused by *Staphylococcus aureus*. Follicles may swell into a red bumps or pimples. The infection may also spread causing swelling, redness, pain, severe tenderness, and production of pus from the infected site.

Hirsutism. Hirsutism is abnormal hair growth in women, particularly in the face, chest, and areolae. Hirsutism is caused by excessive levels of the hormone androgen and/or high sensitivity of hair follicles to androgen. This disorder may be caused by abnormalities in adrenal glands or ovaries.

Keratosis Pilaris. Keratosis pilaris is caused when skin cells—that usually flake off—plug hair follicles causing small painless pimples. Keratosis pilaris is common in teenagers on the upper arms, and babies on their cheeks. There is no tested treatment for keratosis pilaris, which worsens during winter months and humid days, but generally disappears before age 30.

Poliosis. Poliosis is abnormal whitening of hair in small patches that can occur anywhere on the body; on the forehead, it is called a white forelock. Poliosis occurs when hair coloring pigment melanin runs out causing hair discoloration. Poliosis also occurs due to genetic diseases like piebaldism. Most poliosis cases occur in otherwise healthy individuals.

Hair loss. Hair loss is the gradual loss of hair with age seen in both the sexes, but more commonly in men. Hair loss may be caused by diseases, improper hair care, and genetics. Improper treatment of hair with chemicals like dyes, tints, straighteners, bleaches, and permanent waves can cause hair loss if these chemicals are used improperly or excessively. Other causes include shampooing, combing or brushing more often than necessary, and vigorously rubbing wet hair with a towel. The most common cause of hair loss is by genetics—a condition called androgenetic alopecia—resulting in hereditary balding or thinning of hair. Hereditary balding is most obvious around the temples and crown in men, and on top of the head in women. Androgenetic alopecia may be treated with minoxidil-containing products which cause vasodilatation in hair follicles promoting hair growth.

SEE ALSO: Hair Dye; Head Lice; Hormone Replacement Therapy; Hormones.

BIBLIOGRAPHY. Rodney Dawber, *Diseases of the Hair and Scalp* (Blackwell Publishing, 1997); Benjamin Godfrey, *Diseases of Hair* (Churchill, 1872); Jerry Shapiro, *Hair Loss: Principles of Diagnosis and Management of Alopecia* (Taylor & Francis, 2002); Leonard Sperling, *An Atlas of Hair Pathology with Clinical Correlations* (Taylor & Francis, 2003).

Rahul Gladwin, M.D.
University of Health Sciences Antigua

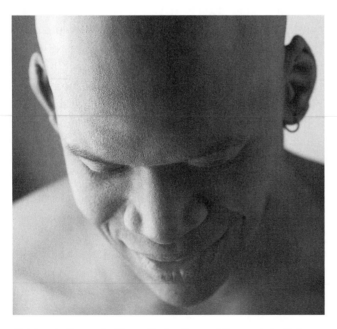

Hair loss is the gradual loss of hair with age; it is seen in both the sexes, but is more common in men.

Hair Dye

Hair coloring products include a wide range of over 5,000 chemical substances, some of which have been reported to be mutagenic and carcinogenic to animals. Hair dye products may be divided into three categories, that is, permanent, semipermanent, and temporary hair colors. Permanent hair colors are the most popular hair dye products. They may be further divided into oxidation hair dyes and progressive hair dyes. Oxidation hair dye products consist of 1.) a solution of dye intermediates, which form hair dyes on chemical reaction, and preformed dyes, which already are dyes and are added to achieve the intended shades, in an aqueous, ammoniacal vehicle containing soap, detergents, and conditioning agents; and 2.) a solution of hydrogen peroxide, usually 6 percent in water.

The prevalence of use of hair dyes is high among women in industrialized countries with more than half of women above age 18 applying hair dyes in Europe and the United States and around 10 percent among males. Consumers use all major types of hair colorants, which may contain aromatic amines, nitro-substituted aromatic amines, high molecular weight complexes, metal salts, and other. The content of hair dye has changed over the years and recent legislation prevents the use of carcinogenic substances in hair dye use.

Some components of hair dyes may cause skin irritation on certain individuals and a preliminary test according to accompanying directions should first be made as it is generally advised by the manufacturers. A major concern on the health effects of hair dyes is, however, the suspicion that they may be linked to cancer. While no clear excess risk of cancer has been observed among hairdressers and barbers, the evaluation of cancer risk among regular users of hair dyes has been poorly evaluated due to lack of adequate data on humans. In 1992, the International Agency for Research on Cancer evaluated hairdressing and barbering as occupations entailing exposures that are probably carcinogenic to humans; personal use of hair colorants could not at that time be evaluated in terms of its carcinogenicity.

Since this last evaluation, several studies have tried to provide human data on regular use of hair dyes. Among the cancer sites that have been most commonly evaluated in association with regular exposure to hair dyes are bladder cancer and lymphomas. Small amounts of

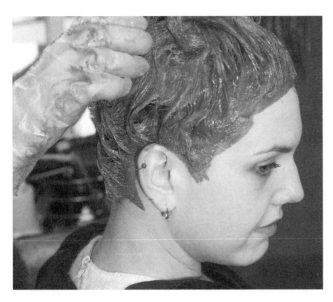

More than half of women in Europe and the United States above the age of 18 use hair dye products.

the bladder carcinogen 4-aminobiphenyl (4-ABP), an aromatic amine, in eight out of the 11 hair dyes tested have been identified. Although an excess risk has been seen in some studies that included information on personal use of permanent hair dyes and bladder cancer risk, the overall results are not yet converging.

Use of hair dyes has been inconsistently associated to the etiology of lymphomas. Recently, Yawei Zhang from Connecticut and Silvia de Sanjose reporting from six European countries have shown that the risk of certain types of lymphomas may increase between 20 to 30 percent among regular users of hair dyes. In both studies, the risk was increased mainly among those women using hair dyes before 1980, but no clear association among those using hair dyes during the last 20 years. This observation suggests that more recent hair dyes may have a safe composition. Further, the evaluation of all available studies in humans estimated a 15 percent increased risk for hematopoietic cancer, 23 percent for Hodgkin's lymphoma, and a 1 percent increased risk for bladder cancer.

New rules are implemented by the European Community Directive on the safe use of ingredients in hair dyes. Twenty-two substances have been added to the list of banned ingredients identified as being potentially carcinogenic.

SEE ALSO: Cancer (General).

BIBLIOGRAPHY. International Agency for Research on Cancer, *Occupational Exposures of Hairdressers and Barbers and Personal Use of Hair Colourants; Some Hair Dyes, Cosmetic Colourants, Industrial Dyestuffs and Aromatic Amines* (International Agency for Research on Cancer, 1993); S. de Sanjose, et al., "Association between Personal Use of Hair Dyes and Lymphoid Neoplasms in Europe," *American Journal of Epidemiology* (v.164/1, 2006); B. Takkouche, M. Etminan, and A. Montes-Martínez, "Personal Use of Hair Dyes and Risk of Cancer. A Meta-Analysis," *Journal of the American Medical Association* (v.293, 2005).

Silvia de Sanjose, M.D., Ph.D.
Catalan Institute of Oncology

Haiti

Haiti is located on the western third of the island of Hispaniola, with the Dominican Republic next door. Plagued by violence and political upheaval throughout its long history, Haiti today has no end to its problems, and it is easily the poorest nation in the western hemisphere. Assaults on the health and welfare for Haitians come from all directions. The population is 8.3 million (2006 estimate), with a growth rate of 2.3 percent annually. The birth rate is 36.44 per 1,000 people and the death rate at 12.17 per 1,000 people. The migration rate is negative, with minus 1.31 migrants per 1,000.

Haiti has virtually no economy and few exports other than people heading for a better life elsewhere. An estimated 70 percent of the population are unemployed. Per capita income is $390 a year. Most food is imported, and therefore expensive, so the average Haitian lives on subsistence diet of 800 calories a day, based on corn, cassava, millet, rice, fruit, beans, goat, pork, and shellfish. There is a shortage of potable water. Access to clean water is 71 percent, but access to sanitary facilities is only 34 percent, even in the urban areas. Massive deforestation in the mountains along the border with the Dominican Republic has left the country vulnerable to storm flooding, mud slides, and soil erosion.

Life expectancy at birth is 51.89 years for males and 54.6 years for female, with healthy life expectancy 43.5 years for men and 44.1 years for women. Infant mortality is high, with 102 of every 1,000 infants dying before the age of 1, and 117 of every 1,000 children dying before the age of 5. Maternal mortality is equally high, with 1,000 deaths per 100,000 live births. Only 24 percent of births are monitored by trained attendants. Seventy-eight percent of women receive at least some prenatal care. Only 27 percent have access to birth control.

The rates of HIV/AIDS are among the highest in the hemisphere, with 5.6 percent of the population, or 280,000 people, already infected with the virus. At least 24,000 Haitians have already died of AIDS. Haiti also has the highest per capita incidence of tuberculosis in Latin America. Tuberculosis alone kills 6,000 Haitians each year.

The tropical climate, poor nutrition, and virtually nonexistent sanitation makes Haiti an excellent breeding ground for a wide variety of diseases, including diarrhea, malaria, typhus, rabies, anthrax, Q fever, brucellosis, hookworm, roundworm, schistosomiasis, and leptospirosis. Diabetes, arising from an unbalanced and nutrition-poor diet, is another growing health problem. In 2000, the World Health Organization tallied 161,000 cases of diabetes in Haiti; by 2030, it expects this number to grow to 401,000. Rates of child immunization are very low, with only 43 percent of children protected against diphtheria, pertussis, tetanus, and polio, and only 54 percent receiving measles vaccination. The AIDS and tuberculosis epidemics have created a generation of orphaned children, who become easy prey for child traffickers. Most schools are closed due to ongoing political violence, with only 50 percent of school-aged children enrolled in programs, and less than 2 percent finishing secondary school.

Sixty percent of the population lack access to basic healthcare. There are 49 hospitals, 217 health centers, and 371 health posts, most of them poorly staffed and poorly equipped. Well over half the population cannot obtain needed medicines. In 1998, the last year for which the World Health Organization has statistics, there were only 1,949 doctors and 834 nurses to serve the entire population.

SEE ALSO: Healthcare, South America.

BIBLIOGRAPHY. Central Intelligence Agency, "The World Factbook: Haiti," www.cia.gov (cited July 2007); World Health Organization, "Haiti," www.who.int cited July 2007).

HEATHER K. MICHON
INDEPENDENT SCHOLAR

Hand Injuries and Disorders

Injuries and disorders of the hand can often cause a person to change his or her entire lifestyle. As time progresses, the human race tends to be increasingly dependent upon their hands for fine coordinated movements, such as typing and dialing numbers on miniature phones. With this dependency upon hands and fingers to maximize technological capability, new hand injuries are emerging, and the existing ones are becoming that much more debilitating. Additionally, because acute hand injury is the leading cause of occupational injury treated in U. S. hospital emergency departments, it is imperative that risk factors for traumatic hand injury are identified and dealt with properly by employers.

CARPAL TUNNEL SYNDROME

The carpal tunnel is a passageway of bones and ligament found at the base of the hand that is sometimes narrowed if swelling occurs. Specifically, carpal tunnel syndrome is caused by compression in the median nerve in the wrist. This may result in pain or a numbness that can extend all the way up the entire length of the arm. Initial symptoms include sensations of itching, burning, and numbness in the fingers and palm of the hand. If untreated, the patient may loose ability to strongly grasp objects or even distinguish between hot and cold by touch. Females are more at risk for developing carpal tunnel syndrome than males. Carpal tunnel syndrome is diagnosed with a physical examination for swelling in the wrists and atrophy of the muscles at the base of the hand. Ultrasound and different electrodiagnostic tests can also be used to diagnose carpal tunnel syndrome. Nonsurgical treatments of carpal tunnel syndrome include prescription medication, exercise, and acupuncture. Surgical treatments include open release surgery and endoscopy.

GANGLION CYSTS

Ganglion cysts are one of the most common types of hand disorders. Ganglion cysts are a swelling due to accumulation of fluid in the back of the hand or wrists. The condition can be frightening as many may wonder if the fluid-filled capsule is cancer. Ganglion cysts are not cancerous, although they may grow as time progresses. While it is unknown what causes the formation of a ganglion, it is known that females

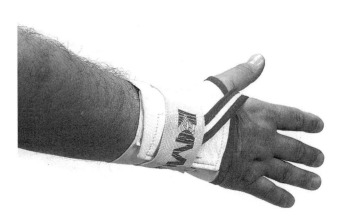

Acute hand injury is the leading cause of occupational injury treated in U. S. hospital emergency departments.

are more likely to be afflicted than males. Depending upon the location of a ganglion cyst, a patient may complain of pain if the ganglion puts pressure upon nerves. To diagnose ganglions, physicians often order X-rays so that conditions such as bone tumors or arthritis can be ruled out. Additionally, if the ganglion is deep under the skin, a magnet resonance imaging (MRI) or ultrasound may also be ordered. Nonsurgical treatment of cysts include immobilization because activity may sometimes worsen symptoms and aspiration of the ganglion with a needle. Nonsurgical treatment of a cyst does not guarantee that the cyst will not return. In surgical treatment of a cyst, the entire ganglion (cyst and outer sac) is removed.

TRIGGER FINGER

Trigger finger is a common hand problem that causes snapping and catching of the fingers as a patient tries to straighten his or her finger. Diagnosis of trigger finger usually includes patient description of symptoms; X-rays and other tests are usually not needed. Trigger finger is common in individuals aged 40–60 and those who are also afflicted by other diseases such as diabetes and rheumatoid arthritis. If catching or popping symptoms are mild, over-the-counter pain medications or resting the finger may be enough to relieve symptoms. Other treatment options include surgery to widen the tunnel in which the finger is getting caught. However, because trigger finger is not a progressive disorder, surgery is only recommended for patients with more severe symptoms.

FINGER FRACTURE

While fractures of the finger are normally considered minor traumas, if untreated, they can cause major problems in an individual's manual dexterity. Finger fractures are most common among athletes and can be identified if the following symptoms persist: swelling, inability to move finger, deformity, and pain when the finger is straight and taps against a surface. Most finger fractures are healed by using a splint to put the broken bone back into place. Often, the fingers adjacent to the fractured ones are used for support. Typically, a splint is worn anywhere from three to six weeks after injury.

TENDONITIS OF THE WRIST

Also known as De Quervain's stenosing tenosynovitis, tendonitis of the wrist occurs when the tendons of the thumb inflame, causing pain and irritation. Occasionally, a lump or thickening can be felt at the base of the hand. It is unknown what causes this inflammation, although overuse is suspected to play a role. The primary symptom of this form of tendonitis is a general sensation of pain over the thumb-side of the hand. Antiinflammatory medication is usually the first course of action. However, if medication is ineffective, surgery may be the only effective option.

OSTEOARTHRITIS OF THE HAND

Osteoarthritis of the hand occurs when the cartilage of the joints in the hand begin to undergo wear and tear due to daily use or traumatic injury and eventually wear out. Osteoarthritis of the hand typically occurs in three locations: at the base of the thumb, at the end joint closest to the finger tip, and at the middle joint of a finger. Swelling, pain, stiffness, and generally diminished grip and pinch strength are all typical symptoms of arthritis of the hand.

Nonsurgical treatment includes medication, resting the fingers and hand, heating pads, splints for overnight use, and cortisone injections.

DUPUYTREN'S DISEASE

Dupuytren's disease is an abnormal thickening of the tissue just beneath the superficial skin of the palm. Initial symptoms often include firm lumps in the palm of the hand, causing fingers to slightly bend. The disease may be noticed when an individual has difficulty shaking hands, placing his or her hand on a flat surface such as a tabletop, and putting his or her hands in his or her pockets. Observation and surgery are the only two treatment methods used for Dupuytren's disease.

Last, one of the common problems that arises with hands, because they are exposed to so many different surfaces, is different types of hand infections. These include Paronychia, Felon, Herpetic Whitlow, osteomyelitis, tendon sheath infections, and mycobacterial infections. Treatment for these different infections vary.

SEE ALSO: Carpal Tunnel Syndrome; Fractures; Osteoarthritis.

BIBLIOGRAPHY. G.M. Alberton, et al., "Extensor Triggering in de Quervain's Stenosing Tenosynovitis," *Journal of Hand Surgery* (v.24, 1999); M. Chammas, et al., "Dupuytren's Disease, Carpal Tunnel Syndrome, Trigger Finger, and Diabetes Mellitus," *ANZ Journal of Surgery* (June 2006); R.P. Hertz and E.A. Emmett, "Risk Factors for Occupational Hand Injury," *Journal of Occupational Medicine* (v.28, 1986); M.C. de Krom, et al., "Carpal Tunnel Syndrome: Prevalence in the General Population," *Journal of Clinical Epidemiology* (v. 282/2, 1992).

MALA GURBANI
UNIVERSITY OF SOUTHERN CALIFORNIA

Haploid

For organisms, such as humans, which carry two copies of each chromosome in somatic (nonreproductive) cells, a haploid cell is one that has only one of each chromosome. The haploid number, N, is the number of chromosomes in a haploid cell. For humans, with 23 pairs of chromosomes in somatic cells, germ cells (sperm and eggs) are haploid cells with 23 unpaired chromosomes each.

The haploid origin of a chromosome is used by scientists to match samples of DNA to individuals in a variety of settings.

Given that a normal human typically has two alleles of each gene (one on each chromosome), it follows that at any given locus only one of the two alleles is represented in a given germ cell. Thus, we might imagine that each locus would determine two haploid germ cells. As reproduction requires the combination of germ cells from two different individuals, human reproduction represents the opportunity for up to four distinct combinations of haploid germ cells.

Once the particular combination of haploid cells is determined during fertilization, though, the maternal or paternal haploid origin of each chromosome will not, except in the case of a select few diseases such as Angelman and Prader-Willi syndromes—the uniparental disomies—be significant in the expression of genes. The relationship between particular loci and their haploid origin is not entirely without value, however. If individual chromosomes, or portions thereof, are sequenced, a genotype for a DNA sequence that came from a single parent can be identified: a haplotype. Shared haplotypes are indicative of relatedness. By comparing haplotypes of sufficient length or haplotypes that are sufficiently rare, it is possible to determine if two individuals share a common ancestor.

SEE ALSO: Base Sequence; Crossing Over.

BIBLIOGRAPHY. Mark Kirkpatrick, ed., *Evolution of Haploid-Diploid Life Cycles: 1993 Symposium on Some Mathematical Questions in Biology* (American Mathematical Society, 1993); R.L. Nussbaum, et al., *Thompson & Thompson: Genetics in Medicine*, 6th ed., revised reprint (Saunders, 2004).

BIMAL P. CHAUDHARI
BOSTON UNIVERSITY

Hardy, James D. (1918–2003)

James D. Hardy was an American surgeon who pioneered transplant operations with three landmark cases: the first human lung transplant in 1963; the first animal-to-human heart transplant in 1964, which caused a heated debate on its ethical and moral consequences; and a double-lung transplant leaving the heart in place in 1987.

Hardy was born on May 14, 1918, the son of a lime plant owner. He grew up in Alabama where he started his premedical studies at the University of Alabama. As that university only had two-year medical programs, Hardy transferred to the University of Pennsylvania where he received the M.D. in 1942. He completed his internship and residence in internal medicine at the Hospital of the University of Pennsylvania, where he became convinced of the importance of combining research and clinical practice. During World War II, Hardy worked in the 81st field hospital in Germany, where he decided to switch from medicine to surgery.

After the war, Hardy again joined the University of Pennsylvania where he received a Damon Runyon Clinical Research Fellowship to study the use of heavy water in the measurement of body fluids. This research earned Hardy the Master of Medical Science in physiological chemistry from the university in 1951. That same year, Hardy moved back to his native South becoming Assistant Professor of Surgery at the University of Tennessee at Memphis and Director of Surgical Research. In 1953, Hardy was appointed Chair of Surgery. Two years later, the university started a four-year medical school in Jackson, and Hardy became the first Chair of Surgery in the new center.

He held this position until 1987 and it was in this capacity that he performed the transplant operations that would make him famous throughout the world. The most controversial of Hardy's transplant was by far the chimpanzee-to-man heart transplant performed in 1964. The operation attracted criticism also from some of Hardy's colleagues. In the long run, Hardy's animal-to-human transplant helped to establish a more secularized vision of the human body rather than the recipient of a man's soul. During his long career, Hardy authored several books on surgery, served as editor in chief of academic surgery journals, and was a member of important surgery associations. He was also the 12th recipient of the prestigious Rudolph Matas Award in Cardiovascular Surgery.

SEE ALSO: Surgery.

BIBLIOGRAPHY. James D. Hardy, *The Academic Surgeon: An Autobiography* (Magnolia Mansions Press, 2003); James D. Hardy, *The World of Surgery, 1945–1985: Memoirs of One Participant* (University of Pennsylvania Press, 1986).

LUCA PRONO
INDEPENDENT SCHOLAR

Hardy-Weinberg Law

The Hardy-Weinberg law is an equation used in genetics that describes the distribution of alleles in a given population. The equation is based on the idea that in sexually reproducing populations, it is possible to mathematically relate the prevalence of alleles of a particular gene to the resulting genotypes (individual combination of alleles). The Hardy-Weinberg law not only describes the frequency of possible genotypic combinations based on allele prevalence, but it also potentially describes the subsequent frequency of the phenotypes predicted by the expression of those alleles.

HARDY-WEINBERG EQUATION

The simplest version of the Hardy-Weinberg law describes the distribution of a non-sex-linked allele with only two variations (which we call "a" and "b") found in a single locus on the chromosome of an organism that sexually reproduces randomly. The equation can be described as follows:

$$q^2 + 2pq + p^2 = 1$$

p = frequency of allele "a"
q = frequency of allele "b"

q^2 describes the frequency of homozygous genotype "aa" (and the resulting phenotype), $2pq$ describes heterozygous genotype "ab," and p^2 describes the frequency of homozygous genotype "bb." The sum of genotype frequencies is always 1.

ASSUMPTIONS

These rules hold constant so long as certain assumptions are met: 1.) The alleles in question do not mutate drastically beyond normal rate over time; 2.) the population is large enough that the allelic distribution is immune to the effects of random genetic mutation (genetic drift); 3.) all individuals have an equal chance of successfully mating with each other; 4.) selection does not occur on the basis of phenotypic expression, and 5.) no migration occurs in or out of the population.

We use the following example to illustrate the principles illustrated in the equation above. If the frequency of allele "a" is known to be 0.8, and the frequency of allele "b" is 0.2, then the frequency of the respective genotypes is per Table 1. The resulting phenotypic frequency depends on whether expression of one of the alleles dominates. If "a" is a dominant allele, then the predicted combined frequency of phenotypes "aa" and "ab" will be 0.96, or 96 percent of the population, while the expression of recessive allele "b" will be only through genotype "bb," which constitutes 0.04, or 4 percent of the population.

Table 1. Hardy-Weinberg Expression Example

Genotype	Hardy-Weinberg Expression	Genotypic Frequency
aa	p^2	$0.8^2 = 0.64$
ab	$2pq$	$2(0.8)(0.2) = 0.32$
bb	q^2	$0.2^2 = 0.04$
Aa + ab + bb	$q^2 + 2pq + p^2$	**0.64 + 0.32 + 0.04 = 1.00**

POTENTIAL MODIFICATIONS

The Hardy-Weinberg equation can be modified to account for more complex patterns, including genes that have more than two alleles or are sex linked.

SEE ALSO: Gene Pool; Genes and Gene Therapy; Genetic Code; Genetics.

BIBLIOGRAPHY. William S. Klug and Michael R. Cummings, *Concepts of Genetics* (Prentice-Hall, 2002) Phillip McClean, "Population and Evolutionary Genetics: The Hardy-Weinberg Law," http://www.ndsu.edu/instruct/mcclean/plsc431/popgen/popgen3.htm (cited July 2007).

Constance W. Liu, M.D.
Case Western Reserve University

Head and Brain Injuries

Around the world each year, over 1 million people die and 1 million more are disabled from head and brain injuries. Despite their status as a global epidemic, head and brain injuries are also considered a silent epidemic. Serious head and brain injury can occur even without a loss of consciousness and can be overlooked following traffic accidents and sports injuries. A lack of understanding about the nature of head and brain injury among the general public, as well as lack of affordable, accessible medical care, prevents people

from seeking treatment after sustaining such trauma. Head injury is a trauma to the head that may or may not involve the brain. Head injuries are classified as internal or external and are further categorized by mechanism, morphology, and severity. Practical prevention and education about head and brain injuries among the general public, as well as effective diagnosis, treatment, and rehabilitation services for affected individuals are of global health importance.

Head injury is a trauma to the head that may or may not involve the brain. Brain injury is often used synonymously with head injury though the latter may not actually involve any neurological complications. Head injuries may be internal or external and can be categorized by mechanism (closed injury or penetrating injury), morphology (fractures, focal intracranial injury, or diffuse intracranial injury), and severity (mild, moderate, or severe). An external head injury is one that does not affect the skull or brain. External injuries may involve a laceration which causes profuse bleeding due to the thousands of blood vessels in the scalp, or trauma which may cause swelling due to fluid or blood buildup beneath the scalp. These injuries can take days or weeks to heal.

Internal head injuries are further classified as closed head injury or penetrating head injury. Closed head injuries include any injury in which the scalp is not broken open. Closed head injury may occur with or without damage to the bones of the skull. For example, if a car stops suddenly and passengers experience whiplash, the brain may be jarred and result in concussion although the skull remains intact. Alternately, if the bones of the skull are smashed into the brain as a result of blunt trauma, but the scalp is not lacerated, this too is categorized as a closed head injury. Penetrating head injury occurs when an object transects the scalp, skull, and brain. A bullet that passes into the brain is an example of a penetrating head injury; wounds of this type can cause skull fragments to pierce the brain tissue and are susceptible to infection.

Skull fractures are the result of any head injury that breaks the bones of the cranium. All skull fractures are internal injuries though they may not be outwardly visible. Symptoms of skull fractures can include: blood or clear fluid leaking from the nose or ear, unequal pupil size, discoloration around the eyes or ears, swelling or indentation of the cranium, loss of consciousness, memory lapse, blurred vision, confusion, irritability, or headache. Skull fractures are categorized as linear, depressed, diastatic, or basilar. Linear fractures are a simple break in the bone that does not require serious medical intervention. Depressed fractures are a dented deformation of the skull that often requires surgical intervention. Diastatic fractures occur along the natural suture lines of the cranial bones causing the space between them to widen. This type of injury is more common among infants prior to fusion of these bones. Basilar fractures occur at the base of the skull and may affect the cribiform plate, occipital, temporal, frontal, and sphenoid bones. This type of injury is rare and requires more force than a cranial vault fracture. However, basilar fractures are generally considered severe as they are more likely to be associated with spinal cord, blood vessel, and nerve damage and are susceptible to meningeal infection.

Focal intracranial injury denotes trauma confined to one area. These injuries may be extra-axial (within the skull but outside the brain), or intra-axial (within the brain). As the latter are specific to brain injuries, extra-axial injuries will be discussed here. Extra-axial focal intracranial injuries include subdural hematoma, epidural hematoma, and subarachnoid hemorrhage. A subdural hematoma is the collection of blood from a ruptured blood vessel between the arachnoid membrane and the dura; an epidural hematoma occurs between the skull and dura. Both subdural and epidural hematoma can be dangerous to brain function as they may increase intracranial pressure and interrupt the flow of cerebrospinal fluid and oxygen. Diffuse intracranial injury often indicates damage to several areas of the white matter of the brain. This typically includes concussion, coma, or diffuse axonal injury.

The severity of a head or brain injury may not always be immediately evident. The most widely used tool in emergency assessment of head and brain trauma is the Glasgow Coma Scale (GCS). This standardized system scores patient competency in eye opening, motor and verbal response; scores between 15 and 13 are considered mild brain injuries, 12 to nine is moderate, and eight to three to are severe. Mild, moderate, and severe are terms used for initial assessment and should not be considered indicators of long-term outcomes. A GCS score can be skewed by shock, intoxication, hypoxemia, metabolic disturbance, spinal cord and orbital injuries, and age. Diagnoses and treatment strategies are based on further physical examination, observation, blood

tests, imaging including X-ray, magnetic resonance imaging (MRI), computed tomography (CT), and/or electroencephalogram (EEG). Treatment will vary by severity of injury and availability of resources.

Foregoing treatment for an initial mild head or brain injury can be risky. After one brain injury has been sustained, the likelihood of recurrence is two to four times greater, placing persons at risk for second impact syndrome or diffuse cerebral swelling. Compared to someone who has never experienced brain injury, the likelihood of recurrence is eightfold after the incurrence of two brain injuries.

A six-year investigation into prevention, diagnosis, and treatment of mild traumatic brain injury by the World Health Organization Collaborating Centre Task Force found that a consensus among experts is lacking. The task force concluded that "clear, comprehensive, evidence-based guidelines dealing with mild traumatic brain injury are urgently needed." Of the reported traumatic brain injuries, approximately 80 percent are classified as mild traumatic brain injuries. As it is extremely challenging to collect reliable data on cases of head and brain injury in the absence of hospitalization, the actual number of persons experiencing mild traumatic brain injury is probably much higher than current data reveals. Practical prevention and education about head and brain injuries among the general public could decrease their occurrence. Effective diagnosis, treatment, and rehabilitation services for affected individuals are of global health importance and can have a profound effect on the quality of life of individuals, families, and communities.

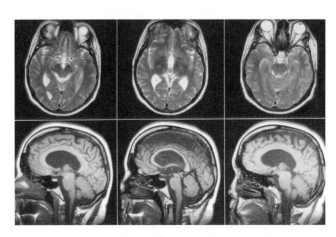

CT scans are used in diagnosing the severity of a head or brain injury, along with X-rays, MRIs, and EEGs.

SEE ALSO: Brain Injuries; Concussion; Neurology; Rehabilitation; Sports Injuries; Stroke.

BIBLIOGRAPHY. Christopher J.L. Murray and Alan D. Lopez, *Global Health Statistics* (Harvard University Press, 1996). Paul Peloso, et al., "Critical Evaluation of the Existing Guidelines on Mild Traumatic Brain Injury," *Journal of Rehabilitation Medicine* (v.36/43, 2004); Ian Roberts, "The CRASH Trial: The First Large-scale, Randomized, Controlled Trial in Head Injury," *Critical Care* (October 2001).

JENNIFER HISSETT
UNIVERSITY OF COLORADO AT DENVER
HEALTH SERVICES CENTER

Head and Brain Malformations

The most relevant head malformation is a condition called craniosynostosis, or the premature fusion of one or more of the head's sutures. The human head is composed of multiple bones held together by several sutures, namely the metopic, coronal, sagittal, and lambdoid sutures. Simple craniosynostosis is when only one suture is involved, while compound craniosynostosis involves two or more sutures. The most common suture affected is the sagittal suture (50 percent of cases), followed by the coronal suture (25 percent), and metopic suture (10 percent). Lambdoid synostosis is very rare, with an incidence of 3 per 100,000 births. The overall prevalence of craniosynostosis is approximately 1 per 2,000 births, or 0.05 percent of children. One-fifth of craniosynostosis cases occur as one of more than 150 different syndromes, while the remainder occur as an isolated, nonsyndromic condition.

The etiology of craniosynostosis is unknown. Several risk factors for the development of this condition have been identified and can be categorized by maternal factors, paternal factors, and infant factors. Maternal factors include white race, advanced age, smoking habits, residence at high altitude, and use of certain medications. Paternal factors include specific occupations, such as in agriculture, forestry, or mechanics. Infant factors include male sex. Genetics also play a role, given that a certain percentage of cases are familial and autosomal dominant in inheritance.

One known genetic mutation is in the gene encoding fibroblast growth factor receptor (FGFR), which is known to be expressed in the cranial sutures. Therefore, if a receptor is produced with a faulty molecular structure or in insufficient quantities, the skull's sutures may not fuse correctly.

Craniosynostosis is diagnosed by physical examination, X-rays, and computed tomography (CT). Physical examination findings may include a misshapen head as well as nonpatent suture lines and fontanelles (soft spots) on the child's head. The signs of craniosynostosis on X-ray include bony bridging across the suture that produces beaking or heaping up of bone; sutures that appear very straight and narrow; and loss of suture clarity. Because CT offers a clearer picture than X-rays, it is the most reliable diagnostic tool.

Craniosynostosis that goes uncorrected may result in increased intracranial pressure (ICP), an asymmetric face, malocclusion (misaligned teeth), and strabismus. Correction, therefore, is surgical and is preferably performed between 3 and 9 months of age by a pediatric neurosurgeon. The different surgical options include strip craniectomy and cranial vault remodeling. Strip craniectomy can now be performed with a minimally invasive, endoscopic technique.

By definition, syndromic craniosynostosis involves multiple organ systems, that is, cardiac, renal, and musculoskeletal. The two most common syndromes are Crouzon's disease and Apert's syndrome, both of which are caused by autosomal dominant mutations on the FGFR2 gene on chromosome 10. The incidence of Crouzon's disease is one per 25,000 and it accounts for 5 percent of craniosynostosis cases. External findings include wide-set and bulging eyes (hypertelorism and proptosis, respectively), beaked nose, and cleft palate. The patient's brain may be affected by hydrocephalus and/or Chiari malformation.

Apert's syndrome affects one per 160,000 and is marked by syndactyly (webbed fingers/toes), hypertelorism, and shallow eye orbits. Intracranial findings in a patient with Apert's syndrome may include megalocephaly and agenesis of the corpus callosum, both of which may contribute to cognitive deficits. Patients may also have cardiac and renal anomalies, such as atrial/ventricular septal defect and hydronephrosis, respectively.

One condition that can be mistaken for craniosynostosis is deformational (positional) plagiocephaly, or flattened head syndrome. This condition has increased in prevalence over the past few decades to about 33 per 10,000 births, or approximately seven times more common than craniosynostosis. The increased prevalence is because of increased efforts to have infants sleep on their backs to prevent sudden infant death syndrome (SIDS), as well as increased awareness of the problem. Plagiocephaly is most commonly caused simply by the passage of the baby's head through the birth canal. Fortunately, plagiocephaly can usually be corrected by alternating the position of the child until the head corrects itself.

SEE ALSO: Brain Malformations; Cleft Lip and Palate; Genetics; Hydrocephalus; Sudden Infant Death Syndrome (SIDS).

BIBLIOGRAPHY. Haidar Kabbani and Talkad S. Raghuveer, "Craniosynostosis," *American Family Physician* (v.69, 2004); P. J. Vinken and G. W. Bruyn, *Congenital Malformations of the Brain and Skull* (Elsevier/North Holland, 1977).

KHOI D. THAN, M.D.
JOHNS HOPKINS UNIVERSITY SCHOOL OF MEDICINE

Head and Neck Cancer

In the United States, cancers of the head and neck are most commonly a result of repeated exposure to toxins, such as cigarette smoke or alcohol. As a matter of fact, the combined effects of exposure to cigarette smoke and alcohol is multiplicative in head and neck cancers (HNCs). Signs and symptoms of possible HNCs include a lump in the throat, a growth in the oral cavity, difficulty swallowing, changes in vocal sound, or changes in skin. Therapies for HNCs typically involve a combination of chemoradiation therapy and surgical resection. Because such procedures would be carried out by a team of otolaryngologists and oncologists, cancers of the brain will not be discussed as that falls under the jurisdiction of neurosurgeons.

NASAL CAVITY

Cancers in the nasal cavity occur around the nasal sinuses, thus termed *paranasal sinus cancers*. The most common presenting symptoms of cancer of the sinuses are facial or dental pain, epistaxis, or frequent nose bleeds, and persistent unilateral nasal obstruction. These cancers have a multitude of causation including occupational exposure to toxic vapors such as formaldehyde. In addition, genomic evidence of the presence of infectious agents such as human papillomavirus 16 and 18 and Epstein-Barr virus in biopsies of paranasal sinus cancers points to virus causality. Finally, cigarette smoke and air pollution are linked to cancers of the nasal cavity.

As in HNCs, the most common cancer of the nasal sinuses is squamous cell carcinoma. They are relatively slow growing and well differentiated.

Esthesioneurblastoma is a rare cancer of the nasal cavity involving the olfactory epithelium. This cancer is believed to derive from uncontrolled proliferation of neural progenitors.

ORAL CAVITY

Squamous cell carcinoma, a cancer that grows exophytically and is ulcerative, is the most common form of cancer found in the oral cavity. These cancers tend to occur later in life. Major predisposing factors leading to squamous cell cancers in the oral cavity include leukoplakia, infection with human papillomavirus (types 16, 18, and 33), alcohol abuse, and mechanical irritation.

It is common place for smokers to switch from cigarettes to chewing tobacco in an attempt to prevent lung cancer. What many do not realize, however, is that they are increasing the probability of inducing cancer of the mouth. Patients who have chewed large amounts of tobacco over long periods can develop leukoplakia, a precancerous lesion that presents as white plaques in the oral mucosa. These plaques are overgrowths of squamous epithelia and are usually dysplastic. Leukoplakia plaques, which are often multifocal, can be found on the vermilion border of the lower lip, buccal mucosa, hard or soft palates, as well as at the bottom of the mouth. While most are a result of long-term tobacco use (including that derived from smoking), they can also be a result of chronic friction (such as from braces or dentures), excessive alcohol consumption, and some foods. About 3 to 6 percent of leukoplakia lesions convert to squamous cell carcinoma.

Gingival cancers typically occur in women on the lower alveolar ridge or gum line around the sixth decade of life. Due to tight adherence between the gum and the mandibular periosteum, these cancers can invade the mandible leading to bone damage.

SALIVARY GLAND

Of the three salivary glands—parotid, submandibular, and sublingual—the cancer most commonly involves the parotid gland (around 70 percent). Of those, about 15 to 25 percent are malignant. Unlike other HNCs, salivary gland cancer is not highly correlated with smoking and excessive alcohol consumption. Instead, exposure to radiation and infectious agents such as Epstein-Barr virus has been linked.

Pleomorphic adenomas are benign encapsulated gland tumors comprised of both epithelial and stromal or supporting cells. Histologically, they appear as collections of spindle and stellate cells. Parotid gland tumors can result in impingement on the CN VII (facial nerve) which is almost always a sign of malignancy. Malignant conversion of pleomorphic adenomas results in malignant mixed salivary gland tumor.

Warthin tumor (papillary cystadenoma lymphomatosum) is a benign encapsulated growth with many cysts. These tumors rarely convert to malignant forms and often occur bilaterally. Intraductal papillomas are benign growths of the submucosa of glandular ducts.

Sjogren's syndrome is a major cause of benign proliferation of the parotid gland. Sjogren's syndrome is an autoimmune disease more commonly affecting women. It is characterized by nontender, enlarged parotid glands which have a higher predisposition for converting into a lymphoma.

LARYNX AND ESOPHAGUS

The larynx is the most common site of HNC occurrence in the United States. Fortunately, detection of laryngeal cancers is able to occur during early stages because these cancers commonly affect the patient's voice, causing hoarseness. Laryngeal cancers arise from environmental factors including asbestos or radiation exposure and long-term tobacco and alcohol use, the effects of which are synergistic. The most common laryngeal cancer is squamous cell carcinoma, which has a pearl-gray appearance on gross examination. Because this cancer can occur on the vocal cords, surgical resection leads to damage or loss of the patient's voice.

Esophageal cancer comes in two forms: squamous cell carcinomas and adenocarcinomas. Usually, squamous cell carcinomas are found in the upper two-thirds of the esophagus, while adenocarcinomas occur in the distal one-third of the esophagus.

Squamous cell carcinoma of the esophagus is believed to be associated with environmental factors including exposure to toxins, such as alcohol consumption and tobacco use, and dietary issues. Deficiency in vitamins A, B_1, B_2, B_6, and C, deficiency in zinc and molybdenum, food contamination with fungi, or high concentration of nitrates in food are common causes of squamous cell carcinoma of the esophagus. Adenocarcinomas typically arise from Barrett esophagus, a complication of long-standing acid reflux. Repeated trauma of stomach acid exposure can lead to metaplasia of the normal distal epithelium of the esophagus from stratified squamous epithelium to columnar epithelium with goblet cells. Diagnosis of HNCs begins with localization of the tumor via imaging techniques such as computed tomography scans followed up with fine-needle aspiration biopsies. Although HNCs result from a large array of causes, the most common treatment for HNCs is surgical resection with and without adjuvant radiation therapy.

SEE ALSO: Cancer (General); Cancer Alternative Therapy; Cancer Chemotherapy; Cancer Radiation Therapy; Cancer—Coping with Cancer.

BIBLIOGRAPHY. H. Mineta, et al., "Human Papilloma Virus (HPV) Type 16 and 18 Detected in Head and Neck Squamous Cell Carcinoma," *Anticancer Research* (v.18/6B, 1998); R.H. Spiro, "Salivary Neoplasms: Overview of a 35-Year Experience with 2,807 Patients," *Head & Neck Surgery* (v.8/3, 1986); M.R. Spitz, "Epidemiology and Risk Factors for Head and Neck Cancer," *Seminars in Oncology* (v.21/3, 1994).

KIMBERLY GOKOFFSKI
UNIVERSITY OF CALIFORNIA, IRVINE

Head Lice

Three species of lice (small, wingless insects) infest humans—*Pediculus humanus capitis* (head lice), *Pediculus humanus corpus* (body lice) and *Phthirus pubis* (pubic lice). Many treatments exist, and patients need to ensure removal of the lice from hair as well as clothing.

Lice live and reproduce only on humans, transmitted by person-to-person contact or clothing, as human lice can survive on fabric for 10 days. Lice cycle through three stages—egg, nymph, and adult. Eggs are deposited on the hair shaft, providing warmth for incubation. The baby louse (nymph) hatches, leaving behind nits (casts of the empty egg)—tiny, yellow/white ovals, firmly cemented to the hair shaft. Visualization of the louse or detection of eggs within five millimeters of scalp permits diagnosis. Nits seen further along the shaft indicate prior infestation and may not need treatment.

Head lice do not transmit disease, only itching. Lice require several blood meals daily and have special mouthpieces for this purpose. Saliva is injected into the feeding site, causing sensitization to foreign antigen, eventually causing itching with repeated bites. Delousing options include chemical treatments with Federal Drug Administration (FDA) approved over-the-counter preparations containing permethrin or pyrethrins, to manual removal. Medications do not kill unhatched embryos; hence, repeat administration must be done after a week to kill newly hatched nymphs. Fine-toothed combs will remove eggs, and hair must be combed daily until there are no further signs of infestation. Vinegar will loosen eggs from the hair shaft, permitting easier removal.

All contacts of the infected individual must be treated simultaneously prevent reinfestation. Bedding and clothes must be washed on the hottest setting. Items unable to be washed should be double-bagged in closed dark trash bags, set aside for three days, then washed. Dry cleaning and ironing will kill lice and eggs. Hair implements should be soaked in a weak bleach solution or rubbing alcohol for one hour. Carpets must be vacuumed and other fabrics treated with insecticides. This entire process must be repeated in five to seven days to prevent reinfestation with newly hatched nymphs.

SEE ALSO: Hair Diseases And Hair Loss; Infant and Toddler Health, Infectious Diseases (General).

BIBLIOGRAPHY. Pediculosis.com, www.pediculosis.com; www.cdc.gov/ncidod/dpd/parasites/lice/default.htm (cited October 2006); A. Goldstein, B. Goldstein, "Pediculosis," www.uptodate.com (cited October 2006).

GAUTAM J. DESAI, D.O.
KAREN H. WENDEL
KANSAS CITY UNIVERSITY OF MEDICINE AND
BIOSCIENCES COLLEGE OF OSTEOPATHIC MEDICINE

Headache and Migraine

Complaints of headache are common making evaluation difficult. Essential to diagnosis and management is working with the patient to determine medical and family medical history in addition to symptoms. Treatment must be based on the cause of the headache. Patients assist in the diagnosis by providing information to describe the pain in relation to intensity (how much it hurts), quality (stabbing, throbbing, ice pick, etc.) site of pain (neck, forehead, localized, on both sides, etc.), associated symptoms (vision disturbances, vertigo, nausea and vomiting, etc.), and duration and frequency of pain.

Sudden onset headache and major complaint of headache without trauma necessitates determining cause and provide immediate treatment for any underlying causes for which the headache may be a secondary symptom. The underlying cause may be vascular, infection, intracranial masses, preeclampsia, carbon monoxide poisoning. In addition to taking vital signs and checking eyes/vision, performing neurological, motor and sensory testing, the physician may also order further tests. Additional tests include blood testing, electrocardiogram, electroencephalogram, computed tomography (CT) scan or magnetic resonance imaging (MRI) will exclude intracranial mass lesion, MR angiography or venography can detect suspected aneurysms and weak areas of vessels. Lumbar puncture will exclude infections.

After determining medical history, physical examination and testing the diagnosis is determined and treatment options considered. The two possible diagnoses for headache are secondary (a symptom of an underlying cause) or primary (tension headache or migraine). Secondary headache pain is a symptom of other illnesses, due to injury, infection, brain malformation, depression, tumors, spinal headache, sinus congestion, aneurysm, giant cell arteritis (inflammation of blood vessels in the head most often seen in elderly patients), cough, hypertension, exertion (exercise including sex), mountain sickness (hypoxia at altitudes 6,560 feet above sea level.

When the diagnosis is primary headache, the headache itself is the illness. The most common and least debilitating primary headache is the ice-cream headache. Other headache triggers include stress, weather or season changes, certain foods and alcohol, and flickering light.

TENSION HEADACHES

The pain has a tight pressing quality, worse with stress or at the end of the day. The pain may be generalized or intense around the neck or back of head. Tension headaches are often triggered by stress, fatigue, noise, and glare.

Treatment includes analgesics and relaxation techniques of massage, hot baths, and biofeedback. When medications such as aspirin, ibuprofen, acetaminophen, and similar drugs fail, using migraine medication may be effective.

Alternative treatments or supportive therapies for tension headache include acupressure, acupuncture, chiropractic, Feldenkrais method (touch to improve movement and movement awareness), hypnotherapy, meditation, myotherapy (deep muscle massage), osteopathic medicine, qigong (Chinese discipline of breathing and exercise), and reflexology (applying pressure to specific points on the foot)

Some headache triggers include stress, weather or season changes, certain foods and alcohol and flickering light.

CLUSTER HEADACHES

Most common in middle-aged males, the pain is excruciating and accompanied by nasal congestion, tears, and red or swollen eyes. Cluster headaches often occur at the same time each day experienced. The pain may be located around the eye, temple, and upper jaw. Cluster headaches are often triggered by alcohol and certain foods. During an acute attack, treatment with sumatriptan or dihydroergotamine can relieve the pain. The recurring nature of these headaches indicates treatment with maintenance medications.

MIGRAINE

While scientists continue to search for specific etiology some studies have connected migraine activity to the neurotransmitter serotonin, brain hyperexcitablilty, the aura is caused by a wave of increased electrical activity and blood flow followed by a loss of electrical activity and decreased blood flow, the area of brain in upper brainstem holds pain sensors, inflammation of the meninges or blood vessels causes throbbing pain, scalp sensitivity to touch and increased pain with bending, straining, or shaking head. Hormonal aspects may trigger migraine either with rising estrogen levels or by taking oral contraceptives or hormone replacement.

Migraines can be chronic occurring more than 15 days per month or episodic occurring less than 15 days per month to as few as one per year. A migraine headache may result in sensitivity to light and have an "aura" followed by severe throbbing unilateral headache lasting from a few hours to one to two days. Migraines are more common in women because of hormonal fluctuations. They start in adolescence and early adulthood and decrease with advancing age. They may occur once a year or as often as one to two times per week, and often after a stressful event.

An aura is associated with an abnormal release of serotonin from platelets and the throbbing headache associated with decrease of platelet and serum serotonin levels. Other chemical triggers include falling estrogen levels and elevated levels of prostaglandin E1.

Persons who experience migraine headaches may experience a common migraine or migraine with aura. Common migraine involves headache on one side, sensitivity to light and/or sound and accompanied by nausea and vomiting. Complete migraine has specific stages: pre-headache, aura, headache, and resolution. The stage before headache includes one or more symptoms of feeling sluggish, depressed, yawning, experiencing mood changes, or irritability. The aura includes visual aura, floaters in front of the eyes, hallucinations, seeing flashing lights, experiencing decreased vision or sensory aura feeling tingling and numbness. Headache is pulsating, throbbing pain. The resolution stage follows the resolution of the pain and feelings or sensations, out of proportion, depression or tiredness, joy, or mania. Two types of rare migraine basilar artery migraine and ophthalmoplegic migraine involve severe visual disturbances along with the throbbing pain. Basilar artery migraine is experienced with blindness, dizziness, ringing in the ears, and facial numbness leading to disturbed consciousness and confusion. In ophthalmoplegic migraine pain around the eye, nausea and vomiting, double vision is due to nerve palsy with the potential to lead to long-term nerve deficiency.

The pathophysiology of migraine appears to include vasomotor mechanism and treatment with medications to relieve arterial pressure and related to the neurotransmitter serotonin. For many years, the common medication for treating migraine was ergot alkaloids. The specific action of these medications also had diagnostic potential, if the medication worked, the headache was migraine. Current treatment during an acute attack includes a variety of fast-acting medications in injectable, nasal and oral forms, with sumatriptan often considered the drug of choice.

Alternative therapies include acupuncture, Alexander technique (inhibition of habitual muscular movement and encouraging the body's natural reflexes to take over), biofeedback, energy medicine (electrical nerve stimulation by electrodes placed near painful site or in proximity to the nerve supplying the painful area), and hypnotherapy. Some physicians experiment with and recommend herbal and mineral remedies to their patients including feverfew, magnesium, and riboflavin.

People who experience frequent headaches may benefit from following a healthy lifestyle including-monitoring their diets, getting enough sleep, and exercising. Patients can take an active part in their healthcare by keeping a journal to record information pertinent to the headaches, which will help their physician with a proper diagnosis and treatment and to establisyh goals for pain management. For additional information, the American Council for Headache Education maintains a Web site at www.achenet.org.

SEE ALSO: Biofeedback; Chiropractic; Osteopathy.

BIBLIOGRAPHY. Michael J. Aminoff, "Nervous System" in *Current Medical Diagnosis & Treatment 2004* (Lange, 2004); David W. Sifton, *The PDR Family Guide to Natural Medicines & Healing Therapies* (Three Rivers Press, 1999); William B. Young, and Stephen D. Silberstein, *Migraine and Other Headaches* (American Academy of Neurology, 2004).

LYN MICHAUD
INDEPENDENT SCHOLAR

Healthcare, Africa

The healthcare system in Africa today varies hugely. In some areas of the continent, diagnosis and treatment is excellent, but there are also many other areas where the system is clearly substandard. Much of this is because of historical reasons, and the systems introduced or neglected by various colonial powers and, after independence, the governments of the respective countries, not having the resources, human or financial, to do everything that was needed to be done.

Prior to the arrival of the colonial powers, there were a range of healthcare systems used in Africa. In Ancient Egypt, surviving clay tablets show that the doctors were often sent to study in Syria and Assyria. It is also clear that they had identified and differentiated between about 200 types of illnesses, with substantial knowledge about the human anatomy, as evident in their embalming processes. The kings of Persia employed Egyptian physicians, and the Greek writer Herodotus describes the specialties of the doctors. These advances in healthcare also influenced the civilizations near Egypt—both in north Africa and in Sudan and Ethiopia.

The Carthaginian Empire tended to draw much of their medical sciences from the Phoenicians and also the Greeks, with Roman healthcare ideas tending to dominate north Africa from the 3rd century B.C.E. These gradually came to see the body as being made up of humors and medical problems being an imbalance of the different humors. With the spread of Arab culture from the 6th and 7th centuries C.E., there was a change in healthcare, with many problems having a more scientific diagnosis. The nature of healthcare was much advanced by the great Arab medical writer Avicenna (980–1037 C.E.) whose ideas were popular in north Africa for many centuries.

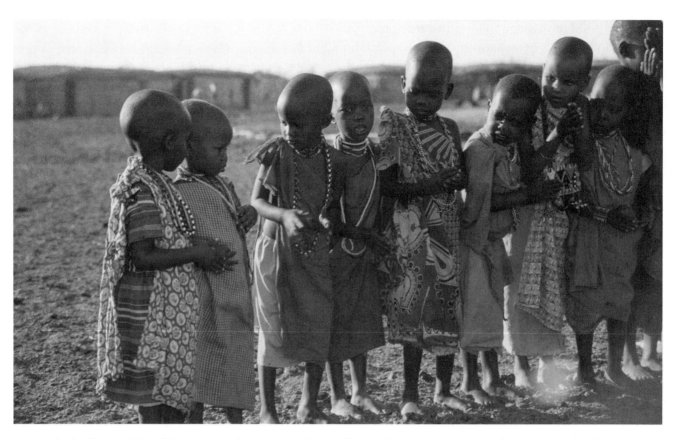

In areas that had large British and European populations, such as South Africa, Southern Rhodesia (modern-day Zimbabwe), and Kenya (pictured above), the level of healthcare was better than in the areas that had small white populations.

In sub-Saharan Africa, healthcare was generally fairly primitive and relied heavily on the use of witch doctors and shamans, as well as on herbal cures and pastes, some of which were effective at dealing with particular ailments. Many of the illnesses which existed during this period remain prevalent with several strains of malaria, yellow fever, typhus, sleeping sickness, "river blindness," cholera, and polio. There have also been problems with leprosy, snakebites, and a host of other medical problems.

The early European colonial powers had to quickly introduce healthcare systems largely because of the number of early sailors and soldiers who died from tropical diseases. In particular, malaria remained a major problem until the 20th century, with a Nigerian nationalist group using the mosquito as their symbol on the basis that it had resulted in the deaths of more Europeans than from any other single cause.

The Portuguese were the first European power to make extensive voyages around the coast of Africa, and the first to establish large numbers of bases on the continent. They drew some of their healthcare ideas from Garcia de Orta (1501/02–68), a Portuguese Jewish physician who was able to work out cures for people suffering from some common tropical diseases, especially cholera. It was not long before the Portuguese established hospitals in their colonial possessions, but these only catered to Europeans and members of the local elite. In most of their colonies, the Europeans suffered most commonly from malaria, with treatment until the early 20th century being difficult until it was proven that the Anopheles mosquito was the vector by which people caught the disease. The Portuguese government sponsored a number of conferences on malaria and other tropical diseases, with a series of stamps issued in their colonies in December 1958 highlighting a Tropical Medicine Congress, and another series in 1962 about an antimalaria campaign, not just for prestige, but also to inform the local population.

Because of centuries of neglect, the healthcare system in most former Portuguese colonies remains poor, although in Angola, there are, on average, some 7.7 doctors and 115 nurses per 100,000 people. It is also estimated that 30 percent of the population can reach hospitals or clinics within an hour. The reason for this might be connected with Agostinho Neto (1922–79), the longtime nationalist leader and the first president after independence being a Lisbon-trained doctor. Much of this progress has also come from considerable expenditure by the present government during the last decade. By contrast in Mozambique, the civil war which wrecked the economy of the country since independence in 1975, there are 0.76 doctors per 100,000 people, and one hospital bed per 1,133 people. The healthcare services in Cape Verde are also poor with 17 doctors and 56 nurses per 100,000 people; with 17 doctors and 109 nurses per 100,000 people in Guinea-Bissau, 47 doctors and 127 nurses per 100,000 people in São Tomé.

Because of a historical agreement with the Portuguese, the Spanish had only a few isolated colonial possessions in Africa. Their original possessions in Morocco were mainly military and trading bases which had only primitive healthcare. The Spanish army, as with other colonial armies, had a number of military doctors and hospitals at their disposal. The settlers also had access to health services that were not made available to the locals. Later, during the early 20th century, in Spanish Morocco there was a great focus on eradicating diseases such as cholera and leprosy, with the Spanish colonial postal authorities issuing large numbers of "semipostal" stamps to raise money for healthcare. Toward the bottom end of the scale, since independence in 1968, the healthcare provisions in Equatorial Guinea remain very poor with only 25 doctors and 40 nurses per 100,000 people.

The first British settlements in Africa were often forts which usually included small garrison hospitals. As the settlements grew, these facilities steadily improved and hospitals were built. Among the many Britons who worked as doctors in Africa was Dr. David Livingstone (1813–73), the missionary and Hugh Lofting (1886–1947) who was also the creator of Doctor Doolittle. In the Sudan, Charles E.G. Beveridge, born in Samoa, and from an Australian family, worked for the Sudan Medical Services for most of his life. In the areas that had large British and European populations, such as South Africa, Southern Rhodesia (modern-day Zimbabwe), and

Kenya, the level of healthcare was better than in the areas that had small white populations. As many of the countries became independent during the 1950s and 1960s, there was a vast improvement in healthcare with help from the World Health Organization. Inoculations and greater health education helped improve life expectancy rates. Gradually, the governments have worked to erode the threat from malnutrition, malaria, cholera, and polio. With more people living longer, liver cancer and some other cancers have become more prevalent. However, during the late 1980s, life expectancy figures fell dramatically with the spread of HIV/AIDS, and the rise in the number of deaths from conditions which were affected by HIV such as pneumonia and Kaposi's sarcoma. With many wars in Africa, and many crises, the work of Médicine sans Frontières has saved the lives of many people, often in appalling conditions, and without much help from governments.

In South Africa, some of the best healthcare in Africa is available, but much of it is restricted to the major cities. The South African surgeon Dr. Christiaan Barnard (1922–2001) performed the first heart transplant operation on December 3, 1967. Areas that were formerly dark-skinned tend to have much lower healthcare available, with the statistics for the entire country being 56 doctors and 472 nurses per 100,000 people, one of the best rates in Africa. Of the former parts of British Africa, the ratios are only higher in Seychelles which as 132 doctors and 468 nurses per 100,000 people. In Namibia, the ratios are 30 doctors and 168 nurses per 100,000, in Botswana, the respective ratios are 24 and 219 per 100,000; the ratios in Nigeria are 19 nurses and 66 doctors.

During British colonial rule, healthcare provisions for Europeans in Southern Rhodesia were very good with Salisbury Hospital and Bulawayo Hospital having much of the equipment which one would have found in hospitals in Europe at the same time. Since independence in 1980, there have been attempts by the government to increase healthcare for the entire population, with a network of hospitals and rural health centers providing increasing levels of care, with Zimbabwe (as it became after 1980) having 14 doctors and 129 nurses per 100,000 people. In Swaziland, there are 15 doctors per 100,000 people; and in Kenya there are 13 doctors and 90 nurses per 100,000 people. Again, like Zimbabwe, Kenya had a significant European population and there are hundreds of hospitals and health centers throughout the country, with the provision of free medical care to all children and adult outpatients. The Kenya Medical Research Institute (KEMRI) was established in 1979 and has done much in recent years to coordinate healthcare. Accounts of the Kenyan medical services have been written by expatriate doctor Christopher Wilson and Canadian nurse Ruth S. Best.

The remainder of former British Africa has fared far worse with Sierra Leone, before the recent fighting, having 7.3 doctors and 33 nurses per 100,000 people, with 45 hospitals throughout the country. For the other countries, the ratio of doctors and nurses per 100,000 people are Zambia 6.9 and 113; Ghana 6.2 and 72; Lesotho 5.4 and 60; Tanzania 4.1 and 85; Gambia 3.5 and 1.3; and Uganda 0.4 and 19. One of the more well-known doctors in Tanzania, Emmanuel N. Ayim, originally from Ghana, is the father of Afro-German scholar May Ayim. The poor figures for Uganda come largely from the civil strife that it faced from the 1970s. Prior to that, the health system was relatively good—for a British African colony—with Denis Parsons Burkitt (1911–93) working there and coming across what became known as Burkitt's lymphoma, a cancer in the lymphatic system. In Malawi (formerly Nyasaland), despite Dr. Hastings Banda (1898–1997), a former doctor in Britain, running the country for the first 31 years after independence, it has only 51 hospitals and clinics and one of the lowest ratio of doctors and nurses 0.9 doctors and 3 nurses per 100,000 people.

In former French colonies in Africa, the two countries that have the best rates of healthcare are Algeria and Tunisia. In the former, the French army doctor Xavier Quatrefarges lived during the 1840s along with his wife Eliza Lynch, later first lady of Paraguay. The great Algerian-French writer Albert Camus (1913-1960), wrote *The Plague* (1947), an allegory described by way of an epidemic in a city in French Algeria. Nowadays, there are 85 doctors and 298 nurses per 100,000 persons, with medical care free for middle- and low-income earners, with healthcare good in the cities but still poor in remote parts of the country.

In Tunisia, there as 70 doctors and 286 nurses per 100,000 people, with massive improvements in healthcare during the 1980s and 1990s. In the rest of former French Africa, the healthcare system has been worse, with Congo having 25 doctors and 185 nurses per 100,000 people, with three general hospitals and over 500 medical centers throughout the country. In Djibouti, there are 14 doctors and 74 nurses per 100,000 people, and in Mauritania, the ratios of 14 doctors and 62 nurses must be seen in the context that there is only one hospital in the entire country, although there are 25 regional health centers.

In Guinea, there are 13 doctors and 56 nurses per 100,000 people, with the ratios in Madagascar being 11 doctors and 22 nurses; in the Cote d'Ivoire, nine doctors and 31 nurses; in Cameroon, 7.6 doctors and 37 nurses; in Togo, 7.6 doctors and 30 nurses; in Senegal, 7.5 doctors and 22 nurses; and in Comoros, 7.4 doctors and 34 nurses. In most of the rest of former French Africa, healthcare is far more rudimentary. There are only 5.7 doctors and 230 nurses per 100,000 in Benin; 4.7 doctors and 13 nurses per 100,000 in Mali; and 3.6 doctors and 37 nurses per 100,000 in Gabon. The healthcare service in Gabon has become most well-known by the work of Dr. Albert Schweitzer (1875-1965), the German doctor who moved to Lambaréné in Gabon where he rebuilt a derelict hospital and ran a leper colony until his death.

The Central African Republic has 3.5 doctors and 8.8 nurses per 100,000 people with few facilities available outside Bangui, the capital. In Niger, with 3.5 doctors and 23 nurses per 100,000 people, there are only two hospitals in the entire country, with only 32 percent of the population within one hour of access to appropriate medical care. Healthcare is even worse in Burkina Faso (formerly Upper Volta), where there are only 3.4 doctors and 20 nurses per 100,000 people, with only a third of the population having access to safe drinking water. In Chad, a third of the children under the age of 5 suffer from malnutrition, and with 3.3 doctors and 15 nurses per 100,000 people belies the fact that most of the health services are concentrated in the south.

The Germans and the Belgians, in their African colonies, provided hospitals for their own settlers and for other Europeans, but little or no healthcare for the local population. After World War I, the German colonies were taken over by the other colonial powers, with the Democratic Republic of Congo (formerly Belgian Congo and later Zaire) now having a reasonably extensive healthcare system with 6.9 doctors and 44 nurses per 100,000 people.

In neighboring Rwanda and Burundi, German colonies and later Belgian colonies, the healthcare system in both countries has been poor in colonial times and since independence. Some of the former Italian colonies have had very poor healthcare, with Alberto Denti di Pirajno's best-selling books, *A Cure for Serpents* (1955) and *A Grave for a Dolphin* (1956), describing the problems facing doctors in the Italian colonies. The system in Somalia—part of which had been an Italian colony, and the other part being British—has all but collapsed during recent civil wars. In Libya, at independence the healthcare system was in a deplorable state, but since the discovery of oil, has seen considerable wealth and it now was 128 doctors and 360 nurses per 100,000 people, with all healthcare, including the provision of medicine, being free.

In Eritrea, there are only three doctors and 16 nurses per 100,000 people, with up to half of all infants dying in their first year. In connection with Eritrea, mention should be made of the Australian doctor Dr. Fred Hollows who established an eye hospital in Asmara. In Ethiopia, briefly an Italian colony, the healthcare service has remained one of the worst in Africa, with only 1.2 doctors and 18 nurses per 100,000 people. However, the Addis Ababa Fistula Hospital, cofounded by Australian Dr. Catherine Hamlin, treats about 1,400 women suffering from obstetric fistula each year. Liberia, the only part of Africa not to be colonized, has 2.3 doctors and 5.9 nurses per 100,000 people, with malaria and leprosy rife.

SEE ALSO: AIDS; Djibouti; Guinea Malaria; South Africa.

BIBLIOGRAPHY. Adelola Adeloye, ed., *African Pioneers of Modern Medicine: Nigerian Doctors of the Nineteenth century* (University Press, Nigeria, 1992); Adelola Adeloye (ed), *Nigerian Pioneers of Modern Medicine* (Ibadan University Press, 1977); J.D. Alsop, "Sea Surgeons, Health and England's Maritime Expansion: the West African trade 1553–1660," *Mariner's Mirror* (v.76/3, 1990); Knud Balslev, *A History of Leprosy in Tanzania* (African Medical & Research Foundation, Nairobi, 1989); Ahmed Bayoumi, *The history of the Sudan Health Services* (African Medical and Research Foundation, Nairobi, 1979); Heather Bell, *Frontiers of Medicine in the Anglo-Egyptian Sudan 1899–1948* (Oxford University Press, 1999); Ann Beck, *A History of the British Medical Administration of East Africa 1900–1950* (Harvard University Press, 1970); Ruth S. Best, *Strawberries All Year Round* (Best, Toronto, 1970); Leonard Bousfield, *Sudan Doctor* (C. Johnson, 1954); Cole P. Dodge and Paul D. Wiebe, eds., *Crisis in Uganda: The Breakdown of Health Services* (Pergamon Press, 1985); Alberto Denti di Pirajno, *A Cure for Serpents: A Doctor in Africa* (Andre Deutsch, 1955); T. Gerald Garry, *African Doctor* (The Book Club, 1939); Michael Gelfand, *A Service to the Sick: A History of the Health Services for Africans in Southern Rhodesia 1890–1953* (Mambo, 1976).

JUSTIN CORFIELD
GEELONG GRAMMAR SCHOOL, AUSTRALIA

Healthcare, Asia and Oceania

Healthcare varies in Asia and Oceania depending on a number of socioeconomic factors. Japan, for instance, has a more sophisticated healthcare delivery system because of its position as a world economic force. In contrast, more isolated and primitive locations such as Papua New Guinea have few, if any, public health service options.

JAPAN

Since World War II, Western biomedicine has dominated Japanese medical care. Public health services, including free screening examinations for particular diseases, prenatal care, and infectious disease control are provided by national and local governments. Payment for personal medical services is offered through a universal medical insurance system that provides relative equality of access, with fees set by a government committee. People without insurance through employers can participate in a national health insurance program administered by local governments. Since the 1970s, all elderly persons have been covered by government-sponsored insurance. Patients are free to select physicians or facilities of their choice. By the turn of the 21st century, there were more than 8,700 general hospitals, more than 1,000 comprehensive hospitals, and approximately 1,000 mental hospitals in Japan with a total capacity of 1.5 million beds. Hospitals provided both outpatient and inpatient care. In addition, 79,000 clinics offered primarily outpatient services, and there were 48,000 dental clinics. Most

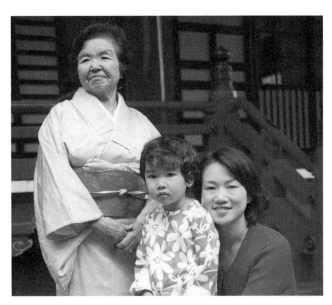

Japan has a more sophisticated healthcare delivery system because of its position as a world economic force.

physicians and hospitals can sell medicine directly to patients, but there are more than 36,000 pharmacies where patients can purchase synthetic or herbal medication.

While national health expenditures have risen in recent years and conditions continue to improve, the system is not perfect. Cost-control problems, excessive paperwork, long waits to see physicians, assembly-line care for outpatients (because few hospitals or clinics make appointments), overmedication, and abuse of the system are some of the traditional ills of the Japanese healthcare system. Another problem is an uneven distribution of health personnel, with cities favored over rural areas.

Recent improvements in the system have been made in an attempt to produce equity between the rural and urban populations, but those in the countryside are still less likely to receive adequate care at all times. With a prevalence rate around .02 percent, Japan is fortunate to be one of the countries that has been the least affected by HIV/AIDS. However, the lack of contact and familiarity with the disease has meant that education about it is somewhat limited. Lack of awareness has resulted in many misperceptions and stigmas about HIV/AIDS in Japanese society. For instance, many view HIV/AIDS as a problem of poor, developing countries rather than something

that is relevant to a nation like Japan. It is thought that HIV/AIDS is a problem caused by and affecting only foreigners. As a result, compared with other countries, HIV/AIDS is of relatively little concern to the Japanese government and population. Therefore, education and awareness campaigns about the disease, while available, are not considered of the utmost importance.

THE PHILIPPINES

Health conditions in the Philippines approximate those in many other southeast Asian countries but lag behind those in the West. The ratio of physicians and hospitals to the total population is similar to those in a number of other countries in the region, but considerably below those of Europe and North America. Most healthcare personnel and facilities are concentrated in urban areas, and periodically, there have been significant migrations of physicians and nurses to the United States. The Philippines has a dual healthcare system consisting of Western biomedicine and traditional medicine. The modern system is based on the germ theory of disease and has scientifically trained practitioners. The traditional approach assumes that illness is caused by a breach of taboos set by supernatural forces. It is not unusual for an individual to alternate between the two forms of medicine. If the benefits of modern medicine are immediately obvious, then they are usually accepted. However, if there is no immediate cure or result, the impulse of many Filipinos to turn to a traditional healer is often strong. In the past, hospital equipment often has not functioned properly because there were not enough technicians capable of effectively maintaining the supply. However by 2000, the Department of Health had apparently addressed at least part of the problem through the establishment of centers for the repair and maintenance of hospital equipment.

Life expectancy in the Philippines has increased over the last several decades and infant deaths have dropped significantly, but again, mortality rates are still higher than those of Western nations. Like many other locales around the world, in the Philippines great healthcare disparities exist between urban and rural areas. Immunization shots for infants and other preventative measures are more prevalent in urban settings than rural, and even though the Department of Health has attempted to develop universal levels of minimum care, the more remote areas inevitably received less attention. While medical treatment has improved and services have expanded, pervasive poverty and lack of access to family planning detracts from the general health of the Philippine people. Much of the population continues to exist below the poverty line, and a high rate of childbirth tends both to deplete family resources and be injurious to the health of the mother.

The main general health hazards are pulmonary, cardiovascular, and gastrointestinal disorders. Although relatively few Filipinos have been infected with AIDS, concern about the disease has caused authorities to give it considerable attention. Since the first cases of HIV/AIDS were reported in 1984, 1,515 HIV infections, including 508 AIDS cases and 196 HIV/AIDS-related deaths, had been reported by June 2001. Overall, the epidemic in the Philippines has been classified as low. As of January 2004, the National Epidemiology Center of the Department of Health recorded 1,979 cases of individuals with HIV/AIDS of which 1,343 (68 percent) were asymptomatic and 636 (32 percent) were AIDS cases at the time of the report. Of the total AIDS cases, 257 (40 percent) had already died as a result of AIDS-related complications.

INDONESIA

Indonesians' greater access to education over the past few decades has translated into an increased adherence to modern forms of healthcare. Life expectancies have risen in many areas and in those same areas the quality of life has improved. However, the distribution of resources for health maintenance and improvement in Indonesia remains unequal. The poor, rural, and uneducated classes generally suffered much higher mortality rates than their more educated counterparts. The overall number of healthcare professionals increased during the period, but many are concentrated in urban areas. Likewise, the better equipped urban hospitals tend to have more physicians and higher central government spending per bed than hospitals in the rural areas. Community and preventative health programs have become a key component of Indonesia's healthcare system.

Community health services are organized in a three-tier system with community health centers at the top. Usually staffed by a physician, these centers provide maternal and child healthcare, general outpatient and preventative healthcare services, pre- and postnatal care, immunization, and communicable

disease control programs. Specialized services are sometimes available at some of the larger clinics. Second-level community health centers include health subcenters consisting of small clinics and maternal and child health centers that are staffed with between one and three nurses and visited weekly or monthly by a physician. The third level of community health services are village-level integrated service posts. These posts are not permanently staffed facilities, but are monthly clinics maintained on donated land, in which a visiting team from the regional health center reinforces local health volunteers. In general, although the community health situation has improving slightly in Indonesia over the last 20 years, the provision of community services remains low by the standards of developing countries.

AUSTRALIA

In Australia, the government, through the Department of Health and Ageing, sets national health policies and subsidizes health services provided by state and territory governments and the private sector. Total expenditure on health by all levels of government and the private sector currently account for almost 10 percent of Australia's Gross Domestic Product. Like other countries, Australia faces growing pressures on health funding because of the aging of the population, technological changes, and increasing patient expectations. The Australian Government funds universal medical services and pharmaceuticals, and gives financial assistance for public hospitals, residential aged care facilities, and home and community care for the elderly. It is also the major source of funds for health research, and provides support for training health professionals and financial assistance to students. State and territory governments have primary responsibility under the Constitution for providing health services, including most acute and psychiatric hospital services. The states and territories also provide a wide range of community and public health services, including school health, dental health, maternal, and child health, occupational health, disease control activities, and a variety of health inspection functions.

The main health responsibilities of local governments in Australia are in environmental control such as garbage disposal, maintenance of clean water, and health inspections. Local government also provides a range of home care and personal preventive services, such as immunization. A universal system of health insurance was introduced in the 1980s and is funded, in part, through a tax on income. The system's three main functions are to cover the cost of medical services, pharmaceuticals, and public hospital care. Under Medicare, all permanent Australian residents are entitled to free public hospital care when choosing to be public patients. Doctors appointed by the hospitals provide the medical treatment. State and territorial governments provide public hospital services and work closely with the Australian government and professional bodies to ensure that the quality of care and appropriate standards are maintained. Australians may elect to be treated as private patients in public hospitals or to use private hospitals. In the private sector, patients can choose to pay directly for medical costs or use private health insurance. The Australian government also subsidises medical, pharmaceutical, and hospital services for veterans and war widows under similar plans administered by the Department of Veterans' Affairs.

Private hospitals provide about a third of all hospital beds in Australia. Private medical practitioners provide most out-of-hospital medical services and perform a large proportion of hospital services alongside salaried doctors. Private practitioners provide most dental services and allied health services such as physiotherapy. About half of all Australians are covered by private health insurance. Forty-three percent of the population are covered by hospital insurance for treatment as a private patient in both public and private hospitals. In almost all cases, coverage also extends to ancillary, nonmedical services provided outside of the hospital or clinical setting such as physiotherapy, dental treatment, and the purchase of eye glasses. Six percent of the population are covered for ancillary services only. The federal government is seeking a better balance between public and private sector involvement in the health sector by encouraging people to take out private health insurance, while preserving Medicare as the universal safety net.

Australia works with international organizations, including the World Health Organization (WHO) and the Organisation for Economic Co-operation and Development (OECD), health ministries in other countries, and with independent research institutes to prevent and control the spread of disease, set international health standards, and support general health promotion activities. International involvement allows Australia and other countries to learn from each other's experiences and also enables Australia to contribute to the international development of health policy. Australia places a special emphasis on the Asia Pacific region, collaborating with international and regional organizations and ministries of health on issues that affect neighboring countries as well as Australia's health policies. Australian academic institutions and health agencies offer international consultant services, on-site training programs, and work placements to strengthen health sector capacity, particularly in the region. Medicare Australia also works with the World Bank, AusAid, and the WHO to provide international consultant services in a range of areas including the development and management of secure online health business solutions; health system financing; health insurance administration; health information systems; pharmaceutical systems design and operations; and training and institutional development.

NEW ZEALAND AND PAPUA NEW GUINEA

New Zealand has a parallel system of public and private health services. Public healthcare is subsidized by the New Zealand government, while private healthcare is paid for by the individual. Individuals who can afford to pay for private health insurance do so, while those who cannot use the public health system. Both systems are of high quality, but there are some advantages to having private health insurance. In New Zealand, health problems are essentially divided into two categories: those associated with accidents and those that are not. Health problems that arise out of an accident are subsidized by the New Zealand government through the Accident Rehabilitation & Compensation Insurance Corporation. The Corporation makes payments to individuals who have suffered injury or disability as the result of an accident. If the individual has health needs or problems that are not related to an accident, then the medical and healthcare required for that individual is still heavily subsidized by the New Zealand government, but not through the Corporation. Regardless, permanent residents of New Zealand are covered under the country's public health system one way or another.

There are public hospitals and private hospitals in New Zealand. Public hospitals are available to any New Zealand resident, while private hospitals are available to anyone who has paid private health insurance premiums, regardless of whether that person is a permanent resident or citizen of New Zealand. The primary advantage of having private health insurance is the individual's ability to receive immediate care at a private hospital while avoiding waiting lists at public hospitals for nonurgent medical situations. Under the public health system, there is no charge for outpatients or overnight visits for New Zealand residents. New Zealand has a reciprocal arrangement with other countries whereby no charge is applied to nonresidents of New Zealand. Otherwise, a nonresident of New Zealand is charged a minimum rate per day for a hospital visit unless their injury is the result of a motor vehicle accident, in which case there is no charge. For New Zealand permanent residents and citizens who suffer injury or disability as the result of an accident, applications may be made to the Accident Rehabilitation and Compensation Insurance Corporation for either loss of earnings due to disability or for the costs of ongoing medical treatment. The claim for loss of earnings due to disability can be made at a rate of 80 percent of the individual's salary. Notwithstanding the public health system subsidies, individuals may choose to purchase their own private health insurance, which they can use to supplement any health services that they receive from the government under the public health system. Under the private healthcare system, anyone may buy health insurance. Those who choose to do so pay an annual premium to an insurance company, and all or part of the individual's health expenses for treatment at private hospitals are paid for by the insurance company. Premiums are set at different levels that coincide with the amount of coverage that the individual requires.

Papua New Guinea's population has suffered significant declines in living standards in recent years due to worsening economic performance. Although the country does not exhibit the widespread abject poverty present in some developing countries, poor health and social indicators show that poverty is a real problem. Papua New Guinea's main social tenets, such as life expectancy and maternal and child mortality rates, show improvements over the last few decades, but are still well below the averages for lower middle income countries. Papua New Guinea still has limited primary healthcare. Infectious diseases claim many lives, and there are serious public health risks from endemic diseases such as malaria, and an emerging HIV/AIDS epidemic. An estimated 1.7 percent of people in the country carry the virus.

SEE ALSO: Australia; China; Chinese Medicine, Traditional; Japan; New Zealand.

BIBLIOGRAPHY. Australian Government, AusAID, www.ausaid.gov.au (cited October 2006); Australian Government, Department of Foreign Affairs and Trade, www.dfat.gov.au/facts/health_care.html (cited October 2006); Australian Government, Department of Health and Aging, www.health.gov.au (cited October 2006); "The Body: HIV and AIDS in Japan," www.thebody.com (cited October 2006); "Country Studies," www.countrystudies.us (cited October 2006); Kundig Associates, "New Zealand's Health System," www.migrate.co.nz/Info/info5.htm (cited October 2006); Milton J. Lewis, *The People's Health: Public Health in Australia, 1950 to the Present* (Praeger, 2003); Fadia Saadah, and James Knowles, *The World Bank Strategy for Health, Nutrition, and Population in the East Asia and Pacific Region* (World Bank Publications, 2001).

BEN WYNNE, PH.D
GAINESVILLE STATE COLLEGE

Healthcare, Europe

As in other parts of the world, lifestyle-related health factors and socio-economic concerns in the European Union (EU) are multi-dimensional and linked to a number of major health problems. The EU is dedicated to dealing with these factors through comprehensive health promotion in various settings such as schools, workplaces, families, and local communities. Communicable diseases such as tuberculosis, measles, and influenza also represent a serious risk to human health in the EU, and contribute to about one-third of all deaths occurring globally. Communicable diseases do not respect national borders and can spread rapidly if actions are not taken to combat them. New diseases emerge and others develop drug-resistant mutations such as multidrug resistant tuberculosis, and methicillin-resistant *Staphylococcus aureus*. In addition to trying to address these concerns, EU researchers are also studying chronic conditions such as cancer, heart diseases, and allergies.

LIFESTYLE FACTORS

In Europe, six out of the seven most important risk factors for premature death (blood pressure, cholesterol, body mass index, inadequate fruit and vegetable intake, physical inactivity, excessive alcohol consumption) relate to how Europeans eat, drink, and move. A balanced diet and regular physical activity, along with refraining from smoking, are important factors in the promotion and maintenance of good health. Moreover, those with lower incomes and education level usually are the most affected by these factors, and therefore are at the greatest risk. Excess weight and obesity are increasing at an alarming rate in Europe. Obesity is one of the most serious public health problems in Europe because it increases significantly the risk of many chronic diseases such as cardiovascular disease, type 2 diabetes and certain cancers. These diseases represent the greatest burden to healthcare systems in Europe and are the leading cause of mortality in EU member states as well as worldwide.

The increase of childhood obesity is of particularly concern. Lifestyle factors, including diet, eating habits, and levels of physical activity and inactivity, are often adopted during the early years of life. As childhood obesity is also strongly linked to obesity in adulthood, the best time to address the problem is early in life. Maintaining normal weight is challenging, particularly in the modern era with its abundance of high calorie foods designed to be rapidly prepared and consumed. The environments that many people live in are conducive to obesity. In many parts of the EU, there is an abundance of energy-rich food that is often poor in nutrients, and at the same time, there are decreasing opportunities for physical activity on the part of the population both at work and during leisure time. Food portion sizes also grow year by year, even though people actually need less and less energy due to the shift toward sedentary lifestyles.

Tobacco is the single largest cause of avoidable death in the EU, accounting for over half a million deaths each year. In the 21st century, it has been estimated that 25 percent of all cancer deaths and 15 percent of all deaths in the EU could be attributed to smoking. In order to curb this epidemic, the European Community is actively developing a comprehensive tobacco control policy that includes legislative measures; the mainstreaming of tobacco control into a range of other Community policies; making sure that the pioneering role of the European Community in many tobacco control areas produces an impact beyond the EU; and establishing the community as a major player in tobacco control at a global level.

Alcohol is also key health factor in European countries that requires constant attention. Europe is the continent where per capita alcohol consumption is the highest in the world. In established market economies such as the EU member states the burden of disease and injury attributable to alcohol is estimated to be almost 10 percent. Combating alcohol-related injuries or health problems therefore is a public health priority in many Member States, and at the EU level. It is not only health consequences in a narrow sense that raise concerns, but also alcohol-related social issues such as violence, crime, domestic problems, social exclusion, difficulties in the workplace, and particularly drunk driving. All of these are areas require political action, and all are being addressed by the member states to one degree or another. In addition, there is agreement among the member states that, beyond individual national efforts, a joint alcohol strategy at the community level should be maintained.

Thousands of acute drug-related deaths are recorded each year throughout the EU, mostly involving young people. National statistics on drug deaths usually refer to acute deaths directly related to drug consumption or overdose, although differences in definitions exist from nation to nation. The actual figure is thought to be considerably higher because of underreporting of deaths related to overdoses and also because of deaths indirectly related to intravenous drug use such as AIDS and other infectious diseases. In addition, drug use as it relates suicide, accidents and violence often goes unreported in drug fatality statistics. Some more inclusive studies have indicated that all of these fatalities could increase the real number of deaths that can be related to drugs as much as three-fold. Various public and private initiatives by EU member states have been designed to decrease risk, although some remain controversial. Needle exchange programs, substitution programs with methadone or related substances for opiate users, and low-threshold and outreach services (for instance walk-in clinics for addicted people irrespective of current drug use) are thought to have had a positive impact in helping decrease the number of drug-related deaths in the EU per annum, although the work is ongoing. Overall, the number of drug-related fatalities has stabilized and even decreased in some areas in recent years.

Cannabis remains the most commonly used illegal substance in Europe, with a high level of variation between countries. Recent studies among 15-year-old students suggest that lifetime prevalence varies from under 10 percent to over 30 percent compared to 1 percent to 10 percent for cocaine (15–34 years). It is difficult to define clear trends that apply to the EU as a whole with regard to drug usage. The use of other drugs is much less common, both among young people and in the general population. Recent use of amphetamines or cocaine is generally found in less than 1 percent of adults. Overall, the increase in the use of ecstasy, which began to occur during the 1990s appears to have stabilized, with only a few countries still reporting an upward trend. Use of synthetic drugs by young people in social settings remains a major concern. Drug users are overrepresented in prisons compared with the general population. Estimates of lifetime prevalence of drug use among prisoners vary between 22 percent and 86 percent, depending on the prison population, detention facility, and country. If the rate of drug use in the EU as a whole is between four and seven cases per 1,000 population aged 15–64, this translates into between 1.2 and 2.1 million problem drug users, of whom around 1 million are active injecting drug users (IDUs). Injecting drug use seems to have fallen since the 1990s; however, it remains a significant concern.

AIDS/HIV RISK

Drug injectors are at very high risk of experiencing adverse consequences such as HIV/hepatitis C virus (HCV) infections. The HIV epidemic is spreading rapidly in some of the new EU countries and their neighbors. Where HIV prevalence has remained high among IDUs, sustained prevention efforts are important to prevent transmission to new users, sexual partners and from mother to child. Injecting drugs use can be a route for the transmission of a range of other infectious diseases such as botulism and tuberculosis. The Directorate General (DG) of Health and Consumer Protection deals with the public health aspects of illegal drug use (as well as legal drugs misuse or abuse), especially prevention programs, education, risk reduction, treatment and the raising of awareness. It cooperates with other agencies with regard to ancillary services of the Commission that deal with the problems created by

drug use such as smuggling, overall increases in crime, and any special needs of law enforcement in these areas. It also cooperates with the European Monitoring Centre for Drugs and Drug Addiction (EMCDDA) in Lisbon and with international organizations, such as the World Health Organization (WHO) and the Pompidou Group of the Council of Europe.

SOCIOECONOMICS AND HEALTH

Socioeconomic factors continue to serve as leading indicators of the quality of health and healthcare in the EU. On average, EU citizens with better jobs, more education or higher incomes have better health and live longer. Differences in life expectancy of five years or more can be found between the most advantaged and least advantaged groups. Such gradients exist within all European countries for many diseases and other general factors contributing to poor health. Limited access to proper healthcare lowers the ability of huge numbers of EU citizens to achieve their potential. As a result, the EU has adopted policies aimed at reducing health inequities. The EU hopes to improve the quality of healthcare afforded the disadvantaged to that of the most advantaged classes in society, and thereby ensure that the health needs of the most disadvantaged are fully addressed as quickly as possible. At the EU level this involves efforts to produce economic, employment and social policy designed to strengthen the European economy and at the same time ensure universal social protection; increase the support of the economies and health infrastructures of countries and regions of the EU which are lagging behind or have special needs; and promote research to identify the causes of socioeconomic health inequalities and develop and evaluate measures to combat them.

An increasing number of patients in the EU receive treatments based on biological substances donated by others. These include blood, tissues, cells, and whole human organs. Such substances are of high therapeutic value, but they also carry risks for the recipients, in particular the risk of transmission of communicable diseases. The community contributes to reducing these risks by adopting legislation on the quality and safety of these substances, and by funding various research projects in this area. Donation of blood and plasma in the EU provides the source material for a wide range of essential, often life-saving, therapeutic substances.

Their universal use in medicine requires the highest achievable level of safety. Human tissues and cells are increasingly used in transplantation, as well as tissue engineering and cell therapy. Due to their biological origins, tissues and cells also carry risks for the transmission of diseases, which obviously poses a concern for those in need of transplants. In the EU, by far the biggest problem with regard to transplants or the use of other biological material is the low number of organ donors, which naturally leads to a severe scarcity of organs. Recently, and in another ongoing efforts, the community has taken steps to help improve the situation by fostering new initiatives at the EU level related to organ donation and the management of biological materials.

The European Center for Disease Prevention and Control (ECDC) is an EU agency that has been created to help strengthen Europe's defenses against infectious diseases, such as influenza, SARS and HIV/AIDS. In the modern era infectious disease outbreaks spread internationally and with alarming speed. Cooperation between national disease control agencies is vital to the process of meeting the increasingly complex health challenges of the 21st century. As a result, the European Parliament and Council passed in 2004 the appropriate legislation creating the ECDC. The organization's mission is to identify, assess and communicate current and emerging threats to human health posed by infectious diseases. In order to achieve this mission, ECDC works in partnership with national health protection bodies across Europe to strengthen and develop continent-wide disease surveillance and early warning systems. By working with experts throughout Europe, the ECDC seeks to pool Europe's health knowledge and, in so doing, to develop authoritative scientific opinions about the risks posed by current and emerging infectious diseases. The ECDC is strategically located in the Tomteboda building in the heart of Stockholm's Karolinska Institute Campus area, near to the Swedish Institute for Infectious Disease Control.

FOOD SAFETY IN EUROPE

Food safety is one of the EU's leading areas of health-related activity. Experience shows that to ensure the safety and reliability of food within the EU and worldwide, the entire food chain has to be evaluated and maintained at an acceptable level. The EU has laws covering how farmers produce food (including what chemicals they may use when growing plants and what they may feed their animals), how food is processed, how food is sold, and what sort of information is provided on food labels. The EU also has laws regulating the safety of food imported into the EU as well as extensive procedures that allow for the tracking of food products coming into member states. The work of keeping the EU's laws on food safety up to date is complemented by the Health and Consumer Protection Directorate-General officials in the Food and Veterinary Office (FVO) based in Grange, Ireland, whose main job is to verify, through inspections that EU countries and other countries exporting food to the EU observe certain rules and regulations. Their work includes working with international organizations and the EU's trading partners on food and farming issues and running the EU's "rapid alert" system on food and feed safety.

Within the EU, having seen the advantages of separating risk assessment from risk management, the European Commission reassigned the work of risk assessment on food safety to a relatively new agency, the European Food Safety Authority (EFSA), in Parma, Italy. The Commission remains responsible, however, for overall risk management. The EU and the United States both have very high standards of food safety, although somewhat different approached to dealing with certain problems related to food and the food supply. In the United States, the Delegation of the European Commission to the United States in Washington works mainly with the U.S. Food & Drug Administration (FDA) within the Department of Health and Human Services, and with the U.S. Department of Agriculture. It also maintains a dialogue with the American food industry and with public interest groups and is available to answer questions that can benefit trade in both directions across the Atlantic Ocean.

PUBLIC HEALTH

Threats to public health are a permanent cause of concern for health authorities all over the world. In order to be prepared to face threats likely to affect public health in the EU, the Commission collaborates with EU member states to develop preparedness activities and plans. A generic preparedness plan has been issued by the commission to address generically different types of health threats. More specific plans have been issued both at national and at the community level to address the issues of pandemic influenza, SARS, smallpox, and bioterrorism. Under new programs developed in the first decade of the 21st century, actions and support measures in the field of noncommunicable diseases have been focused on developing strategies and mechanisms for preventing, exchanging information on, and responding to noncommunicable disease threats, including gender-specific health threats and rare diseases.

During the late 1990s, a significant debate developed over how to organize surveillance for infectious diseases in the EU culminating in the decision by the European Parliament and Council to create a plan for a decentralized health networks as opposed to constructing a large central European surveillance center. According to the plan, institutions in member states received funding to organize European surveillance for one or more related infectious pathogens. Using an approach based on risk and hazard analysis, studies identified common control points and concluded that the networking approach was successful but needed augmentation under a framework of improving existing organizational, financial, and legal factors. An important contributor to the networks' success has been the high level of participation by national public health institutes, in large part because these institutions have had an active role in running the networks themselves. The networks' start-up costs have been low because existing physical infrastructures in the participating institutions are utilized. These networks, combined with European infrastructures such as the European Program of Intervention Epidemiology Training, and publications such as *Eurosurveillance* and *Eurosurveillance Weekly*, have accelerated the development of the elements needed for effective control of communicable diseases at the European level. For example, surveillance systems and epidemiological response capacities have been improved, surveillance and laboratory methods are increasingly cross-referenced, published forums for sharing experiences related to control measures now exist, and a group of highly trained field epidemiologists has been formed and is functioning.

In the modern era, health systems and health policies across the EU have become more interconnected than at any other time in history. This is the case because of a number of factors, including the in-creased mobility of patients and professionals around the EU, growing common public expectations across Europe, greater dissemination of new medical technologies and techniques, and the enlargement of the union itself. This increased interconnection raises many health policy issues, including those related to the quality of, and access to, cross-border care; information requirements for patients, health professionals and policy makers; the nature of cooperation on health matters among the member nations; and the ability to reconcile national policies with the obligations of the EU's internal concerns.

Rights to healthcare are recognized in the Charter of Fundamental Rights of the EU, and high-quality health services have become a priority issue for European citizens. The European Court of Justice has made it clear that treaty provisions on free movement apply to health services, regardless of how they are organized or financed at the national level. However, many healthcare stakeholders have asked for greater clarity with regard to what community law means as it applies to health services. The European Commission therefore continues to develop a community framework for safe, high quality and efficient health services by reinforcing cooperation between member states and by ensuring equal application of Community law to health services and healthcare. In general, the commission sets the standard for health functions based on a foundation of legal certainty and the pledged support of member states. Legal certainty is critical tenet of the process as it serves to significantly boost the confidence of citizens as well as national and local health professionals. Across Europe, there has traditionally been a need to address the wider application of European Court of Justice rulings regarding treaty provisions on the free movement of patients, professionals and health services. This focuses in particular on cross-border care, although cross-border care has consequences for all health services, whether provided across borders or not. Of equal import is the support for member states in areas where European action can add value to national action on healthcare services.

Discussions about "patient mobility" at the EU level were prompted in the late 1990s after several judgments of the European Court of Justice. Until then, the mechanisms within the EU enabling patients to receive treatment abroad (other than patients paying for the treatment themselves) were limited. However, one important ruling made it clear that as health services are provided for remuneration, they must be regarded as services within the meaning of EU Treaty and thus relevant provisions on the free movement of services apply. On the basis of this and subsequent decisions, any nonhospital care to which individuals are entitled in the individual's own member state may be sought in any other member state without prior authorization, and be reimbursed up to the level of reimbursement provided by individual's own system. This also extends to hospital care. To track the potential needs of the EU along these lines, the European Commission has launched public health reporting projects that will continue well into the 21st century. The reports deal with topical public health issues that provide the basis for further policy developments. The aim of launching the effort was to bring together top European scientists and officials in the field of public health and statistics from all EU countries so that they could contribute collectively to the creation of the European Health Information and Knowledge System.

The dissemination of health information to different users throughout the EU has changed dramatically over the last few decades. A great deal of effort has been put into the compilation of data, the development of indicators and new technologies for the analysis and presentation of health data, and the evaluation of the effectiveness of health reporting. However, health reporting traditionally has been a public health issue discussed widely among health professionals at the local, regional and national levels. The objective of the EU Public Health Program is to provide member states with appropriate health information in order to support their national health policies. For a growing number of member states, health status analysis and reporting has become an important instrument to support national health policy cycles. Basically, such health reporting supports the preparation, planning, implementation and evaluation of health policy including programs and at the community level and at the member state level. General health policy within the EU deals with priority settings for health policy and with the past and possible future effects of health policy programs.

EUROPEAN HEALTH GOALS

One of the European Commission's aims is to produce comparable information on health and health-related behavior of the populations of member states, and on diseases and their effect on health systems as a whole. This information is based on common indicators agreed to by member states. Most of the research and policy supported by the Program of Community Action in the Field of Public Health are related to the development of indicators in various health fields in order to facilitate and improve the collection of data. An initial set of European Community Health Indicators (ECHI) has been produced and widely disseminated. The work is ongoing with existing indicators undergoing constant scrutiny, and with new indicators periodically being added to the mix. The objective is to produce as complete a list of ECHIs as possible to serve as the foundation for the European Health Information and Knowledge System. This and other related programs have also funded the production of regular European health reports that disseminate critical information to member states.

Currently, and most likely for the foreseeable future, work on indicators and data collection will be conducted in coordination with a variety of organizations and task forces in hopes of creating a prototype for future health monitoring. The tasks of those involved will cover all five phases of data management: the analysis of data needs in their respective areas; definition of indicators and quality assurance; technical support for national efforts; data collection at the EU level; reporting and analysis; and the promotion of the results. Within this framework collaboration and close coordination with Eurostat and its partnership groups is a very important part of the process. The objective is to complete the ECHIs list that will serve as a foundation for the European Health Information and Knowledge System.

The ECHI project has already developed a comprehensive list of indicators, in close cooperation with many of the other projects under the program. As of June 2006, the general list contained approximately 400 items or indicators, although there is a push among some in the European Commission to develop a shortlist in order to prioritize needs and streamline data collection among the member states. To this end, ECHI has undertaken the task of selecting the indicators for the shortlist in close collaboration with the project leaders and the Commission departments that are affected.

SEE ALSO: European Association for the Study of Obesity (EASO); European Public Health Alliance (EPHA); European Public Health Association (EUPHA).

BIBLIOGRAPHY. Country Studies, www.countrystudies. us (cited October 2006); European Centre for Disease Prevention and Control (ECDC), www.ecdc.eu.int (cited October 2006); Richard Freeman, *The Politics of Health in Europe* (Manchester University Press, 2000); Wilhelm Kirch, *Public Health in Europe: 10 Years European Public Health Association* (Springer, 2004); Martin McKee, Laura MacLehose, and Ellen Nolte, *Health Policy and European Union Enlargement* (Open University Press, 2004); Elias Mossialos, Anna Dixon, and Josep Figueras, eds., *Funding Health Care: Options for Europe* (Open University Press, 2002).

BEN WYNNE, PH.D.
GAINESVILLE STATE COLLEGE

Healthcare, South America

Because it covers a vast area and includes an estimated population of almost 400 million, healthcare on the South American continent varies widely. In some areas, great strides have recently been made in improving health and healthcare systems, while in other, more primitive areas, there are few, if any, significant healthcare options.

BRAZIL

Brazil is by far the largest and most populous country in South America. Its strong industrial and agricultural sectors make it South America's leading economic power. The Brazilian constitution of 1988 and the Organic Health Law of 1990 universalized access to medical care, unified the public health system supported by the Ministry of Health and the National Institute for Medical Assistance and Social Security, and decentralized the management and organization of health services from the federal to the state and municipal levels. Many of the sweeping health reforms that were initiated during the period attempted to extend coverage to those outside the social security system.

The constitution grants all Brazilian citizens the right to free medical assistance from public as well as private providers reimbursed by the government. While the public domain oversees basic and preventive healthcare, the private nonprofit and for-profit healthcare sector delivers the bulk of medical services, including government-subsidized inpatient care. This publicly financed, privately provided health system continues to intensify its focus on high-cost curative care, driving hospital costs steadily upward. Therapeutic treatment in hospitals tends to dominate funding at the expense of health promotion and disease prevention programs. Not only have basic and preventive health services for the entire population diminished, but the public health system also subsidizes expensive, high-technology medical procedures that consume 30 to 40 percent of health resources and often end up being used to attend affluent segments of the society.

Although states and municipalities have rapidly acquired more responsibility in administering health funds and facilities, the federal government in Brazil retains the role of financing public health outlays. As stipulated by the constitution, government subsidies for health services are derived from the social security budget, which is predominantly based on earmarked taxes and contributions from employee payroll and business profits. Private sources finance half of total health expenditures. Perceptions of inefficiency in the government reimbursement schedule and deterioration in service quality of the public health system spurred a rapid growth in the private financing of healthcare beginning in the 1980s, particularly in economically advanced areas. The private sector covers roughly 20 percent of the Brazilian population and consists of several hundred firms offering four principal types of medical plans: private health insurance, prepaid group practice, medical cooperatives, and company health plans. The group medical plans rank Brazil as the largest health maintenance organization (HMO) provider in Latin America.

BOLIVIA

From the mid-1970s to the mid-1980s, Bolivia made slow but steady progress in improving the health conditions of its population. Overall life expectancy rose, and the mortality rate dropped for both adults and children. Despite these improvements, however, Bolivia's health indicators remain among the worst in the western hemisphere. Health conditions vary significantly across regions, within regions, and by urban or rural residence. Infants in rural areas have a far greater probability of dying than those in urban settings. Similarly, mortality rates for rural children up to the age of 5 are nearly double those found in children residing in the cities. Studies also note disparities in rates among ethnic groups. Rates are highest among children of mothers who speak only an indigenous language, intermediate among bilingual mothers, and lowest among monolingual Spanish-speaking mothers. Bolivian health specialists also confront a variety of diseases that affect the general population. In the past, the government has organized mass campaigns in an effort to deal with malaria epidemics, and relatively aggressive vaccination programs to combat yellow fever and jungle fever. Pulmonary tuberculosis and silicosis remain serious concerns. Toward the end of the 20th century, the government began restructuring its healthcare system to allow for more effective delivery. Bolivia's health network traditionally had been characterized by a high degree of fragmentation and duplication of services. Although the Ministry of Social Services and Public Health had overall responsibility for the system, 10 separate social security funds offered health services to members insured through their place of employment. In addition to wasting scarce resources, this approach had a heavy urban bias. The new approach called for a unified system under the control of the Ministry of Social Services and Public Health, with emphasis on preventive rather than curative medicine.

CHILE

By the early 1970s, the state-run health programs in Chile faced a financial crisis, and as a result, policy makers in the 1980s redesigned the nation's existing healthcare institutions. The end result was a system that contains essentially five components, the most prominent being the National System of Health Services (SNSS). The SNSS organizes and implements broad public health programs in areas such as inoculations and maternal-infant care. It provides periodic preventive medical care to all children less than 6 years of age not enrolled in alternative medical plans. Through this program, which has broad national coverage, low-income mothers can receive supplemental nutritional assistance for their children and for themselves if they are pregnant or nursing.

As a result, the incidence of moderate-to-severe childhood malnutrition among those participating in the program was reduced to negligible levels. While the SNSS remains the largest healthcare provider in the country, other components of the Chilean health system include the National Health Fund, the Security Assistance Institutions, private insurance companies, and private medicine, which includes both private hospitals and clinics. In the 21st century, Chilean health indicators are much closer to those of industrial nations than to those of the developing world. The SNSS still handles the vast majority of all medical visits and almost all births occur with professional assistance in hospitals or maternity clinics. In rural areas where women might need to travel greater distances to give birth, they can spend the last 10 to 15 days of pregnancy in special hostels. Inoculations of infants and children are virtually universal for tuberculosis, diphtheria, pertussis, tetanus, poliomyelitis, and measles.

ECUADOR

In Ecuador, both the public and the private sectors provide health services. Most public healthcare comes under the direction of the Ministry of Public Health, although the armed forces, the Ecuadorian Social Security Institute (IESS), and a number of other autonomous agencies also contribute. The Ministry of Health covers the vast majority of the population and the IESS approximately 10 percent. The Ministry of Public Health has organized a multitiered system of healthcare in Ecuador. Auxiliary healthcare personnel staff posts that serve small rural settlements with populations of less than 1,500, and more significant health centers staffed with healthcare professionals service communities of 1,500 to 5,000 inhabitants. Provincial and national hospitals are located in the largest cities.

By the turn of the 21st century, there were more than 2,000 health establishments nationwide with the Ministry of Public Health running well over half of those. However, the limited numbers of healthcare professionals in the country and their lack of training continues to hamper public healthcare efforts. These deficiencies are most apparent with regard to medical specialists, technicians, and nurses. Infant mortality rates in Ecuador have improved over the past few decades although recent rates remain a serious concern, and infant mortality can vary greatly by region and socioeconomic status. Childhood mortality rates have generally decreased as a result of immunization campaigns and attempts to control diarrheal diseases. In Ecuador, the main causes of death among adults are motor vehicle accidents, coronary heart disease, cerebrovascular disease, cancer, and tuberculosis. A number of tropical diseases also concern health officials, including onchocerciasis (river blindness) which is found in a number of isolated areas, Chagas disease (a parasitic infection), leishmaniasis (also a parasitic infection), and malaria.

URUGUAY

Uruguay has been described as South America's "first welfare state" due to its pioneering efforts in the fields of healthcare as well as public education and social security. Starting with the progressive reforms of the early part of the 20th century, the state has taken a leading role in providing healthcare, particularly to the lower classes, although private medicine remains the preferred option of the middle and upper social divisions. During the first half of the 20th century, Uruguay and Argentina led Latin America in advanced standards of medical care, and into the 1990s, the University of the Republic's medical school had a high international reputation and attracted students from other countries in South America. However, in recent years, standards of care in public hospitals and clinics have been adversely affected by budget restrictions.

Uruguay's welfare state has declined a great deal in the standards of protection that it affords the mass of the population. Still, spending on healthcare equipment is significant and health standards in general in Uruguay remain relatively high when compared to other countries in Central and South America. A significant effort has been made to increase the proportion of infants receiving inoculations against diseases such as whooping cough and measles, and the average life expectancy at birth is around 70 years for men and 76 years for women, only slightly behind Chile and Argentina. The leading causes of death in the country are circulatory disease, tumors, trauma, respiratory disorders and infections, perinatal complications, infectious diseases, suicide, and cirrhosis of the liver.

COLOMBIA

In the new century, most Colombians enjoy significantly better healthcare and nutrition than previous generations. The country had risen from the ranks of the poorest nations in Latin America during the 1950s and 1960s to an intermediate status based on leading health and economic indicators. These improvements are the result of rapid socioeconomic modernization, which was accompanied by improvements in education and working conditions; greater access to urban healthcare facilities; running water and sewerage systems; and, in general, more modern attitudes toward sexuality, medicine, disease prevention, nutrition, and exercise. There were also explicit state policies designed to improve access to and availability of healthcare and medical services. Beginning in the 1980s, Colombia developed a public and private infrastructure of hospitals and other healthcare facilities, a widespread network of medical schools, and a specialized set of institutions responsible for formulating and handling public policy in the health sector.

Despite general improvement, the benefits of better healthcare are not evenly distributed among the different strata of Colombian society, or from region to region. In urban areas, the upper and middle classes and many blue-collar workers enjoy above-average health conditions. In contrast, the rural and urban poor suffer from higher mortality and morbidity rates because of inadequate or inaccessible medical services, housing, and food. As a result, Colombian health policy-makers continue to be faced with the task of improving services to the least-favored segments of society, while improving the quality and overall performance of the national healthcare system

VENEZUELA

Venezuela has had, by Latin American standards, an enviable record in health and social welfare and one that has shown tremendous progress through the years. In 1940, the overall life expectancy at birth was 43 years. By the end of the century, that figure had risen to over 70 years (71 years for males and 77 for females, both among the highest in Latin America). This reflects generally improving health conditions in recent decades, and the increase in preventive public health measures undertaken by the government. For example, successful inoculation programs have decreased the incidence of a number of contagious diseases.

On the other hand, comparisons between causes of mortality 50 years ago and in the modern era show that Venezuela, a rapidly industrializing country, has become more prone to causes of death usually associated with urban and industrialized countries and a faster pace of life. These include heart disease, accidents, cancer, certain respiratory illnesses, and so forth. Infant mortality has also declined because of better public health measures, prenatal care, and national immunization campaigns. Overall, healthcare facilities have grown in number and in quality, and at the same time, the population had become more urban and better educated.

There has been an increase in the number of medical facilities and personnel offering healthcare. Immunization campaigns have systematically improved children's health, and regular campaigns to destroy disease-bearing insects and to improve water and sanitary facilities have all boosted Venezuela's health. However, the availability of care in rural areas represents a gap in the healthcare delivery system. Doctors tend to concentrate in the large cities, especially Caracas, leaving many smaller provincial towns without adequate medical personnel. Private medical facilities, operated for profit, enjoy greater prestige than public institutions. Charitable organizations, especially the Roman Catholic Church, operate some health facilities. The bulk of the population, however, relies on the Venezuelan Social Security Institute, which operates its own hospitals, covering its costs out of social security funds.

PERU

Beginning in the early 1990s, Peru was hit by a cholera epidemic that highlighted long-standing healthcare problems in the country. A number of studies amply illustrate Peru's vulnerability to disease and the uneven distribution of resources to combat illness. Most health facilities and the leading health facilities are concentrated in metropolitan Lima, followed by the principal older coastal cities. Whereas Lima has approximately one doctor for every 400 persons on average, and other coastal areas have a ratio of one doctor for every 2,000, rural areas consistently have only one doctor for about every 12,000 persons.

The same levels of inequity apply with respect to hospital beds, nurses, and all the medical specialties. Even in the modern era, a significant portion of urban residents and most rural Peruvians lack basic potable water and sewerage. As a result, the population has been exposed to a wide variety of waterborne diseases, which in turn further reflect the inequities evidenced in Peru's healthcare system. The leading causes of death by infectious diseases have varied from year to year, but invariably, the principal ones are respiratory infections, gastroenteritis, common colds, malaria, tuberculosis, influenza, measles, chicken pox, and whooping cough. Many important health and social issues in Peru are interrelated with the country's steadily worsening environmental conditions. The high levels of pollution in large sectors of Lima, Chimbote, and other coastal centers are the result of the unregulated dumping of industrial, automotive, and domestic wastes. The loss of irrigated coastal farmland to urban sprawl, erosion of highland farms, and the clear-cutting of Amazonian forest have all conspired to impoverish the nation's most valuable natural resources and further exacerbate social conditions. Unfortunately, while Peru is endowed with perhaps the widest range of resources in South America, somehow they have never been coherently or effectively utilized to construct a balanced and progressive society.

ARGENTINA

Argentina offers both a public and private healthcare system. About 18 million Argentineans have health insurance through their unions and go to clinics called *obras sociales* for medical care. About 4 million people from the middle and upper classes are privately insured. Some large private health insurance companies have their own hospitals. About a third of the population does not have health insurance, and of these, almost half are children. Those without health insurance go to public hospitals for treatment. These hospitals are equipped to handle emergencies but may not have the facilities for more involved forms of treatment. Government cuts to the public health system have left many poorer Argentineans without access to needed healthcare services.

Although most areas have a safe water supply and, in general, healthy living conditions, in certain interior regions, particularly in the north, and in poverty-stricken areas in the cities, living conditions are far from ideal. Many homes in these areas have no running water, sewage system, or electricity, and there may be no healthcare facilities nearby. AIDS-related diseases are growing, and cholera and tuberculosis have reappeared in some regions. Medical care in Buenos Aires is generally good, but care varies in quality outside the capital, and in some parts of Argentina, the hospitals do not have the most up-to-date equipment. Serious medical problems requiring hospitalization or perhaps even medical evacuation to the United States can cost thousands of dollars or more, and doctors and hospitals often expect immediate cash payment for health services.

Like the rest of the world, South America has not escaped exposure to the HIV/AIDS epidemic. By far the largest and most populous country on the continent, Brazil suffers under a diverse epidemic that has penetrated all 26 states in the country. Although national HIV prevalence among pregnant women has remained low, a growing share of new HIV infections are among women, and those living in deprived circumstances appear to be disproportionately at risk of infection. In Brazil's cities, the contribution of injecting drug use to HIV transmission appears to have declined due to a variety of programs designed to reduce the risk of exposure. Official estimates show that three-quarters of the estimated 200,000 drug injectors in Brazil now use sterile syringes. In Argentina, most new infections have been occurring during unprotected heterosexual intercourse, with increasing numbers of women acquiring HIV. The male-to-female ratio among reported AIDS cases shrank from 15:1 in 1988 to 3:1 in 2004. Injecting drug use and unsafe sex between men continue to provide impetus to the spread of HIV in Argentina, especially in the urban areas of Buenos Aires, Cordoba, and Santa Fe provinces, where an estimated 80 percent of AIDS cases have occurred. When tested in the city of Buenos Aires, some 44 percent of drug injectors were HIV positive, while in other studies HIV prevalence of 7 to 15 percent has been found among men who have sex with men. HIV has penetrated rural parts of Paraguay, especially along the borders with Argentina and Brazil. Bolivia's epidemic remains small and appears to be driven largely by commercial sex and sex between men, much of it concentrated in urban areas. Infection levels in groups of men who have sex with men have reached 15 percent in La Paz and almost 24 percent in Santa Cruz. A study in the city of Cochabamba has shown that 3.5 percent of the surveyed street youth were living with HIV, and most had been infected sexually. Sex between men appears to be a prominent factor also in Ecuador's growing epidemic, where new reports of HIV cases have almost doubled in the last decade. In Colombia, HIV initially affected mostly men, so much so that they comprise 83 percent of all AIDS cases reported to the national health authorities to date. However, a significant proportion of men who have sex with men also maintain sexual relationships with women. As a result, increasing numbers of women are becoming infected.

SEE ALSO: Argentina; Brazil; Peru.

BIBLIOGRAPHY. Anabela Abreu, et al., eds., HIV/AIDS in Latin American Countries: An Assessment of National Capacity (World Bank, 2003); AVERT, www.avert.org (cited October 2006); Country Studies, www.countrystudies.us (cited October 2006); Cultural Profiles Project, www.cp-pc.ca/english/index.html (cited October 2006); Family Health International, www.fhi.org/en/index.htm (cited October 2006); Sonia Fleury, Susana Belmartino, and Enis Baris, eds., *Reshaping Health Care in Latin America: A Comparative Analysis of Health Care Reform in Argentina, Brazil, and Mexico* (IDRC, 2001); Transparency International, *Global Corruption Report 2006: Special Focus: Corruption and Health* (Pluto Press, 2006).

BEN WYNNE, PH.D.
GAINESVILLE STATE COLLEGE

Healthcare, U.S. and Canada

While Canada and the United States had quite similar healthcare systems in the 1960s, the two neighbors now stand in marked contrast in terms of healthcare system provision and payment. The United States features a market-based system of delivery and payment, while healthcare delivery is organized in Canada by provincial governments, which also are responsible for most healthcare expenditures. One of the biggest differences between the two is that the United States is one of only a few industrialized countries not to guarantee healthcare for all of its citizens, while Canada represents an example of a country with universal healthcare guaranteed due to the heavy involvement of the government in providing funding for care.

Although the United States' healthcare system is largely characterized by private provision, federal and state governments still play a substantial role in providing the funding for healthcare services, especially via large national entitlement programs, Medicare, Medicaid, and State Children's Health Insurance Program (SCHIP). Medicare provides direct payments from the federal government to private providers for physician and hospital services, and recently expanded to include funding for prescription drugs. Generally available to individuals over the age of 65, as well as certain other categories of people (such as those officially classified as disabled), Medicare and other public programs account for approximately 50 percent of all healthcare expenditures in the United States, and is funded via payroll taxes into a trust fund, one which is slated to run out of funds at some time in the 21st century without substantial overhaul of the program.

GOVERNMENT-SPONSORED PROGRAMS

Medicaid also provides direct payments from state and federal governments to providers, often via state Medicaid programs. While Medicaid eligibility is determined at the state level, this program is largely limited to poor, pregnant women, children, and elderly persons needing long-term care assistance. SCHIP generally covers children up to the age of 18 whose families make too much money to qualify for Medicaid but who are still considered "low income" according to state guidelines. A handful of states have extended SCHIP to all uninsured children in the state, regardless of family income. Other smaller government programs provide for direct provision of care for certain categories of people, such as military veterans and Native Americans. The federal government and many state governments also provide health insurance to employees, as do many municipal governments. In recent years, a growing number of providers have stopped accepting patients insured by Medicaid and even Medicare, citing burdensome administrative requirements and low reimbursement rates.

Individuals who are not eligible for Medicare, Medicaid, or SCHIP in the United States must purchase health insurance or healthcare on the private market. Many Americans are provided with subsidized health insurance as a fringe benefit of employment, although the percentage of employers offering health insurance to workers and, especially, workers' dependents, is shrinking every year due to higher health insurance premiums. Small and family-owned businesses are particularly unlikely to offer health insurance, as these firms are too small to negotiate attractive premiums. Likewise, part-time or freelance workers are usually not offered health insurance plans by their employers. Decreasing coverage by employers has fueled a recent rise in the number of Americans without health insurance in the early 21st century. Individuals can purchase insurance premiums, but these premiums are often prohibitively expensive. In 2004, an estimated 15 percent of the total population, or about 45 million Americans, lacked health insurance. While critics of increased government funding for healthcare often indicate that a government program may reduce choice, it is important to note that most privately insured Americans now belong to an HMO plan, which restricts choice of providers to certain networks if patients want full reimbursement of expenses. These providers are those that have negotiated with the insurance company for a certain price, in exchange for referrals for business. Thus, the market is already restricting choice of provider.

HEALTH INSURANCE

One myth regarding healthcare in the United States is that health insurance is required for access to care. The federal Emergency Medical Treatment and Labor Act (EMTALA) states that hospitals and providers accepting Medicare payments must provide emergency medical care, including providing a medical intake exam, stabilizing an emergency condition, or allowing a pregnant woman to deliver, regardless of ability to pay. This law applies to all individuals regardless of United States citizenship or immigration status, and thus has become a primary means of obtaining medical care for illegal immigrants, who often have no access to either government programs or employer-sponsored insurance. The costs of providing care for uninsured individuals in emergency rooms is often passed on to other consumers in the form of higher charges and premiums, which often induces employers or other funders to drop coverage, leading to more uninsured patients. Many free clinics also exist, as well as community-based health clinics that charge low-income patients special rates. Still, consistently accessing primary care via free or community-based clinics can be difficult and time consuming.

Another problem related to health insurance affordability is the problem of underinsurance. Many of those with health insurance are only insured against catastrophic losses, and must pay high deductibles, coinsurance, or copayments for pharmaceuticals, primary care physician visits, and procedures that cost below a certain minimum value. These extra charges can be quite financially burdensome, especially for low-income families; an estimated 50 percent of those who file for bankruptcy do so because of an inability to pay medical bills. A majority of these 50 percent had some sort of insurance. Furthermore, the burden of these charges means that many of those with health insurance still go without needed care because they cannot afford to pay the unsubsidized bill.

The problems of uninsurance, underinsurance, and lack of access to care have all contributed to health disparities in the United States between racial groups and social classes, with low-income minorities suffering particularly poor health outcomes relative to other segments of the population. While many argue that these disparities are due to innate health behaviors, a distrust of the medical system among minority patients, and population health factors such as obesity rates, nutritional practices, language barriers, and smoking and other substance abuse, lack of access to affordable care certainly seems to play a role in perpetuating these disparities, particularly in terms of alleviating disabilities and chronic conditions such as diabetes and hypertension.

In contrast to the United States, most Canadians receive healthcare free at the point of service, although healthcare is still largely provided privately, rather than in state-owned clinics and hospitals as with Great Britain's National Health Service. Physicians also generally receive a fee per service, rather than acting as government employees. The federal and provincial governments provide almost all of the money for physicians and inpatient services. The largest public program in Canada is also called Medicare, which are all run according to common principles set out in the Canada Health Act, but are administered by different provinces, much as Medicaid is administered by each state in the United States. Patients within the Medicare system are free to choose their own providers, who are then reimbursed. Medicare at the federal level operates largely via block grants to the provinces, in conjunction with funding for other social programs; this arrangement can lead to significant differences in the types of care and means of accessing care across provinces. The largest federal program outside of Medicare provides for care for the First Nations people, directly reimbursing providers for their care. As in the United States, veterans and prison inmates are provided for by their own programs. Canada funds the Medicare and other health programs via payroll taxes on employers, as well as user premiums in some provinces.

Canada's healthcare plan does not cover certain services, including dental care for anyone over 14, optometry services (in some areas), or prescription drugs. Many Canadians have supplementary health insurance to cover these items, as do many elderly Americans who do not want to rely on Medicare as the sole means of insurance. Canadians also purchase health insurance on the private market in order to access care more quickly. Canada does prohibit direct purchase of services within Canada, so citizens have a difficult time "opting out" of the system unless they travel to the United States or another country. As in the United States, a right to healthcare does not always result in access to care, or access in a timely fashion, although little rigorous data exist evaluating how harmful wait lists and other access delays are to patients. Wait times for hospital procedures or office appointments can stretch weeks or months, fueled partially by a chronic shortage of physicians.

Nonetheless, despite access problems and some limits on services, the Canadian state guarantees a much higher level of medical services free at the point of use than the United States does, and thus comparative health policy analysts and advocates for (and opponents of) American universal health coverage often use the United States' and Canada's healthcare systems to illustrate the relative merits of a market-based health system (albeit one with substantial state involvement) and a government-sponsored, single-payer health system. Although cross-country comparisons of health outcomes are difficult, proponents of universal healthcare in the United States will usually point out that while the United States spends an estimated 15 percent of its Gross National Product (GNP) on healthcare, while Canada spends only approximately 9.5 percent, population health statistics are often better for Canadians than for Americans, indicating that the United

States is getting less "value for money" for healthcare expenditures than Canadians are. According to the World Health Organization (WHO) in 2005, Canadians had a higher life expectancy (79.3 years vs. 77.0 years), lower infant mortality rates (5.6/1,000 live births to 6.4/1,000 live births), and lower rates of under-5 child mortality (6/1,000 live births to 8/1,000 live births) than the United States.

Many hypotheses have been advanced to explain these differences, especially those that argue either for or against the United States expanding federal and state funding for the health system. One reason why health outcomes in the United States might be worse than in Canada is due to population health reasons. Drugs, violence, war wounds, alcohol abuse, and obesity are all more common in the United States than in Canada (although Canadians are slightly more likely to smoke), all of which place a burden on the health system. The United States has more illegal immigrants, who are more likely to use expensive emergency rooms for primary care in lieu of relatively inexpensive outpatient clinics. Yet, both countries face the problem of caring for aging populations, so demographics alone likely does not explain all of the cost difference between the two countries.

One reason proposed as to why the United States spends more on healthcare with poorer results is because there are so many uninsured Americans who lack access to preventive care as well as primary care, diagnosis, and treatment, and thus present in emergency rooms only when they have already progressed to an advanced stage of an illness or surgical problem that is then more difficult and costly to treat. Access to primary care, however, also seems to be somewhat a problem in Canada, albeit not as extensive a problem as in the United States. The 2003 Canadian Community Health Survey indicated that up to 1.2 million Canadians do not have a primary care doctor, either because they could not find one or had not yet looked. Those without a primary doctor, as in the United States, are more likely to visit an emergency room. Wait lists also contribute to delayed care in Canada. Thus, this problem of access to primary care seems to plague both nations, only the problem is more severe in the United States.

There are also some expenditure differences in specific areas that may also help drive the differential in spending between the two countries. Because Canada's system of payments is more homogenous than the United States' system of reimbursement from several different private and public sources, Canada also has a lower percentage of total healthcare expenditures going toward administrative costs. Administrators and physicians are also paid more, on average, in the United States, which is one reason why Canada faces a chronic physician shortage, as many are lured south of the border. There is more direct-to-consumer marketing in the United States of health plans and pharmaceuticals, costs that eventually reach payers. Research and development spending on pharmaceuticals and other technologies is also higher in the United States. Some argue that without the profit motivation, innovation in healthcare would falter should the United States move toward more of a state-funded medical system.

It is difficult to know using Canada as an example, since the Canadian government might be unable to afford greater technological spending, or it could be choosing to spend less because it also benefits from innovations discovered in and funded by the United States. Finally, the United States' infamous malpractice litigation suits often increase costs in healthcare, both in terms of malpractice insurance premiums from physicians and also because of "defensive medicine," whereby physicians order tests and procedures that are probably not necessary but will protect them against a lawsuit, should a negative outcome occur.

Particularly cited by opponents of moving away from a market-based system in the United States is the argument that U.S. healthcare costs more because it is of higher quality. The United States leads the world in terms of advanced diagnostic equipment, such as magnetic resonance imaging (MRI) and computed tomography (CT) scanners. Canadians seeking these services have often crossed the border to pay out-of-pocket rather than wait in long lines at home, anecdotes that critics of universal health insurance in the United States cite as proof that the United States' system is superior. Yet, because Canada funds treatments that are proven most cost-effective, some argue that Canada offers superior treatment because it is more likely to yield results. Numerous comparative studies examining mortality outcomes from cancer show that while Americans are more likely to develop certain types of cancers, such as breast and prostate cancer, the overall mortality rate in the two countries is about the same, indicating that Canada's health system might perform better in terms of cancer care.

The two approaches to healthcare both have economic consequences. Canada's publicly funded system requires higher income taxes, which can suppress economic growth. Yet, in the United States, individuals often face "job lock," whereby they fear changing employment lest they lose affordable healthcare coverage. This "job lock" can suppress labor market flexibility. Furthermore, companies that pay high premiums for employee care are often at a competitive disadvantage in the global economy, because of this relatively high cost of labor. This disadvantage has been particularly prevalent in industries such as the auto industry, which faces highly unionized workforces and heavy "legacy" costs—health benefits promised to previous generations of workers who are now retired. Both countries face the challenge of increasing medical costs due to higher utilization rates of expensive technology, as well as aging populations.

Recently, in the United States, some states and municipalities have started universal access programs of their own, tired of waiting for federal reform. The City of San Francisco and the State of Oregon have both recently moved toward covering all uninsured citizens, as has the State of Massachusetts. Proposals range from forcing companies to cover more of their part-time workers to expanding Medicaid and SCHIP to all uninsured. Yet, these reformers face strong opposition to universal health insurance from the hospital and health insurance industry, and in many cases from physicians and health workers themselves, who fear lower incomes and reduced autonomy. Reform proposals in Canada generally focus on increasing the amount of funding for reimbursements to providers, rather than dismantling the system of public health insurance altogether. Canadians seem to take pride in their universal health system, in part because, by being based on fairness and equity, it is distinct from the United States' market-based system.

SEE ALSO: Medicaid; Medicare.

BIBLIOGRAPHY. Steffie Woolhandler Terry Campbell, and David U. Himmelstein, "Costs of Health Care Administra-

tion in the United States and Canada," *New England Journal of Medicine,* (August 21, 2003); U.E. Reinhardt, et. al., "U.S. Health Care Spending In An International Context," *Health Affairs,* (v.23/3, 2004).

ANNIE DUDE
UNIVERSITY OF CHICAGO

Health Insurance Portability and Accountability Act (HIPAA)

BACKGROUND

The Health Insurance Portability and Accountability Act (HIPAA), enacted by the United States Congress in 1996 (Public Law 104-191), is the most significant federal legislation affecting the U.S. healthcare industry since the creation of Medicare and Medicaid in 1965. Over time, the greater utilization of and wider access to personal health information (PHI) in conjunction with insufficient confidentiality protection procedures amplified the potential for unauthorized use and disclosure of individual's PHI. These trends placed substantial pressure on traditional confidentiality protections and consequently lead to the development of HIPAA legislation.

HIPAA was designed to improve the portability and continuity of health insurance coverage; combat waste, fraud and abuse in healthcare; simplify the administration of health insurance; protect the privacy and security of patients' medical information; and standardize electronic healthcare transactions. HIPAA's impacts penetrate into all facets of the U.S. healthcare system, most notably on the practices of medical care and clinical research.

COMPONENTS

The Healthcare Access, Portability, and Renewability provisions (Title I) regulate the availability and scope of health insurance plans in order to protect the stability of coverage for employees (and their families). The Title also prohibits health plans from creating eligibility rules or assessing premiums based on an individual's health status, medical history, genetic information, or disability and restricts the limitations on benefits health plans can impose based on an individual's preexisting conditions.

The Administrative Simplification provisions (Title II) augment the efficiency and effectiveness of the healthcare system by regulating the exchange of electronic healthcare data. The U.S. Department of Health and Human Services, charged with the task of implementing Title II, instituted five regulations applicable to covered entities (health plans, clearinghouses, and providers) that transmit PHI data.

The Standards for Privacy of Individually Identifiable Health Information (Privacy Rule) establishes, for the first time, comprehensive protections for the use and the disclosure of PHI. The Privacy Rule guarantees that health data are properly insulated while simultaneously allowing the exchange of health information necessary for ensuring quality healthcare and protecting the public's health. It also assures the confidentiality and documentation of any PHI disclosure and mandates notification to individuals regarding any use of their PHI. The provisions are comprehensive and designed to strike a balance between permitting critical uses of information and securing individuals' privacy.

The Transactions and Code Set Rules institute uniform standards for electronic healthcare transactions involving the transfer of PHI and establish consistent code sets and identifiers for electronic data interchange. The Security Rule establishes standardized security requirements for administrative, technical, and physical procedures to ensure confidentiality during the use and dissemination of PHI. The Unique Identifiers Rule institutes consistent standards for electronic transactions by requiring employers and healthcare providers to obtain and use a unique identifier code for all electronic transactions. Last, the Enforcement Rule outlines offenses, monetary penalties, investigation procedures, and hearings for violations. Covered entities that knowingly and improperly disclose identifiable PHI are subject to civil penalties (up to $25,000 annually) and criminal penalties (up to $250,000 and 10 years imprisonment).

IMPLICATIONS

The complex legalities and potential penalties associated with HIPAA as well as the increase in paperwork and the cost of implementation have necessitated significant changes in the way healthcare providers

and researchers operate. HIPAA restrictions limit, if not eliminate, retrospective chart-based research and researchers' ability to prospectively recruit research subjects. HIPAA regulations require that covered entities obtain patients' signed authorization to use or disclose PHI for research purposes. Such research modifications have also significantly increased the cost of performing clinical research.

SEE ALSO: Department of Health and Human Services (DHHS); Institute of Medicine (IOM); Institutional Review Board (IRB); Insurance.

BIBLIOGRAPHY. B. C. Fuchs, et al., *The Health Insurance Portability and Accountability Act (HIPAA) of 1996: Guidance on Frequently Asked Questions* (CRS, 1998); D. Shalowitz and D. Wendler, "Informed Consent for Research and Authorization under the Health Insurance Portability and Accountability Act Privacy Rule: An Integrated Approach," *Annals of Internal Medicine (v.*144/9, 2006); G. M. Stevens, *A Brief Summary of the HIPAA Medical Privacy Rule* (CRS, 2003); U.S. Department of Health and Human Services, *Summary of the HIPAA Privacy Rule* (Office for Civil Rights, 2003); J. F. Wilson, "Health Insurance Portability and Accountability Act Privacy Rule Causes Ongoing Concerns among Clinicians and Researchers," *Annals of Internal Medicine* (v.145/4, 2006).

REBEKAH M. ZINCAVAGE
DUANE R. NEFF
BRANDEIS UNIVERSITY

Health Maintenance Organization (HMO)

A health management organization is type of medical service in which members prepay a monthly or annual fee for their healthcare needs, including hospitalization. The term was coined by a health policy analyst, Dr. Paul Ellwood, in the early 1970s. At the time, Ellwood and some of his like-minded colleagues regarded Medicare as the advent of a disturbing trend toward socialized medicine. Because of this, he intended to introduce the "health maintenance organization" (HMO) as a better alternative to a socialized system. Ellwood's goal was to initiate a new direction in healthcare which would not only provide quality service to the public, but would also contain escalating healthcare costs by preventing disease and also maintain good health in the population. Most HMOs involve physicians engaged in group practice. Because costs to patients are fixed in advance, preventive medicine is stressed to avoid costly hospitalization. One criticism of HMOs is that patients can use only doctors and specialists who are associated with the organization. Many people who have had a long-standing relationship with a family doctor or specialist have balked at what they see as a limitation of choice. "Open-ended" HMOs offer members the option of seeing a doctor who is not part of the HMO, but the patient must pay additional costs. Proponents of HMOs say that they make healthcare available to more people and that their emphasis on prevention results in earlier diagnosis and increased healthcare savings. Numerous complaints (and lawsuits) have arisen, however, over HMOs' refusals to approve various treatments, and over the concern that the organizations skimp on care in order to realize profits.

An HMO enters into contractual arrangements with healthcare providers (e.g., physicians, hospitals, and other healthcare professionals) who together form a "provider network." In simple terms, a contracted provider is one who provides services to health plan members at discounted rates in exchange for receiving health plan referrals. Unlike traditional indemnity insurance, healthcare provided by an HMO generally follows a set of care guidelines provided through the HMO's network of providers. Under this model, providers contract with an HMO to receive more patients and in return usually agree to provide services at a discount. This arrangement allows the HMO to charge a lower monthly premium, which is an advantage over indemnity insurance, provided that its members are willing to abide by the additional restrictions.Members are required to see only providers within this network to have their healthcare paid for by the HMO. If the member receives care from a provider who isn't in the network, the HMO won't pay for care unless it was pre-authorized by the HMO or deemed an emergency. Members select a primary care physician (PCP), often called a "gatekeeper," who provides, arranges, coordinates, and authorizes all aspects of the member's healthcare. PCPs are usually family doctors, internal medicine doctors, general

practitioners, pediatricians, and obstetricians/gynecologists. In a typical HMO, most medical needs must first go through the PCP, who authorizes referrals to specialists or other doctors if deemed necessary. Emergency medical care does not require prior authorization from a PCP, and many plans allow women to select an obstetrician/gynecoogist (OB/GYN) in addition to a PCP, whom they may see without a referral. Members can only see a specialist (e.g., cardiologist, dermatologist, rheumatologist) if this is authorized by the PCP. If the member sees a specialist without a referral, the HMO won't pay for the care. HMOs are the most restrictive type of health plan because they give members the least choice in selecting a healthcare provider. However, HMOs typically provide members with a greater range of health benefits for the lowest out-of-pocket expenses, such as either no or a very low copayment (the amount of money a member is required to pay the provider in addition to what the HMO pays. It often must be paid prior to services being rendered.

HMOs also manage care through utilization review. The amount of utilization is usually expressed as a number of visits or services or a dollar amount per member per month. Utilization review is intended to identify providers providing an unusually high amount of services, in which case some services may not be medically necessary, or an unusually low amount of services, in which case patients may not be receiving appropriate care and are in danger of worsening a condition. HMOs often provide preventive care for a lower copayment or for free, in order to keep members from developing a preventable condition that would require a great deal of medical services. When HMOs were coming into existence, indemnity plans often did not cover preventive services, such as immunizations, well-baby checkups, mammograms, or physicals.

It is this inclusion of services intended to maintain a member's health that gave the HMO its name. Some services, such as outpatient mental healthcare, are often provided on a limited basis, and more costly forms of care, diagnosis, or treatment may not be covered. Experimental treatments and elective services that are not medically necessary (such as elective plastic surgery) are almost never covered. Other methods for managing care are case management, in which patients with catastrophic cases are identified, or disease management, in which patients with certain chronic diseases like diabetes, asthma, or some forms of cancer are identified. In either case, the HMO takes a greater level of involvement in the patient's care, assigning a case manager to the patient or a group of patients to ensure that no two providers provide overlapping care, and to ensure that the patient is receiving appropriate treatment, so that the condition does not get worse beyond what can be helped. HMOs often shift some financial risk to providers through a system called capitation, where certain providers (usually PCPs) receive a fixed payment per member per month and in return provide certain services for free.

Under this arrangement, the provider does not have the incentive to provide unnecessary care, as he will not receive any additional payment for the care. Some plans offer a bonus to providers whose care meets a predetermined level of quality. Some critics regard HMOs as monopolies that distort the market for healthcare. They argue that HMOs were supposed to be a stopgap solution, and perhaps even set up for ultimate failure so the public would demand that the federal government would take over with a national healthcare system.

SEE ALSO: Health Insurance Portability and Accountability Act (HIPAA); Medicaid.

BIBLIOGRAPHY. American Heart Association, www. americanheart.org (cited October 2006); Ellyn Spragins, "Beware Your HMO," *Newsweek* (October 23, 1995); John E. Kralewski, Roger Feldman, Bryan Dowd, and Janet Shapiro, *"Strategies Employed by HMOs to Achieve Hospital Discounts: A Case Study of Seven HMOs" Health Care Management Review* (v.16/1, 1991); Huey L. Mays, Jerald Katzoff, and Marc L. Rivo, "Managed Health Care: Implications for the Physician Workforce and Medical Education," *Journal of American Medical Association* (v.274/9, 1995); William MacMillan Rodney, "Health Care Reform: Does Primary Care Mean, 'Whoever Gets There First?'" *American Family Physician,* (v.50/2, 1994); Linda S. Widra and Myron D. Fottler, "Determinants of HMO Success: The Case of Complete Health," *Health Care Manage Review,* (v.17/2,1992).

BEN WYNNE, PH.D
GAINESVILLE STATE COLLEGE

Health Resource and Services Administration (HRSA)

Created through the 1982 merger of the Health Resources Administration and the Health Services Administration, the Health Resource and Services Administration (HRSA) is an agency of the United States Department of Health and Human Services. It is the primary federal agency for improving access to healthcare services for those who are uninsured, isolated, or medically vulnerable. The HRSA provides national leadership, program resources, and services needed to improve access to culturally competent, quality health care.

Focusing on those with the most need, the agency has as its goals the overall improvement of the nation's access to healthcare, the improvement of healthcare outcomes, the improvement of the quality of healthcare, the elimination of health disparities, the improvement of public healthcare systems, the improvement of responses to emergency situations, and overall excellence in management practices.

The HRSA has six operating components. The Bureau of Health Professions (BHPr) provides national leadership in coordinating, evaluating, and supporting the development and utilization of the Nation's health personnel. The Bureau of Primary Health Care (BPHC) provides national leadership in assessing the nation's healthcare needs of underserved populations and in assisting communities to provide primary healthcare services to the underserved in moving toward eliminating health disparities.

The Bureau also administers the Black Lung Clinics program, the Native Hawaiian Health Care Program, the Healthy Communities Access Program, the Radiation Exposure Screening and Education Program, and the National Hansen's Disease Program. Healthcare Systems Bureau (HSB) provides national leadership and direction in several key functional areas, including the procurement, allocation and transplantation of human organs and blood stem cell; the facilitation of the development of state, territorial, and municipal preparedness programs to enhance the capacity of the nation's hospitals and other healthcare entities to respond to mass casualty incidents caused by terrorism and other public health emergencies; the provision of programmatic, financial and architectural/engineering support for healthcare facilities construction/renovation programs; the reduction in numbers of uninsured persons through the State Planning Grants Program; and the management and operation of the national programs for childhood vaccine and smallpox vaccine injury compensation.

The HIV/AIDS Bureau (HAB) provides leadership in the delivery of high-quality clinical care and supporting services for uninsured and underinsured individuals living with and families affected by HIV/AIDS. It includes the Office for Advancement of Telehealth, the HRSA-wide developer of telehealth, including the use of electronic information and telecommunications technologies for all types of health-related activities. It also includes HRSA's Center for Quality which strengthens and improves the quality of health care, especially related to agency programs and service populations.

The Maternal and Child Health Bureau (MCHB) provides national leadership, in partnership with key stakeholders, to improve the physical and mental health, safety and well-being of the maternal and child health (MCH) population. The MCH population includes all of the Nation's women, infants, children, adolescents, and their families (including fathers), and children with special healthcare needs.

The Bureau also manages the HRSA Office of Women's Health. The Office of Rural Health Policy (ORHP) serves as a focal point within the department and as a principle source of advice to the administrator and secretary for coordinating efforts to strengthen and improve the delivery of health services to populations in the nation's rural areas and border areas.

SEE ALSO: Department of Health and Human Services (DHHS).

BIBLIOGRAPHY. Health Resources and Services Administration, www.hrsa.gov (cited September 2006); Health Resources and Administration HIV/AIDS Bureau, hab.hrsa.gov/history.htm (cited September 2006); United States Department of Health and Human Services, www.hhs.gov (cited September 2006).

Ben Wynne, Ph.D
Gainesville State College

Hearing Problems in Children

Most children are able to hear the minute they are born. However, two or three out of every 1,000 children in the United States are born without the ability to hear. Hearing problems such as hearing loss can be a significant life-changing event to a newborn baby or child and to his or her family. Among the wide range of hearing disabilities, there are two different types of permanent hearing loss and a condition of temporary hearing impairment that can be seen commonly among children. Treatment options are available to resolve reversible hearing problems and understanding if your child is experiencing hearing difficulties can help the treatment process be more effective.

Temporary hearing loss in children can be caused by a variety of problems. These include a collection of wax in the ear canal, a foreign object stuck in the ear, excess mucus that accompanies a cold and sits in the Eustachian tube, or an ear infection such as otitis media (infection of the middle ear). Children can also develop hearing problems from specific diseases such as meningitis. Although there are many causes of temporary hearing loss, permanent hearing impairment is also possible.

Permanent deafness can fall into one of two categories. The first type is a hearing condition where the auditory nerve (cranial nerve 8) in the inner ear is damaged. This damage cannot be reversed. The other

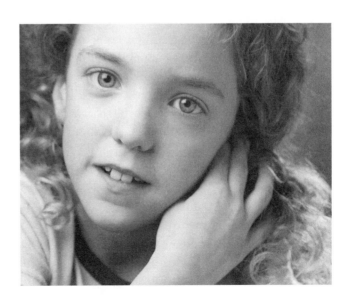

Two or three out of every 1,000 children in the United States are born without the ability to hear.

type of hearing loss is where external sound waves are unable to reach the inner ear. This can be caused by numerous problems such as earwax buildup, fluid collection, or even a punctured eardrum that cannot be fixed. Hearing problems that go without the proper treatment and care progressively get worse until they disappear completely. Treatment options include hearing aids, special training, specific medications, and certain surgical procedures. Because of the problems that can arise without early treatment of hearing impairment, it is imperative that you take note of your child's daily activities and look for signs that might indicate some difficulty in hearing. Some of these signs include when a child fails to respond when called, complains of hearing ringing in his or her ears, speaks loudly at inappropriate times, watches television at an abnormally high volume, pronounces words incorrectly, comes across as inattentive, and is highly prone to daydreaming. If any of these indications are noted, it is crucial that action be taken immediately.

The mechanism of the process of hearing and the reasoning behind hearing impairment is an important concept necessary to learn to develop a strong understanding of this disability. Unfortunately, sound does not travel properly through fluid or cerumen (earwax), and because of this, children who develop ear infections may experience difficulties in hearing. Normal speech tends to sound soft spoken like a whisper, so these children are inclined to feel the need to speak much louder. This hearing impairment only exists so long as the infection is present. It has no connection with any permanent hearing deficits. Nevertheless, if the child were to develop constant recurrent middle ear infections, it is likely that this child will experience a delay in his or her speech development only because he or she is unable to hear properly.

Hearing problems that arise at birth can be difficult to diagnose. They might not be too obvious until the baby reaches the age of 12 to 18 months, the time when children start saying their first words. Prior to this age, children with hearing loss have a tendency to respond to their surroundings by utilizing their senses such as their eyes and sense of touch. This method of reacting to their environment can actually cover any underlying hearing difficulty the child might have.

SEE ALSO: Acoustic Neuroma; Child Development; Deafness; Ear Disorders.

BIBLIOGRAPHY. Better Health, "Ear Problems in Children," www.betterhealth.vic.gov (cited May 2007); Better Health, "Hearing Problems in Children," www.betterhealth.vic.gov (cited May 2007); MedlinePlus, "Hearing Disorders and Deafness," www.nlm.nih.gov/medlineplus (cited May 2007); World Health Organization, "World Health Organization Fact Sheet on Deafness and Hearing Impairment," http://www.who.int/mediacentre/factsheets/fs300/en/ (cited May 2007).

AKTA SEHGAL
UNIVERSITY OF MISSOURI, KANSAS CITY
SCHOOL OF MEDICINE

Heart Attack

Cardiovascular disease (comprised mainly of heart disease and stroke) represents the leading cause of mortality and morbidity globally. In the United States, heart attacks make up about half of the prevalence of all coronary heart disease.

DEFINITION AND MEDICAL DIAGNOSIS

A heart attack, known in medical terms as an acute myocardial infarction, refers to the death of heart tissue following the rupture of atherosclerotic plaque in the wall of a coronary artery that causes a blood clot to block the flow of blood and supply of oxygen through the artery downstream to that area. The rupture of the atherosclerotic plaque is often triggered within a few hours by factors such as physical exertion (particularly for people not normally active), emotional stress, anger, and excitement. A heart attack can be life threatening, and typically requires hospitalization. Common symptoms of a heart attack include chest pain, sweating, and shortness of breath, although heart attacks can also occur without any symptoms (so-called "silent" heart attacks). A diagnosis of heart attack is made according to criteria of a positive history, electrocardiogram, and heart enzymes measured in the blood, as set out by the World Health Organization. "Probable" and "definite" diagnoses of a heart attack require that two and all three of these criteria are met, respectively.

RISK FACTORS

Established risk factors for coronary artery atherosclerosis (and thus heart attacks) include age, male gender, cigarette smoking, elevated low-density lipoprotein (LDL) cholesterol, low high-density lipoprotein (HDL) cholesterol, hypertension, diabetes, physical inactivity, obesity, and low socioeconomic status (as measured by income and education). Risk factors for which there is less consensus among scientists include novel markers of systemic inflammation such as C-reactive protein, elevated homocysteine and lipoprotein(a) levels, psychological factors such as depression and hostility, and physical and social environmental factors such as living in a poor neighborhood.

The average age at which a first heart attack occurs is 66 years in men and 70 years in women. In general, higher rates of a first heart attack occur among blacks than among those of other races/ethnicities. The average rates for a first heart attack per 1,000 population in nonblack women during the 1990s were estimated at 6.8, 14.2, and 33.2 for ages 65 to 74, 75 to 84, and 85 and older, respectively. Among black women, the average rates per 1,000 for these same age groups were higher at 8.6, 17.6, and 24.8, respectively. These discrepancies are in keeping with the higher prevalence of heart disease risk factors also found among blacks.

Based on a study spanning 52 countries, nine modifiable risk factors (including smoking, abnormal lipid levels, hypertension, and diabetes) account for more than 90 percent of the risk of a first heart attack. This suggests a tremendous potential to reduce heart attack risk and the burden of heart disease through these risk factors. The associations were consistent between men and women, between racial/ethnic groups, and across geographic regions, such that these findings should be applicable worldwide.

In recent years, research studies have increasingly explored associations between the socioeconomic environments of neighborhoods in which one lives and the risk of a heart attack. In a four-year follow-up study of the entire Swedish population aged 40 to 64 years, researchers looked at the relationship between the level of neighborhood socioeconomic deprivation and the risk of being admitted to hospital with a nonfatal heart attack, controlling for one's age and income. Both women and men living in the poorest versus richest neighborhoods had 1.9 and 1.4 times higher odds of a nonfatal heart attack, respectively.

TREATMENTS AND MEDICAL CONSEQUENCES

After a diagnosis of heart attack is made, medical treatments while in hospital include clot-dissolving medications (thrombolysis), angioplasty, and coronary bypass surgery. If not already on them, patients are started on medications including aspirin, beta-blockers, and statins, and are recommended to make changes to lifestyle risk factors, to lower their risk of future cardiovascular events. Based on data from the Framingham Heart Study, those who survive a heart attack are estimated to have 1.5 to 15 times higher risks of illness and death than those in the general population. Within six years of a heart attack, 18 percent of men and 35 percent are estimated to experience another heart attack, 8 percent of men and 11 percent of women to suffer a stroke, and 7 percent of men and 6 percent of women to have a sudden death. Studies are also ongoing as to the extent to which psychosocial factors, including social support, may help to improve long-term survival among heart attack patients. A heart attack is a life-threatening condition that contributes to substantial morbidity and mortality worldwide. A variety of risk factors for heart attacks have been established, while other risk factors have emerged and continue to be investigated. Many of the established risk factors are modifiable, such that intervening on these risk factors could have a major impact on the overall burden of heart attacks and cardiovascular disease. A number of treatments have also been developed to limit medical consequences among heart attack patients.

SEE ALSO: Cholesterol; Diabetes; Heart Diseases (General); Heart Diseases—Prevention; High Blood Pressure.

BIBLIOGRAPHY. P.C. Strike and A. Steptoe, "Behavioral and Emotional Triggers of Acute Coronary Syndromes: A Systematic Review and Critique," *Psychosomatic Medicine* (v.67, 2005); K. Sundquist, M. Malmstrom, and S.E. Johannson, "Neighborhood Deprivation and Incidence of Coronary Heart Disease: A Multilevel Study of 2.6 Million Women and Men in Sweden," *Journal of Epidemiology and Community Health* (v.58, 2004); T. Thom, et al., "Heart Disease and Stroke Statistics—2006 Update: A Report from the American Heart Association Statistics Committee and Stroke Statistics Subcommittee," *Circulation* (v.113, 2006).

DANIEL KIM, M.D., M.P.H., M.SC.
HARVARD SCHOOL OF PUBLIC HEALTH

Heart Bypass Surgery

Heart bypass surgery, also known as coronary artery bypass graft surgery (CABG), is the most commonly performed surgical procedure performed on the heart to bypass the obstructed artery (the coronary artery) of the heart and improve blood flow to the heart. The coronary arteries supply oxygen and nutrients to the cardiac muscles; due to the small size of the arteries, they are often prone to accumulation of fats and cholesterol which can lead to plaque formation and the development of atherosclerosis. If these arteries are blocked there is also a risk of developing ischemic heart disease or coronary artery disease leading to the development of angina. Factors increasing plaque accumulation include high blood pressure, increased cholesterol levels, smoking and the presence of diabetes. The increase in age (greater than 55 years for women and 45 years for men) also increases the risk as does a positive family history for early heart disease. To determine the presence of coronary artery disease, a stress test accompanied by electrocardiogram monitoring of the heart and cardiac catheterisation is performed. The latter is performed by insertion of a catheter through the artery in the groin or arm to the heart, with injection of contrast medium into the arteries.

CABGs are generally performed to relieve the chest pain and reduce the risk of death from coronary artery disease. A CABG generally takes four to six hours to complete. There are many techniques of performing a CABG; a detour is created to bypass the obstructed artery. Various arteries and veins may be used as grafts, these conduits include the saphenous vein, the internal thoracic artery (internal mammary artery) and the radial artery. Before the surgery the surgeon will use a coronary angiogram to identify the blockages. The surgical procedure begins with an incision of the middle of the chest followed by a median sternotomy (cutting of sternum). Through this incision the surgeon is able to view the heart and the aorta. To achieve the cardiopulmonary bypass tubes are inserted into the right atrium of the heart which will collect venous blood from the body to the membrane oxygenator in the bypass pump (heart-lung machine) thus enabling circulation of oxugenated blood to other parts of the body. The aorta is cross claped to allow bypasses to be connected to the aorta. The heart is stopped using a mixture of chemicals called cardioplegia.

Standard CABG surgery may be associated with concerns over neurological and inflammatory complications related to the bypass and thus many patients receive the off-pump CABG (OPCABG). This technique is used to perform the bypass without the use of the bypass pump. The advantage of this type of surgery is that it may be perfomed whilst the heart is still beating, thus reducing the risk of loss of memory. OPCABG has been reported to be superior in terms of length of stay in hospital following surgery and incidence of stroke; however it associated with a higher rate of mediastinal infection than CABG surgery. A technique known as minimally invasive direct coronary artery bypass (MIDCAB) is also used where the normal action of incision of the chest during the other techniques is avoided.

Heart bypasses differ in the numbers of coronary arteries bypassed in the procedure. There may be single bypass (one coronoary artery bypassed), double (two), triple (three), quadruple (four), and quintiple (five). For the coronary arteries to be bypassed, it must be ensured that the arteries are not too small, not heavily calcified, and not located within the heart muscle (intramycocardial). The recovery period after CABG (the first four to eight weeks after the surgery) is associated with higher risks of complications and hospital readmission. CABGs are associated with several risks; they are associated with significant postoperative cardiovascular morbidity and mortality in high-risk patients. Possible risks in receiving a CABG are myocardial infarctions which occur in five to 10 percent of patients. Stroke occurs in one to two percent, primarily in elderly patient. Depression is common after surgery, but is generally improved with the use of cognitive behavioral therapy. Research suggests that risks of CABG are worse in women than men. Overall mortality related to CABG is three to four percent. Mortality may be higher in women, primarily due to their advanced age at the time of CABG surgery and smaller coronary arteries as women are generally smaller than men. Mortality and complications increase with factors such as age (older than 70 years), kidney failure and presence of other diseases such as diabetes mellitus. Approximately 25 to 30 percent of patients undergoing CABG have diabetes mellitus, these patients have increased risk due to respiratory, renal and cerebral complications, and wound infections. Diabetes mellitus represents an independent risk factor for late graft failure and mortality from cardiac causes. CABGs are however performed on these patients as it results in better quality of life in the diabetic patient with severe coronary artery disease, as compared to medical treatment and the use of other surgical procedures such as percutaneous coronary angioplasty.

The long-term results after CABG surgery include possible blockage of vein grafts after surgery due to blood clotting. After a successful CABG, a patient's anginal chest pain generally resolves; however they may experience chest discomfort due to the incision of the chest prior to the bypass. In general, the success rate of CABG is approximately 90 percent; many of these patients experience significant improvements after the surgery.

SEE ALSO: Heart Attack; Heart Diseases (General).

BIBLIOGRAPHY. A. Jalal, et al., "Coronary Artery Bypass Grafting on Beating Heart. Does it Provide Superior Myocardial Preservation than Conventional Technique?" *Saudi Medical Journal* (v.28/6, 2001).

FARHANA AKTER
KING'S COLLEGE, LONDON

Heart Diseases (General)

Heart disease is the leading cause of death and disability worldwide. Approximately 16.7 million people die from heart disease each year, with coronary heart disease killing more than 7 million people. Heart disease can affect any component of the cardiovascular system, which includes the heart muscle, valves, conduction system, coronary arteries and veins, as well as systemic arteries and veins. Coronary artery heart disease, alone, accounts for roughly 2.3 million cases of heart disease annually. There are a variety of types of heart disease that affect a wide range of age groups and ultimately may lead to heart failure. Congenital heart disease, valvular heart disease, cardiomyopathies, and coronary artery disease are examples of heart disease. The severity of these diseases is dependant upon the degree to which they affect the ability of the heart to adequately pump blood throughout the body to meet nutritional demands.

Coronary artery disease (CAD) is the most common form of heart disease. CAD is the number one killer worldwide for those older than 60 years of age, and is the second leading cause of death, behind HIV/AIDS, for those 15 to 59 years old. Each year, 3.8 million men and 3.4 million women worldwide die from CAD. Currently, in the United States it is estimated that one out of every 2,000 people are affected by CAD. Although genetics play a role in the development of CAD, 80 to 90 percent of people who die of CAD have one or more risk factors influenced by an unhealthy lifestyle. CAD occurs when the arteries that supply blood to the heart muscle become hardened and narrowed.

This process is due to a buildup consisting mostly of fat, cholesterol, and calcium that circulate in the blood. The buildup of material is referred to as a plaque and leads to a condition known as atherosclerosis. As the plaque grows in size, the amount of blood passing through the vessels decreases and heart muscle does not receive adequate oxygen needed to survive. The development of atherosclerosis is a process that develops over time, often beginning in childhood and gradually increasing with age. CAD varies in severity and its presentation can range from asymptomatic to chest pain associated with exertion (angina), heart attack, and sudden cardiac death. Acute coronary syndrome refers to the symptoms associated with acute myocardial ischemia due to CAD. Of all people who die within the first month of experiencing CAD symptoms, approximately two-thirds of these people die before reaching the hospital. This highlights the importance of prevention and early recognition of CAD symptoms.

Risk factors for CAD in developed countries are divided into two groups: modifiable and nonmodifiable. Modifiable risk factors include high blood pressure, high cholesterol, smoking, diabetes, excess weight, and sedentary lifestyle. Nonmodifiable risk factors include family history, increased age, and male gender. Approximately 75 percent of heart disease can be attributed to conventional risk factors. Some less recognized risk factors include low socioeconomic status, mental illness, stress, alcohol, excess blood homocysteine, and inflammation. Those in developing countries face an even greater burden of risk factors in the fact that they also have to contend with low birth weight and folate deficiency due to malnutrition and communicable diseases, as well as the other risk factors.

As the name implies, modifiable risk factors are those factors that an individual can change in his or her daily lifestyle. High blood pressure, also known as hypertension, is a very common factor leading to CAD. It is estimated that by the time that a person reaches 60 years old, he or she has a greater than 60 percent chance that they are living with high blood pressure. Of that number, 31 percent of those people are unaware of the condition and are not experiencing any signs or symptoms. High cholesterol is most frequently a result of the food we eat; however genetics play an important role in determining cholesterol levels.

Cholesterol can be made by the body or obtained from the foods high in cholesterol (i.e., meat, fish, eggs). Foods that do not contain cholesterol but are high in saturated fats and trans fats also lead to elevated levels of cholesterol production and increase risk of heart disease. Cholesterol is divided into four different types. Increased levels of total cholesterol, triglycerides, and low-density lipoprotein (LDL) are responsible for increased risk, and an estimated one-third of all cardiovascular disease worldwide is attributed to high cholesterol. High-density lipoprotein (HDL) is the final type of cholesterol and has been shown to have a protective effect on the arteries of the body; therefore, decreased HDL levels leads to increased risk of heart disease. Therefore control of cholesterol is an important consideration in the attempt to decrease the risk of developing CAD.

LIFESTYLE HEART RISKS

Concerning smoking, cigarette smokers are 60 percent more likely to develop CAD due to toxins damaging the inner layer of the blood vessel walls. Even though there is an increased incidence of CAD in smokers, approximately 20 percent of adult men and 22 percent of adult women continue to smoke cigarettes. Healthcare costs directly related to smoking result in a global net loss of $200 billion per year, with one-third of those losses occurring in developing countries. Diabetes is a disease characterized by elevated blood sugar levels, and is primarily caused by decreased insulin production (type 1) or decreased responsiveness of tissues to insulin (type 2). Insulin is a hormone produced by the pancreas, and functions to transport sugars from the bloodstream to various

tissues for nutrition and storage. Another risk factor is excess weight, which leads to increased workload of the heart and is a key factor in the development of high blood pressure. Body mass index (BMI) is a method to calculate the degree of excess weight, and takes into account the weight and height of the individual. Healthy people have a BMI in the range of 18.4 to 24.9, while an index of 25 to 29.9 is considered overweight and an index of more than 30 is considered obese. Studies have shown that a decrease in weight by 11 to 22 pounds can reduce the risk of developing high blood pressure by over 25 percent. It has been proven that physical activity improves the ability of the heart and lungs to pump blood more effectively. Subjects with a sedentary lifestyle have a twofold increased risk of having a fatal heart attack compared to active people of the same age with equal risk factors. Exercise on a regular basis also helps to decrease all of the other aforementioned modifiable risk factors.

Prevention strategies, such as lifestyle modifications, are the first step to decreasing the risk of heart disease. Recommendations to a healthier lifestyle include 30 minutes of moderate physical activity four or more days a week, smoking cessation, and diets rich in fruits, vegetables, and potassium that avoid saturated fats and high-calorie meals. Decreasing body weight and avoiding stresses of daily life can reduce the demand on the heart. CAD typically occurs in middle-aged people, but risk factors are determined by lifestyle behaviors in childhood and early adulthood. Worldwide, 18 million children under 5 years are overweight, and 14 percent of 13- to 15-year-olds smoke cigarettes. This highlights the importance of healthy lifestyle choices early on to significantly decrease risk of heart disease in the future.

Congenital heart disease refers to defects of the heart that are present at birth, and most commonly affect the chambers of the heart, heart valves, and the arteries and veins in close proximity of the heart. Examples of the most common defects include atrial septal defect (ASD), ventricular septal defect (VSD), and patent ductus arteriosus (PDA), with VSD being the most common congenital defect. In the United States, in approximately six to eight of every 1,000 live births, the baby will be born with a congenital heart defect. Congenital diseases of the heart may be a consequence of genetic factors or adverse exposures during pregnancy such as maternal alcohol use, certain medications (e.g., warfarin, angiotensin converting enzymes) used by the expectant mother, maternal malnutrition, and maternal infections such as rubella. Although many of these defects will be detected at birth, many patients present for the first time in adulthood. It is estimated that more than 750,000 adults in the United States are currently living with congenital heart disease. This number is expected to increase by approximately 9,000 adults per year.

CONGENITAL FACTORS

Another category of heart disease involves the valves within the heart. These valves help direct the flow of blood by opening and closing with contraction and relaxation of the heart. The two types of valvular abnormalities involve difficultly opening valves (stenosis) and the inability to tightly close valves (regurgitation). These abnormalities can lead to decreased ability of the heart to efficiently pump blood and can eventually lead to heart failure. Within the heart, there are four valves: the aortic, mitral, tricuspid, and the pulmonic valves. The aortic valve, located in the left ventricle and leads to the aorta, and the mitral valve, located between the left atrium and left ventricle and regulates blood flow within the heart and are key in any discussion concerning valvular abnormalities. There are two types of aortic stenosis that are not congenital in nature; these include aortic stenosis due to calcium deposits and rheumatic aortic stenosis due to old rheumatic fever.

Calcific aortic stenosis has a high correlation with coronary artery disease. The most common etiology for congenital aortic stenosis is bicuspid aortic valve. Stenosis decreases the size of the outlet from the heart, thus the heart muscle must work harder to pump out the same amount of blood as a normal heart. This increased workload causes the heart muscle to thicken, and eventually the muscle will not be able to maintain the workload and it will ultimately result in heart failure. Regurgitation is the development of backflow through valves that are unable to tightly close. This additional blood that leaks back causes the heart muscle to stretch and the chambers of the heart to become dilated, leading to decreased efficiency and potentially heart failure. Regurgitation most commonly occurs in three of the four valves of the heart: the aortic, mitral, and tricuspid valves. The cause of this regurgitation can be related to aging, infection, genetics (e.g., Marfan's

syndrome), and autoimmune diseases (e.g., systemic lupus erythematosus). Concerning mitral stenosis, the majority of cases are secondary to rheumatic heart disease, and predominantly affect women. Mitral valve stenosis and regurgitation affect blood flow between the left atrium and left ventricle, and are attributed to the same factors as aortic stenosis and regurgitation. Mitral valve prolapse, most commonly diagnosed valvular abnormality, is a condition where the mitral valve bulges into the left atrium. Prolapse is a direct result of insufficient or lax fibrous bands, called chordae tendenae, which anchor the valve to the left ventricle. The tricuspid and pulmonic valves are also susceptible to stenosis and regurgitation; however, this occurs with less frequency than the aortic and mitral valves. Therapies for valvular dysfunctions vary from medical management to treat the symptoms or surgical intervention to replace or repair the valve itself.

ILLNESS AND HEART DISEASE

Rheumatic fever can develop following a bacterial infection in the blood, and results in an inflammatory illness that can lead to disability or death. Rheumatic fever and rheumatic heart disease affects 15.6 million people globally, including 2.4 million children. It is the most common cardiac disease in children and young adults. There are an estimated 500,000 new cases each year, 300,000 of which are from Africa. Rheumatic fever is due to bacterial invasion by *Streptococcus pyogenes* and is typically preceded by a sore throat and fever that is left untreated. The aortic and mitral valves are the most commonly affected; however, the tricuspid and pulmonic valves are not immune to damage. Ultimately, acute rheumatic fever can lead to scarring of the heart valves. Theses valves that are affected by rheumatic heart disease are more susceptible to colonization by other bacteria, and can progress to infective endocarditis.

Cardiomyopathies are diseases of the heart muscle that alter the ability of the heart to pump adequate blood throughout the body. An estimated 50,000 Americans are affected by cardiomyopathies, and they are the leading cause of heart failure leading to transplantation. The three main categories of cardiomyopathy include genetic, mixed, and acquired cardiomyopathies. The most important causes of genetic abnormalities include hypertrophic cardiomyopathy. Hypertrophic cardiomyopathy involves the thickening of the heart muscle, which causes outflow obstruction and inadequate filling of the heart chambers with blood. This condition is inherited in half the cases, and affects one out of 500 live births in the United States.

Hypertrophic cardiomyopathy is the second leading cause of heart disease, and the most common cause of sudden death in young, otherwise healthy athletes. Examples of mixed cardiomyopathies include dilated and restrictive cardiomyopathy. In dilated cardiomyopathy, the heart muscle becomes stretched and loses its ability to contract, and can be due to a virus, excessive alcohol intake, or due to unknown causes. It is also the third most common cause of heart failure and the most frequent cause of heart transplantation. Restrictive cardiomyopathy hinders the ability of the muscle to contract and relax due to scarring or abnormal deposits in the muscle, but in most cases the cause remains unknown. Chest radiation, chemotherapy, and connective tissue diseases can lead to scarring and fibrosis, while amyloidosis and hemochromatosis are responsible for abnormal deposits. The final classification, acquired cardiomyopathy, can be due to inflammation (myocarditis), stress, or chronically elevated heart rates.

It is important to recognize the extent and impact of heart disease among the worldwide population. The incidence continues to rise in developing countries as the average life expectancy increases. Genetics plays a minor role in the development of heart disease, leaving unhealthy lifestyle decisions to be the greatest predictor of the development of heart disease. There are many decisions one can make to decrease the risk of heart disease such as smoking cessation, diets low in cholesterol and high in fruits and vegetables, and regular exercise. Proper education for children concerning healthy lifestyles should be taught at a young age to reduce the incidence of heart disease in adulthood. There have been great strides made in diagnostic technology and the treatment of heart disease; however, the fundamental message concerning heart disease is that the greatest reduction in death and disability can be seen with prevention and not cure.

SEE ALSO: Heart Attack; Heart Bypass Surgery; Heart Disease—Prevention; Heart Transplantation..

BIBLIOGRAPHY. Bernard J. Gersh, *The Ultimate Guide to Heart Health: Mayo Clinic Heart Book* (William Morrow, 2000); "Heart Disease," www.cdc.gov (cited September 2006); "Heart Disease," www.who.org (cited October 2006); Dennis L. Kasper, *Harrison's Principles of Internal Medicine* (McGraw-Hill, 2005); Barry J. Maron, et al., "Contemporary Definitions and Classification of the Cardiomyopathies: An American Heart Association Scientific Statement from the Council on Clinical Cardiology, Heart Failure and Transplantation Committee; Quality of Care and Outcomes Research and Functional Genomics and Translational Biology Interdisciplinary Working Groups; and Council on Epidemiology and Prevention," *Circulation* (v.113, 2006).

HAMID GHANBARI
INDEPENDENT SCHOLAR

Heart Diseases—Prevention

According to the World Health Organization (WHO), an estimated 17 million people die of cardiovascular diseases (CVD) every year worldwide. The two leading types of CVD are coronary heart disease and stroke, both of which the death rates are declining in developed regions such as North America and western European countries, but rising steadily in still developing countries. This decline has been attributed to a combination between advances in diagnosis and treatment, and most importantly on aggressive public health policies on preventive measures that minimize the role modifiable risk factors in CVD progression.

In the worldwide INTERHEART study, which comprised of 52 countries and 30,000 study subjects, nine potential modifiable risk factors were found to be contributing to over 90 percentof the population risk for a first myocardial infarction (MI). These factors consisted on physical activity, diet and consumption of fruits and vegetables, alcohol consumption, psychosocial factors, smoking, hypertension, diabetes, dyslipidemia, and abdominal obesity.

PHYSICAL ACTIVITY

It should come as no surprise that physical activity is directly related to lowering the risk of CVD. The mechanism for lowering cardiovascular risk is due to improved oxygen transport and reduced myocardial oxygen demand due to lowered systolic blood pressure and decreased resting heart rate. The effect of physical activity appears to be graded, that is, the risk of coronary disease decreases in a stepwise fashion as the intensity of the activity is increased. General consensus defines adequate physical activity as lasting 20 minutes or more of brisk walking, for about five times a week without pauses.

DIET AND ALCOHOL

It has been shown in multiple studies that a diet high in fruits and vegetables contribute to a lower risk of cardiovascular disease, namely MI and stroke. Also, a high fiber diet can substantially reduce the risk of cardiovascular complications. Dietary fat is also an important contributor to CVD, and it appears that the type of fat ingested is more important than the total amount of fat. Trans fatty acids are associated with a higher incidence of coronary heart disease, while polyunsaturated fat and monounsaturated fat decreases this incidence. Fish consumption, due to its high amount of omega-3 fatty acids, also has been shown in randomized trials to lower the incidence of cardiovascular disease. Recent news has focused on the role of alcohol in lowering CVD risk. Moderate consumption of alcohol, that is one drink per day for women and two drinks per day for men have shown to decrease cardiovascular mortality. As should be expected, excessive intake of alcohol substantially increases the risk of stroke.

PSYCHOSOCIAL FACTORS

A reduction in the psychosocial stressors in life contributed to a reduction in cardiovascular risk. These factors included depression, stress at work or home, financial stress, and feeling of control.

SMOKING

Multiple studies and meta-analysis have shown the importance of smoking cessation in preventing cardiovascular disease, making smoking the largest preventable cause of death. Smoking not only increases blood pressure and heart rate, but at the biological level, it causes endothelial injury, platelet activation and coronary plaque destabilization. Significant benefits are seen after smoking cessation at one year, decreasing the risk of MI and death from cardiovascular disease by one-half; while cessation at three years equals the cardiovascular risk from that of a nonsmoker.

HYPERTENSION

Aggressive blood pressure control is essential in reducing cardiovascular risk. The Seventh Joint National Committee (JNC 7) provides important guidelines for therapy based on concomitant diseases as well as the degree of hypertension. Systolic blood pressure control is just as important as diastolic blood pressure. Hypertension is defined as blood pressure greater than 140/90 in two separate readings taken at more than two office visits. Tighter blood pressure control (< 130/80) is aimed at patients with hypertension and other comorbid diseases such as diabetes, renal insufficiency and heart failure. First-line agents for initiation of drug therapy should be a thiazide diuretic or a beta-blocker based on the ALLHAT study. Other choices to consider are ACE inhibitors, angiotensin-receptor blockers, and calcium channel blockers, depending on their other comorbidities. Additionally, it is important to stress the importance of lifestyle modifications which are essentially very similar if not identical to the cardiovascular modifiable risk factors.

DIABETES

The role of tight glycemic control cannot be overemphasized. Diabetes is now considered a coronary artery disease (CAD) equivalent, which should come as no surprise since the presence of diabetes allows for more severe CAD as well as more diffuse coronary disease.

A subanalysis of the United Kingdom Prostective Diabetes Study found that a 1 percent reduction in HbA1C was associated with an 18 percent reduction in MI as well as 15 percent reduction in stroke. In addition, tight glycemic control has clear and significant benefits on microvascular complications such as neuropathy, nephropathy, and retinopathy.

DYSLIPIDEMIA

Appropriate management of dyslipidemia leads to the slowing of the progression of atherosclerosis. Statins have become the mainstay of lipid lowering therapy but its mechanism of action appears to be more pleomorphic than previously thought. Additional benefits of statins include improved endothelial function, decreased platelet thrombus formation, and decreased vascular inflammation by decreasing CRP levels, a marker of active inflammation. Current guidelines for the treatment of dyslipidemia are based on the Adult Treatment Panel III (ATP III) and it involves a nine-step process.

SEE ALSO: Heart Attack; Heart Bypass Surgery; Heart Diseases (General); Heart Valve Diseases.

BIBLIOGRAPHY. Bernard J. Gersh, *The Ultimate Guide to Heart Health: Mayo Clinic Heart Book* (William Morrow, 2000); "Heart Disease," www.cdc.gov (cited September 2006); "Heart Disease," www.who.org (cited October 2006); Dennis L. Kasper, *Harrison's Principles of Internal Medicine* (McGraw-Hill, 2005).

MICHAEL YEUNG
INDEPENDENT SCHOLAR

Heart Transplantation

Heart transplantation is a surgical procedure to implant a healthy heart into a patient with heart failure. Heart transplantation is usually the last option on a list of treatments for heart diseases. The primary diagnoses of patients receiving heart transplants are coronary artery disease, cardiomyopathy, and congenital diseases. The first heart transplant was performed by Professor Christiaan Barnard at Groote Schuur Hospital in South Africa in December 1967. A major barrier to transplantation is the process of rejection in which the recipient's immune system recognizes the graft being foreign and attacks it. The antigens responsible for this reaction are the HLA system. The HLA genes are highly polymorphic and any two individuals (except identical twins) will express different HLA proteins.

The three organ rejection reactions are hyperacute, acute, and chronic. Hyperacute rejection occurs within minutes or hours of transplantation and can be recognized by the surgeon just after the graft vasculature is anastomosed to the recipient's. This process occurs when preformed antidonor antibodies are present in the circulation of the recipient. An acute rejection occurs within days of transplantation in an untreated recipient or may occur months or years later when the immunosuppression has ended. Acute rejection is a combined process in which cellular and humoral parts of the immune system contribute. Chronic re-

jection presents in patients over a period of four to six months. It is usually irreversible and is the single largest cause of organ transplant rejection.

Mechanisms for increasing graft survival are to match more of the HLA genes between the recipient and the donor. Also, patients are given immunosuppressive drugs to prevent attack of the transplanted organ by the transplant recipient's immune system. Common drugs are cyclosporine, azathioprine, steroids, rapamycin, and mycophenolate mofetil. A common side effect of immunosuppressive treatment is for the recipient to be more susceptible to opportunistic infections most likely by fungal or viral organisms. Also, these patients are at a higher risk for cancers that are caused by viruses. Current research to overcome this obstacle of immunosuppression is looking at inducing donor-specific tolerance in host T lymphocyte cells.

The United Network for Organ Sharing (UNOS) is a private, nonprofit organization that matches available organ donors with waiting transplant recipients through the national Organ Procurement and Transplantation Network (OPTN). Organ procurement is dependent on recipient time on waiting list, severity of disease, ABO blood type, and body size. Contraindications specific to heart transplants are if the patient has an active infection, pulmonary hypertension, untreatable liver or kidney disease, chronic lung disease, mental illnesses, disease of the blood vessels in the brain, and continued alcohol or drug abuse.

In general, the two forms of heart procedures are orthotopic or heterotopic. In an orthotopic procedure, the patient's heart is removed leaving portions of the left and right atrium, pulmonary vein, and aorta. The new heart is then modeled to fit the recipient's chest and the different chambers and vessels are anastomosed together. In a heterotopic procedure, the patient's own heart is not removed before implanting the donor heart. The two hearts are connected together to form a "double heart." This way, the patient's own heart may recover from the decreased workload and be able to function normally in the future. This procedure is also done if the donor heart is large enough to sustain the patient's body or if the donor heart is too weak. In both procedures, the donor heart is stimulated to maintain a regular beat through medications or a pacemaker. After the surgery, the patient usually remains in the intensive care unit for 24 to 72 hours. Also for the next few months following the surgery, the patient revisits the transplant center for weekly physical examinations.

According to 2000 data from the Registry of the International Society for Heart and Lung Transplantation (ISHLT), 81 percent of transplant recipients survive one year. During the first year, infection and acute rejection are the leading causes of death. A constant 4 percent decrease occurs yearly after the first year as the incidence of coronary allograft vascular disease increases. Pediatric patients less than 1 year of age are least likely to reject the donor heart, but 30 percent of older pediatric patients succumb to transplant rejection.

SEE ALSO: Heart Attack; Heart Bypass Surgery; Heart Diseases; Organ Donation; Organ Transplantation.

BIBLIOGRAPHY. Vinay Kumar, et al., *Pathologic Basis of Disease* (Elsevier Saunders, 2005); Mary C. Mancini, "Heart Transplantation," www.emedicine.com (cited January 2006); Medline Plus, "Heart Transplant," www.nlm.nih.gov (cited January 2006); United Network for Organ Sharing, "How the Transplant System Works: Matching Organ Donors and Recipients," www.unos.org (cited January 2006).

PAVAN BHATRAJU
UNIVERSITY OF LOUISVILLE

Heart Valve Diseases

Heart valve disease refers to a group of conditions affecting the mobility and closure of the heart's four valves. Anatomically, the heart is divided into four chambers. Deoxygenated blood returns from the periphery of our body through the inferior and superior vena cava into the right atrium. The tricuspid valve serves as the gateway from the right atrium into the right ventricle. The pulmonic valve, in turn, regulates the flux of the blood from the right ventricle into the pulmonary arteries. Blood then enters the pulmonary circulation for oxygenation, and return to the left atrium. From the left atrium, blood transverses the mitral valve to reach the left ventricle, and ultimately is pumped to the aorta leading to our systemic circulation through the aortic valve.

Heart valve diseases arise as a result of congenital abnormalities or acquired conditions such as infections or degenerative processes, which in turn change the hemodynamic blood patterns that flow through the heart valves. These abnormalities often lead to narrowing or stenosis, or it can also lead to leakage, which is also called regurgitation. Valvular murmurs can often be picked up through auscultation, and the degree of severity is formally quantified by the use of transthoracic echocardiogram. Below is a review of the most common valvular conditions.

AORTIC VALVE STENOSIS

Aortic stenosis occurs from a narrowing of the aortic valve, often caused by either progressive calcification of the valve or rheumatic heart disease. It is important to note that rheumatic aortic valve is often accompanied by mitral valve disease as well. There are also congenital conditions such as unicuspid and most commonly bicuspid aortic valve which changes the properties of the valve and predisposes it to early narrowing.

The natural history of aortic stenosis is characterized by asymptomatic progression until the valve area is narrowed enough to elicit the classical symptoms of angina, syncope, and exertional dyspnea. Severe aortic stenosis is suggested by an aortic jet velocity greater than 4 m/s, a mean transvalvular gradient greater than 50 mmHg, and an aortic valve area of less than 1 cm². Severe aortic stenosis warrants surgical intervention with aortic valve replacement. In Heyde's syndrome, a subgroup of patients with aortic stenosis are also found to have concomitant gastrointestinal bleeding. This is thought to be due to defective von Willebrand factors from disruptive passage across the narrow valve in the background of arteriovenous malformations.

AORTIC VALVE INSUFFICIENCY

Aortic valve insufficiency may occur from an abnormality of the aortic valve or a dilatation of the aortic root, causing diastolic regurgitant flow from the aorta back into the left ventricle. This backflow of blood causes increased left ventricular pressure, dilatation, and hypertrophy. Causes for this dilatation include bicuspid aortic valve, aortic aneurysms, and Marfan's syndrome. Of importance, patients with aortic insufficiency who develop severe left ventricular dilatation are at increased risk of sudden cardiac death (SCD), and serial annual echocardiograms are warranted in order to monitor the progression of disease. Medical therapy with afterload reducers such as nifedipine or angiotensin-converting enzyme (ACE) inhibitors can delay the progression of aortic insufficiency. Surgical replacement of the aortic valve should be considered when the left ventricular end-systolic diameter reaches 55 mm or if the ejection fraction is less than 60 percent.

MITRAL VALVE STENOSIS

Mitral stenosis is often associated with prior history of rheumatic heart disease, with more women affected than men in a 2:1 ratio. Of note, the sequelae of rheumatic fever presents at different age groups depending on the geographic area. For example, in Africa, the sequelae of rheumatic mitral stenosis occurs during their teenage years, as opposed to patients in Asia who often present in their 20s, and patients from the United States and Europe, who become symptomatic during their 50s.

The initial presentation of severe mitral stenosis is dyspnea, often during exertion or exercise. Cough and occasionally hemoptysis are also findings consistent with this condition. Some female patients may also present with pulmonary congestion symptoms during their pregnancy due to increase blood flow and volume through a stenotic mitral valve. Severe mitral stenosis is suggested by a mitral valve area <1 cm², a transvalvular diastolic pressure gradient >10 mm Hg, or severe pulmonary hypertension >60 mm Hg. It is also important to note that severe increases in left atrial pressure due to the stenotic valve, predisposes left atrial enlargement, and subsequent development of atrial fibrillation.

Management of mitral stenosis in asymptomatic patients involves avoidance of factors that may increase left atrial pressure such as vigorous exercise, fevers, or tachycardia. Anticoagulation is indicated for patients with mitral stenosis and atrial fibrillation due to the higher incidence of thromboembolism. Interventions for severe mitral stenosis include mitral valve repair by percutaneous valvotomy or mitral valve replacement. Percutaneous valvotomy is an appropriate alternative to surgery, but it requires a transesophageal echocardiogram in order to rule out the presence of a left atrial appendage thrombus and also ensure that mitral regurgitation is less than moderate in severity. Most common complications of valvotomy include severe mitral regurgitation, systemic embolization of thrombus, and pericardial tamponade. Surgical commissurotomy or mitral valve replacement is indicated if percutaneous valvotomy cannot be performed safely. Comparison of percutaneous versus surgical approaches has yielded similar success rates.

MITRAL VALVE REGURGITATION

Chronic mitral valve regurgitation is mostly caused by myxomatous disease such as Marfan's or Ehlers-Danlos, mitral valve prolapse, infective endocarditis, or rheumatic heart disease. Mitral regurgitation should be followed by a cardiologist for serial echocardiograms and clinical evaluation in order to determine the timing of intervention. Mitral valve repair is the procedure of choice when appropriate, and it avoids the complications of open heart surgery as well as chronic anticoagulation.

It is important to differentiate acute versus chronic mitral regurgitation because the former can be a medical emergency. Acute mitral regurgitation is often seen with rupture of the chordae tendineae due to endocarditis or myocardial infarction. This leads to severe dyspnea and pulmonary edema, and may require surgical intervention.

SEE ALSO: Heart Attack; Heart Bypass Surgery; Heart Diseases (General).

BIBLIOGRAPHY. Bernard J. Gersh, *The Ultimate Guide to Heart Health: Mayo Clinic Heart Book* (William Morrow, 2000); "Heart Disease," www.cdc.gov (cited September 2006); "Heart Disease," www.who.org (cited October 2006).

MICHAEL YEUNG
INDEPENDENT SCHOLAR

Heat Index

Heat index is the ambient or environmental temperature as perceived by the human body. The heat index is based on both raw air temperature values and the relative humidity or moisture that is present in the air. The heat index offers a value that expresses how the climate "feels" on the body in an objective and universal manner. Heat and heat-related injuries across the developing world are a significant cause of occupational injuries and hazards and are a preventable illness. Heat-related injuries affect millions in both mild and severe climates each year.

The body is able to release heat by fluctuating the rate and depth of blood circulation in the periphery, by liberating water through the skin and sweat glands, and through respiration. These described compensatory mechanisms are very important for maintaining normal body temperature. More specifically, sweating cools the body with evaporating water off the skin and taking with it some of the heat the body holds. However, if the humidity in the air is high, it cannot easily release this water and therefore, cannot easily release heat. In very humid climates, such as regions along the equator, it is difficult for the body to compensate and to lose heat in an efficient manner. This leads to heat injury and illness.

These compensatory mechanisms start acting when the environment is cooler or warmer than normal body temperature (37.0 degrees C or 98.6 degrees F). The ability to maintain body temperature within these limits is described as thermoregulation. Deviation too far from these normal limits can cause unconsciousness and death. A high heat index is indicative of high ambient air temperatures and high humidity. A low heat index are low ambient air temperatures and low relative humidity. A high heat index can also exacerbate other underlying disease such as respiratory illness as asthma and chronic obstructive pulmonary disease (COPD).

Measurements have been taken based on subjective descriptions of how hot subjects feel for a given temperature and humidity, allowing an index to be made which corresponds a temperature and humidity combination to a higher temperature in dry air. Calculation for heat index in Celsius takes into account vapor pressure, relative humidity, and temperature:

Heat index = $T + 5/9 \times (e - 10)$;

where $e = V \times [(6.112 \times 10 \char`\^((7.5T / 237.7) + T)] \times (R / 100)$; where V = vapor pressure; R = relative humidity, and T = temperature. A table exists that correlates heat and relative humidity in this heat index for easy observation of dangerous heat conditions.

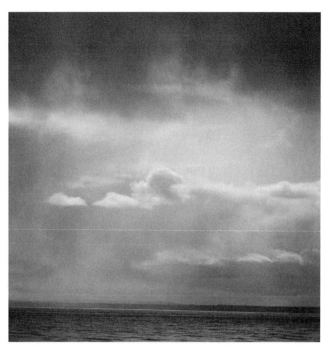

The heat index is based on both raw air temperature values and the relative humidity or moisture that is present in the air.

For example, if it is 27 degrees C ambient temperature with relative humidity of 95 percent it will "feel" like 31.3 degrees C. Maintaining normal body temperature requires much of the energy we get from food consumption. If the body does not have enough fat stores, calorie consumption, or clean drinkable water, thermoregulation becomes compromised and heat illness and injury may occur. Clean potable water sources and consequent consumption is a major threat to much of the developing world where the heat index remains high for much of the year and heat illness inflicts many.

SEE ALSO: Drinking Water; Oral Rehydration Therapy; Sun Exposure.

BIBLIOGRAPHY. Christopher C. Burt, *Extreme Weather: A Guide and Record Book* (Norton, 2004); M. Khogali, "Heat-Related Illness" *Middle East Journal of Anesthesiology* (v.12/6, 1995); D. Tek, J.S. Olshaker, "Heat Illness." *Emergency Medicine Clinics of North America* (v.10/2, 1992); Jack Williams, *The Weather Book*, (Vintage Books, 1997).

JOHN MICHAEL QUINN V, MPH
UNIVERSITY OF ILLINOIS AT CHICAGO

Hematologist

Disorders of the blood and their related body organs are vast and complex disease processes. Doctors who treat them require special medical training to ensure people with these diseases are able to receive proper treatment. However, not all blood diseases need to be treated by a hematologist. The term *hematology* is defined as the study of one particular branch of medicine concerned with blood, the blood-forming organs, and blood diseases. Hematology includes the study of etiology, diagnosis, treatment, prognosis, and prevention of blood diseases. A doctor who specializes in this diagnosing and treating is called a hematologist.

Work for hematologists may range from the management of a hematology laboratory, work at a microscope viewing blood and bone marrow slides, to interpretation of various other blood test results. By viewing blood under the microscope, a doctor is able to visually see if the cells are of normal shape, size, and number. Variation in any of these from what is considered "normal" may indicate a blood disease is present. Sometimes, parasites can even be seen in blood cells and lead to the diagnosis of malaria, for example. Besides looking at blood, some other tests involve reacting blood with specific chemicals to see how the blood behaves. For example to check if a person has a bleeding disorder, a chemical is added to the blood which causes it to react and form a blood clot. The amount of time necessary for blood to clot is recorded. Normal times have been established through experiments, thus by comparing the test person's time to the normal test value, a hematologist can determine if a bleeding disorder is present. This is just one example of hundreds of blood tests performed.

Examples of common diseases treated by hematologists are anemia, disorders of blood clotting, and leukemia. Anemia is simply a decrease in the number of red blood cells, also known as the oxygen carying cells of the human body. Without these cells, we would not be able to get oxygen to the rest of our body. Causes of anemia are great, but most commonly, it is simply a decreased amount of iron in the body which is necessary for red blood cell function. Anemia can also be caused by destruction of blood cells by parasites like those that cause malaria (plasmodium falciparum, for example). One of the many other causes of anemia worthy of mention is because of vitamin defficiency or failure of proper resorption of vitamins required in the steps of making red blood cells. A hematologist must explore all of these possibilities of causes of anemia including, but not mentioned above, leukemia or blood cancer in order to help resolve a patient's underlying cause of anemia.

Hemophilia is a disease that results from lack of certain blood-clotting factors. There are different types based on which factor is missing. A well-known person with hemophilia in recent past was Ryan White. He may be better known from his fight for civil rights of those with HIV. Ryan White contracted HIV through a blood transfusion as part of his treatment for hemophilia. This is not very common anymore due to screening and a better understanding of the AIDS virus, but in the 1980s, there was a poor understanding of this virus.

While hemophilia is a disease characterized by the decreased ability to form a blood clot, several other diseases result from decreased or total lack of clot formation. An example is von Willebrand's disease, which results from a related but different blood clotting factor. A hematologist must carefully analyze several tests designed to determine the missing or decreased factors to determine the type of bleeding disorder. Only then can the proper treatment and precautions for the patient be determined.

Blood cancers or leukemias and lymphomas are also a major part of the work of hematologists. These doctors are called hematologist/oncologists, where oncology means cancer. Many different types of leukemias exist. Examples of leukemias commonly seen are acute lymphoblastic leukemia and chronic lymphoblastic leukemia. Many of the leukemias and lymphomas are derived from white blood cells. White blood cells, like any other cell in the body, start out as immature cells and mature into their final form. As a mature cell, they are mostly responsible for fighting infections in one way or another. Disturbance in the maturation or development causes the formation of cells that do not function properly, which is then called a leukemic or lymphoma cell, depending on the origin of the cell. It is the job of a hematologist to examine these cells under a microscope and analyze cells with special equipment, such as flow cytometry, to determine exactly what type of cell is causing the leukemia or lymphoma. Only after the cell type and origin are determined can the proper treatment be rendered. This is because different chemotherapeutic agents are aimed at treating different types of leukemias.

Hematologists are specialists of medicine who work in conjunction with other physicians to treat patients with blood diseases. It is only after a hematologist has determined the underlying cause of the blood disorder that the proper treatment can be determined. The decision to give a blood transusion, hormones, nutritional supplements, bone marrow transfusions, or even chemotherapy depends on the expertise of the hematologist and testing/analysis of blood and related organs. Hematologists serve to diagnose and treat many blood disorders that range from very common and not life threatening like iron deficiency anemia to rare but deadly forms of leukemia.

SEE ALSO: Anemia; Hematology; Leukemia.

BIBLIOGRAPHY. Robert Hillman, and Kenneth A. Ault, *Hematology in Clinical Practice* (McGraw Hill, 2002); Kumar Vinay, et al., *Robbins and Cotran Pathologic Basis of Disease* (Elsevier Saunders, 2005).

Angela Garner, M.D.
University of Missouri–Kansas City

the lymphatic system. Following the success of blood transfusions since the 17th century, hematology has become heavily concerned with ensuring that transfusions are done as safely as possible. This involves ensuring that the blood plasma from the donor is free of infection or disease, and that it has been stored properly and categorized into the correct group. This has become particularly important from the mid-1980s with the problems over HIV-infected blood, and later with blood which may be infected with bovine spongiform encephalopathy ("mad cow disease") or other related complaints.

In addition to mainstream hematology, there are also specialities such as dealing with bleeding disorders including hemophilia, treating hematological malignancies including leukemia and lymphoma, and also treating hemoglobinopathies. There are a number of different classes of hematologic diseases: hemoglobinopathies, anemias, problems involving a decreased number of blood cells, myeloproliferative disorders (with an increased number of cells), hematological malignancies, coagulopathies, and other miscellaneous issues.

The study of hemoglobinopathies involves covering areas where there is a congenital abnormality of the hemoglobin molecule or in the rate of hemo-

Hematology

Hematology is a branch of physiology and biology that is concerned with the study of human blood, the human organs concerned with blood, and also diseases of the blood. It also involves a study of the etiology, treatment, prognosis, and prevention of blood diseases, with work carried out by medical professionals known as hematologists. The word *hema* comes from the Greek word for "blood," with *logos* from the Greek meaning "study."

As a basic medical science, hematology is concerned with dealing with blood, blood cells, and blood vessels. This involves working with blood tests, blood poisoning, venipunctures, and related issues. It also is concerned with other related aspects of medicine such as dealing with problems concerned with the reticuloendothelial system, including bone marrow, the spleen, liver complaints, and also problems with

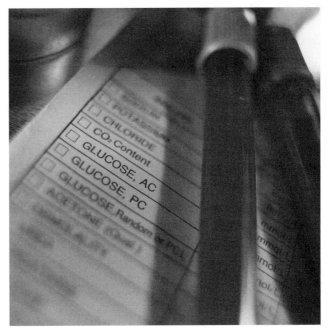

Hematology involves treatment, prognosis, and prevention of diseases by testing blood and blood cells.

globin synthesis. This includes sickle-cell diseases which come from genetic disorders of sickle hemoglobin. Other related diseases include thalassemia, an inherited disease affecting red blood cells; and methemoglobinemia which is characterized by a high level of methemoglobin in the blood.

With anemias, there is a wide range of potential diseases ranging from some that result from an iron deficiency in the body—often preventable by taking iron supplements and/or eating more red meat, especially kidney. Megaloblastic anemia comes from a B12 deficiency of a folate deficiency, the latter being a particularly important issue for pregnant women. There are also a large number of diseases involving the destruction of red blood cells, collectively called Hemolytic anemias. A number of these are genetic, but others might be induced by drugs, especially a high dose of penicillin. Some are concerned with the membrane of red blood cells, while others are more concerned with their metabolism or direct physical damage to them. Mention should also be made of aplastic anemia whereby bone marrow does not produce enough cells to replenish blood cells in the body. Varieties of this disorder include Fanconi anemia, named after the Swiss pediatrician Guide Fanconi; Diamond-Blackfan anemia, a congenitcal erythroid aplasia; and the acquired pure red cell aplasia.

A number of hematologic diseases also arise from a person having a decreased number of blood cells for a whole range of reasons from myelodysplastic syndrome, myelofibrosis, neutropenia, agranulocytosis, glanzmann's thrombastehenia, and thrombocytopenia.

Myeloproliferative disorders, which involve an increased number of cells, can come from polycythemia vera, whereby there is an increase in the number of cells in general; leukocytosis, which involves an increase in the number of white blood cells; thrombocytosis where there is an increase in the number of platelets and various myeloproliferative disorders.

There are also a number of hematological malignancies which involve lymphomas, myelomas, plasmacytoma, and leukemias. The lymphomas include Hodgkin's disease, the non-Hodgkin's lymphoma, Burkitt's lymphoma, anaplastic large cell lymphoma, and splenic marginal zone lymphoma. The first three of these are generally classified as cancers which affect lymphocytes and, occasionally, histiocytes. For myelomas, there is multiple myeloma and also Aldernström

macroglobulinemia. Plasmacytoma occurs where a malignant monoclonal plasma cell tumor can grow in the bone or in soft tissue. For leukemias, there is a range: acute lymphocytic leukemia (ALL), chronic lymphocytic leukemia (CLL), acute myelogenous leukemia (AML), chronic myelogenous leukemia (CML), T-cell prolymphocytic leukemia (T-PLL), chronic neutrophilic leukemia (CNL), hairy cell leukemia (HCL), T-cell large granular lymphocyte leukemia (T-LGL), and aggressive NK-cell leukemia.

Disorders of bleeding and coagulation are known as coagulopathies, with the most widely known being those which involve the disorders in clotting proteins such as hemophilia (hemophilia A, hemophilia B, and hemophilia C). In addition there is von Willebrand disease, disseminated intravascular coagulation, protein S deficiency, and antiphosphlipid syndrome. The three main diseases connected with the disorders of platelets are thrombocytopenia, Glanzmann's thrombasthenia, and Wiskott-Aldricj syndrome. Other disorders of bleeding and coagulation include thrombocytosis, recurrent thrombosis, and disseminated intravascular coagulation. The last category of hematological problems include some disorders such as hemochromatosis, asplenia, hypersplenism, monoclonal gammopathy, and also a number of hematological changes which are secondary to nonhematological disorders such as AIDS, malaris and leishmaniasis.

SEE ALSO: AIDS; Anemia; Leukemia.

BIBLIOGRAPHY. Laurent Degos, David C. Linch, and Bob Löwenberg, eds., *Textbook of Malignant Haematology* (Taylor & Francis, 2005); William G. Finn and LoAnn C. Peterson, *Hematopathology in Oncology* (Kluwer Academic Publishers, 2004); A.V. Hoffbrand, J.E. Pettit, and P.A.H. Moss, *Essential Haematology* (Blackwell Science, 2002); Martin R. Howard and Peter J. Hamilton, *Haematology: An Illustrated Colour Text* (Churchill Livingstone, 1997); Atul B. Mehta and A. Victor Hoffbrand, *Haematology at a Glance* (Blackwell, 2005); Reinhold Munker, Erhard Hiller, and Ronald Paquette, *Modern Hematology: Biology and Clinical Management* (Humana Press, 2000); Chris Pallister, *Blood Physiology and Pathophysiology* (Butterworth-Heinemann, 1994).

JUSTIN CORFIELD
GEELONG GRAMMAR SCHOOL, AUSTRALIA

Hemizygous

A cell or organism is hemizygous at a locus (a fixed position on a chromosome, such as the position of a gene) if it possesses only one allele for a given trait. In humans, males are hemizygous for alleles expressed on the sex chromosomes as they have only one of each. Contrast this with females who have two copies of the X chromosome and are thus either homozygous or heterozygous at loci on the sex chromosomes. The classic example of hemizygous inheritance is hemophilia.

Classic hemophilia (hemophilia A) is an X-linked, recessive disorder caused by mutations affecting the factor VIII gene, located on the long arm of the X chromosome but nowhere on the Y chromosome. Thus, men with only one mutant allele for the factor VIII gene show a diseased phenotype because the Y chromosome does not have an allele capable of expressing wildtype factor VIII. Women, on the other hand, are not hemizygous at the locus of the factor VIII gene. As only one wildtype allele is necessary to prevent a diseased state, women who are heterozygous at the factor VIII locus will usually not show signs of disease. Only women who are homozygous for the mutant genotype (or are heterozygous with two different, mutant phenotypes) will show signs of disease. The prevalence of hemophilia (and all X-linked recessive diseases) is thus much higher in men than in women.

The hemizygous nature of men also has consequences for the inheritance of X-linked disease. In the case of X-linked recessive diseases, a man with the disease state will pass on the mutant allele to all of his daughters and none of his sons (because all sons receive the Y chromosome). The fate of both the sons and daughters of a man with the mutant allele thus depends on the status of the mother. On the other hand, consider a man with the wildtype allele at the locus in question. While the status of his sons still depends on the status of the mother, the man can be confident that virtually none of his daughters will be affected because they are guaranteed to inherit a wildtype allele from him.

Not all hemizygous traits are X-linked recessive. Although much less common, certain traits are X-linked dominant and there also some Y-linked disease states. The general considerations for inheritance of X-linked dominant traits are similar to those for X-linked recessive traits. However, because dominant inheritance only requires one mutant allele to be present for disease to manifest itself, all of the daughters of an affected father will be affected, whereas affected mothers stand only a 50 percent chance of passing on an affected allele, regardless of the sex of the offspring. It should also be noted that many X-linked dominant disorders are much more prevalent among women than men, even more so than simple probability would suggest. The most common explanation for this is that hemizygosity for a dominant mutant allele is lethal during gestation. This does not seem to be the case with Y-linked alleles, the inheritance of which is always dominant. Males who carry mutations on Y-linked genes may suffer from infertility but seldom suffer a serious disease state that is incompatible with life.

SEE ALSO: Allele; Heterozygote; Homozygote.

BIBLIOGRAPHY. S, Callejas, et al., "Hemizygous Subtelomeres of an African Trypanosome Chromosome May Account for over 75% of Chromosome Length," *Genome Research (v.16/9,* 2006); R. L. Nussbaum, et al., *Thompson & Thompson: Genetics in Medicine,* 6th ed., revised reprint (Saunders, 2004).

BIMAL P. CHAUDHARI
BOSTON UNIVERSITY

Hemochromatosis

Hemochromatosis is a disorder that interferes with iron metabolism, which results in the excessive accumulation of iron in the body. This abnormal buildup of iron is toxic to the body and can cause damage to the organs. Hereditary hemochromatosis is one of the most common genetic disorders in the United States. It is estimated that one out of 200 to 300 individuals are affected. Hemochromatosis is more common in Caucasians of European descent.

CAUSES

There are two main causes of hemochromatosis: primary (hereditary) or secondary. Primary hemochromatosis is inherited as a homozygous-recessive genetic disorder. An individual who inherits the defective gene from both parents may develop hemochromatosis. Not all individuals who inherit both defective genes will develop manifestations of hemochromatosis. The carrier state, individual with one copy of the defective gene, is estimated to be one out of every nine individuals. The gene affected is called HFE, which is located on chromosome 6. The HFE gene codes for a molecule that regulates the intestinal absorption of dietary iron. The body closely regulates and balances the amount of iron absorbed in the intestines with the amount of iron lost daily. When two copies of the defective HFE gene are inherited, the result is abnormal regulation of intestinal absorption of dietary iron. This leads to excess accumulation of iron in the body. Secondary hemochromatosis is usually due to an underlying disease or condition; it can also be due to blood transfusions. Hemolytic anemias such as thalassemia or sideroblastic anemia are the most common cause of secondary hemochromatosis. Blood transfusions to manage aplastic anemia and sickle cell disease can also lead to iron overload.

CLINICAL SYMPTOMS

The symptoms of hemochromatosis usually appear between ages 30 and 50 and are more frequent in males. Males present symptoms at an earlier age than females because of the physiologic iron loss during menstruation and pregnancy. Principal clinical manifestations include abdominal pain, fatigue, darkening of the skin pigmentation, joint pain, testicular atrophy, and loss of sexual desire. Hemochromatosis causes a buildup of iron in the body, especially in the liver, heart, and pancreas. Hemochromatosis can lead to liver enlargement, cirrhosis (scarring of the liver causing dysfunction), liver failure, or cancer of the liver (hepatocellular carcinoma). Iron buildup in cardiac tissue can cause irregular heart rate or rhythm (arrhythmia) and lead to heart failure. Hemochromatosis can cause damage to the pancreas and lead to diabetes mellitus.

SCREENING AND TREATMENT

Screening for hemochromatosis involves blood tests to evaluate serum iron levels and ferritin levels. Screening family members is important for primary hemochromatosis. Treatment is necessary to remove the excess iron in the body and to prevent organ damage from toxic levels of iron. Patients are treated by phlebotomy (removal of blood).

SEE ALSO: Anemia; Sickle Cell Disease.

BIBILOGRAPHY: Centers for Disease Control and Prevention, "Hemochromatosis," www.cdc.gov (cited April 25, 2007); "Hemochromatosis," *ADAM Medical Encyclopedia*, www.nlm.nih.gov/medlineplus (cited April 25, 2007); V. Kumar, A. K. Abbas, and N. Fausto, *Robbins and Coltran Pathologic Basis of Disease*, 7th ed. (Saunders, 2005); National Institutes of Health, National Heart, Lung, and Blood Institute, "Hemochromatosis," www.nhlbi.nih.gov (cited April 2007).

ANGELA J. GARNER, MD
MELISSA MEINERS
UNIVERSITY OF MISSOURI-KANSAS CITY

Hemorrhagic Fever

Hemorrhagic fevers (HFs) are diseases characterized by raised body temperature (fever) and rapid blood loss (hemorrhage), which may be either internal or external. They are often referred to as viral hemorrhagic fevers (VHFs) because most are caused by a virus from one of four families: Filoviridae, Arenaviridae, Bunyaviridae, or Flaviviridae. Well-known HFs include Ebola HF, Marpurg HF, Lassa fever, and Rift Valley fever.

VHFs are zoonotic and reside in an animal reservoir host or arthropod. Because VHFs are dependent on their animal or insect hosts, outbreaks are generally restricted to areas where the hosts live; this is why many VHFs include a geographic designation in their name. This risk of VHFs, therefore, varies by location: Carriers of some diseases exist in very limited geographic areas, and the risk of contracting those VHF is also limited to those areas.

However, other carriers (such as the common rat) exist throughout the world, and thus some VHFs themselves are widely distributed. In addition, VHFs may be spread through transportation of infected animals (Marpurg virus was introduced to Germany and Yugoslavia by infected lab monkeys, for instance) and some, including Ebola, Marpurg, Lassa, and Crimean-Congo Fevers, can also be transmitted from an infected human to another human, or through contact with the blood or other body fluids of an infected person.

Signs and symptoms common to VHFs include fever, fatigue, dizziness, muscle aches, and weakness and exhaustion. There may be signs of bleeding under the skin or from body orifices, and severe cases may show shock, coma, or seizures. Some VHFs cause only mild illness, while others can be life threatening. Renal failure is associated with some VHFs, and Ebola HF is believed to be fatal in 50 to 90 percent of clinically ill cases, for instance. There is no cure for most VHFs, and no treatment other than supportive care; exceptions include Ribavarin, which has been used to treat Lassa fever, and convalescent-phase plasma, which has been used to treat Argentine HF.

SEE ALSO: Dengue; Fever; Sudan; Tropical Medicine.

BIBLIOGRAPHY. Centers for Disease Control and Prevention, "Viral Hemorrhagic Fevers Fact Sheet," www.cdc.gov (cited March 2007); World Health Organization, "Infection Control for Viral Haemorrhagic Fevers in the African Health Care Setting," www.who.int (cited March 2007).

SARAH BOSLAUGH
BJC HEALTHCARE

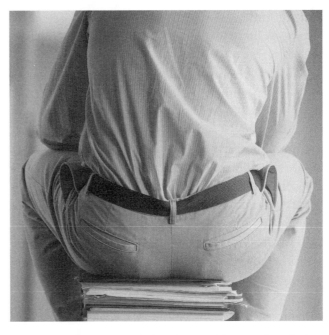

Each year, about 500,000 people in the United States seek medical treatment for hemorrhoids.

Hemorrhoids

A hemorrhoid, also known collectively as emerods or piles, was first so described during the 16th century and the word is derived from the Greek for "the discharging of blood." It is a swelling and inflammation of veins which can occur in the rectum or anal channel. Essentially, it can be formed by a distension of the vein network under the mucous membrane around the anal channel, or under the skin around the nearby external area. As such, it is a form of varicose vein which can develop from an infection or leads from an increase in the intraabdominal pressure which can occur when lifting very heavy objects, the channel suffering extra strain, or during pregnancy. At its worst, it may result from complications connected with chronic liver disease or the presence of tumors.

The presence of hemorrhoids is actually extremely common with some surveys showing that as many as 50 percent of all Americans have had hemorrhoids at some stage during their life before they reach the age of 50. Each year, about 500,000 people in the United States seek medical treatment for this condition, with about 15 percent of these—generally the ones with the worst cases—needing some kind of surgery. It can, therefore, be shown the vast majority of the people who suffer do not seek treatment either because it does not pose much of a medical problem or the condition quickly reverses.

There has been a range of research into the causes of hemorrhoids, with a definite genetic link, and some families are often more predisposed to this condition. This can come from a weakness in the vessel wall which means that a condition which results in the higher risk of having hemorrhoids for some people may well be inherited. Additional factors come from obesity and also the increasing sedentary lifestyle, meaning that hemorrhoids are a greater factor in developed countries than in the third world. The British novelist Anthony Burgess, who suffered from hemorrhoids over many years, called the condition "Writer's Evil," presumably on the basis that one of the causes comes from the long periods of sedentary activity undertaken by most writers. Another person who also suffered from hemorrhoids was Emperor Napoleon I who, according to his physician, had a bad attack during the Battle of Waterloo in 1815, which made it difficult for him to ride a horse during the battle, and even took him away from the battlefield, costing him the battle, his throne, and his empire.

Some of the obvious causes come from postponing of bowel movement, constipation, chronic diarrhea, sustained low-fiber diets, poor bathroom habits, and also pregnancy. It has been suggested that people using the modern lavatory increases the risk of suffering from hemorrhoids, with squat toilets engendering a lower predisposition. However, there has only been limited research on this. A more obvious cause comes from dietary reasons. People who do not drink enough fluid or use too many diuretics (which includes consumption of coffee or colas) can result in harder bowel movements and hence harder stools, leading to irritation which can lead to hemorrhoids. As a result, a diet with increased fiber or hydration, the use of nonirritating laxatives, and baths can be used for treating some types of mild hemorrhoids, with more serious cases requiring medical examination. The most extreme cases are treated by hemorrhoidectomy which involves surgery to excise and remove the hemorrhoid.

SEE ALSO: Gastroenterologist; Gastroenterology.

BIBLIOGRAPHY. Barbara Becker, *Relief from Chronic Hemorrhoids* (Dell, 1992); Steven Peikin, *Gastrointestinal Health* (HarperCollins, 1999); Sidney E. Wanderman and Betty Rothbart, *Hemorrhoids* (Consumer Reports Books, 1991).

Justin Corfield
Geelong Grammar School, Australia

Hepatitis

The liver is an abdominal organ that is responsible for an array of vital functions. Hepatitis is a general term used to refer to inflammation of the liver, which can be acute or chronic with a wide variety of causes. Understanding the severity of hepatitis requires an appreciation for the normal synthetic and metabolic functions of the liver.

The liver synthesizes proteins, carbohydrates, and fats. The major site for production of proteins for blood clotting is the liver. In addition, maintenance of sugar balance requires liver function. Liver cells create glucose from pyruvate and lactate in the blood, and can use blood sugars to generate amino acids, fatty acids, or can store excess glucose in the form of glycogen. The liver also regulates production of fatty acids and cholesterol, and produces bile that is important in the metabolism of fats. Last, detoxification of a large number of drugs is accomplished by liver cells, as is the removal of ammonia from the blood.

Acute viral hepatitis is a general term used to describe the liver inflammation caused by at least five different, unrelated viruses. The five known hepatitis viruses are hepatitis A, B, C, D (or delta), and E. Hepatitis A and E are spread through a fecal-oral route secondary to poor sanitary conditions. They are highly contagious and can occur in outbreaks but do not have long-term health consequences. Hepatitis B, C, and D are spread via infected blood and sexual contact. While hepatitis B, C, and D do not cause outbreaks, they can lead to chronic hepatitis, which causes cirrhosis and liver cancer (hepatocellular carcinoma).

Symptoms of acute hepatitis are varied. There are prodromal symptoms that often precede acute hepatitis, such as a skin rash, painful swollen joints, and fever. Acute hepatitis produces symptoms such as anorexia and nausea. One of the most noticeable signs of hepatitis is jaundice, or yellowing of the skin. The normal liver eliminates a compound caused bilirubin, but hepatic dysfunction leads to a backup of bilirubin into the circulation, and accumulation of this yellow compound in the skin, conjunctiva and mucous membranes. In the cases of hepatitis A and C, these symptoms resolve; however, with hepatitis B, C, and D, there is often progression to chronic liver disease.

Chronic hepatitis can be caused by viral illness and also by medications, alcohol, metabolic abnormalities, and autoimmune disorders. Medications that may potentially cause drug-induced liver disease include isoniazid, nonsteroidal antiinflammatory medications, methyldopa, nitrofurantoin, and many others. Indications of chronic hepatitis are vague, and include fatigue, sleep disorders, pain under the right rib cage, and enlarge liver and spleen, redness (erythema) of the palms and spider angiomata, or dilated blood vessels visible on the skin. Chronic hepatitis can eventually lead to cirrhosis of the liver, or a state of scarring and fibrosis. Patients are often fatigued and susceptible to infection, and may lose weight and become malnourished due to malabsorption. Poor absorption of vitamin A and D lead to vision impairment and osteopenia (thinning of bones), respectively. In addition, liver cirrhosis can lead to gynecomastia (swelling of breast tissue) and atrophic testicles.

If cirrhosis progresses to advanced cirrhosis or chronic liver failure, individuals may develop portal hypertension. This occurs when the liver becomes too fibrotic and scarred to adequately filter and transport blood, causing a backup of blood from the portal venous system into the systemic venous system. This can cause fluid retention and edema (swelling), acites (fluid retention in the abdomen), and a backup of blood into veins around the umbilicus, rectum, and lower esophagus. If the backup of blood becomes severe, patients can experience severe bleeding, exacerbated by the lack of clotting factors secondary to cirrhosis. Because portal hypertension prevents sufficient detoxification of ammonia and other metabolites, patients can experience encephalopathy leading to confusion and coma. The backup of blood into the spleen can cause splenomegaly, or spleen enlargement and splenic dysfunction, anemia (decreased red blood cells), leukopenia (decreased white blood cells), and thrombocytopenia (decreased platelets).

Prevention of hepatitis is of utmost importance given the significant morbidity and mortality associated with acute and chronic hepatitis. Vaccines exist for both hepatitis A and B. In addition, avoidance of medicines known to cause liver inflammation as well as alcohol can prevent drug- and alcohol-induced hepatitis. Treatment of hepatitis is largely dependent on the cause of liver inflammation, and can range from supportive care in mild cases to liver transplantation when there is severe cirrhosis and liver failure.

SEE ALSO: Hepatitis C.

BIBLIOGRAPHY. Elaine A. Moore, *Hepatitis: Causes, Treatments and Resources* (McFarland, 2006); Jing-Hsiung James Ou, ed., *Hepatitis Viruses* (Kluwer Academic Publishers, 2001).

CHRISTINE CURRY
INDEPENDENT SCHOLAR

Hepatitis C

Hepatitis C is inflammation of the liver caused by a bloodborne pathogen, the hepatitis C virus (HCV). Hepatitis C is only one of many viruses of the hepatitis family that causes viral liver disease; others include hepatitis A, B, D, and E. HCV causes both acute hepatitis, characterized by jaundice, fatigue, abdominal pain, and loss of appetite, as well as long-term liver diseases such as liver cancer and cirrhosis. Symptoms generally appear after an incubation period of 15 to 150 days, although the majority (70 percent) of those infected are asymptomatic. Chronic infection occurs in approximately 55 to 85 percent of infected persons, and about one to five percent of those chronically infected will eventually die from chronic liver diseases. In countries where liver transplants are available, cirrhotic HCV patients often represent the majority of recipients of donated livers. Patients infected with HCV are often also infected with HIV or hepatitis B, both of which can worsen HCV disease prognosis, as can high alcohol consumption.

Transmission of HCV is via direct contact with infected blood, and transmission is often a result of contaminated blood transfusions, the use of contaminated syringes, or contaminated circumcision, tattooing, or piercing equipment. Sharing of syringes among intravenous drug injectors in prisons has led to outbreaks. Patients on kidney dialysis, transplant recipients, and hemophiliacs have also been infected in the past. Sexual transmission is possible, although rarer, and transmission rates are enhanced when individuals are coinfected with other sexually transmitted diseases or are sexually assaulted. Healthcare workers face a risk of infection from workplace injuries. The virus can also be transmitted from a mother to a baby during childbirth in approximately 4 percent of cases, although the transmission probability rises if a mother is coinfected with HIV. Hepatitis C is not spread via casual contact, sneezing, coughing, breastfeeding, food, or water, although it can be spread via sharing common items such as razors and toothbrushes if they contain contaminated blood.

Globally, approximately 170 million people are infected with hepatitis C, and thus it statistically affects about four to five times as many people as those currently infected with HIV. Approximately three to 4 million new infections occur annually. Individuals are often coinfected with HIV or hepatitis B. Areas of the world with the highest prevalence rates include Africa, southeast and eastern Asia, and the eastern Mediterranean region. Countries that have a larger-than-average reservoir of chronically infected HCV patients, such as Italy, Pakistan, Egypt, and Japan, often have a history of widespread injection-based prophylaxis treatments against other infectious diseases, suggesting that sterilization of injection equipment is essential when implementing population-based vaccination and treatment programs. Public awareness of the disease is often not as high as of other infectious diseases, such as HIV, and as patients are often asymptomatic, even those infected are often not aware of their illness until they present with long-term liver complications. Medical awareness of HCV is also lower than for HIV, and many patients at high risk of HCV infection go undetected even by medical personnel.

There is no vaccine against HCV, and developing vaccines and treatments has proved challenging because HCV is highly variable and mutates rapidly. Interferon, either alone or in combination with ribavirin, is used to treat HCV infection. The combination treatment proves effective in approximately half of infected persons, although this success rate varies widely depending on which genotype of the virus the patient is infected with. These drugs can also cause serious side effects: Ribavirin can cause severe anemia and interferon treatment can result in depression, seizures, or flu-like symptoms. Treatment is recommended for individuals whose infection does not resolve within two months (approximately 60 percent of all those infected). Women who are pregnant should not be treated with either drug. There is no postexposure prophylaxis for HCV.

Preventing new infections is much more economically feasible than providing long-term treatment for chronically infected patients, because treatments such as liver transplants and the interferon/ribavirin regimes are quite costly. Preventative measures often include screening of blood donors, organ donors, and the blood supply; viral inactivation of plasma products; and implementing preventative measures in healthcare settings, including sterilizing injection equipment. As the majority of new infections in the developing world occur among intravenous drug users, promoting safe injecting behaviors in high-risk populations is particularly important in reducing new infections. Also, in addition to maintaining safe injection practices in medical settings, noninjection-based methods of drug delivery, such as pills or liquids, should be promoted when possible.

SEE ALSO: Hepatitis.

BIBLIOGRAPHY. M. Dolan, *The Hepatitis C Handbook,* (North Atlantic Books, 1999); H. Worman, *The Hepatitis C SourceBook* (NTC Publishing, 2002).

ANNIE DUDE
UNIVERSITY OF CHICAGO

Herbal Medicine

For as long as humankind has suffered from illnesses, it has looked for substances to alleviate its symptoms. Since the early 20th century, those medicines have tended to be the standardized synthetic drugs found behind any pharmacist's counter; before that, however, the nature and practice of prescription was different. The medicinal use of herbs dates back thousands of years and is common to all cultures, and in fact, many current prescription medications are derived from botanicals. There is a cultural element to the use of traditional remedies that may confound a nonintegrated approach; treatments are recommended by friends at least as often as by physicians, and users show a remarkable amount of resolve—one study indicated that 72 percent would continue use even after a scientific study with negative results. There is a push toward evidence-based medicine in the United States, and many herbal products are undergoing clinical trials to determine their efficacy with mixed results. Patients may seek out herbal products, feeling they are safer than prescription products, as they are natural. Many examples of adverse events exist in the medical literature, at times due to interactions with prescription medication. Through the education of the public as well as healthcare workers, some of these adverse events may be avoided.

The foreword to the *Physician's Desk Reference on Herbal Medicines* (3rd ed.), defines herbal medicine as preparations derived from naturally occurring plants with medicinal or preventive properties. Natural remedies are popular throughout the planet, although their use is often manifested differently depending upon the prevailing healing traditions of the given culture. In America, the use of alternative or complementary avenues of healthcare—often including herbal medicines—is on the rise.

The lack of a strong foundation of empirical data regarding their efficacy, and poor communication between conventional healthcare providers and their herb-taking patients produces a strained and potentially dangerous environment, but the potential benefits of this and other complementary and alternative medicine (CAM) modalities have prompted many modern physicians to seek a fruitful integration of botanicals and pharmaceuticals. Many patients will not tell their physician, even if asked about herbal use, as they feel the physician may be scornful, or may not know about herbal products. Many physicians fail to ask patients about the use of these products, possibly leading the patient to believe their use is unimportant. Medical schools traditionally do not educate students about CAM modalities, although this is beginning to change.

WORLDWIDE USE OF HERBAL MEDICINE

Herbs continue to be used medicinally by people around the world. In some developing countries, the use of an herbal remedy is still inextricably tied to rituals of healing with supernatural/spiritual overtones. In others, the preponderant use of herbs is the result of economic factors—some natural remedies require neither a doctor to prescribe nor a pharmacist to prepare them. The traditional healers of China regularly use herbs along with other techniques considered CAM in the Western model of healthcare, such as acupuncture and therapeutic massage. Their use goes back at least 5,000 years and as far back as the Ming Dynasty (1386–1644 A.D.), Li Shizhen catalogued medicinally used botanical products in the still-popular text *Compendium of Materia Medica.* In India, over 80 percent of the population takes at least one of the 6,000 herbal combinations used in ayurvedic tradition.

In the European Union (EU), herbal medicine (or phytotherapy) is often highly integrated into what is considered mainstream medical care, and the use is regulated in a similar manner to conventional drugs everywhere except the United Kingdom and the Netherlands. Two-thirds of the general public in Germany uses herbal remedies, which accounts for 50 percent of the $7 billion spent on herbal medicines by the EU in 1996. Accordingly, all German physicians are required to train and be tested over the proper use of herbs before they may be licensed. Roughly 80 percent of those doctors go on to prescribe herbal medicine to their patients.

DOMESTIC USE OF HERBAL MEDICINE

In the United States, the use of natural remedies is on the upswing (nearly one in five people reported having used at least one such product in 2002) after a significant decline following the spread of synthetic pharmaceuticals, which provided larger effects and profits. This resurgence may be attributed to a variety of factors, such as a desire among some people to seek out unconventional and "natural" paths, the inability of conventional medicine to cure chronic conditions (such as arthritis, depression, and memory loss), a loss of faith in the pharmaceutical companies and/or the government, and misleading advertising on the part of some herbal supplement providers.

While it is incorrect and unsafe to assume that all natural remedies are inherently beneficial and innocuous, some herbs have been proven to possess qualities that do promote health or treat illness when used properly. Similarly, while many believe that synthetic drug manufacturers strive to marginalize the use of herbal supplements (and therefore are suspicious of government-funded studies that seem to discredit alternative medicine), it is important to note that those supplements are largely deregulated and some suppliers will use this uncertainty to their own advantage ("10 Natural Cures *They* Don't Want You to Know About", etc.).

DOMESTIC REGULATION OF HERBAL MEDICINE

The increased public interest in natural healthcare that began in the 1960s prompted Congress to establish the National Institutes of Health Office of Alternative Medicine in 1992, which became the National Center for Complementary and Alternative Medicine (NCCAM) six years later. Thirty years after the Kefauver-Harris

Drug Amendment of 1962 relegated herbal remedies to the laxly monitored classification of food supplements, the Food and Drug Administration (FDA) tried to develop a more stringent set of regulations but was opposed, resulting in the 1994 passage of the Dietary Supplement Health and Education Act (DSHEA) which failed to require supplement manufacturers to prove that a product was either safe or efficacious prior to release. Due to the FDA's lack of premarket involvement, supplements must state on the label "This statement has not been evaluated by the FDA. This product is not intended to diagnose, treat, cure, or prevent any disease" although the labels may still claim that the herbs "improve memory" or "support digestive health".

National surveys show that 81 percent of Americans believe a supplement should not be sold without proven safety, but 70 percent believe the FDA currently tests and regulates all herbal products on the market. As recently as November 9, 2004, the FDA announced major initiatives to improve the transparency and standardization of dietary supplements (as herbal remedies must be called under DSHEA), but all Good Manufacturing Practices (GMPs) proposed thus far are purely voluntary on the part of the supplier.

Beyond the legal red tape, herbal medicine has proven more difficult to regulate than its synthetic counterpart. The quality of an herbal product is dependent upon a host of interrelated factors, many of which are not easily isolated and studied. Some examples of these mitigating factors include the fact that plants are often mislabeled, the specific species used for the extraction vary, and the methods of harvesting and processing differ greatly. Numerous studies have shown wide discrepancies between the advertised amount of active ingredient in many commercially available nutraceutical and the actual content. Furthermore, prescription medications have been found in ostensibly natural products, and heavy metals with the potential to cause arsenic or lead poisoning are occasionally discovered in products imported from Asia. The inclusion of the metals is at times intentional, as they are believed to accelerate the healing process, and at times reflects the factory parts where the product is made.

Due to the lack of regulatory structure for herbal medications, there tends to be dramatic variation in the quality of available products. This can have huge implications in the safety and efficacy of these products. Quality of herbal products is determined by many variables, all of which can affect their clinical use and safety. Plant species, parts used, harvesting, storage conditions, processing and accuracy of labeling all can have a huge impact on the consistency and standardization of herbs.

The pharmacologic potency of herbs may be dependent on how and where it was harvested, storage length and condition and by processing techniques. This leads to variation of similar products even within manufacturing plants. There are also many reports of inaccurate labeling and lack of product standardization and content. One study found that close to 40 percent of products were insufficiently or inconsistently labeled and that there were huge variations in recommended dosing.

While controlled trials have demonstrated the superiority of some natural remedies when compared to placebo, some have led to adverse effects. One of the most-documented examples of this is the herb ephedra, or *Ma Huang*. A compound with similar properties to amphetamine, ephedra is often combined with guarana (caffeine) to promote weight loss or to boost athletic ability. Ephedra was also the primary ingredient in herbal Fen-Phen, marketed as a natural alternative to the antiobesity drugs fenfluramine and phentermine. Between 1994 and 1997, the FDA investigated over 800 claims of adverse effects, including death, myocardial infarctions, and cerebrovascular accidents, and in 2004 the sale of ephedra-containing products was banned (this was later overturned in court by the manufacturer, who argued successfully that the FDA did not have jurisdiction in herbal products, and needed to prove ephedra was unsafe).

Not all adverse effects are as easily documented, however. While research is ongoing, evidence of traditional and conventional medicines interacting has surfaced through case reports and in vitro studies. St. John's wort, while proven efficacious as an antidepressant in treatment of mild to moderate depression, appears to interact with oral contraceptives, anticoagulants, digoxin, antiviral agents, and cyclosporine, as well as anesthetic agents used prior to surgery. The challenge faced by the modern physician lies in reconciling the growing use of herbal remedies by the public with the lack of a sufficient set of data regarding their efficacy and potential adverse effects and interactions.

INTEGRATING HERBAL AND CONVENTIONAL MEDICINE

Combining traditional herbal remedies with modern scientific advances is not a new concept for American physicians. The first *United States Pharmacopoeia*, published in 1820, was comprised of over 65 percent natural substances. As those medicines became increasingly replaced by modern pharmaceuticals, however, a comprehensive knowledge of their effects and uses was no longer seen to be a necessary part of a medical education. Currently the divide between the two forms of healthcare is sufficiently wide that a recent survey found most primary care providers unaware of their patient's herbal intake and most patients unlikely to discuss their use of alternative remedies with their doctor even in the event of an adverse experience.

In an effort to close this gap, some medical schools have begun to offer courses in CAM modalities. The 2002 White House Commission on Complementary and Alternative Medicine Policy (WHCCAMP) recommended increased funding and incentives for CAM research and improved protections for participants in those studies; WHCCAMP also specifically noted the importance of an open and integrative dialogue between traditional and conventional medical practitioners.

POPULAR HERBAL REMEDIES

According to the 2002 National Health Interview Survey (NHIS), the most frequently used herbal medicines were echinacea, ginseng, ginkgo biloba, garlic, St. John's wort, peppermint, ginger root, and soy. The following section discusses *purported* (not all have been proven efficacious) uses of several products. This should not be taken as medical advice to treat a medical condition, and is for informational purposes only.

ECHINACEA

The 2002 NHIS rated echinacea as the most popular herbal remedy, and its domestic sales totaled $70 million in 1998. There are nine species of the plant, including *Echinacea purpurea*, *E. pallida*, and *E. angustifolia*, commonly utilized to treat or prevent the common cold. A large NCCAM study recently did not reveal echinacea to be of benefit to reduce symptoms of the common cold, but research continues. The roots are part of the pharmacologically active part of the plant, and their consumption is thought to stimulate the immune system through a higher macrophage production rate. Echinacea is also used as a local anesthetic and antiinflammatory agent when applied topically. Doctors should discourage the use of this plant by patients with allergies, asthma, atopy, autoimmune disorders, or transplants, as there is a theoretical risk worsening those conditions, or precipitating an attack on the newly transplanted organ.

GINSENG

The second most popular herbal remedy according the 2002 NIHS, ginseng stimulates the central nervous system and increases glycogen storage. The World Health Organization (WHO) has approved its use as an agent to combat fatigue and stress, and the results of small studies of its effectiveness have been promising but inconclusive. Studies continue for the use of ginseng in patients with diabetes. There are many reports of mislabeling of ginseng, and some products on the market labeled as ginseng do not contain any active product.

GINKGO BILOBA

This medicine accounted for the highest sales figure in the 1998 study ($151 million). The leaf is the active part of the plant, and many distributors claim that its ingestion will increase blood fluidity and improve memory function. A recent test involving a 230-person trial group found no improvement in memory, learning, attention, or concentration compared to a placebo, but other studies have indicated that ginkgo helps reverse the effects of tinnitus. It may be of use in mild-moderate dementia, as it works by improving blood flow to the brain. This effect is also responsible for the side effect of bleeding.

GARLIC

Garlic is often advertised as an immune enhancer and a check against high cholesterol levels. While the WHO, among other groups, has sanctioned its use in the treatment of hyperlipidemia, other studies have been mixed. Garlic supplements should not be taken in extremely large doses within the week prior to a surgery due to potential platelet inhibition. Usual dietary doses are unlikely to have an adverse bleeding effect.

ST. JOHN'S WORT

St. John's wort accounted for nearly $140 million in sales in 1998, and the history of its use stretches back at least as far as Hippocrates' account from the 5th century B.C.E. Its active ingredients (hypericin and hyperforin) help to combat depression. Over a dozen clinical trials have shown it to be significantly more effective than a placebo and comparable in effect to imipramine. While the current body of evidence implies that its use is fairly safe, St. John's wort should not be taken in conjunction with other antidepressants, and the usual precautions that are taken to assess the patient for bipolar disorder must be adhered to as well in order to avoid precipitating a manic state.

PEPPERMINT

The use of peppermint oil (primarily composed of menthol and menthone) may aid in the treatment of shingles, gingivitis, and indigestion. When combined with caraway oils, multiple double-blind trials have indicated that it can reduce the negative effects of irritable bowel syndrome. Its use is generally safe, but patients with gallstones, liver damage, or chronic heartburn should be wary.

GINGER

The rhizome (stem) of the ginger plant has achieved widespread use as a spice and as a remedy for a variety of ills. Studies have found the ingestion of ginger to be helpful in the treatment of motion sickness and osteoarthritis, and when used in conjunction with other natural substances it may help fight epilepsy and various kinds of nausea, especially the nausea and vomiting associated with pregnancy.

SOY

Soy has gained popularity as a milk substitute, and it is commonly used in the prevention of osteoporosis and the treatment of high blood pressure or cholesterol, although results of studies for these purposes are mixed. In addition, patients would have to drink a lot (five to 10 glasses) of soymilk or eat a lot (two and a half cups) of tofu in order to obtain the same effects as a 0.3 mg pill of conjugated estrogen. Some research has indicated that soy may help prevent the onset of cancer, but results are inconclusive.

SAW PALMETTO

Saw palmetto has been used to treat urinary disorders for over 17,000 years. In Germany, a patient with mild-moderate benign prostatic hyperplasia (BPH) would be

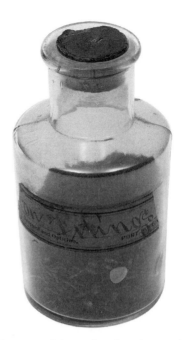

Twenty to 30 percent of the medicinal products in the United States are derived from botanicals.

more likely to be advised to take saw palmetto than a traditional prescription medication. Studies have shown it is efficacious for the short-term treatment of mild-moderate BPH, and often with fewer side effects than some prescription medications used for this purpose. As the push toward evidence based medicine drives further research into the use, efficacy, side effects, interactions and safety of herbal medications, physicians and consumers will be able to more confidently utilize these as another tool in the fight against disease. Problems remain, as herbal products cannot be patented, hence, corporations may be unwilling to spend millions of research dollars to prove the efficacy of these products and not see a return on investment. Also, the lack of standardization remains a problem , as patients may receive varying amounts of active ingredients from month to month.

SEE ALSO: Herbal Remedy; National Center for Complementary and Alternative Medicine (NCCAM); Pharmacology.

BIBLIOGRAPHY. E. Ernst, *Harmless herbs? A review of recent literature.* American Journal of Medicine (v.104, 1998); C.A. Newall, L.A. Anderson, and J.D. Phillipson, *Herbal Medicines. A Guide for Healthcare Professional* (The Pharmaceutical Press, 1996); Robert Saper, "Overview of Herbal

Medicine," www.uptodate.com (cited October 17, 2006); U.M. Thatte, et al., *The Flip Side of Ayurveda. Journal of Postgraduate Medicine* (v.39, 1993).

GAUTAM J. DESAI, D.O.
INGRID Y. MADJAR
KANSAS CITY UNIVERSITY OF MEDICINE AND
BIOSCIENCES COLLEGE OF OSTEOPATHIC MEDICINE
SHAMOLI KHANDERIA, D.O., PHARM.D.
PRIVATE PRACTICE PHYSICIAN

Herbal Remedy

Many Americans turn to herbal remedies, either in conjunction with, or in place of, prescription medication, to treat various ailments. These products are advertised in the popular media, as well as in health food stores. The purity and efficacy of many remedies remain in question, as research is only now commencing in earnest on many herbal products in the United States.

Over 80 percent of the medicinal products in the United States during the early 1800s were derived from botanicals; today, this number is only 20 to 30 percent. The use of plant extracts for medicinal purposes is termed phytotherapy, and there are various formulations of herbal remedies, including liquid, dry, powdered, distillations, and fresh parts of the herb. Herbal remedies may be ingested or applied topically. Various portions of the plant may be used, including the flowers, leaves, roots, and stems, depending on the species and intended use.

Often, closely related species are included in common herbal products, which may cause problems in the intended use. There are nine species of the herb echinacea—commercial products often contain three or more species, each with distinct pharmacologic properties. Variation in active ingredient between bottles may cause a change in clinical effects based on the product used, even if from the same manufacturer. Different plant parts (roots, stems, leaves) from the same herb also may have variable properties and are rarely differentiated in herbal products.

Special populations that must take care when using herbal remedies are geriatric patients, children, and pregnant/breastfeeding patients. The elderly may be on multiple medications, which can increase their chances of an interaction. Children are more susceptible to toxins, as they are still developing. Few studies exist on pregnant or lactating patients regarding the use of herbal products and their effects on the fetus/newborn.

Examples of herbal remedies and their *purported* uses (some of which have not been verified through research) include:

1. Saw Palmetto: benign prostatic hypertrophy
2. St. John's wort: mild depression
3. Ginger root: nausea and vomiting of pregnancy
4. Echinacea: to enhance the immune system

Examples of herbal remedies and possible side effects/interactions include: ginkgo biloba interacting with warfarin to cause easier bleeding, and St. John's wort interacting with anesthetics prior to surgery.

Unlike prescription medication, herbal medicines are not tested by the Food and Drug Administration (FDA) for purity, efficacy, or content. Often, testing of herbal products reveals less active ingredient than is advertised on the label. Even within samples produced by the same manufacturer, the amount of active ingredient may vary, which may have an effect on the purported use, so the public needs to be aware of the risk/benefit ratio prior to choosing a herbal remedy. This is especially true for those at higher risk for an adverse reaction/interaction—the young, elderly, and breastfeeding/pregnant patients.

SEE ALSO: Herbal Medicine; National Center for Complementary and Alternative Medicine (NCCAM); Pharmacology.

BIBLIOGRAPHY. Ellen Hughes, Bradly Jacobs, and Brian Berman, *Current Medical Diagnosis and Treatment, Complementary and Alternative Medicine 2006*, www.accessmedicine.com (cited October 2006); Robert Saper, "An Overview of Herbal Medicine," www.uptodate.com (cited October 2006).

GAUTAM J. DESAI, D.O.
PINAKI N. PATEL, MS III
KANSAS CITY UNIVERSITY OF MEDICINE AND
BIOSCIENCES COLLEGE OF OSTEOPATHIC MEDICINE
SHAMOLI KHANDERIA, D.O., PHARM.D.
PRIVATE PRACTICE PHYSICIAN, DENVER, COLORADO
SHELLEY L. ALEXANDER, D.O.
UNIVERSITY OF MISSOURI–KANSAS CITY
SCHOOL OF MEDICINE

Herbalism

Herbal medical practice in North America draws primarily on traditions from native healers of this continent and Europe, and secondarily from eastern Asia and the Indian subcontinent. Much less common in North America are those herbal traditions native to Africa, Australia, or the various island kingdoms. All herbal traditions use plants variously prepared to treat patient symptoms.

EUROPEAN TRADITION

An archaeological find in present-day Iraq from a 60,000-year-old burial site shows drawings of *Althea* and *Achillea*, botanicals used today. Cuneiform tablets from Iraq dating to 4000 B.C.E. show such medicines as *Glycyrrhiza, Papaver, Thymus,* and *Brassica.* An Egyptian papyrus from the 16th century B.C.E contains some 800 recipes and over 700 plants, treatments for diabetes, and the use of mudpacks for open sores. Hippocrates, the Greek father of medicine, wrote in 400 B.C.E about the medical use of over 300 plants. Theophrastus (371–287 B.C.E) wrote *Inquiry into Plants* and *Growth of Plants*, describing over 550 plants and their uses. The Greek physician Dioscorides in the 1st century C.E. authored *De Materia Medica*, cataloging the medical use of over 600 plants, 35 animals, and 90 minerals. Naturalist and botanist Pietro Mattioli of Venice reprinted it in 1544. Between 400 and 1500 C.E., the Catholic Church controlled medical knowledge and herbal medicines were grown administered by the clergy and knowledgeable laypeople. This changed with Church decrees that forced the clergy to focus on saving souls, and medical and herbal education to become a part of the early universities.

English herbal tradition was legalized under Henry VIII in 1541 under the Herbalist Charter. It preserved the use of herbs for the King and all of his subjects. The best lexicon of these plants was *The Herbal (The English Physitian* [Physician]*)* of 1652 produced by Nicholas Culpeper (1616–54) who began his herbal practice as a physician in 1640. It described various botanicals, their harvesting, preparation, and use with a view to the astrological chart. A modern update to Culpeper that borrowed heavily without credit from King's American Dispensatory was Maud Grieve's *A Modern Herbal* published in 1931. It provided information on the medicinal, culinary, cosmetic, cultiva-

tion, and economic uses of some 800 herbs. Between Culpeper and Grieves was Carl von Linne (1701–78) who set about to categorize every plant, animal, and mineral. He established botanical taxonomy and the use of a Latin binomial consisting of genus and species (e.g., *Echinacea angustifolia, Taraxacum officinale*) to describe every plant. This system has become a universal language for naming all plants (and animals) including those used in herbalism.

ECLECTIC TRADITION

Constantine Rafinesque (1784–1841), a botanist and advocate of herbs as medicines, explored the Mississippi River Valley learning from the various American Indian communities what plants were used, how they were prepared, and for what conditions. He is credited as the first to use the term *eclectic* meaning "to adopt into practice what is beneficial." Explorers, trappers, and early settlers traveling west along the Oregon Trail and other routes adopted from the various Indian tribes many more herbs (e.g., *Artemisia, Arctostaphylos, Lomatium, Vaccinium*, etc.) and used them daily. An estimated 90 percent of the North American medicinal herbs used here and in Europe came from east of the Mississippi River with 75 percent from the Appalachian forests. Botanical diversity in the Mississippi drainage and regions to the east is greater than that of the Rocky Mountains and lands to the west. Native American traditions were mainly oral, so few texts exist. The single best reference on Native American herbs and their use is by Moerman. This reference is organized alphabetically by species, indicating its use as a drug, food, fiber, dye, and other uses, and within these categories by tribe and how they specifically used the plant. This text includes over 4,000 plants, from 1,200 genera and their use by 291 different societies from the North American Arctic to Mexico.

Wooster Beach (1794–1868) apprenticed with Jacob Tidd, a German herbal doctor, until Tidd's death and then graduated from Barclay Street Medical University, New York. He wanted to reform the then-current heroic medical treatments of bleeding and mercury chloride (calomel) to the use of herbal medicines. His enthusiastic efforts led him to being ostracized by the New York State Medical Society and it was their political clout that helped deny him the necessary charter to establish a college and grant legitimate medical diplomas in the state of New York. Worthington College, Worthington, Ohio, was a financially ailing chartered school that he transformed into the Reformed Medical College in 1831. In 1855, it moved and became the Eclectic Medical Institute of Cincinnati, Ohio. This institution graduated its last class in 1939 as World War II was beginning. The eclectic tradition with respect to use of botanical medicines was adopted by naturopathic medicine which now has four-year full-time colleges in Canada (two schools), United States (five schools), and England, and three-year full-time colleges in South Africa, Australia, India, and New Zealand. The World Health Organization is preparing a monograph on naturopathic medical education and how botanical medicine is incorporated into its training and clinical practice.

The Eclectic School was responsible through the effort of John Uri Lloyd (1849–1936) in advancing pharmacognosy, the study of plant constituents and their use as medicines. Lloyd published over 5,000 papers mainly on plant constituents and held 16 patents, inventing devices for botanical extraction and preparation. *King's American Dispensatory*, first published in 1855 by John King, was a detailed catalogue of constituents, actions, indications, doses, and more on the hundreds of plants used by eclectic physicians. The revised edition was edited by Harvey Wickes Felter and Lloyd and released as a two-volume reference in 1898 and reprinted in 1983. Today's popular botanicals, *Echinacea, Crataegus, Hypericum, Hydrastis*, and so forth, and many lesser known herbs, *Ampelopsis, Aspidosperma, Menispermum, Sterculias*, and so forth, were described with detail in *King's*. John Milton Scudder (1829–94) undertook an ambitious project to publish the specific patient signs and symptoms and clinical indications for these plants, leaving aside any effect not directly attributed to the action of the botanical medicine.

THOMSON AND PHYSIOMEDICAL TRADITION

Samuel Thomson (1769–1843), a poor New Hampshire farmer, claimed to have learned herbal medicine from the local Indians. His theories were largely his own and led to the Thomsonian system with an underlying philosophy of self-treatment. Thomson published *New Guide to Health* in 1822 and sold it plus a kit of medicines for home or family use under patent protection for $20; he claimed 100,000 families purchased the kit. Alva Curtis, MD (1797–1881), worked as editor for the *Thomson Recorder*, another of his publications, but viewed the ill-effects of the large doses of powerful emetics (*Lobelia inflata*) and warming herbs (*Capsicum frutescens*) as too strong. She left and formed physiomedicalism.

The tenets of physiomedicalism were 1.) cure of disease must conform to the laws of life and assist nature, 2.) no poisonous substance could be used in treatment, 3.) practitioners should be scientifically educated (unlike Thomson), and 4.) botanical medicines should be studied to determine their effect. The Physio-Medical Institute, Cincinnati, Ohio, was short lived, but its philosophy survived in England, becoming the basis of the National Institute of Medical Herbalist, now a four-year full-time course at the University of Wales. The physiomedical philosophy blended well with the strong British herbal tradition. The British use of herbs dates back to the Druids and before and is a blend with the herbal traditions brought by various invaders of the British Isles including the Vikings and the Romans.

ASIAN TRADITIONS

Chinese medicine, arguably one of the oldest, most systematized medicines of the world, is based on a distinct philosophy of the human body and how it interacts or reacts to its environment with respect to its overall health. Important to the medicine are 1.) yin and yang (philosophical polar constructs representing cold, rest, darkness or passive, interior and hot, activity, light or vigor exterior, respectively); 2.) fundamental substances such as qi (matter on the verge of becoming energy), blood (a circulating yin fluid that nourishes, moistens, and maintains the body), jing (congenital essence inherited from parents and vitality from ingested food), and body fluids (nonblood fluids such as saliva, gastric juices, urine); 3.) organs, heart, spleen, triple warmer (similar but not always identical to our Western definition), and so forth; 4.) meridians (channels that carry blood, but not blood vessels, and chi through the body connecting the organs); and 5.) conditions that cause disharmony (disease) such as wind (a yang phenomenon that generates movement, change, and urgency), heat (a yang phenomenon in which the patient is hot), cold (a yin phenomenon in which the patient is cold), dampness (a yin phenomenon producing heaviness, discharges, or obstructions to the movement of qi), and so forth.

Shan Ching from 250 B.C.E. and *Hai Ching* from 120 B.C.E are their oldest extant medical texts with 52 diseases and 283 prescriptions using 247 drugs, mostly plants; all are still used today. A copy of *Shen Nung Pen Tsao Ching* from 500 C.E. enumerated 365 herbs, *Hsin Hsiu Pen Tsao* from 659 C.E. contained 850 medicinal substances in 27 volumes, *Kai Pao Pen Tsao* of 973 C.E. listed 984 herbs, its 1057 C.E. edition 1,084 herbs, and the 1590 C.E. edition 1,518 medicines including 374 new herbs. *Chung Yao Ta Tsu Tien*, the People's Republic of China's dictionary of Chinese herb drugs, lists 5,767 different medicinal substances, mostly plants of which 235 species are used commonly and almost daily. Herbal combinations (including mineral and animal substances) are prescribed to counter the patient's conditions or diagnosis as well as for building up the patient's resistance to his or her diagnosis/condition. The kampo formulas and medical philosophy of Japan and other Asian medical systems (Tibet, Korea, Thailand, Vietnam) are similar but distinct from traditional Chinese medicine.

AYURVEDIC TRADITION

Ayurvedic medicine, the traditional medicine of the Indian subcontinent, is similar in age to Chinese medicine and provides healthcare to about 70 percent of the population. It was built on an oral tradition where medical students had to memorize over 45,000 verses until *Atreya Samhita* was written in Sanskrit circa 500 B.C.E. Ayurvedic medicine has eight major disciplines including internal medicine, surgery, gynecology and pediatrics, gerontology, psychiatry, sexology/fertility, toxicology of medicinal substances, and medicine and surgery of the head. The materia medica consists of over 1,000 plants plus minerals and animal substances. The principles of Vata (movement, breathing, animation, activity), Pitta (energy released from biochemical processes, digestion, vision), and Kapha (stability, form, cohesion, mental strength, disease resistance) aid in patient diagnosis and prescriptions to evacuate (parasites), stop elimination (hemostatics, diarrhea), modify the temperament, and effect the disease.

SUMMARY

Each of these herbal traditions thrives within a multicultural North America. Occasionally, the plants used will overlap traditional boundaries with slightly different indications (e.g., *Allium, Zingiber, Glycyrrhiza, Arctium*, etc.). Within each tradition, the herbalist writes a formula of one to 10 herbs specific to the patient's diagnosis. The herbal practitioner may prepare the formula or give directions to the patient for its preparation and administration. Many herbalists still grow or wild-craft their herbs. These methods of herbal administration may include infusions, decoctions, tinctures, fluid extracts, salves, ointments, suppositories, vapors, essential oils, encapsulations, standardized extracts, or constituent extracts. Some herbal practitioners will also use traditional or "patent" formula with a long history of use that are described in older texts, while others will prepare a specific formula for a specific patient and his or her condition.

Each herbal tradition was also very aware of poisonous plants and how to avoid them or prepare for use in a nontoxic manner (e.g., *Aconitum napellus, Digitalis* spp., *Atropa belladonna, Datura stramonium*). In addition, the herbalist must be aware of real or potential negative and positive interactions between the herbal prescription and any prescribed or over-the-counter medications the patient is taking. The rich tradition of herbalism has provided us with many currently used drugs (e.g., reserpine, digoxin, taxol, vincristine) and will no doubt lead to future discoveries that will benefit humankind.

SEE ALSO: Alternative Medicine; Chinese Medicine, Traditional.

BIBLIOGRAPHY. H.A. Baer, "The Potential Rejuvenation of American Naturopathy as a Consequence of the Holistic Health Movement," *Medical Anthropology* (v.13, 1992); D. Bensky and A. Gamble, *Chinese Herbal Medicine Materia Medica*, rev. ed. (Eastland Press, 1993); W. Boyle, *Herb Doctors: Pioneers in Nineteenth Century Botanical Medicine* (Buckeye Naturopathic Press, 1988); F. Brinker, *Herb Contraindications and Drug Interactions* (Eclectic Medical Publications, 2001); F. Brinker, *Native Healing Gifts: Rediscovering Indigenous Plant Medicines of the Greater Southwest* (Eclectic Medical Publications, 1995); F. Brinker, *Pioneers, Plants and Medicines along the Oregon Trail* (Eclectic Medical Publications, 1993); H.G.M. Chishti, *The Traditional Healer* (Healing Arts Press, 1988); G. Cody, "History of Naturopathic Medicine," in J. Pizzorno and M. Murray, eds., *Textbook of Natural Medicine* (Bastyr University Press, 1985); W. H. Cook, *The Physiomedical Dispensatory* (Eclectic Medical Publications, 1998); N. Culpeper, *Culpeper's Complete Herbal* (Foulsham, 1640); I. N. Dobelis, *Magic and Medicine of Plants* (Reader's Digest Association, 1986); F. W. Felter and J. U. Lloyd, *King's American Dispensatory*, 18th ed. (Eclectic Medical Publications, 1983); J. Filliozat, *The Classical Doctrine of Indian Medicine* (B. Jain, 1964); M. Grieve, *A Modern Herbal* (Tiger Books, 1931); B. Griggs, *Green Pharmacy* (Jill, Norman and Hobhouse, 1981); B. Heyn, *Ayurvedic Medicine* (Thorson's, 1987).

PAUL RICHARD SAUNDERS, PH.D., N.D., DHANP
CANADIAN COLLEGE OF NATUROPATHIC MEDICINE

Herbalist

A herbalist is a person who prescribes primarily herbal remedies for various medical ailments. The practice is very old and may be dated to two millennia B.C.E in Egypt and China. It continues to be popular in China and east Asian countries, although from the time of the Industrial Revolution, the practice became increasingly discredited in Western countries as new scientific techniques seized the imagination of people in those countries.

In modern times, herbalists have received something of an upturn in fortunes because many people have come to feel that Western medicine is too reliant on chemical sciences which cannot be trusted and which are mediated by pharmaceutical companies that have dubious intentions. Nevertheless, at the heart of herbalism is a belief in the restorative or curative powers of herbs which, in many cases, has no verifiable basis and, in other cases, obscures potentially dangerous side effects.

Because a herbalist is required to be able to recognize a wide range of plants and to identify their specific uses, it as customary in preindustrial societies for the herbalist, possibly in addition to other religious or sacred duties, to spend years studying the art, perhaps as an apprentice to an older herbalist. In some societies, women were able to enter the profession, perhaps as part of duties which also included midwifery. At a basic level, the herbalist would have been required to identify safe and unsafe wild plants and to advise on pain relief and health-giving preparations. In countries where poppies grew, opium became known as a method of pain relief and other examples exist of herbal remedies actually performing the functions required of them, although they may have undesirable side effects and other issues. In other cases, societies became dependent on particular herbs and attributed great power to them even though no scientific evidence for their efficacy exists.

An example of this is the use of ginseng in Korea, which is prescribed for a very wide range of ailments and generally believed to have numerous benefits, although these have yet to be substantiated in laboratories. In other cases still, herbalists used items that have subsequently come to be used in different but genuinely efficacious ways. The impact of quinine on preventing the spread of malaria, for example, has become well known.

Irrespective of the demonstrated ability of herbalists to prescribe effective treatments, it is certainly true that the decoupling of many people from the land on which they live has led to a number of negative impacts, not least of which is loss of knowledge about local plants and flowers. Local wisdom may still be useful in the modern world and, as the pace of global climate change and environmental degradation intensifies, it would be unfortunate if knowledge of plants becomes extinct, as well as the plants themselves.

Western medicine should be chosen over the prescriptions of herbalists because evidence exists of its effectiveness, which may be repeated in laboratory conditions and because of the study of side effects or interactions with other substances. Furthermore, medicine deriving from companies that adhere to strict government regulations is much more likely to have strict quality-control issues which ensure that it is of the same, advertised strength and quality on a consistent basis.

SEE ALSO: Herbal Medicine; Herbal Remedy; Herbalism.

BIBLIOGRAPHY. W. Boyle, *Herb Doctors: Pioneers in Nineteenth Century Botanical Medicine* (Buckeye Naturopathic Press, 1988); Robert Saper, "An Overview of Herbal Medicine," www.uptodate.com (cited June 2007).

JOHN WALSH
SHINAWATRA UNIVERSITY

Hernia

The term *hernia* is used to describe the protrusion of a body part or organ through an opening or defect in the fascia, muscle, or wall of a cavity. The fibrous lining of the abdominal cavity that supports, separates, and unites the muscles and tissues is known as fascia. In a hernia, the involved body part or organ is usually contained within the confines of the cavity, and upon herniation, is considered out of place. Hernias are generally found in the abdominal cavity, and can be asymptomatic or may produce a lump, ache, pain, or bulge at rest or with straining. A defect or opening in fascia can be congenital or acquired. Hernias can be lined or covered with tissue and this is known as a hernia sac.

Activities and conditions that increase the intraabdominal pressure such as heavy lifting, pregnancy, and obesity can lead to or accentuate an abdominal wall weakness manifesting itself as a hernia. There are several descriptive terms used to further classify hernias. A reducible hernia is one that returns to the cavity where it belongs via an application of pressure to it, or from a positional change. An incarcerated hernia is one that becomes trapped and cannot be reduced or returned to the cavity. When an incarcerated hernia becomes squeezed in such a way that blood supply to the organ or body part is compromised, it is known as a strangulated hernia. This is a condition that requires immediate surgical intervention.

Hernias are also described by their anatomic location. For example, a scrotal hernia describes a protrusion into the scrotum. Hernias of the lower abdominal wall can occur in the groin and are known as either inguinal or femoral hernias, depending on specific anatomical location. Femoral hernias are more common in women than men.

Groin hernias are the most common type of hernia. Inguinal hernias are further classified as direct or indirect based again on specific anatomical considerations, and how and where the protrusion occurs. Congenital and acquired umbilical hernias occur at the umbilicus due to a defect in the ventral abdominal wall and are commonly seen in obese people and pregnant women. Umbilical hernias can resolve spontaneously in children without sequelae, but frequently incarcerate or strangulate in adults. A hernia that appears at the area of a previous surgical site is known as an incisional hernia. A phrenic hernia occurs when an organ protrudes through the diaphragm. The hiatus (opening) of the diaphragm where the esophagus passes through can be the site of a hernia. The stomach may herniate or protrude through this opening resulting in a hiatal hernia. This type of hernia is considered a sliding hernia if it returns or slides back into the cavity where it belongs. Other types of abdominal hernias may also be sliding hernias.

Hernias can contain part or all of an organ inside the abnormal protrusion. For example, a Richter's hernia describes a hernia in the abdominal cavity where only part of the bowel circumference is involved. If the brain protrudes where it does not belong, it is called a cerebral hernia. Hernias are also named for the organ that is out of place. For example, an ovarian hernia contains an ovary as the misplaced and protruding organ.

The only way to correct a hernia is with surgery, and this is known as herniorrhaphy. There are several different techniques used to repair abdominal wall and groin hernias such as various suture methods, surgical mesh placement, and laparoscopic repair. The best surgical technique for hernia repair remains controversial. Herniorrhaphy is one of the most frequently performed general surgery procedures.

The diagnosis of hernia is frequently made clinically based on physical examination, but imaging modalities do exist to confirm, elaborate, and aid in diagnosis. Complications associated with hernia repair include recurrence, infection, bleeding, and pain. Complications associated with not repairing abdominal wall and groin hernias include a small risk of incarceration and strangulation and thus a surgical emergency. The surgical correction of an uncomplicated, asymptomatic hernia versus watchful waiting remains a decision between the surgeon and the informed patient.

SEE ALSO: Gastroesophageal Reflux/Hiatal Hernia.

BIBLIOGRAPHY. David C. Brooks, "Abdominal Wall and Groin Hernias," www.utdol.com (cited January 19, 2006); Karen E. Deveney, "Chapter 32. Hernias and Other Lesions of the Abdominal Wall," www.accessmedicine.com (cited 2006); Donald Venes, ed., *Taber's Cyclopedic Medical Dictionary*, 20th ed. (F. A. Davis, 2005).

W. Joshua Cox, D.O.
Kansas City University of Medicine
and Biosciences

Heroin Abuse

The illicit use of heroin is an important international health concern, especially in light of evidence showing that unsafe drug injection practices lead to transmission of the human immunodeficiency virus (HIV), the virus causing the acquired immunodeficiency syndrome (AIDS), as well as other deadly diseases. Heroin is a semisynthesized drug that is processed from morphine, a natural derivative of the poppy seed plant, and is readily produced and distributed in multiple countries worldwide. Globally, approximately 11 million people are estimated to abuse heroin.

In the United States, heroin use is illegal and is classified as a Drug Enforcement Agency (DEA) Schedule I drug, meaning that heroin has a high potential for abuse, is available for research purposes only, and has no approved medical indication. The drug is sold on the street as a white or brown powder, or as a thick, black, tacky substance. Often, the drug is not pure but is mixed or "cut" with other substances such as sugar, starch, milk, quinine, or other drugs. Therefore, the actual potency of illegally acquired heroin varies widely, placing the user at risk of overdose and death.

Heroin can be injected intravenously, snorted nasally, or smoked. Injection is usually the most common route of administration, although in some locations, inhalation occurs more frequently. In general, intravenous injection produces a more intense pleasurable feeling and exhibits quicker onset of drug effect than sniffing or smoking.

DRUG EFFECTS

After a single dose of heroin, the user experiences a surge of euphoria or a "rush," as well as a warm flushing of the skin. Profound relief of pain, if any is present, takes place. The mouth becomes dry and the extremities begin to feel heavy. Pupils become very small, respiratory rate decreases, and gastrointestinal motility slows, causing constipation. Central nervous system effects include drowsiness and confusion, and in overdose, can progress to unconsciousness, coma, and ultimately, death. Alternating wakeful and drowsy states can also occur, a phenomenon known as being "on the nod."

Immediate and long-term risks are associated with heroin use. The most important of these is overdose. The practice of injection is also inherently dangerous, because poorly dissolved additives present in street heroin can travel through the blood stream, embolizing in the lungs, liver, kidneys, or brain, causing tissues in these organs to infarct, or die. The veins of repeated injectors can become collapsed, causing the user to seek out other veins, sometimes including those of the neck. There is a high risk of infection associated with injection because sterile needles are not often available, and endocarditis (infection of the heart lining and valves), pneumonia, bone and joint infections, and abscesses of the skin and other organs can occur. Users who share needles with others can acquire and transmit bloodborne viruses such as HIV and the hepatitis viruses B and C, which can cause long-standing liver disease, cirrhosis, and ultimately, liver failure requiring transplantation.

Addiction to heroin is marked by tolerance and withdrawal. Tolerance is achieving less drug effect after taking a dose similar to previous administrations, or stated another way, requiring more drug to experience the same effect as before. Withdrawal is a syndrome of physiological effects that the user experiences after taking heroin for a long period of time, then stopping. It is marked by craving, restlessness, muscle and bone pain, insomnia, diarrhea, vomiting, kicking movements, cold flashes, and goose bumps. It is based on this constellation of effects that the terms "kicking the habit" and "going cold turkey" were coined. Although intensely unpleasurable for the addict, heroin withdrawal, unlike withdrawal from alcohol or barbiturate abuse, is generally not fatal.

TREATMENT

Acutely intoxicated users at risk of overdose can be administered naloxone or naltrexone, compounds that block the effects of opiates in the body. These compounds do little to treat addiction, however. Heroin users represent close to 15 percent of admissions to publicly funded substance abuse treatment programs in the United States. It is important to realize that no single treatment is appropriate for all individuals, and drug users often relapse into their old habits, requiring multiple attempts at treatment. The process can take months to years, and must carefully address the multiple needs of the user, not just his or her addiction.

The first step in treatment is often detoxification, a process in which the patient is safely weaned from his

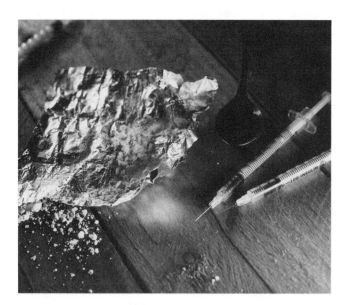

It is estimated that approximately 11 million people abuse heroin, which can be injected intravenously, snorted nasally, or smoked.

or her addiction while minimizing or alleviating the symptoms of withdrawal. By itself, detoxification is not treatment. After, a combined therapy is generally employed in which medication, cognitive behavioral therapy, and social support are central components.

The most common medications for heroin addiction include methadone and buprenorphine. These compounds partially block the receptors within the body on which heroin normally acts. The net effect, therefore, is to reduce withdrawal symptoms (especially craving) while also blocking the effects of continued heroin usage among those who do continue to abuse the drug. These compounds have some addiction potential, causing some to argue that they should not be used, but they can be safely tapered off over a period of time to avoid this effect. Methadone and buprenorphine can be safely used in pregnancy, although newborns exposed in utero to these compounds may require careful treatment for withdrawal from them.

Effective cognitive behavioral therapy is also important to the recovering heroin user, and includes residential and outpatient approaches. Cognitive behavioral therapy helps patients appreciate the circumstances that often lead them to use heroin, and helps them safely avoid these situations or effectively cope with them. Counselors are also trained to help patients modify their attitudes and behaviors about drug use and to teach effective life skills. Family therapy in which abuse is confronted by the entire family of an adolescent heroin user, may also be employed.

SOCIETAL/GLOBAL IMPACT

In the United States, more than half of drug-related costs to society are attributed to crime associated with drug use. The immediate costs of crime include the price of police, legal and correction services, and federal drug traffic control, as well as less immediate consequences, such as lost productivity of perpetrators and victims, and importantly, healthcare expenditures for intentional and unintentional injuries.

The burden of injection drug use-related disease is high. As mentioned earlier, needle sharing can lead to transmission of HIV and hepatitis B and C, diseases with important public health consequences. For example, in the United States, 70 to 80 percent of new cases of hepatitis C, the most common reason for end-stage liver disease requiring transplantation, are attributable to unsafe injection drug use. Minority groups, including African Americans and Hispanics, are particularly vulnerable and show higher rates of disease than other members of the population.

It is believed that worldwide, production of heroin has more than doubled or even tripled since 1985. Three major production and trafficking routes exist: (1) from Afghanistan to nearby countries in the Middle East and eastern Europe; (2) from Burma and Laos to China and Oceania (especially Australia); and (3) from Latin America, including Mexico, Colombia, and Peru, to North America. Of the nations in which heroin is illegally produced, Afghanistan is the leader worldwide, followed by Burma and Laos. Following years of variable growth, illicit opium poppy cultivation decreased in 2005.

Globally, 16 million people abuse opiates, and 11 million abuse heroin. More than half of these users live in Asia, and the highest rates of abuse are found along trafficking routes originating in Afghanistan. Although Afghanistan and eastern and southeast Europe showed increases in the prevalence of heroin use, the global trend leveled off in the early 21st century. This was predominately due to falling levels of opiate abuse in east and southeast Asia and Oceania. Nonetheless, unsafe injection drug use represents an important and often neglected cause of HIV transmission, especially in Asia.

Harm reduction is a philosophically different and practical approach that aims to mitigate the dangers of drug use. Proponents argue that often little can be done to decrease the actual prevalence of drug use, but much can be done to decrease the harms of usage. For example, making available sterile syringes for heroin injectors decreases the transmission of blood-borne disease by reducing the need for needle sharing. Opponents of harm reduction believe that such activities facilitate and promote drug use.

North America's first supervised injection site was opened in Vancouver, Canada, in September 2003, and offers a safe environment for users to inject drugs and connect with healthcare professionals and addiction services. Heroin abuse remains a public health crisis worldwide. When compared to age-matched controls, heroin users worldwide demonstrate 20 to 30 times higher all-cause mortality, a fact that highlights the need for effective and innovative interventions that address the complexities of addiction and human behavior.

SEE ALSO: AIDS; Drug Abuse; Hepatitis; Pregnancy and Substance Abuse.

BIBLIOGRAPHY. "NIDA—Research Report Series—Heroin Abuse and Addiction," www.nida.nih.gov (cited September 2006); "World Drug Report 2006—Executive Summary," www.unodc.org (cited September 2006).

SCOTT E. HADLAND, M.D., M.P.H.
WASHINGTON UNIVERSITY SCHOOL OF MEDICINE

Herpes Simplex

Herpes simplex virus (HSV) is a common virus affecting humans. It is perhaps best known as the cause of cold sores, the facial blisters that sometimes occur following a cold or fever. There are two types of herpes simplex viruses. Type 1 primarily involves the face and eyes and type 2 primarily causes genital infections. Each year in the United States, approximately 25 million people have flare-ups of facial herpes, and 5 million develop genital herpes. There are about 500,000 people in the United States with a history of herpetic eye disease. Transmission is via contact of infected secretions (saliva or genital) with mucous membranes or with open skin. HSV-2 is spread primarily sexually, and its rates are variable among different adult populations, depending on sexual behavior.

After exposure, the virus replicates locally in the epithelial cells, causing lysis of the infected cells and producing an inflammatory response. This response results in the characteristic rash, which consists of small, thin-walled vesicles on an erythematous base. Continued replication results in viremia in immuno-compromised hosts but rarely in normal hosts. Following primary infection, the virus becomes latent in a sensory nerve ganglion.

Gingivostomatitis and pharyngitis are the most frequent clinical manifestations of first-episode HSV-1 infection, while recurrent herpes labialis is the most frequent clinical manifestation of reactivation HSV infection. HSV pharyngitis and gingivostomatitis usually result from primary infection and clinical symptoms and signs include fever, malaise, myalgias, inability to eat, irritability, and cervical adenopathy. Recurrent oral lesions occur in 60 to 90 percent of infected individuals, are usually milder, and generally occur on the lower lip at the outer vermilion border. The recurrences often are triggered by local trauma, sunburn, or stress.

First-episode primary genital herpes is characterized by fever, headache, malaise, and myalgias. Pain, itching, dysuria, vaginal and urethral discharge, and tender inguinal lymphadenopathy are the predominant local symptoms. Widely spaced bilateral lesions of the external genitalia are characteristic. Lesions may be present in varying stages, including vesicles, pustules, or painful erythematous ulcers. The clinical courses of acute first-episode genital herpes among patients with HSV-1 and HSV-2 infections are similar. However, the recurrence rates of genital disease differ with the viral subtype: the 12-month recurrence rates among patients with first-episode HSV-2 and HSV-1 infections are 90 percent and 55 percent, respectively.

HSV infection of the eye is the most frequent cause of corneal blindness in the United States. HSV keratitis presents with an acute onset of pain, blurring of vision, chemosis, conjunctivitis, and characteristic dendritic lesions of the cornea. Debridement, topical antiviral treatment, and/or interferon therapy hastens healing. However, recurrences are common, and the deeper structures of the eye may sustain immunopathologic injury. Chorioretinitis, usually a manifestation of disseminated HSV infection, may occur in neonates or in patients with human immunodeficiency virus (HIV) infection. Many aspects of mucocutaneous and visceral HSV infections are amenable to antiviral chemotherapy, such as acyclovir, valacyclovir, and famciclovir.

SEE ALSO: Eye Diseases (General); Sexually Transmitted Diseases.

BIBLIOGRAPHY. A.G.M. Langenberg, et al., "A Prospective Study of New Infections with Herpes Simplex Virus Type 1 and Herpes Simplex Virus Type 2," *New England Journal of Medicine* (v.341, 1999).

Nakul Gupta
Ross University School of Medicine

Heterosexual

Heterosexuality is applied to the phenomenon of physical, aesthetical, or platonic attraction between people of different genders (mainly women and men, but because gender and sex are not the same, the spectrum of variables became wider). It is also used

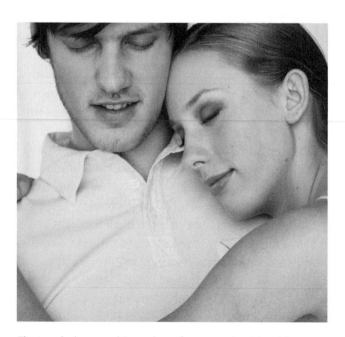

The term heterosexual *is used to refer to sexual activity with another person of the opposite sex.*

to refer to the sexual activity with another person of the opposite sex. Therefore, heterosexual is the person whose sexual preferences, orientation, practices, and feelings were developed in the framework of his or her heterosexuality.

TERMINOLOGY

The term comes from the Greek *heteros*, which means *different*. It was explicitly used for the first time at the end of the 19th century in opposition to homosexuality, because, also for the first time, heterosexual behavior was no longer perceived as the main model of intimate human relationships but as a possible identity among many other identities.

HETEROSEXUALITY IN OLD CULTURES

Heterosexuality originates a vision of the sexuality understood in hierarchical terms: It was not a mutual feeling between equals but rather a relationship between an individual (usually a man) and his object of desire (usually a woman but not exclusively). Nevertheless, in the later Hellenistic period and in Roman times, there was a higher degree of freedom for women and it was observed in the production of objects destined for the pleasure of both, male and female, and simultaneously, it also became obvious in the erotic representations of heterosexual couples as equals, enjoying the same comfort and the same intense emotions.

However, the main feature in heterosexual relationships from old times onward is its institutionalization and, therefore, the existence of an institutionalized inequality consisting in role differences and power distribution. In old mythology, females are submitted to the will of men and gods, and they only exist to be a recipient of their seeds and give children to them. Aristotle believed that only male seed could procreate; women were just mere receptacles.

HETEROSEXUALITY AS THE MAIN ACCEPTED SEXUAL

All current experts, with no exception, agree that heterosexual behavior used to be a compulsory rule of behavior (based on the assumption that men and women are innately attracted to each other) and, therefore, the common pattern of sexual normality. For that same reason, there is no reliable statistics on it and heterosexuality was only in recent times a real object of study. Its basis and main purpose was procreation. First of all, because there was an implicit analogy with the animal world where sexual reproduction and the continuity of the species were natural results of heterosexual coitus. And second, because heterosexual relationships have always been closely linked to religions, and for most of them, it was important to guarantee the fertility of human beings. On the other hand, all mythologies strengthen that idea by offering a large variety of metaphors about the polarization of sexes. In that sense, we can see here what some experts call ritualized behavior built on polar role definition.

However, in our times, heterosexuality is no longer the only rule to be followed but an option among many others, which means that even the idea of normality has changed. A heterosexual relationship goes beyond the coitus—something excluded from the perspectives on the topic in the 19th century—and it also involves an emotional context where pleasure, desire, the consent in terms of giving and receiving emotions, and so forth, are expressed. Currently, sexuality and reproduction have been decoupled. In many ancient cultures, such as in Greece, heterosexuality was mandatory only to secure procreation, but the field of pleasure and emotions was reserved for homosexual intimacy.

SEE ALSO: Bisexual; Homosexual; Lesbian.

BIBLIOGRAPHY. Chrys Ingraham, ed., *Thinking Straight: The Power, the Promise and the Paradox of Heterosexuality* (Taylor & Francis, 2004); Anita L. Nelson and Jo Ann Woodward, eds., *Sexually Transmitted Diseases: A Practical Guide for Primary Care (Current Clinical Practice)* (Humana Press, 2007).

NATALIA FERNANDEZ DIAZ
INDEPENDENT SCHOLAR

Heterozygote

An individual is heterozygous at a given locus if he has different alleles on both homologous chromosomes within the 22 autosomal chromosomes or the paired sex chromosomes of a female (males, with two different sex chromosomes, are classified as hemizygous at the sex chromosome). Heterozygosity is determined on a locus-by-locus basis and is not used to characterize a whole genome or individual. In terms of human disease, when the wildtype phenotype is determined by a dominant allele, heterozygotes show the wildtype phenotype and disease states are characterized by the loss of heterozygosity. When the wildtype allele is recessive, heterozygotes with one disease causing allele show the diseased phenotype.

There are many physiological functions that do not require wildtype gene products to be expressed from both alleles for normal functioning. In such cases, heterozygosity at the given locus is correlated to wildtype phenotype. Disease states that alter these functions must therefore feature the loss of heterozygosity. Such inheritance is typically termed *recessive inheritance*. A classic example of autosomal recessive inheritance is cystic fibrosis. The wildtype allele codes for the CFTR protein that regulates ion transport and helps maintain body fluids. Although most people without cystic fibrosis have two wildtype alleles, only one is needed to prevent cystic fibrosis. Cystic fibrosis develops when both alleles are mutated. If each allele was subject to a different mutation, the subject is termed a *compound heterozygote* at the locus, otherwise the subject is deemed homozygous for a disease-causing allele. In practice, compound heterozygotes are often (erroneously) referred to as homozygous recessive so long as each of their mutations is associated with the same disease state.

Certain physiological functions require two functional alleles of a given gene. In such cases, heterozygotes produce a decreased level of wildtype protein synthesis in addition to potentially producing some disease associated proteins. Such inheritance is typically termed *dominant inheritance*. A classic example of such a disease state is Huntington's disease. Briefly, a mutation of the Huntington gene produces an extended form of the mutant Huntington protein which causes cell death in selective areas of the brain. In this disease state, acquisition of heterozygous genotype is the key: individuals homozygous for the mutant allele are no worse off than individuals heterozygous at the locus.

SEE ALSO: Allele; Hemizygous; Homozygote.

BIBLIOGRAPHY. R.L. Nussbaum, et al., *Thompson & Thompson: Genetics in Medicine,* 6th ed., revised reprint (Saunders, 2004).

BIMAL P. CHAUDHARI
BOSTON UNIVERSITY

High Blood Pressure

High blood pressure or hypertension is an increase in the lateral pressure exerted on the walls of the arteries above normal level (ideally 120/80 mm Hg). There is no rigidly defined threshold level of blood pressure which defines risk from safety and the standards vary with age, sex, geographical distribution, height, weight, diet especially sodium intake, hormonal factors, and so forth. Regardless, the current international standards is set on a diastolic pressure greater than or equal to 90 mm Hg or a systolic pressure of greater than or equal to 140 mm Hg is considered to constitute high blood pressure or more aptly hypertension. Systolic blood pressure is the recording taken when the heart is in a state of contraction, while diastolic blood pressure is taken when the heart is relaxed.

Screening programs reveal that 800 million individuals worldwide are affected by hypertension, constituting about 25 percent of general population. The prevalence and vulnerability to complications increases with age. For obscure reasons, the incidence is high in African Americans. It accounts for 20 to 50 percent of all deaths. Epidemiological data reveal that systolic blood pressure is more important than diastolic blood pressure as a risk factor for cardiovascular diseases, except for young patients.

Hypertension is one of the chronic diseases that has shown the largest decline in mortality over the past four decades. Although the number of deaths in women exceeds those in men, the rate of fall is similar in both sexes. This fall is attributable to the introduction of effective drugs during the past 15 to 20 years.

The cardiovascular system is a very dynamic system facing normal variations in blood pressure during course of the day, variations in emotions, excitement, stress, environment, and so forth because normal blood pressure is the outcome of interplay of many factors. For example, blood pressure is at its peak early morning just before waking up due to a surge of adrenocorticoid hormone. However, such a variation during time of the day (diurnal variation) is considered essentially normal and not as part of any disease process. Similarly, an anxious examinee might show an exaggerated elevation in blood pressure—so-called "white coat" hypertension. Repeated measurements, made on separate occasions, in a stress-free environment are required for a definitive diagnosis of hypertension.

High blood pressure is not only one of the major risk factors for most forms of cardiovascular disease, but it is also a condition with its own risk factors. The World Health Organization (WHO) has reviewed the risk factors for essential hypertension as nonmodifiable and modifiable risk factors. Age, gender, genetic factors, and ethnicity are those risk factors that are beyond human manipulation. However, those contributing entities that can be artfully tailored according to personal requirements are weight, salt intake, and low consumption of saturated fat, alcohol, and oral contraceptives, which are an important cause of increased arterial pressure in females. Use of unrefined foods including more fiber and bran, active lifestyle, avoidance of stress, and improvement of socioeconomic status in monetarily deprived countries are important preventive strategies unanimously devised by researchers and practitioners.

Hypertension is a complex, multifactorial disease that has both genetic and environmental determinants. More than 95 percent of people have no known cause for high blood pressure, called essential hypertension. Essential, primary, or benign hypertension is a diag-

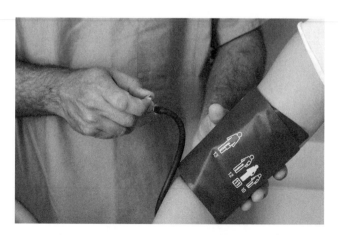

Screening programs reveal that 800 million individuals worldwide are affected by hypertension.

nosis of exclusion because it is often familial, and may be precipitated by alcohol abuse and obesity. This type of high pressure does not cause short-term problems, and for it, most course remains asymptomatic and thus undiagnosed. It is compatible with a long life, but later in life, it can cause complications such as myocardial infarction (MI), brain stroke, or others.

A minority of people, 5 percent or so, develop accelerated or malignant hypertension having a rapidly rising blood pressure and, if untreated, leads to death in a couple of years. The secondary causes of elevated blood pressure are chronic kidney disease or a constriction of blood supply to the kidneys (renal artery stenosis) and tumors of the adrenal glands which secretes high levels of catecholamines (phaeochromocytoma). Other secondary causes include Cushing's disease and Conn's syndrome and coarctation of the aorta.

Hypertension is a fairly common health problem and its prevalence increases with age. It often remains silent until late in its course. It has no specific symptoms. More than one-fourth of its victims remain unaware of their hypertension, and it remains poorly controlled in those who are diagnosed. Gentle as it seems at its onset, if untreated it can lead to death or morbidity from heart failure, cerebrovascular accident (brain stroke), or kidney failure. It is a major risk factor for coronary heart disease, involving constriction of the vessels of the heart, impinging on its oxygen and nutrient supply. Clinical assessment of a patient with high blood pressure has four aims:

- To identify an underlying cause
- To assess the severity of the condition and devise a suitable treatment
- To identify end organ damage, that is, involvement of heart, brain, kidneys, and eyes
- To assess risk of cardiovascular disease involving the heart and adjoining vessels, in context of other risk factors

Because hypertension is correlated with increased morbidity and mortality, it is important to define its causes and to be able to initiate appropriate programs to prevent or manage it. Behavioral and dietary changes are the initial therapeutic strategies. Exercise and active lifestyle have a positive role in long-term prevention of hypertension.

The choice of drug treatment is influenced by the presence or absence of complications. Beta-blockers and calcium channel blockers (CCBs) are useful in patients with angina (complaints of pain in left side of chest and left arm) because of the dual action of these drugs. Similarly, angiotensin converting enzyme (ACE) inhibitors are especially useful if there is any associated dysfunction of the left ventricle.

Intensive research aiming at control of hypertension at individual and community level has already provided valuable results. However, much needs to be learned about the underlying mechanisms culminating in essential hypertension and its devastating complications. Many countries in the world still need to invest in this field and launch nationwide programs for awareness, prevention, management, and treatment of hypertension.

SEE ALSO: Heart Attack; Stroke.

BIBLIOGRAPHY. Vinay Kumar, Abul K. Abbas, and Nelson Fausto, *Robbins and Cotran Pathologic Basis of Disease,,* 7th ed., (Saunders, 2004); J.E. Park, *Textbook of Preventive and Social Medicine* (M/S Banarsidas Bhanot, 1986); Nicholas Boon, *Davidson's Textbook of Medicine* (Churchill Livingstone, 2006).

Sidrah Farooq
Independent Scholar

High-Risk Pregnancy

High-risk pregnancy is defined as one in which there is a possibility that the mother, fetus, or newborn could be at risk of serious illness or even death prior to, during, or after delivery. There are many preexisting and coexisting factors that may contribute to this increased risk including those relating to the health of the mother, obstetric abnormalities, and fetal illness. These risk factors can be identified early during pregnancy and given appropriate consideration by a prenatal care provider. Some complex conditions may require the involvement of a specialist in maternal and child health, geneticist, or pediatrician, anesthesiologist, or other medical specialist in the medical evaluation, counseling, and care of the expecting mother. Leading causes of maternal mortality include thromboembolic disease, hypertensive disease, hemorrhage, infection,

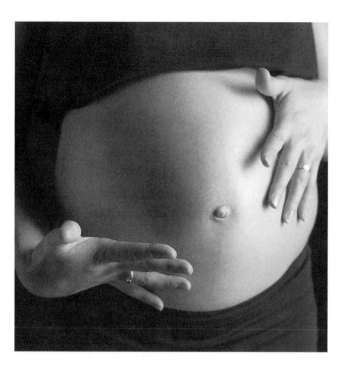

There are many preexisting and coexisting factors that may contribute to a high-risk pregnancy.

and ectopic pregnancy. Infant mortality is defined as death from birth to 1 year of age and includes as causes congenital malformations and conditions related to premature birth. Appropriate and timely prenatal care is essential in ensuring the best possible outcome for both mother and infant.

DIAGNOSTIC CRITERIA AND ASSESSMENT

Women who are high risk can be identified as such during an early prenatal care evaluation to assess the health status of both mother and fetus, to estimate the latter's gestational age, and to outline a plan for continued prenatal care. Prenatal care should include a thorough medical history to identify specific risk factors, a complete physical examination, routing laboratory screenings for common disorders, and follow-up maternal and fetal assessments over the course of the pregnancy to attempt to minimize risk.

EPIDEMIOLOGY AND RISK FACTORS

Preterm labor is the leading cause of perinatal morbidity and infant (neonatal) mortality.

Risk factors for preterm labor include younger or older maternal age (below 16 or over 35 years); low socioeconomic status; poor maternal nutrition; low

maternal weight (below 110 lb); uterine, placental, or cervical abnormalities; smoking; substance abuse; infection; anemia; multiple gestation (being pregnant with more than one baby); and previous complications in pregnancy. Other preexisting health conditions such as gestational diabetes, heart disease, cancer, sexually transmitted diseases, chronic hypertension, or human immunodeficiency virus (HIV) may cause a high-risk pregnancy.

Gestational diabetes occurs exclusively in pregnant women and occurs in about five percent of all pregnancies in the United States. Although most women are able to control their diabetes through a careful regimen of diet, exercise, and monitored weight and blood sugar and give birth to healthy babies, untreated gestational diabetes can result in jaundice, hypoglycemia, mineral deficiencies, or respiratory distress in the infant.

Preeclampsia is a condition that causes hypertension and proteinuria (large amounts of protein being secreted in the urine) and occurs in about seven percent of pregnant women in the United States. Preeclampsia typically occurs midway through pregnancy and may be accompanied by swelling in the face and hands, abdominal pain, headache, and blurred vision. If left untreated, preeclampsia progresses to eclampsia, a more severe condition characterized by seizures that can be fatal. Although there is no cure for preeclampsia, in severe cases, delivery of the fetus is the only resolution. In more mild cases of preeclampsia, home treatment of bedrest and frequent assessment by a care provider may be recommended.

PREVENTION STRATEGIES: PRECONCEPTION AND PRENATAL CARE

There is increasing attention to care given in family planning and gynecology centers, as these settings provide an opportunity to address issues of importance to a potential pregnancy, such as existing medical problems, social habits (e.g., alcohol or substance abuse, diet, and exercise), or genetic issues. Additionally, preconception care includes a recommendation of folic acid to prevent against neural tube defects in the developing fetus and control of existing medical problems in the mother such as diabetes.

The initial prenatal visit is ripe with opportunity to screen for many of the risk factors that can cause preterm labor or additional complications during pregnancy. It is recommended that the first prenatal visit take place in the first trimester or pregnancy and that information on maternal health, particularly past medical and obstetric history, is noted. Some diseases and disorders that could complicate pregnancy are chronic hypertension, heart disease, diabetes, cancer, genetic diseases such as sickle cell anemia, pulmonary disorders, cancer, substance abuse, epilepsy, anemia, pelvic injury, and psychiatric disorders, particularly eating disorders. Women who suffer from anorexia nervosa or bulimia nervosa are significantly more likely to suffer miscarriages and to have infants with lower birth weights than those in the general population.

Screening for domestic violence during the prenatal visit is recommended. With the possible exception of preeclampsia, domestic violence is more prevalent than any other significant medical condition screened for during prenatal visits.

SEE ALSO: Eating Disorders; Postpartum Depression; Preeclampsia; Pregnancy; Pregnancy and Substance Abuse; Premature Babies; Prenatal Care.

BIBLIOGRAPHY. American Academy of Pediatrics and the American College of Obstetrics and Gynecologists, *Guidelines to Perinatal Care*, 5th ed. (American Academy of Pediatrics, 2002); N. Micali, E. Simonoff, and J. Treasure, "Risk of Major Adverse Perinatal Outcomes in Women with Eating Disorders," *British Journal of Psychiatry* (v.190, 2007); S.H. Mehta, et al., eds., *Current Diagnosis & Treatment Obstetrics & Gynecology*, 10th ed. (McGraw-Hill, 2007); Medline Plus, National Institutes of Health and National Library of Medicine, "High Risk Pregnancy," www.nlm.nih.gov/medlineplus/highriskpregnancy.html (cited April 2007).

Lareina Nadine La Flair, M.P.H.
Harvard Medical School

Hip Disorders and Injuries

The hip is a complex joint formed by the articulation of several bones surrounded by muscular attachments and ligaments to form what is known as a ball and socket joint. The complexity provides for tremendous strength but lends to disease susceptibility especially in the event of mechanical stress that may result in debilitating injury. Given the musculoskeletal and supporting structural relations any assortment of disorders is possible. In general, the most common disorders plaguing the hip joint can be classified and further differentiated based on the age of onset, supporting tissue origin of the disorder, bony fracture involvement, and/ or the arthritic components of the ailment. Discussion of the basic principles, functional terminology and anatomical relations will provide the foundation for the overview to follow.

The hip forms the essential connection between the lower limb and the bony structures of the pelvic girdle. The hip represents a ball and socket joint, providing a strong and stable foundation, which allows movement to occur in a number of axes. With the femoral head representing the ball and the acetabulum the socket, the round head of the femur articulates with the cup like acetabulum of the hipbone. Most of the head of the femur is covered with articlar cartilage, which is thickest over weight bearing areas. The acetabulum, a semicircular depression in the lateral portion of the hipbone is formed by the fusion of three bony contributions, the ileum, ischium and pubis. The hip is designed for stability over a wide range of movements essential for daily function and ambulation. Functional necessity is evidenced by the fact that during a standing position the entire weight of the upper body is transmitted through the hipbones down into the head and neck of the communicating femurs. Injury and disorders account for extreme impairment in functioning.

INJURIES AND DISORDERS IN CHILDREN

Congenital dislocation of the hip, also referred to as developmental dysplasia, is an ancient term for a disorder of the hip that has been recognized for several hundred years. The disorder may manifest itself on the day of birth or may follow a more insidious course through the first few years of life. The exact cause is unknown but it is believed that some children may be born with a shallow acetabulum. This may provide a predisposed period in which unusual positioning or a short period of ligamentous laxity may result in a hip joint that will demonstrate insecurity. Diagnosis is often made by physical exam alone.

The examination finding is revealed with the Ortolani maneuver. The examiner's thumb is placed over the patient's inner thigh, and the index finger is gently placed over the outer thigh. The hip is rotated externally, and gentle pressure is placed over the outer thigh. The examiner will feel a "clunk" when the femoral head is rotated in and out of the acetabulum. In the absence of physical exam findings an X ray will not suffice as an additional diagnostic tool based on the lack of bony calcification at this point in skeletal maturation, a sonogram may be required to confirm a suspected diagnosis.Permanent disability will result without treatment. Treatment is initiated with braced abduction with a harness or in a less sophisticated environment the wearing of "double diapers" can be worn for six months to keep the legs abducted. Should conservative measures fail, surgery may need to be considered as an option based on the patient's age and prior treatment attempts.

Children in the age range of approximately four to 12 years of age are susceptible to Legg-Calve-Perthes disease, the name which is given to the idiopathic osteonecrosis of the capital femoral epiphysial head, possibly resulting from an interruption in the blood supply to the developing bone. One in 1,200 children will be plagued by such a disorder with the first signs being that of hip or groin pain. The child is likely to walk with a limp and a decreased hip range of motion may be noted on physical examination. Knee pain on the same side as the effected hip is likely to be present as well. Knee pain in a child must be considered as a potential indicator of a hip injury/disorder, as pain from the hip is referred to the knee and communicated as pain in the region.

Standard radiographic studies can be diagnostic in such a disorder. Physical examination findings may consist of the Roll Test: with patient lying in on their back, the examiner rolls the hip of the affected extremity into external and internal rotation. This test should invoke involuntary contraction, guarding or spasm, especially with internal rotation. Treatment is controversial, but generally the goal of treatment is to avoid severe degenerative arthritis.

Slipped capital femoral epiphysis is the most common hip abnormality presenting in adolescence. In addition the disorder represents a principal cause of early osteoarthritis. Stress around the hip results in a force of a shearing nature to be applied at the maturing and actively growing region of the femur. Trauma plays a role in the appearance of the fracture, but an inherent weakness of the immature cartilage also is present. Early treatment leads to better outcome. Unfortunately, slipped capital femoral epiphysis is frequently misdiagnosed, as this disorder has symptoms that can be confusing. Clinical presentation is often misleading, with only 50 percent of patients presenting with hip pain and 25 percent presenting with knee pain. The inconsistency of symptom presentation results in frequent delays in diagnosis.

The incidence is one per 100,000 people. Slipped capital femoral epiphysis occurs most commonly in adolescents, with a slightly greater incidence in males than in females. The disorder typically manifests just after the onset of puberty, frequently in overweight children. Diagnosis is made using anteroposterior (AP) pelvis and lateral frog-leg radiographs. The treatment includes stabilization of the hip. Fixation of the joint may be completed with the use of pins, screws, or wires crossing the immature region of cartilage and stabilizing the joint, with the ultimate goal of avoiding further damage to the penetrating vessels by stabilizing the fracture.

OSTEOARTHRITIS OF THE HIP

A common articular complication is that of arthritis derived from either an osteopathic or rheumatologic origin. Osteoarthritis, commonly referred to as degenerative joint disease, is one of the most common causes of disability in the developed world. Individuals younger than 55 years of age have an equal distribution of effected joints regardless of gender; in older individuals, hip osteoarthritis is more common in men. Racial differences exist in the incidence of hip osteoarthritis as well with a greater incidence in whites as compared to the Chinese of Hong Kong, for example. The principal pathological feature of osteoarthritis is the progressive erosion articular cartilage. The cartilage will then become soft, frayed, and progressively thinned. Eventually the exposed bone (subchondral) will convert to a more dense substance with a smooth surface, a process known as eburnation. Simultaneously there will be bony protuberant outgrowths known as osteophytes from the bone margins ultimately leading to pain and loss of function as a result.

Osteoarthritis mainly affects weight-bearing joints, and is more common in overweight and older persons. Whilst the most prominent of the changes take place in the load-bearing areas of the cartilage, smaller joints may be affected that may not have served as predominant load absorbing joints. Despite the fact that these alterations take place at a macroscopic level, the disorder involves not only the cartilage, but involvement of the entire synovial joint is observed, in which all of the surrounding (synovium) and supporting tissues (ligaments) are affected. The joint pain of osteoarthritis of the hip is described as a deep aching sensation present in the involved joint. Generally, movement of the involved hip joint provokes the pain and rest will usually relieve the pain. With progression of the disease the pain may become persistent. Such advanced disease may be responsible for nocturnal pain and sleep interference, particularly in advanced osteoarthritis of the hip.

RHEUMATOID ARTHRITIS OF THE HIP

Rheumatoid arthritis is a systemic disease of unknown origin. The disease is more prevalent in women and predominantly affects connective tissue; arthritis is the dominant clinical manifestation. This form of arthritis frequently involves many joints. Arthritis of the hip is likely to be present with multiple joint involvements, especially those of the hands and feet.

The pathology of rheumatoid arthritis varies from that of osteoarthritis with the former representing an inflammatory process and the latter representing a non-inflammatory condition. In addition, osteoarthritis created a thinning of connective articular membranes where rheumatoid arthritis will be accompanied by thickening of articular soft tissue, with extension of synovial tissue over articular cartilages, which become eroded; the course is variable but often is chronic and progressive, leading to deformities and disability.

BURSITIS

The bursa, a closed sac or envelope lined with synovial membrane and containing fluid becomes irritated and inflamed. Bursae as functional units are usually found or formed in areas subject to friction. These fluid-filled sacs that functions as a gliding surface to reduce friction between tissues of the hip joint. There are two major bursa of the hip, both of which can be associated with stiffness and pain around the hip joint. Bursitis of the hip refers to the inflammation of the bursa. Pain will be present with movements at the hip joint usually subsiding while the leg is not placed in such a position so a to flex or extend the hip. Range

of motion will be limited by pain and muscle strength testing will demonstrate mild weakness.

FRACTURE

A common form of nonarticular complication involving the hip joint is that of fracture or trauma to the region. Hip fracture and dislocation constitute a major problem due to the disabling nature of these injuries, largely due to the inability to ambulate without surgical intervention following such an injury. Hip fractures primarily occur in the elderly. While relatively few in number, requiring predisposing conditions and significant trauma to provide adequate stress, hip fractures account for millions of hospital days. In addition prompt intervention is required to avoid the frequent complication of death in the elderly following hip fracture (20 to 30 percent of elderly patients in the first year after fracture).

Any component of the hip joint may suffer fracture when placed under adequate stress as a result of a trauma or accidental fall. Commonly the integrity of the bony structures may be compromised due to an underlying arthritic condition such as osteoarthritis that may predispose to fracture under normally sustainable forces. Of the bony structures that articulate to form the hip, the femoral neck may fracture most commonly in individuals older than fifty. While these fractures are usually treated surgically with no complications, the unique blood supply to the region leaves the individual at a high risk for avascular necrosis of the femoral head.

COMPLICATION OF FRACTURE, AVASCULAR NECROSIS

Avascular necrosis may result following fracture of the femoral neck. The potential disruption of the circulation following fracture is high. If such a compromise should occur the femoral head would be forced to rely on a secondary and possibly compromised circulatory supply. Secondary avascular necrosis of all or a portion of the femoral head may result from the disrupted supply of nutrient and inadequate removal of metabolic waste. Avascular necrosis is not unique to fracture as a complication. Any disorder or injury of adequate severity to interrupt blood supply may result in such a complication.

DISLOCATION

The potential for dislocation of the hip joint is highest as a result of trauma and may occur with or without fracture. Unless there is preexisting disease in the joint region complete dislocation of the femoral head from the acetabulum (a cup-shaped depression on the external surface of the hip bone, with which the head of the femur articulates) is extremely difficult outside of a high-energy trauma situation. Complications include avascular necrosis with the disruption of arterial supply to the region as well as infection with the compromised supply of immune defenses. Confounding factors include the duration and severity of dislocation and the incidence of complication increases linearly with the interval of dislocation.

TREATMENT OF ARTICULAR VERSUS NON-ARTICULAR INJURIES AND DISORDERS

Articular complications such as osteoarthritis are aimed at maintaining mobility reducing pain and minimizing disability in the effected individual. The intensity of the therapy will be guided by the severity of the condition in the individual patient. For example an individual with mild disease may only require occasional analgesic. For advanced disease, particularly of the hip, the required treatment will consist of an assortment of nonpharmacologic measures to be supplemented by analgesic and or nonsteroidal antiinflammatory therapy. For example, the application of heat to an osteoarthritic joint may reduce pain and stiffness. Most importantly participation in conditioning and exercise programs can be done safely to improve fitness and health without increasing joint pain or the need for analgesic medications.

Rheumatoid arthritis creates an incredibly complicated treatment challenge given that the pathophysiology is not completely delineated. Any treatment guidelines further than basic principles are beyond the scope of this selection. The basic goals of therapy include the reduction in inflammation, relief of pain, and the maintenance of function. Treatment is directed at suppressing the inflammatory and immunologic processes that underlie the pathology of the disorder. Improving symptoms and slowing the progressive damage to the surrounding articular structures hopefully follow a conservative approach.

Basic pharmacologic therapy initially includes the use of nonsteroidal antiinflammatory medication, except aspirin.

Clinical experience has lead to the realization that a group of medications known as disease-modifying antirheumatic drugs (DMARD) have the capacity to alter the course of rheumatoid arthritis. These drugs are to be started as soon as a diagnosis of rheumatoid arthritis is established, especially in those with evidence suggestive of aggressive disease with a poor prognosis. Immunosuppressive therapy plays a role in pharmacologic therapy as well and in the management of severely damaged joints total joint replacements can be done with the highest success occurring in the replacement of hips, knees, and shoulders.

SURGICAL INTERVENTION

Surgical treatment for joint disorders is a region where therapies overlap in the distinction of articular and nonarticular disorders. Surgery plays a role in the management of severely damaged joints, with the goal of pain relief and a reduction in disability. Hip arthroplasty may be indicated in the event of progressive disease leading to incapacitating arthritis (osteogenic or rheumatologic), limiting movement, hindering activities of daily living and requiring pain medication stronger than aspirin.

Surgical intervention may be required in the nonarticular hip disorders based on individual circumstances and confounding factors. A femoral neck fracture in an individual in which avascular necrosis is highly likely, in an elderly patient for example, surgery may be warranted as a means of treatment. A hip joint that has suffered preexisting disease and then encounters dislocation may require total arthroplasty.

SEE ALSO: Arthritis; Fractures; Surgery.

BIBLIOGRAPHY. Brent Adler, "Slipped Capital Femoral Epiphysis," www.emedicine.com (cited July 2004); D. L. Kasper, et al., *Harrison's Principles of Internal Medicine*, 16th ed., (McGraw-Hill, 2005); Keith L. Moorse and Arthur F. Dailey, *Clinically Oriented Anatomy*, 5th ed. (Lippincott Williams and Wilkins, 2006); Robert A. Novelline, *Squires Fundamentals of Radiology*, 6th ed. (Harvard University Press, 2004).

DONALD W. HOHMAN JR.
ST. GEORGE'S UNIVERSITY

Hispanic American Health

In the past two decades, epidemiological research has examined the so-called Hispanic paradox, wherein the Hispanic American population displays a level of population health above what would be expected, given its socioeconomically disadvantaged position. A Hispanic American advantage has been observed using mortality and morbidity data, and a number of plausible hypotheses are being tested in the epidemiological and medical sociological literatures. These hypotheses include the "healthy immigrant" hypothesis and the "salmon bias" hypothesis. While a consensus has not emerged about these hypotheses, research on Hispanic American health has the potential to contribute to the literature on health inequalities and the social determinants of health. More specifically, research on Hispanic American health may highlight the importance of contextual factors (e.g., the quality of community ties, including levels of social capital and social cohesion) and, importantly, may identify pathways through which the health effects of relative socioeconomic deprivation may be alleviated.

EXPLAINING THE HISPANIC PARADOX

The causes of the paradox are poorly understood, but a number of viable hypotheses have been developed in the literature. These include the "healthy immigrant" hypothesis wherein Hispanic Americans display a health advantage because of disproportionate migration by people with good health in comparison to those in poor health. In this scenario, the observed health advantage is a statistical artifact resulting from self-selection. Additionally, researchers have sought to test the "salmon bias" hypothesis, wherein the health advantage displayed at the population level by Hispanic Americans is a result of less healthy Hispanics returning to their original home countries, thereby lowering the mortality rate of those remaining. Another explanation of the Hispanic paradox suggests that the observed patterns of population health are the result of data artifacts, or data problems including issues with ethnic identification in social surveys and official records.

Explanations of the health advantage enjoyed by Hispanic Americans have also incorporated insights from the study of the social determinants of health, including the concepts of social capital/social cohesion and acculturation. Indeed, the Hispanic paradox offers important research grounds on which to investigate social and cultural factors which may influence levels of population health, including the concept of social capital. This is a debated topic within social science, but in health research, it has typically been defined as the quality of social networks and/or community levels of reciprocity and trust. It is plausible that the Hispanic paradox is at least partly attributable to high levels of social capital in communities with a high percentage of Hispanic residents; such communities may generate higher levels of social support, encourage health-enhancing community interaction, and compensate for health risks associated with relative material deprivation. Studies examining acculturation have involved time-series or longitudinal analysis of how the Hispanic paradox may change over time in the United States. It is likely that myriad factors underlie the Hispanic paradox, and the healthy immigrant and salmon bias hypotheses are not necessarily contradictory; they may both be true, though perhaps stronger for some groups than others.

HEALTH INDICATORS

Death rates for Hispanic Americans differ greatly from death rates for African Americans and non-Hispanic white Americans. According to recent analyses published by the National Center for Health Statistics, death rates (per 100,000) were lower for Hispanic Americans than non-Hispanic white Americans for sex and age group except females under age 5 and males aged 15 to 24. The age-adjusted death rate for Hispanic American males was 818.1, while for non-Hispanic white American males, it was 1,035.4 and for African American males, it was 1,403.5. For Hispanic American females, the age-adjusted death rate was 546.0, while for non-Hispanic white American females it was 721.5 and for African American females, it was 927.6. Mortality differences in favor of Hispanic Americans have also been reported using data from the U.S. National Longitudinal Mortality Study and the U.S. National Health Interview Survey–Multiple Cause of Death data sets. In an analysis of the U.S. National Health Interview Survey–Multiple Cause of Death data set published by Alberto Palloni and Elizabeth Arias, the difference in mortality amounted to approximately five to eight years of additional life expectancy at age 45 (excluding Puerto Ricans and Cubans, who did not display the paradoxical advantage). The evidence base for the Hispanic paradox is dominated by mortality data. However, recent results indicate that the paradox may also be observable with measures of stroke, cancer, heart attack, hip fracture, hypertension, and diabetes mellitus.

SOCIAL INEQUALITIES IN HEALTH

A large field in social epidemiology and medical sociology has investigated social inequalities in health within the framework of the social determinants of health. The basis of this framework is that health is produced not only by access to medical treatment, but also by the cumulative experience of social conditions over the life course. As such, social conditions may be seen as the fundamental causes of illness, or the "causes of the causes." A fundamental building block of the social determinants of health model is the social gradient in health, or the patterning of morbidity and mortality by socioeconomic position. Importantly, this gradient does not typically display a threshold effect; that is, health differences run throughout the income spectrum, from the very bottom to the very top. Research on Hispanic American health is important to this tradition because it 1.) represents a paradox, because the health of Hispanic Americans is better than would be expected given the relatively socially disadvantaged position, and 2.) highlights the important role of social and cultural factors as determinants of health.

CHALLENGES AND OPPORTUNITIES

Relatively few studies of Hispanic American health have been conducted at the national level, despite the growing size of the Hispanic population in the United States. However, over the past few years, a number of studies have been published and the Hispanic paradox has attracted more attention. These studies have highlighted important challenges, including problems of data quality in national health surveys and official records. Ethnic classification is particularly difficult to measure in social surveys and its measurement in official vital statistics is also problematic. Research has also been limited by an overemphasis on the Hispanic population as an aggregated whole, rather than its many diverse groups. Contemporary research on Hispanic American health is attempting to disaggregate the analysis by country of origin, and preliminary results indicate that the paradox may be most detectable among Mexican Americans and not at all present for Puerto Ricans and Cubans. This underscores the heterogeneity present in the Hispanic American population and offers an important avenue for future empirical research.

Overall, research on Hispanic American health holds the potential to significantly contribute to epidemiological and medical sociological knowledge on the social determinants of health. The apparent paradox wherein the Hispanic population enjoys a higher level of health status than would be predicted given its relatively socioeconomically deprived position lends credence to the importance of social and cultural determinants of health, while at the same time, warns researchers of the dangers associated with an overly reductionist approach to health inequalities that focuses solely on individual-level income.

SEE ALSO: African American Health; Asian American Health.

BIBLIOGRAPHY. Karl Eschobach, et al., "Neighborhood Context and Mortality among Older Mexican Americans: Is There a Barrio Advantage?" *American Journal of Public Health* (v.94/10 2004); L. Franzini, J. Ribble, and A. M. Keddie, "Understanding the Hispanic Paradox," *Ethnicity and Disease* (v.11, 2001); National Center for Health Statistics, *National Vital Statistics Reports* (v.51/5, 2003); Alberto Palloni and Elizabeth Arias, "Paradox Lost: Explaining the Hispanic Adult Mortality Advantage," *Demography* (v.41/3, 2004).

FERNANDO DE MAIO, PH.D.
SIMON FRASER UNIVERSITY

Histology

Histology is the study of microscopic anatomy using slides of tissue sections. It is a crucial aspect of determining diagnosis and prognosis for many diseases, as well as an educational tool for understanding the structure of the human body and the mechanisms of disease. When histology is used to study diseased tissue, it is called histopathology.

There are many techniques for getting the tissue specimen from the body to the microscope slide. The first step is fixation, whereby the tissue is soaked in a chemical that stops all metabolic processes. The most commonly used fixative is formalin, which contains formaldehyde and phosphate-buffered saline. The sample is then washed, put in multiple solutions of progressively more concentrated alcohol to remove the water, and washed with an organic solvent to remove the alcohol. The second step is embedding, whereby the specimen is impregnated with melted paraffin wax and set to cool. The washing and embedding process takes at least 12 hours when using standard procedures. The tissue-containing paraffin block is then cut into very thin slices of two to eight micrometers and mounted on slides. In the final step, the slide is stained with a dye so the tissue can be visualized.

There are several dyes that are used to highlight different features of the cells. The most commonly used one is hematoxylin and eosin (H&E). Hematoxylin stains the nuclei of cells blue while eosin stains the cytoplasm pink. Other dyes include crystal violet, which stains gram-positive bacteria dark blue, and periodic acid Schiff (PAS), which stains carbohydrates pink. Masson's trichrome stains keratin red, collagen and bone blue-green, cytoplasm pink, and nuclei black. Silver staining is used to highlight DNA and proteins like type III collagen. To highlight fat, Sudan stain is used. To localize specific proteins or antigens, the tissue is exposed to antigen-specific antibodies conjugated to a fluorescent dye.

Alternative techniques of fixation and embedding are sometimes when they are needed. For example, to retain membrane structures for electron microscopy, histologists use fixatives containing heavy metals that bind to phospholipids. Tissue can also be frozen and cut using a cryostat. This technique is called cryosection, and is used when the analysis of a specimen needs to be performed quickly. Cryosection is used during intraoperative consultation, which is when during a surgery, histology is used to look at tissue that has been removed to determine how to proceed. For example, if a cancer is suspected to have spread, a sample of the suspected metastasis (spreading cancer) is given to a pathologist to determine if it is cancer. If so, the surgry is usually not curative, and the surgeon will choose a less aggressive surgery.

Another use of histology is to determine the nature of infectious agents, for example whether a bacterial infection is gram-positive or gram-negative will allow the more proper choice of antibiotic. Histological mechanisms are also used to screen for diseases, such as the analysis of cervical scrapings collected during a Pap smear to determine if the endothelium is progressing toward cervical cancer.

SEE ALSO: Cervical Cancer; Diagnostic Tests.

BIBLIOGRAPHY. Abraham Kierszenbaum, *Histology and Cell Biology: An Introduction to Pathology* (Elsevier Health Sciences, 2006); Michael H. Ross, *Histology: A Text and Atlas* (Lippincott Williams & Wilkins, 2003).

LAURA JANNECK
CASE WESTERN RESERVE UNIVERSITY
SCHOOL OF MEDICINE

Hodgkin's Lymphoma

Lymphoma is a cancer of the lymphatic system, which is composed of the lymph nodes and other immunological and blood-forming organs. Hodgkin's lymphoma (HL) is a subtype of lymphoma with unique characteristics. Dr. Thomas Hodgkins, an English physician and pathologist first described this disease in 1832.

The National Cancer Institute estimates that there are 78,00 new cases of Hodgkin's lymphoma per year in the United States and 62,329 new cases in the world each year. It is more common in men than women and more common in whites than in Asians. New cases occur most frequently in young people and individuals older than 50.

Patients with Hodgkin's lymphoma may have a number of signs and symptoms, including enlarged lymph nodes, unexplained weight loss, fever, night sweats, itching, and intermittent fever. On examination, they may have an enlarged spleen or enlarged liver. Less common but also seen are chest pain, cough, shortness of breath, coughing of blood, and nervous system problems.

While the cause of this cancer is unknown, the Epstein-Barr virus is thought to have some relationship with the lymphoma. Patients with HIV infection also have a higher incidence of Hodgkin's lymphoma than the general population. A thorough history, physical examination, and laboratory studies of the blood and imaging techniques may direct a physician toward the diagnosis of Hodgkin's lymphoma, but the definitive diagnosis must be made with examination of the cancer tissue. This may be obtained from a biopsy of a lymph node. All Hodgkin's lymphoma tissue reveals characteristic Reed-Sternberg cells when the cancer tissue is examined under the microscope.

The World Health Organization (WHO) classifies HL into five types based on tissue findings. Sixty to 80 percent of all cases are nodular sclerosing type, 15-30 percent are the mixed-cellularity type, less than one percent are lymphocyte depleted, five percent are lymphocyte rich, and five percent are nodular lymphocyte-predominant type. The nodular sclerosing type is frequently observed in adolescents and young adults.

Staging of Hodgkins lymphoma is most commonly done clinically with the Ann Arbor classification. Stage 1 denotes cancer involving a single lymph node area or single extranodal site. Stage 2 is cancer involving two or more lymph node areas on the same side of the diaphragm. Stage 3 denotes lymph node areas on both sides of the diaphragm involved. Stage IV indicates disseminated or multiple involvement of extranodal organs. "A" or "B" designations indicate the absence or presence of B symptoms. B designation signifies the presence of either fever or unexplained loss of more than 10 percent of body weight in the last six months. A designation is the absence of any B symptoms. The stage of HL correlates indirectly with prognosis; in other words, the farther the spread of the disease, the poorer the prognosis.

Treatment options for HL include radiation therapy, chemotherapy, and high-dose chemotherapy with transplantation. There are several possible combinations of chemotherapy, but the standard regimen now in use is ABVD (adriamycin, bleomycin, vinblastine, and dacarbazine).

Prognosis of patients with HL is dependent on the staging of the cancer. The statistic "five-year survival" indicates the percentage of people who are alive five years after their diagnosis. The five-year survival rate for patients with stage I and II Hodgkins lymphoma is 90 percent, for stage III is 84 percent, and for stage IV is 65 percent.

SEE ALSO: Cancer (General); Lymphoma; Non-Hodgkin's Lymphoma.

BIBLIOGRAPHY. A. Jemal, et al., "Cancer Statistics," *CA: A Cancer Journal for Clinicians* (v. 56/2, 2006); T.A. Lister, et al., "Report of a Committee Convened to Discuss the Evaluation and Staging of Patients with Hodgkin's Disease: Cotswolds Meeting," *Journal of Clinical Oncology* (v.8, 1990); SEER: "Surveillance Epidemiology and End Results Cancer Statistics Review, 1975–2002," http://seer.cancer.gov/ (cited July 2007).

RACHANA POTRU
MICHIGAN STATE UNIVERSITY
COLLEGE OF HUMAN MEDICINE

Homeopathy

Homeopathy is a system of therapeutic thought based on the concept that "like cures like." It was developed at the end of the 18th century by the German physician Samuel Hahnemann. Using as evidence the effect of quinine on himself that it produced symptoms that resembled those of malaria, he developed the concept of the "law of similars." This law supposes that diseases should be treated by drugs that produce in healthy people the types of symptoms of the disease which it is hoped to be remedied. Homeopathy was welcomed at the time as a positive and innovative manner of thinking and to be preferred to other methods such as bleeding and purging which were then still widespread. However, in the 20th century and beyond, homeopathy began to be treated with some disdain by scientists because it did not cohere with the methods then being developed and extended.

Modern homeopaths are likely to concentrate on the correct identification of the disease to be treated on which considerable care is likely to be spent. For many symptoms or combinations of symptoms, many possible diseases or causes might be responsible. The homeopath is likely to rely on self-description by patients and personal experience to identify the correct cause and hence to select the appropriate cure. There is also the issue of identifying a suitable remedy for each disease or problem. Thousands of these exist, but most have become part of the homeopathic canon either through reliance on previous wisdom or on personal experience and experimentation. The large-scale resources available in many cases to develop new pharmaceuticals have not been available to homeopaths generally speaking and documentation of the efficacy of treatment and possibility of side effects is also lacking. In the absence of rigorous quality-control standards which are transparent and enforceable by state law agencies, there is also the potential problem of inconsistency of supply and variability in potency of drug used.

Once the homeopath has determined the nature of the medical cause of symptoms and determined, therefore, an appropriate treatment, it is necessary to dilute the treatment in a much larger volume of water. One drug alone is used and the dilution may be more than one part of effective agent to one trillion parts of water. According to scientific theory, such a low level of active agent can have no possible impact upon any cure that might subsequently eventuate. Nevertheless, homeopathy continues to have many adherents and it strikes a chord with many people who believe that the nature of the modern developed world relies too much upon artificial or unnatural substances and that chemical pharmaceuticals are inherently undesirable. Medical research has not found compelling evidence for the efficacy of homeopathy but it has not dismissed it completely either. There are cases in which people suffering from hay fever or some kinds of asthma and flu have obtained relief from homeopathic remedies. However, distinguishing between positive results from homeopathy and those arising from placebo effects has also not yet been fully achieved. On a realistic note, homeopathic remedies are not likely to do any actual harm because the patient will almost certainly be drinking nothing other than plain water.

A number of homeopathy clinics are supported by the National Health Service in the United Kingdom and have been since 1948, although this has been controversial in some cases. Homeopathic treatments are dispensed in these cases by qualified medical practitioners and they and their patients may choose to use homeopathy more or less at their discretion. Non-medically qualified homeopaths also exist and are obliged to be registered with the appropriate society before they can legally offer consultation. Homeopathy is particularly popular in India, where the ayurvedic tradition has a number of similarities with its approach, as well as in some European countries. It is much less popular in the United States and its popularity continues to decline.

SEE ALSO: Alternative Medicine; Herbal Medicine.

BIBLIOGRAPHY. D. Edward, *The American Institute of Homeopathy Handbook for Parents: A Guide to Healthy Treatment for Everything from Colds and Allergies to ADHD, Obesity, and Depression* (Jossey-Bass, 2005); Eliza O'Driscoll, "With Complements," *Occupational Health* (v.56/11, 2004).

John Walsh
Shinawatra University

Homicide

The term *homicide* refers to the act of killing another human being and comes from the Latin word *homo* for a human being, and *–cide* from the Latin *caedere* meaning "to kill." The term *homicide* is used as a criminal offense in the United States, whereas in Britain, the criminal offense is usually referred to as murder, with manslaughter referring to the taking of human life in a manner, at law, less culpable than murder.

There are several derivative terms that come from the word *homicide*, including parricide (killing of one's parents), patricide (killing of one's father), matricide (killing of one's mother), mariticide (killing of one's spouse), uxorcide (killing of one's wife), filicide (killing of one's children), fratricide (killing of one's brother or a friend in battle), sororicide (killing of one's sister), infanticide (killing of an infant), regicide (killing of a monarch), genocide (killing of a race), and suicide (killing of oneself).

Although nowadays the laws in most countries are the same regardless of the person killed, throughout history there have been laws governing these, often involving harsher punishments for some types of homicide. For example, in Rome, the offense of parricide resulted in one of the harshest punishments involving flogging and eventually drowning at sea with the culprit sewn, along with a dog and a rooster, into a leather sack symbolizing the womb. However, since medieval times, the punishments for most types of homicides have been the same, except for regicide, for which horrendous punishments were often prescribed. Following the restoration of King Charles II in 1660, the new royal government sought to arrest the "Regicides"—those who had been involved in the trial and execution of the king's father, King Charles I, in 1649. This resulted in the tracking down of all the judges involved in the trial of Charles I, and their imprisonment or execution, or their murder. Those involved in the execution of King Louis XVI of France in 1793 were also known as Regicides although they did not gain the same notoriety as those in Britain. The criminal code generally divides homicidal crimes into three different fields: murder, manslaughter, and criminal homicide. The first includes felony murder and capital murder. Manslaughter includes voluntary manslaughter, involuntary manslaughter, intoxication manslaughter, death by dangerous driving, and reckless manslaughter. Criminal homicide includes culpable homicide in Scottish law, with negligent homicide in some criminal jurisdictions, and criminally negligent homicide.

There has regularly been a difficult legal problem concerning suicide. For religious reasons, it is often regarded as a criminal offence, and during the Middle Ages and early modern Europe, attempted suicide was often regarded as attempted murder. There has also been a complicated legal area concerning assisting someone else committing suicide, with it being regarded as a criminal offense in most parts of the world.

There have been many books on the topic of homicide, with a number concentrating on the forensic or medical aspects of the various cases, some providing psychological information on the people concerned, and others dealing with the cases from a legal angle.

SEE ALSO: Suicide.

BIBLIOGRAPHY. Robert Asher, Lawrence B. Goodheart, and Alan Rogers, eds., *Murder on Trial: 1620–2002* (State University of New York Press, 2005); Bruce L. Danto, John Bruhns, and Austin H. Kutscher, eds., *The Human Side of Homicide* (Columbia University Press, 1982); Terance D. Miethe and Wendy C. Regoeczi, with Kriss A. Drass, *Rethinking Homicide: Exploring the Structure and Process Underlying Deadly Situations* (Cambridge University Press, 2004); Gini Graham Scott, *Homicide by the Rich and Famous: A Century of Prominent Killers* (Praeger, 2005).

JUSTIN CORFIELD
GEELONG GRAMMAR SCHOOL, AUSTRALIA

Homosexuality

The term *homosexual* was coined in the 19th century by combining the Greek prefix *homo-*, meaning

same, and the Latin root *sex-*, meaning sex or gender; it first appeared in print in a 1869 German pamphlet published anonymously by the journalist and social reformer Karl-Maria Kertbeny (1824–82). However, sexual relationships between members of the same sex have existed since ancient times in many different cultures and societies. It is difficult to make general statements about the prevalence of homosexual relationships or about people who engage in such relationships because of the differing ways intimate relationships are perceived and discussed in different cultures and historical periods, and because such behavior may remain covert because it is taboo within a particular society.

DEFINING AND MEASURING HOMOSEXUALITY

The term *homosexual* is both a noun and an adjective: one may refer to an individual as a homosexual, or refer to homosexual behavior or homosexual activity. In practice the terms *gay* for men and *lesbian* for women are often used instead, along with other terms such as *queer*, while the term *straight* is often used interchangeably with heterosexual. Defining a sexual act as heterosexual or homosexual is fairly simple in most cases, because it depends on the biological sex of the individuals involved (although there are complicating factors such as how to classify transgender and hermaphroditic individuals). However, defining what constitutes a sexual act is less simple, particularly when one considers cases such as the "romantic friendships" common among women in 19th-century America.

It is much more problematic to attempt to classify individuals into single categories of sexual behavior or preference, for instance, by asking respondents to a survey to check one box describing themselves from among "homosexual," "heterosexual," or "bisexual." While some individuals live their entire lives having had sexual desire for, and sexual relations with, members of one sex, many others have a more varied experience, and behavior, desire, and identification may not coincide. For this reason, any discussion of homosexuality must include an acknowledgment of definition and measurement issues.

The modern, scientific study of sexuality began in Germany in the mid-19th century, and two differing conceptions of homosexuality were presented from the beginning. Karl Heinrich Ulrichs (1825–95) believed in the discrete categorization of human sexuality, and conceived of homosexuals as constituting a "third sex" alongside heterosexual males and heterosexual females. In contrast, Magnus Hirschfeld (1868–1935) developed a theory of "intermediate steps" which posited that every person was a unique combination of male and female characteristics. Alfred Kinsey (1824–1956), the pioneering American sex researcher, agreed with Hirschfeld that people could be a mix of homosexual and heterosexual proclivities, and classified them on a seven-point scale from 0 (exclusively heterosexual) to six (exclusively homosexual).

There are four major approaches to measuring and classifying homosexuality are evident in contemporary surveys:

1. focusing on identity or sexual orientation, for instance, asking people if they consider themselves to be gay, straight, or bisexual;
2. focusing on sexual behavior, for instance, asking people if in the last 12 months they have had sexual contact with men, women, both, or neither;
3. focusing on sexual attraction, for instance, asking people if they are exclusively or primarily attracted to males, females, both, or neither;
4. focusing on how they are perceived by others, for instance, asking if people have been harassed or threatened because they were perceived to be lesbian, gay, or bisexual.

Of course the approach used, and the period of time involved, will make a difference in the number of people classified as homosexual: for instance, more people have engaged in homosexual behavior over their lifetime than have had such experiences in the previous year. Smith presents a summary of a number of surveys of sexual behavior in the United States: he found that no contemporary survey has come close to Kinsey's estimate that 10 percent of the adult United States population is homosexual, and that typically two to three percent of sexually active men and one to two percent of sexually active women are classified as currently homosexual.

HOMOSEXUALITY AND HEALTH

Because of the measurement issues discussed above, and the fact that questions about sexual preference or sexual behavior have not consistently been included in major U.S. health surveys, it is difficult to make definitive statements about the health of homosexuals or their specific health needs. However, several general statements can be made.

It is true that some health risks, including those related to sexual practices, differ for homosexuals: for instance, gay men are at higher risk for contracting many sexually transmitted diseases, including HIV/AIDS, than lesbians or most heterosexuals. In fact, AIDS was originally called Gay-Related Immune Deficiency or GRID, because the first U.S. cases were identified in gay men. Balancing this point is the fact that gay men and lesbians have most of the same health risks and needs as do straight men and women, a fact which may be obscured if discussion of gay and lesbian health focuses exclusively on sexually transmitted diseases. This is a particularly important consideration because, due to discrimination, alienation or lack of understanding of their health needs, gay men and women do not always receive the routine screening and preventive health services recommended for all men and women. For instance, the report issued by the Institute of Medicine's Committee of Lesbian Health Research Priorities in 1999 found that lesbians were less likely to receive Pap smears than heterosexual women, although they have equal need for this screening procedure. A third consideration is that the lack of legal recognition of gay partnerships on an equal basis with marriage affects gay and lesbian access to healthcare, because while many married people receive their health insurance through their spouse's employer, gay and lesbian partners do not have this option. A final point is that gay men and lesbians have been found to have higher rates of psychiatric disorders and of health risk behaviors such as alcohol and substance abuse and smoking, and the risk of suicide attempts among gay and lesbian youth has been found to be much higher than among heterosexual youth. These results are usually attributed to stress caused by antigay discrimination.

SEE ALSO: Lesbian; Sexually Transmitted Diseases.

BIBLIOGRAPHY. L. Faderman, *Surpassing the Love of Men: Romantic Friendship and Love between Women from the Renaissance to the Present* (Morrow, 1981); GayData, www.gaydata.org (cited October 25, 2006); J.E. Heck, R.L. Sell, S.S. Gorin, "Health Care Access among Individuals

Involved in Same-Sex Relationships," *American Journal of Public Health* (v.96/6, 2006); A.C. Kinsey, W. B. Pomeroy, and C.E. Martin, *Sexual Behavior in the Human Male* (Saunders, 1948); A.C. Kinsey, et al., *Sexual Behavior in the Human Female*, (Saunders, 1953); T.G.M. Sandfort, et al., "Same-Sex Sexual Behavior and Psychiatric Disorders: Findings from the Netherlands Mental Health Survey and Incidence Study (NEMESIS)," *Archives of General Psychiatry* (v.58, 2001); T. W. Smith, *American Sexual Behavior: Trends, Socio-Demographic Differences, and Risk Behavior*, GSS Topical Report No. 25 (National Opinion Research Center, 1998); A.L. Solarz, ed., *Lesbian Health: Current Assessment and Directions for the Future* (Academy Press, 1999).

SARAH BOSLAUGH, PH.D., M.P.H.
BJC HEALTHCARE

Homozygote

A homozygote is an individual with two identical alleles at a given locus within the 22 autosomal chromosomes or the paired sex chromosomes of a female (males, with two different sex chromosomes, are classified as hemizygous at the sex chromosome). Homozygosity is determined on a locus-by-locus basis and is not used to characterize a whole genome. In terms of human disease, all diseases of genetic origin (as well as many diseases in which genetic predisposition is a key factor) require or are promoted by a loss of wildtype homozygosity. Further, some diseases and states require the gain of a mutant homozygosity. These two pathways to disease broadly correspond to the concepts of dominant and recessive inheritance of disease, although there are some caveats.

Certain physiological functions require two functional alleles of a given gene. In such cases, the loss of homozygosity caused by mutation to either of the alleles leads to a decreased level of wildtype protein synthesis and/or expression of protein coded for by the mutant allele. Such inheritance is typically termed *dominant inheritance*. A classic example of such a disease state is Huntington's disease. Briefly, a mutation of the Huntington gene produces an extended form of the mutant Huntington pro-

tein which causes cell death in selective areas of the brain. In this disease state, loss of homozygous wildtype is the key: Individuals homozygous for the mutant allele are no worse off than individuals who have one mutant allele and one wildtype allele.

There are many physiological functions that do not require wildtype gene products to be expressed from both alleles for normal functioning. Disease states that alter these functions must, therefore, feature the total loss of wildtype allele expression. Furthermore, certain disease states require not only the loss of wildtype expression, but the expression of two mutant alleles coding for the same protein. In practice, such conditions are exceedingly rare and not currently of clinical significance. These so-called recessive gain of function mutations primarily have been found to affect channels and membrane proteins responsible for signaling pathways.

SEE ALSO: Allele; Hemizygous; Heterozygote.

BIBLIOGRAPHY. H.A. Lester and A. Karschin, "Gain of Function Mutants: Ion Channels and G Protein-Coupled Receptors," *Annual Review of Neuroscience* (v.23, 2000); R. L. Nussbaum, et al., *Thompson & Thompson: Genetics in Medicine*, 6th ed., revised reprint (Saunders, 2004).

BIMAL P. CHAUDHARI
BOSTON UNIVERSITY

Honduras

Honduras is located in the heart of central America, between Nicaragua, El Salvador, and Guatemala. The country won independence from Spain in 1821 and has managed to stay largely clear of the endless civil wars that have plagued its neighbors, but it has never prospered in its relative freedom, and most of its citizens struggle to stay afloat.

The population is 7.3 million (2006 estimate) and is growing at 2.16 percent annually. The birth rate is 28.24 per 1,000 people, the death rate 5.28 per 1,000, and the migration rate is in the negative column, with minus 1.39 migrants per 1,000 people. Hundreds of thousands of Hondurans have left the country in recent years, most traveling north to find work in the

United States. It is simply more profitable. In 2002 alone, these economic immigrants wired home some $700 million in remittances.

Honduras is largely covered by mountains, with just a few lowlands along the coast and the river valleys. Between 40 and 50 percent of the population lives in urban areas. Population density is 64 people per square kilometer. Only 9.53 percent of the land is arable, but for many decades, most of the country's slim Gross Domestic Product has come from agricultural exports such as bananas and coffee and fully one-third of Hondurans work in agribusiness. The national economy was decimated in 1998 in the aftermath of Hurricane Mitch. That devastating storm took the lives of 5,600 Hondurans and caused several billions of dollars in damage.

The government has recently opened the door to *maquiladoras*, foreign-owned factories taking advantage of free-trade arrangements. However, neither agribusiness, mining, nor *maquiladoras* have done much to improve the lot of most Hondurans. Per capita income is $1,030 a year, and 21 percent of the population gets by on less than $1 a day.

The average diet is based on beans, rice, tortillas, plantains, meat, potatoes, and cheese. Rates of malnutrition are high, particularly among the poor. About 90 percent of the people have access to clean water and 68 percent have access to sanitary facilities, but access drops significantly outside the cities. Honduras has the highest rate of parasitic infection in the western hemisphere. Hookworm is common, as are malaria and hepatitis. Life expectancy at birth is 67.75 for men and 70.98 for women, but healthy life expectancy is much lower at 56.3 for men and 60.5 for women. Infant mortality is 25.82 per 1,000 live births. The mortality rate for children between the ages of 1 and 5 years is 41 per 1,000. The average woman has 3.59 children and the maternal mortality rate is 220 deaths per 100,000 live births. Only 56 percent of births are monitored by trained attendants.

The HIV/AIDS rate is 1.8 percent, with an estimated 63,000 living with the virus in 2003 and at least 4,100 AIDS-related deaths. This, along with other factors, has contributed to a large population of orphans, with more than 180,000 children under the age of 17 having lost one or both parents.

Violent crime is rampant in the cities, with murder, rape, assault, and kidnapping for profit now common. Gang violence has flourished almost unchecked.

Honduras spends about $41 per capita annually on healthcare. Medical care outside the main cities of Tegucigalpa and San Pedro Sula are sketchy and hard to come by; ambulance service from the outlying regions is rare. The World Health Organization counted 3,676 doctors and 8,333 nurses serving a population of 7.3 million.

SEE ALSO: Healthcare, South America.

BIBLIOGRAPHY. Central Intelligence Agency, "The World Factbook—Honduras, www.cia.gov (cited June 2007); World Health Organization, Honduras, www.who.int (cited June 2007).

HEATHER K. MICHON
INDEPENDENT SCHOLAR

Hormone Replacement Therapy

Hormones are a set of chemical substances which exist inside the body and regulate a number of critical life functions. As a result of various changes in bodily condition, the responsible organs may fail to produce sufficient or any hormones and this can result in negative health outcomes. For example, menopause inhibits the production of estrogen and this can result in hot flushes and more serious symptoms. In certain cases, medical practitioners will recommend replacement of the hormone from an external source as a means of treating the undesirable symptoms. The production of hormones has generally resulted from synthesizing cognate hormones from animals and treating them appropriately before introducing them into the patient's body.

However, improvements in scientific and pharmaceutical technology make it possible for entirely artificially created hormones to be used in the future. Hormone replacement therapy (HRT) overall represents a large economic opportunity for pharmaceutical companies to exploit and, consequently, there has been some controversy concerning the motivations for some medical practitioners to prescribe HRT and the incentives they might be receiving to influence their decisions.

HRT most commonly takes the form of a combination of estrogen and progestin. The purpose of the treatment is generally to reduce the symptoms of postmenopausal health, but the operations of hormones within the body are so complex and multivalent that the reintroduction of hormones can have many different and often unpredictable effects. These may be either positive or negative. Positive side effects can include strengthening of the bones and reduction of the risk of colon cancer. Negative side effects include elevated risks of cardiovascular disease and breast and other types of cancer, stroke, blood clots, and dementia. Some of the promised positive side effects of HRT, which include better self-esteem through enhanced beauty and sex life have not fully materialized. Some research has also shown that postmenopausal symptoms may have been overstated and that those women who do suffer from them may not obtain the level of relief that had been promised. As a result, many doctors now follow the policy that only HRT should only be prescribed when the woman concerned is suffering symptoms of vaginal dryness, hot flushes, or insomnia to such an extent that they significantly affect quality of life. An alternative prescription may also be offered if the risk of osteoporosis is deemed to be sufficient.

However, there are many occasions on which the woman is left without a clear direction, because symptoms might be present but bearable, at least periodically, while the risks of the treatment may appear possibly worse. In these cases, the woman may have to bear the responsibility for the decision personally and this might be an onerous burden, especially if the woman feels intimidated by the medical experts and the other aspects of the environment. The revelations of the research findings which occurred over the past few years have proved to be rather disturbing to those who have been receiving HRT or had been considering doing so. Trust in the medical profession has been shaken to some extent and the reputation of the pharmaceutical industry has also been further affected.

HRT has become a sociological as well as a medical issue. A number of authors have argued that the process of menopause, for example, is one that is natural and which women are in general terms quite capable of dealing with through their own resources. However, medical practitioners have, so it is argued, changed the perception of this natural procedure so that it has become regarded as a medical process and an event which requires the intervention of experts and their scientific products. In other words, women are disempowered because their bodies betray them by becoming the scene of an inherent weakness which only outsiders and drugs can manage. Since women's bodies are so often the battleground for controversy over political and religious debate, this argument has become not just impassioned but powerful as well. After all, it is clear that there are powerful incentives for medical practitioners to prescribe expensive regimes of drugs and medicines and to ensure that all citizens believe themselves to be necessarily patients for much of their lives.

Consequently, it may be concluded by some that the treatment of menopause is part of a system aimed at trapping women and their carers in a world of commerce in which they must continually yield their money to maintain good health and subvert the problems their bodies continually cause them.

SEE ALSO: Hormones; Menopause; Menstruation and Premenstrual Syndrome.

BIBLIOGRAPHY. Amy Allina, and Cynthia Pearson, "The Great Hormone Hoax," *Multinational Monitor* (July/August, 2002); Elizabeth Barrett-Connor, and Deborah Grady, "Hormone Replacement Therapy, Heart Disease, and Other Considerations," *Annual Review of Public Health*, (v.19, 1998); National Women's Health Network, *The Truth about Hormone Replacement Therapy: How to Break Free from the Medical Myths of Menopause* (Prima Lifestyles, 2002).

JOHN WALSH,
SHINAWATRA UNIVERSITY

Hormones

The word *hormone* is derived from a Greek word meaning "to arouse to activity." Endocrinologists are physicians who specialize in the study of the endocrine system, which generates hormones. This system was first identified by French physician Claude Bernard (1813–78) in the mid-19th century. The word *endocrine* is also Greek in origin and means "separated within," which describes the actions by which hormonal activity is aroused in the cells of origin (autocrine) as well as in the surrounding cells (paracrine). Once hormones are secreted, they enter into the blood stream to perform specific functions, thereby keeping the body in working order as they interact with the brain, heart, liver, kidneys, digestive system, nervous system, immune system, and other parts and systems of the body. As they perform their assigned functions, hormones regulate the rate of chemical reactions in specific cells and influence the way in which substances in the body are transported through cell membranes. Once hormones perform their specific functions, they are eliminated through the kidneys.

Hormones also play a major role in growth and development. Malfunctions of growth hormones may lead to either dwarfism or gigantism. During conception, hormones influence the formation of sex organs. After birth, hormone levels decline. During puberty, which generally begins in industrialized nations between the ages of 12 and 14 years, hormone levels rise rapidly. Puberty may be delayed in poorer countries as a result of poor nutrition. If malfunctions occur in the production of sex hormones, individuals may not develop the secondary sex characteristics that lead to male and female characteristics in adulthood. During puberty, females normally start to menstruate as their bodies begin producing eggs in preparation for motherhood. Subsequently, fluctuating hormonal levels may result in pre-menstrual syndrome (PMS), which is associated with a variety of symptoms such as pain, bloating, and wide mood swings. Delayed or absent menstruation or abnormal menstrual pain are indicative of possible problems.

Male hormones released during puberty result in the appearance of facial and body hair, deepened voices, elongation of the long bones of limbs, and increased aggression and libido. Male and female hormones during puberty are also responsible for teenage acne and for the infamous moodiness of teenagers. Because hormones exercise some neural controls over emotions, they also determine how humans of all ages deal with stress and emotions such as aggression and fear.

The major female hormone, estrogen, and the major male hormone, testosterone, activate the sex drive and control fertility, ensuring that the human race will survive through procreation. Once a female becomes pregnant, estrogen and progesterone prepare her body for motherhood. When she reaches the end of her childbearing years, levels of "female" hormones drop, and a woman enters menopause. In one percent of females, premature ovarian failure occurs when a woman under the age of 40 stops producing estrogen and enters menopause. The physical protections that estrogen provides have been well documented, and hormone replacement therapy (HRT) has been widely used to offset the loss of estrogen during and after menopause. However, a number of studies have linked HRT to cancer, particularly breast cancer, and many women have sought alternative methods of dealing with estrogen loss. In males, some studies have revealed a link between high testosterone levels, which may be associated with high dietary fat intake, and prostate cancer. However, the exact causes of such cancers are unknown.

There are six major glands of the endocrine system—pituitary, thyroid, parathyroid, pancreas, adrenal, and gonads—as well as a number of minor glands. Each has its own particular function designed to ensure good health. The pituitary gland is considered the leader of the endocrine system. The hypothalamus conducts the hormones secreted by the pituitary gland to target areas. Together, they work with the brain to control other endocrine glands. Hormones are divided into two classes: amino acid and peptide hormones, which are not liquid soluble, and the steroid hormones, which are highly liquid soluble.

A hormone imbalance occurs when hormone levels are either too aggressive or deficient, leading to a variety of medical conditions. For instance, insulin is a polypeptide hormone secreted by the pancreas. If the liver does not perform its task of producing insulin in appropriate amounts, a person may become diabetic. This condition is associated with a number of other disorders such as blindness, cataracts, cardiovascular disease, and even death. Women of childbearing age who have hormonal imbalances as a result of bouts with infectious diseases or as a result of cancer treatments may experience fertility problems. Many cancers are fed by naturally occurring hormones such as estrogen, which produces granulose cell tumors, and androgen progen, which is responsible for leydig cell tumors.

A number of noted endocrinologists have enhanced the study of hormonal abnormalities. American neurologist and surgeon Harvey Cushing (1869–1939), for instance, studied the functions of the pituitary gland, leading to the identification of Cushing's disease, which results from a malfunction in the secretion of the hormones affecting carbohydrate metabolism. The chief function of thyroid hormones is to increase basal metabolic rate and control growth and development. Hyperthyroidism was first identified by Irish physician Robert Graves (1797–1853). Grave's disease affects one percent of the total population and is more often found in females (2 percent) than in males (0.2 percent). The condition known as Addison's disease, an abnormality of the adrenal cortex glands, was identified by British physician Thomas Addison (1795–1860).

In addition to naturally produced hormones, artificial hormones, such as birth control pills, may be voluntarily taken to mitigate or block the effects of hormones produced by the body. Environmentalists contend that many of the artificial hormones that are inherent in certain chemicals are associated with cancer, infertility, endometriosis, fibroids, and immunosystem and thyroid disorders. Chemical-based hormones have also been blamed for learning and behavioral disorders, hyperactivity, and lower than average intelligence. Consequently, the United States Environmental Protection Agency (EPA) has been charged with researching chemicals suspected of disrupting human hormones.

SEE ALSO: Birth Defects; Cancer (General); Diabetes; Endocrine Diseases (General); Environmental Protection Agency (EPA); Gastroenterology; Gynecology; Kidneys; Liver Diseases (General); Menopause; Pregnancy.

BIBLIOGRAPHY. Lindsey Berkson, *Hormone Deception: How Everyday Foods and Products Are Disrupting Your Hormones* (McGraw-Hill, 2000); Sue Ann Binkley, *Endocrinology* (Harper Collins, 1995); George Fried and George J. Hademenos, *Schaum's Outline of Theory and Problems of Biology* (McGraw-Hill Professional, 1999); Paul Gard, *Human Endocrinology* (Taylor and Francis, 1998); M.E. Hadley, *Gastrointestinal Hormones* (Prentice-Hall, 1992); David McKay Hart, Jane Norman, *Gynaecology Illustrated* (Churchill Livingstone, 2000); Christopher K Herwill. and John D. Flack, *Endocrine Toxicology* (Cambridge University Press, 1992); John F. Laycock, and Peter H. Wise, *Essential Endocrinology* (Oxford University Press, 1996).

ELIZABETH R. PURDY, PH.D.
INDEPENDENT SCHOLAR

Hounsfield, Godfrey (1919–2004)

British electrical engineer who was awarded a share in the Nobel Prize in Physiology or Medicine in 1979 for his contributions to the creation of the computerized axial tomography (CAT or CT) scanner. Hounsfield's invention combined X-ray images with the aid of a computer to generate cross-sectional views and three-dimensional images of the internal organs and structures of the body. CAT scanners can be used, for example, to examine the head to identify traumatic injuries (such as blood clots or skull fractures), tumors, and infections. CAT scan methods can also be used to calculate the density of bone in the evaluation of osteoporosis. Hounsfield's name is inextricably linked to his creation as the Hounsfield scale defines a quantitative measure of radiodensity used in assessing CAT scans.

Hounsfield was born in Nottinghamshire, England, on August 28, 1919, the youngest of five children. He was fascinated with electronics from an early age, and in school, he had excellent results in physics and maths, but by his own admission, lacked interest in the other subjects offered at the Newark Magnus Grammar School. During World War II, he volunteered to join the Royal Air Force (RAF) as a reservist, which gave him the chance to learn the basic principles of electronics.

While in the RAF, Hounsfield quickly became a radio mechanic instructor. One of his superiors noticed Hounsfield's electronic skills and recommended him to the Faraday House Electrical Engineering College in London, where he obtained his diploma. After the war, he started working at EMI in Middlesex on radar and guided weapons. His personal interests, however, soon led him to research computers, which in the 1950s, were still in their primitive stages. Together with his team, Hounsfield designed the first all-transistor computer to be constructed in Britain, the EMIDEC 1100.

It was in the late 1960s that Hounsfield began working on the project that would eventually lead to the creation of the CAT scanner. The first prototype of Hounsfield's CAT scanner was designed to examine the head and, as the Nobel Committee's statement pointed out, before that, "ordinary X-ray examinations of the head had shown the skull bones, but the brain had remained a gray, undifferentiated fog. Now, suddenly, the fog had cleared." Hounsfield continued his research to perfect the scanner after the Nobel and he also successfully designed a whole-body scanner. Because of his invention, Hounsfield received many awards. In 1975, he was elected to the Royal Society. The following year, he was appointed Commander of the British Empire and, in 1981, he was knighted. Hounsfield died on August 12, 2004.

SEE ALSO: Diagnostic Imaging; Diagnostic Tests.

BIBLIOGRAPHY. Caroline Richmond, "Sir Godfrey Hounsfield," *British Medical Journal* (v.329, 2004); Susan Zonnos, *Godfrey Hounsfield and the Invention of Cat Scans* (Lane Publishers, 2002).

LUCA PRONO
INDEPENDENT SCHOLAR

Household Poisons

Poisonings are an unfortunate but common worldwide occurrence. A poison is defined as a substance that through its chemical action usually kills, injures, or impairs an organism. Poisoning from household substances is sometimes because of children's curiosity, although adults are also frequently poisoned as well, either accidentally or intentionally. Poison exposure is largely by ingestion, but may be through dermal, inhalational, or ocular routes. Poisoning from household substances is avoidable, thus it is imperative to educate the public, especially parents, of the dangers of common items. If poisoning is suspected, rapid emergency treatment is mandated, and should be done utilizing a Poison Control Center.

The National Capital Poison Center lists the most common substances responsible for poisoning children—cosmetics, cleaning substances, medications, antiseptics, plants, vitamins, pesticides, and foreign objects such as coins. Although other, more dangerous items exist, household substances are readily available to children, and special precautions should be taken to keep them out of reach. In adults, the most common substances include pain medicines, sedatives, cleaning substances, antidepressants, alcohol, and cardiovascular drugs. The most toxic substances to humans are iron pills, cleaning products, hydrocarbons (gas, oil, and lighter fluid), pesticides, alcohol, windshield wiper fluid, and antifreeze.

Iron pills (which resemble candy) are a common and especially fatal threat to children. The recommended dose for children less than 6 years of age is 10 milligrams/day. Supplements range from 18 to 150 milligrams/pill and as little as 600 milligrams is harmful to a small child. Signs and symptoms of iron poisoning include nausea/vomiting, gastrointestinal bleeding, shock, and coma. Death can ensue within hours. The Food and Drug Administration has taken precautions in dosing and packaging requirements to try to reduce the number of iron poisonings in children. Medications, both prescription and over the counter, should *always* be kept in childproof containers.

Cleaning products are dangerous to children and adults alike due to their strong acid or base content. These include drain openers, toilet bowl cleaners, rust remover, and oven cleaner. They cause chemical burns, both internally and externally, and may damage the lungs after a long exposure in a poorly ventilated area, usually in adults who are cleaning using these products.

Antifreeze and windshield wiper fluid often cause accidental poisonings. Antifreeze is especially attractive to children due to the sweet smell and taste of ethylene glycol, the main ingredient. If ingested, antifreeze can damage the nervous system, cardiovascular system, and kidneys. The patient may have a rapid heart rate, confusion, dizziness, seizures, and coma. The main toxin in wiper fluid is methanol. Pure concentrated methanol is extremely toxic and two tablespoons is fatal to a child. Six to eight ounces is harmful to an adult. Ingestion of wiper fluid, which contains a diluted solution of methanol, can cause blindness and death, and is a medical emergency.

Many household plants such as aloe, holly, mistletoe, and azaleas, are poisonous to humans. Plants usually do not pose a problem unless the household has a young child who puts everything in his or her mouth. Aloe, a succulent houseplant used topically to treat minor cuts and burns, causes abdominal pain, diarrhea, and possible kidney damage if ingested. Mistletoe is a popular holiday decoration that can cause inflammation of the gastrointestinal tract. Holly berries contain toxins called saponins. Ingestion of two or three berries will cause gastroenteritis; 20 to 30 berries can be fatal. Azaleas are potentially fatal. If ingested, symptoms include decreased heart rate, decreased blood pressure, and paralysis.

Alcohol is very dangerous—in small children, minimal amounts of liquor, beer, or wine can quickly lead to intoxication, followed by seizures, coma, and death. Mouthwash, colognes, and other household products also pose a threat. Previously, parents were encouraged to keep syrup of ipecac in case of accidental poisoning. Syrup of ipecac works by inducing emesis (vomiting). The medical community now discourages this practice. There is no evidence for the use of syrup of ipecac; it was just *assumed* that inducing vomiting would rapidly remove the poison and be of benefit. Emergency rooms today may use activated charcoal, which binds to and prevents the absorption of substances into the bloodstream. Additionally, patients with eating disorders may utilize syrup of ipecac for weight loss.

If a poisoning is suspected, rapid medical attention is necessary to prevent long-term damage or death. Poison Control Centers are excellent resources in suspected poisoning, and are available nationally through a toll-free number (currently 1-800-222-1222). They are staffed by toxicologists, pharmacists, and other professionals who can give guidance as to whether a hospital trip is necessary, and are a resource available free of charge to both healthcare workers as well as the general public. This number should *only* be used in the case of a poisoning emergency, but if the patient is not conscious, 911 should be called first. Prevention is a better option, and many poisonings can be avoided by simply knowing which substances are dangerous and storing them properly.

SEE ALSO: Poisoning; Environmental Toxicology; Agency for Toxic Substances and Disease Registry; Mercury

BIBLIOGRAPHY. American Academy of Pediatrics, *Q and A: Poison Treatment in the Home,* www.aap.org (cited October 2006); A.D.A.M. Medical Encyclopedia, *Windshield Washer Fluid,* www.nlm.nih.gov/medlineplus (cited 10 2006); Audrey Hingley, *FDA Consumer: Preventing Childhood Poisoning,* www.cfsan.fda.gov (cited October 2006); Mark Hostetler and Sandra Schneider, *Emergency Medicine: A Comprehensive Study Guide,* 6th ed., Access Medicine, www.accessmedicine.com (cited October 2006).

GAUTAM J. DESAI, D.O.
ELLY K. HUGHES, MS II
KANSAS CITY UNIVERSITY OF MEDICINE AND
BIOSCIENCES COLLEGE OF OSTEOPATHIC MEDICINE

Hughlings Jackson, John (1835–1911)

John Hughlings Jackson was a leading physician, thinker, and writer who became known for his studies of epilepsy, speech defects, and nervous system disorders arising from injury to the brain and spinal cord. He has been called the "father" of English neurology, and pioneered the development of neurology as a medical specialty.

Born on March 4, 1835, in Providence, Green Hammerton, Yorkshire, in England, he was the son of Samuel Jackson, a British yeoman, and Sarah Hughlings, the daughter of a Welsh revenue collector.

During his career as a physician, he worked at the London Hospital (1859–94) and later in the National Hospital for Paralysis and Epilepsy (1862–1906), which was located in Regent's Park, and was later moved to Queen Square, and renamed to what is today known as the National Hospital for Neurology and Neurosurgery.

He was one of the first people to make the association between structural brain damage and abnormal mental states. He was the first to describe in 1863 a type of epilepsy known today as Jacksonian epilepsy or Jacksonian seizures, after observing his wife's epileptic seizures, which would always follow a similar pattern. They would start at one of her hands, progress to her wrist, then move to her shoulder, and finally to her face. Finally, they would affect the leg on the same side of her body, and ultimately stop. He thus went on in 1875 to attribute the seizures to the motor region of the cerebral cortex (the external layer of the brain). In 1881, he was also the first to describe a type of epilepsy now known as temporal lobe epilepsy. His work on epilepsy paved the way to the development of modern methods to find brain lesions and the investigation of localized brain functions.

Besides his comprehensive studies on epilepsy, he was also one of the first to recognize the pattern of disease of the cerebellum (the part of the brain which coordinates, among other functions, balance and posture), and also developed research in the realm of aphasia (a speech disorder) and neuro-ophtalmology. In 1864, he confirmed the discovery by Paul Broca (a French surgeon) that the speech centre in right-handed persons was located in the left hemisphere and vice versa.

He was elected a Fellow of the Royal Society of London for the Improvement of Natural Knowledge in 1878. He was also one of the founders of the renowned British specialist journal *Brain*, along with David Ferrier and James Crichton-Browne, two friends who were prominent neurologists at the time. The journal, which is still published today, covered the interaction between experimental and clinical neurology. He died in London on October 7, 1911.

SEE ALSO: Epilepsy; Neurologist; Neurology; Neurologic Diseases.

BIBLIOGRAPHY. Macdonald and Eileen A. Critchley, *John Hughlings Jackson: Father of English Neurology* (Oxford University Press, 1998).

Tiago Villanueva
Centro Hospitalar de Lisboa-zona central

Human Genome Organization, The (HUGO)

The Human Genome Organization (HUGO) was established by a group of scientists in 1989 to promote and sustain international collaboration in the field of human genetics. The organization's primary objectives are to investigate the nature, structure, function, and interaction of the genes, genomic elements, and genomes of humans and relevant pathogenic and model organisms; to characterize the nature, distribution, and evolution of genetic variation in humans and other relevant organisms; to study the relationship between genetic variation and the environment in the origins and characteristics of human populations and the causes, diagnoses, treatments, and prevention of disease; to foster the interaction, coordination, and dissemination of information and technology between investigators and the global society in genomics, proteomics, bioinformatics, systems biology, and the clinical sciences by promoting quality education, comprehensive communication, and accurate, comprehensive, and accessible knowledge resources for genes, genomes, and disease; and, to sponsor factually grounded dialogues on the social, legal, and ethical issues related to genetic and genomic information and championing the regionally appropriate, ethical utilization of this information for the good of the individual and the society.

Membership is open to all persons concerned with the human genome or related scientific fields. HUGO is governed by a General Assembly of its membership that convenes once a year to set, steer, and evaluate policy. The Assembly elects officers and an 18-member Executive Council to serve the day-to-day operational needs of the organization. HUGO is incorporated in Geneva, Switzerland, and has three regional offices: the North American office in Bethesda, Maryland, the European office in London, and the Pacific office in Osaka, Japan. Funding for the organization comes from a number of nongovernmental foundations including the Howard Hughes Medical Institute, the Lucille P. Markey Charitable Trust, and the Wesley Foundation.

Each year HUGO holds its annual Human Genome Meeting (HGM) designed to update and increase knowledge in the ever-evolving field of human genome research. The meetings center on a stimulating and interesting program of plenary lectures, symposia, workshops, and include poster presentations and social events which all help to make any HGM the ideal forum to share information and results with researchers in both science and industry.

The organization also sponsors a number of other meetings and workshops throughout the year to disseminate information on specific topics, and publishes a newsletter, the *Genome Digest*. HUGO's Travel Awards Program is intended to encourage and assist younger scientists involved in the analysis of the human genome. Specifically, the program is designed to enable young investigators to travel from their country of residence to a laboratory in another country for the purpose of learning a new method or technique which can then be brought back and introduced to their home laboratory; and to facilitate collaborative research among laboratories involved in the analysis of the human genome.

SEE ALSO: Genetics; Genomic Library.

BIBLIOGRAPHY. Centre for Life, www.life.org.uk (cited September 2006); Rodney Loeppky, *Encoding Capital: The Political Economy of the Human Genome Project* (Routledge, 2005); The Human Genome Organization, www.hugo-international.org/index.htm (cited September 2006); Human Genome Project Information, www.ornl.gov/sci/techresources/Human_Genome/home.shtml; World Health Organization: Genetics Resource Center, www.who.int/genomics/en (cited September 2006).

BEN WYNNE, PH.D
GAINESVILLE STATE COLLEGE

Human Development Report ranks Hungary 35th in the world on overall quality-of-life issues.

The Health Insurance Fund (HIF) is responsible for providing healthcare in Hungary, and local governments receive grants from the central government to administer the health program. Governments negotiate contracts with various providers to provide coverage for most of the population. The National Public Health Program has been implemented to improve general health, and the government has established goals that include increasing life expectancy by three years and slashing rates of major illnesses and injuries. Targeted areas include reducing the smoking rate, preventing and treating alcohol and drug abuse, promoting better diet and lifestyles, expanding sex education programs, improving the environment, and preventing epidemics. Social security is funded by employee and employer contributions supplemented by the government. The program covers workers, the self-employed, apprentices, entertainers, attorneys, civil servants, ministers, and the unemployed. Other Hungarians can buy into the pension plan.

The government spends an average of six percent of the total budget on healthcare. In international dollars, $1,269 is allotted per capita, and the government earmarks 8.4 percent of the Gross Domestic Product

Hungary

The central European nation of Hungary has one of the two strongest economies of all transition countries, and the per capita income of $16,300 is one-half that of the Big Four nations. Hungary is considered the 62nd richest nation in the world. Growth continues to be strong (4.1 percent). Despite a number of economic gains, the government has been beset by unsustainable budgets, current account deficits, inflation (14 percent) and unemployment (7.2 percent). Labor participation is low at only 57 percent. Hungary has a poverty rate of 8.6 percent of the population. The Gini coefficient is 24.4, and the richest 10 percent of Hungarians hold 20.5 percent of resources as compared to 4.1 percent for the poorest 10 percent. The overall standard of living is relatively high, and the United Nations Development Programme's (UNDP)

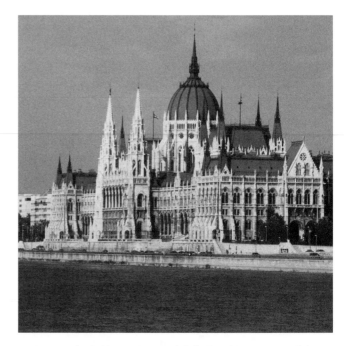

In Hungary, $1,269 in international dollars and 8.4 percent of the Gross Domestic Product (GDP) are allocated for healthcare.

(GDP) for health. Government spending accounts for 72.4 percent of all government expenditures in Hungary, and 83.4 percent of that spending is directed toward social security programs. The private sector supplies 27.6 percent of all health funding, and 88.90 of private spending is generated by out-of-pocket expenses. There are 3.33 physicians, 8.85 nurses, 0.21 midwives, 0.54 dentists, and 0.52 pharmacists per 1,000 population in Hungary.

The population of 9.981,334 Hungarians experiences a life expectancy of 72.77 years, with females outliving males an average of nine years. Literacy is widespread, and less than three percent of the population over the age of 15 are unable to read and write. All of the relevant population is enrolled in primary and secondary school. While all urban residents have sustained access to safe drinking water and improved sanitation, two percent of rural residents lack access to safe drinking water and 15 percent lack access to proper sanitation. Around 77 percent of Hungarian women use some method of birth control, and Hungarian women have the 14th lowest fertility rate in the world, giving birth at a rate of 1.32 children each. All births are attended by trained personnel, and the adjusted maternal mortality rate is 16 deaths per 100,000 live births.

Between 1990 and 2004, both infant and under-five mortality were more than halved, dropping from 15 to seven and from 17 to eight deaths per 1,000 live births respectively. Currently, infant mortality is reported at 8.39 deaths per 1,000 live births. Nine percent of infants are underweight at birth. Two percent of under-5 are moderately underweight, and two percent suffer from wasting diseases. Three percent are moderately to severely stunted. Infant immunization rates are reported at 99 percent for diphtheria, pertussis, and tetanus (DPT1 and DPT3), tuberculosis, polio, and measles.

Environmentally, Hungary has been left with many problems common to former Soviet bloc nations, and government resources have been strained as officials endeavor to reduce air, soil, and water pollution to meet European Union (EU) guidelines. Hungary has a 0.1 percent adult prevalence rate of HIV/AIDS. Around 2,800 people currently have the disease, but it has proved fatal to less than 100 people. Meningococcal disease was reported in Hungary in January 1999. Circulatory diseases, cancer, and accidents are the three leading causes of death.

SEE ALSO: European Public Health Alliance (EPHA) Healthcare, Europe.

BIBLIOGRAPHY. William H. Berqquist, *Freedom: Narratives of Change in Hungary and Estonia* (Jossey-Bass, 1994); Central Intelligence Agency, "Hungary," *World Factbook*, www.cia.gov (cited July 2007); Commission on the Status of Women, "Hungary," www.un.org (cited July 2007); Martin A. Levin and Martin Shapiro, eds., *Transatlantic Policymaking in an Age of Austerity: Diversity and Drift* (Georgetown University Press, 2004); UNICEF, "Hungary," Social Security Administration, "Hungary," www.ssa.gov (cited July 2007).

ELIZABETH R. PURDY, PH.D.
INDEPENDENT SCHOLAR

Huntington's Disease

The brain is a complex organ with numerous connections and interconnections that both aid in its study and confound it. Because of the intricate network of connections between brain cells, a disease that leads to degeneration of a specific population of brain cells can have a drastic effect on the brain as well as on the patient as a whole. There are many examples of neurological disorders; one prominent example is Huntington's disease (HD).

Within the brain, there are regions that control specific facets of brain function. For example, there is a region where all somatosensory information is ultimately processed, and another region where smells are processed. There is also a brain region that sends a signal to initiate body movement. Many brain functions integrate information from various brain regions. Movement is one such example. A major brain region that has important feedback on movement is the basal ganglia. The basal ganglia is itself made up of several distinct brain regions. The two most common disorders of the basal ganglia are Parkinson's disease (PD) and Huntington's disease. A person affected with PD will not be able to move as much as a healthy person, whereas someone with HD will exhibit excess, uncontrolled movements. A characteristic movement is a ballismus, or large forceful movement that usually occurs in the arms.

The brain is composed of two main types of cells, neurons and glia. Neurons are cells that send electrical signals within the brain or down to the spinal cord. Glia are the support cells. Within the neurons, there are multiple subtypes. One such subtype is called the medium spiny neurons. They are medium in size, relative to other neurons, and have spiny-appearing projections from the cell body by which they send and receive electrical signals. Medium spiny neurons reside in the basal ganglia, and these cells degenerate in HD. Along with movement disorders, HD can cause intellectual degeneration as well as emotional disorders.

There is currently no known treatment or cure for HD. The only medications used can alleviate some movement or emotional problems. Research is focused on the genetic cause of HD, which is a mutation in the huntingtin gene. This gene encodes the huntingtin protein, which as of yet has no known effect in brain cells. The type of mutation in the huntingtin gene is called a trinucleotide repeat expansion. When DNA encodes a protein, every three nucleotides of the coding DNA stand for one particular amino acid to be added to the protein.

Certain rare arrangements of nucleotides make a gene prone to trinucleotide repeat expansion, or abnormal multiple repeats of the trinucleotide segment. In HD, the trinucleotide repeat occurs in the coding region of the huntingtin gene; therefore, the resulting protein has an excessive string of one amino acid within the central region of the protein, resulting in a mutant protein of altered shape and size which can no longer function as normal. In the case of huntingtin, the mutated protein takes on a new toxic function, unrelated to the normal protein's function. The excess amino acid is glutamine.

The mutated huntingtin protein leads to death of the medium spiny neurons and subsequently HD. The mutation is dominant; only one of the two copies of the gene need be mutated in order to get the disease. Thus a child of an HD parent has a 50-percent chance of inheriting HD.

The disease usually manifests itself around the age of 40 or 50 years. Until then, a person may live a normal healthy lifestyle. In rare cases, an individual begins to exhibit HD symptoms before the age of 20. This early HD is called juvenile Huntington's disease. Generally, a person with the mutated huntingtin gene will develop HD at the same age as the affected parent. Genetic testing can be carried out to determine if an individual will have HD even before symptoms occur; because

knowledge of the impending disease may cause severe anxiety and stress, and there is currently no treatment, such testing is not typically recommended unless in the case of family planning. In the vast majority of HD patients, the mutated gene is inherited from a parent. In about 2 percent of the cases, the disease results from a spontaneous mutation in the huntingtin gene.

The name Huntington's disease dates back to 1872, when Dr. George Huntington of Ohio first described it in a medical paper. The disease was initially called Huntington's chorea or chorea major, due to the dance-like movements of HD patients. HD is rare, affecting approximately 8 people in 100,000 globally. It is more common in western Europeans, and nearly unseen in Asians and Africans.

SEE ALSO: Brain Diseases; Diagnostic Tests; Genetic Brain Disorders; Genetic Code; Genetic Disorders; Genetic Testing/Counseling; Genetics; Gerontology; National Institute of Mental Health (NIMH); National Institute of Neurological Disorders and Stroke (NINDS); National Institute on Aging (NIA); Neurological Diseases (General); Parkinson's Disease; Tremor.

BIBLIOGRAPHY. Jean Barema, *The Test: Living in the Shadow of Huntington's Disease* (Franklin Square Press, 2005); ICON Health Publications, *The Official Patient's Sourcebook on Huntington's Disease: A Revised and Updated Directory for the Internet Age* (ICON Health Publications, 2002); Richard R. Karlen, *Devil's Dance* (Ironbound Press, 1998); Oliver Quarrell, *Huntington's Disease: The Facts* (Oxford University Press, 1999).

CLAUDIA WINOGRAD
UNIVERSITY OF ILLINOIS AT URBANA-CHAMPAIGN

Hydrocephalus

The word *hydrocephalus* is derived from the Greek words meaning "water" and "head," and thus is defined as the accumulation of cerebrospinal fluid (CSF) in the ventricles of the brain, causing their enlargement and swelling. The estimated prevalence worldwide is 1 to 1.5 percent, or approximately 60 million individuals. It is one of the most common neurologic problems that affect humankind.

There are two major types of hydrocephalus: obstructive (noncommunicating) and nonobstructive (communicating). Obstructive hydrocephalus occurs when the normal circulation of CSF is blocked (obstructed), usually between the third and fourth ventricles at the aqueduct of Sylvius. Nonobstructive hydrocephalus is a result of poor absorption of CSF at the level of the arachnoid granulations; the flow of CSF in nonobstructive hydrocephalus is otherwise normal. Hydrocephalus can also be caused by excessive CSF production, such as with a choroid plexus papilloma.

An example of nonobstructive hydrocephalus is normal pressure hydrocephalus (NPH), a common neurologic problem that afflicts the elderly. Patients are usually older than 60 years and males are affected slightly more often than women. The classic clinical triad is dementia, gait disturbance, and urinary incontinence. The hydrocephalus is termed *normal pressure* because the opening pressure on lumbar puncture is nonelevated.

Other specific types of hydrocephalus include hydrocephalus ex vacuo (enlargement of the ventricles due to loss of cerebral tissue, that is, cortical atrophy, which can occur naturally with age), hydranencephaly (absence of a substantial amount of brain tissue), external hydrocephalus (enlarged subarachnoid spaces over the frontal lobes), arrested hydrocephalus (hydrocephalus without symptoms), and entrapped fourth ventricle (a fourth ventricle that does not communicate with the third ventricle).

Etiologies of hydrocephalus can be divided into two broad categories: congenital and acquired. Congenital causes of hydrocephalus include neural tube defects, Chiari malformations, aqueductal stenosis, aqueductal gliosis, Dandy-Walker malformations, X-linked inherited disorders, and intrauterine infection. Acquired causes of hydrocephalus include infections (i.e., meningitis, cysticercosis), hemorrhage (i.e., subarachnoid hemorrhage, intraventricular hemorrhage), masses, postoperative changes, neurosarcoidosis, and spinal tumors.

The signs and symptoms of active hydrocephalus in young children include an enlarging cranium, irritability, poor head control, nausea and vomiting, enlargement and engorgement of scalp veins, cranial nerve VI (abducens) palsy, upward gaze palsy, hyperactive reflexes, and irregular respirations. In older children and adults, other symptoms include papilledema (swelling of the optic nerves on ophthalmologic examination), headaches, and gait changes.

The treatment of hydrocephalus can be procedural, medical, or surgical. Procedural treatment of hydrocephalus is accomplished with spinal taps (lumbar puncture), which drains out CSF. Medical treatment is accomplished with diuretics, particularly acetazolamide; this, however, is only a temporary measure. The definitive treatment of hydrocephalus is surgical, of which there are four options. Choroid plexectomy is a procedure that targets the choroid plexus, which is present in the brain's ventricles and produces CSF. Another option is to open a narrowed Sylvian aqueduct. Third ventriculostomy is a surgical procedure in which holes are made in the floor of the third ventricle, allowing CSF to drain into the basal cisterns of the brain. This procedure is typically done endoscopically and recent studies have shown it to be more beneficial in younger patients. Last, the most common surgical option is shunting.

There are three main different kinds of shunts used in practice today: ventriculoperitoneal (VP), ventriculoatrial (VA), and lumboperitoneal (LP). VP shunts are the most common type of shunt used and divert CSF from the lateral ventricle to the abdominal peritoneum. VA shunts divert CSF from the ventricles to the right atrium of the heart, and are the treatment of choice when abdominal abnormalities are present in the patient. The prevalence of shunts in the United States is greater than 125,000.

Although shunts are the most important intervention in the treatment of hydrocephalus, they are associated with complications. Some of the most common problems that occur with shunts include undershunting, overshunting, infection, seizures, and skin breakdown. Shunts can also become obstructed or disconnected, and cause peritonitis, hydrocele, ascites, volvulus, or intestinal strangulation. A rare but serious complication of shunt malfunction or hydrocephalus is blindness. This can occur via three mechanisms: occlusion of the posterior cerebral arteries caused by herniation of the brain, chronic papilledema, and/or dilatation of the third ventricle with compression of the optic chiasm.

People will always suffer from hydrocephalus, and survival is poor if the condition is left untreated. Fortunately, different organizations from developed countries travel abroad to help those in third world countries with limited access to neurosurgeons. The most notable of these is Project Shunt, based out of the University of Michigan, which travels to Guatemala annually to operate on those in need. Hopefully, the options for treatment of this serious disorder will continue to improve, with minimal side effects or complications.

SEE ALSO: Blindness; Brain Cancer; Meningitis; Sarcoidosis; Spinal Cord Diseases.

BIBLIOGRAPHY. Mark S. Greenberg, *Handbook of Neurosurgery*, 5th ed. (Thieme, 2001); Chuck Toporek and Kellie Robinson, *Hydrocephalus: A Guide for Patients, Families and Friends* (Patient-Centered Guides, 1999).

KHOI D. THAN, M.D.
JOHNS HOPKINS UNIVERSITY SCHOOL OF MEDICINE

Hygiene

The development of hygiene and hygienic practices has been fundamental in preventing infections through cleanliness, and has also been very important in helping patients recover from ailments. On a personal level, it involves washing hands and the body with clean water. Domestic hygiene demands having a clean house environment, with occupational hygiene meaning that workers have a clean workplace. The word itself is derived from Hygieia, the Greek goddess of health and sanitation, who was known as Salus in the Roman Empire. As a word, it first appeared in French as *hygiaine* in 1597, and Salmon in 1671 noted that there were three speculative parts in medicine: physiology, hygiene, and pathology.

Knowledge about hygiene and cleanliness and the need for it was clearly evident in ancient times with references to it in a number of ancient Hindu texts such as the *Hausmriti* and the *Vishnu Purana*. Indeed bathing is one of the daily duties of Hindus, with the custom of washing in the Ganges River at Benares and elsewhere having great symbolic importance. Washing was also practiced by large numbers of ancient peoples with the Romans constructing large public bath houses, while wealthy Romans had their own private bath houses. These often involved a range of pools, some with hot water, and some with cool water, while there were also facilities for massage with oil or scraping the skin with a metal "strigil." The water was kept fresh by use of the aqueduct. The most impressive of the baths in the Roman Empire were the Baths of Caracalla, in Rome, built from 216 C.E., to accommodate 1,600 bathers. In the New Testament of the Bible, the concept of baptism involves total immersion in water to cleanse one of sins, with Jesus also being involved in the washing of the feet, a practice that has continued into modern times in the Christian Church on Maundy Thursday (the last Thursday before Easter), with the Pope washing the feet of the subdeacons. The Koran prescribes a number of customs surrounding good hygiene, and Muslims wash their faces under running water, and their feet and hands at mosques.

As well as personal cleanliness, the cleaning of wounds has been found to be essential in helping them heal quickly. In Anglo-Saxon times in Britain and some parts of Europe, there was a custom of using honey to treat wounds, but by medieval times, it would found that the wound would heal much faster if washed in clean water.

Although it is now regarded as a healthy and hygienic practice to wash regularly, with many people having a shower at least once a day, this has not always been the case, and was not possible in much of the world where people did not have ready access to fresh water. Although people living near the sea and rivers were able to bathe easily, with the increase in population around the world, and the growth of cities, increasingly more people had to rely on water which was often not fresh. This led to outbreaks of disease such as cholera.

During Elizabethan times in England, Queen Elizabeth I (reigned 1558–1603) and some other wealthy people took up bathing in seawater which was regarded as more hygienic by many people. To do this, bathing boxes were constructed, with the box moved into the seawater, and the person able to bathe inside the box. However there were some people who claimed that washing would remove a protective layer of skin

With increasing interest in personal hygiene, and the growth of cities with consequent overcrowding, and also problems with removal of human waste, the hygiene of buildings became important during Victorian England. In November 1871, Edward, the

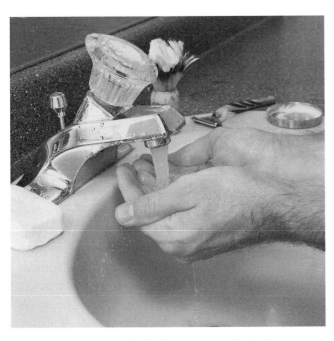

Most primary schools teach children to observe hygienic practices including washing one's hands after going to the lavatory.

Prince of Wales (later Edward VII) fell ill at Londes-borough Lodge, Scarborough, after having contract-ed typhoid fever. After huge public concern about what had happened, a medical doctor, William Henry Corfield (1843–1903) attached to University College London, writing to *The Times* newspaper was able to narrow the problem down to poor house sanitation. This led to new design standards being introduced for public buildings, and the doctor con-cerned wrote 32 books and treatises on aspects of hygiene in buildings.

In the late 19th century, and the early 20th cen-tury, there was an increasing emphasis on workplace hygiene. Hospitals and public buildings, especially schools, were regularly cleaned with disinfectant. However, many factories and mines continued to have people working in unhygienic conditions. The English writer D.H. Lawrence (1885–1930) wrote often of his father returning from the coal mine covered in coal dust. This led to regular demands for the provision of facilities at mines and in factories to allow workers to wash, and have ample and clean lavatories. These basic requirements were gradually introduced from the 1930s, although some mines and factories in less developed countries often have people working in un-hygienic conditions, even now.

Nowadays, most primary schools around the world teach children to observe hygienic practices. This in-volves, at its most basic, washing one's hands after go-ing to the lavatory, or touching animals, washing the body and hair frequently, and washing of hands be-fore eating. To this is added oral hygiene, with regular brushing of teeth, frequently washing hands, wrists and faces, and the regular washing of clothes and the wearing of clean clothes, as well as living in a clean environment. They are also taught to wash wounds, and not to share cutlery, as well as wash plates after meals and throw out uneaten food.

SEE ALSO: Food Safety; Foodborne Diseases.

BIBLIOGRAPHY. A. Leslie Banks and J.A. Hislop, *Health and Hygiene* (University of Tutorial Press, 1965); L.B. Es-critt and Sidney F. Rich, *The Work of the Sanitary Engi-neer* (Macdonald & Evans, 1949); Michael Hau, *The Cult of Health and Beauty in Germany: A Social History 1890–1930* (University of Chicago Press, 2003); Heikki Mikkeli, *Hygiene in the Early Modern Medical Tradition* (Academia Scientiarum Fennica, 1999); Henry E. Sigerust, Landmarks in the History of Hygiene (Oxford University Press, 1956); Leonie Mosel Williams, *Health, Life and Living* (Heine-mann, 1998).

JUSTIN CORFIELD
GEELONG GRAMMAR SCHOOL, AUSTRALIA

Hyperactivity

Hyperactivity is a condition where people become abnormally excitable and exuberant. Although the condition must have existed for thousands of years, the word itself is relatively new, being first used in its present context in the 20th century.

Some people show symptoms of hyperactivity natu-rally, with the condition varying considerably from one person to another. It is generally believed to be com-mon for children who have a very short concentration span and want to constantly be involved in a form of activity. Often, it may involve strong emotional reac-tions, and may show itself in symptoms such as fidg-eting, constant movement, and an inability to concen-trate for long. At its worst, hyperactivity can become serious because it can inhibit learning in schools, the following of emergency instructions, or getting along with colleagues in the workplace, and can, on occasions, be harmful to themselves and/or others.

Medical research in hyperactivity is generally connected with what has been called attention deficit hyperactivity disorder (ADHD), with experts disputing the level of its prevalence in society. Under normal circumstances, young children can be lively and have short attention spans. Similarly, teenage children can also, at times, have short attention spans through puberty. Boredom and suffering from mental conflict such as problems at home can also lead to hyperactivity. This often reflects itself on children being unsettled at school, or an inability to read for any substantial period, and with children being keen to involve themselves in activities including those that are antisocial. At home, it also reflects itself in not being able to concentrate on any specific task, watching television, and constantly changing between channels, or being unable to maintain a reasonable posture throughout a meal or other family occasion.

There have been many views as to how hyperactivity can be caused. Popular beliefs involve the consumption of too much sugar, either through red-colored cordial, or more often, through large-scale consumption of sugary soft drinks, especially those that contain caffeine, certain chocolate confections, and the like. Teachers and parents often claim that eating particular food or drinking specific drinks do result in children becoming far more rowdy, excitable, and energetic, and this has led to some schools trying to change the food children eat either by providing healthier food for school lunches or trying to influence their choices by not making certain items available. In recent years, there have been a number of books that have been published which seek to answer problems raised by parents and teachers.

SEE ALSO: Attention Deficit Disorder with Hyperactivity.

BIBLIOGRAPHY. Robert V. Kail, *Children and Their Development* (Pearson Prentice Hall, 2007); Gwnedd Lloyd, Joan Stead, and David Cohen, eds., *Critical New Perspectives on ADHD* (Routledge, 2006); Richard A. Lougy, Silvia L. DeRuvo, and David K. Rosenthal, *Teaching Young Children with ADHD: Successful Strategies and Practical Interventions for PreK–3* (Sage, 2007); Sami Timini, *Naughty Boys: Anti-Social Behavior, ADHD and the Role of Culture* (Palgrave Macmillan, 2005).

JUSTIN CORFIELD
GEELONG GRAMMAR SCHOOL, AUSTRALIA

Hypoglycemia

Hypoglycemia is a clinical syndrome characterized by episodes of low blood glucose (sugar). These episodes can be accompanied by marked autonomic manifestations. There are no specific symptoms of hypoglycemia, but they may include hunger, feelings of anxiety, sweating, nausea, trembling, dizziness, visual disturbances, drowsiness, difficulty speaking, fatigue, palpitations, confusion, and headache. Serum glucose is measured and classified as being low, normal, or elevated. Currently, 70 to 100 mg/dL is considered to be normal. Symptoms of hypoglycemia usually occur when blood glucose levels are less than 50 to 60 mg/dL. Hypoglycemia is a syndrome with diverse etiologies; therefore, treatment should be aimed toward the specific etiology.

Glucose is a form of sugar that the body uses as fuel. Carbohydrates are the main dietary sources of glucose. After a meal, glucose is absorbed into the bloodstream and distributed to the body's cells where it is used for energy. Blood glucose homeostasis involves complex interactions between the central nervous system and the endocrine system. The primary glucoregulatory organs are the liver, pancreas, adrenal glands, and pituitary gland. These organs regulate glucose through the release of hormones including insulin, glucagon, epinephrine, norepinephrine, glucocorticoids, and growth hormone.

Insulin is the primary regulator of glucose metabolism; it acts predominantly on the liver, skeletal muscle, and adipose (fat) tissue. Insulin is produced by the pancreas and acts to suppress endogenous glucose production, stimulates glucose use, and promotes conversion to glycogen for storage. Ultimately, it acts to lower the blood glucose levels. When hypoglycemia occurs, the body acts in defense by decreasing insulin secretion. Glucagon and epinephrine also protect the body from acute hypoglycemia by stimulating the release of glucose from the liver. They do this through two processes: glycogenolysis and gluconeogenesis. The former process is the breakdown of glycogen into glucose for immediate use. The latter is generation of new glucose. Other hormones such as growth hormone and cortisol protect from hypoglycemia over prolonged periods of time.

Evaluating a patient with hypoglycemia can be quite complex. Koch's postulates of hypoglycemia underlines the steps to evaluating patients with hypoglycemia. First, recognize the patient's symptoms could be caused by hypoglycemia. Second, document that the patient's serum glucose concentrations are low while the patient is symptomatic. Third, show that the symptoms can be relieved by the administration of glucose. The goal is to diagnose hypoglycemia and any other clinically relevant associated diseases.

A patient with serum glucose less than 60 should be evaluated for a hypoglycemic disorder. A patient with low blood glucose in the absence of symptoms does not need further evaluation. However, repeated episodes of hypoglycemia necessitate evaluation. In healthy persons, isolated episodes of hypoglycemia may result from accidental or intentional drug ingestion such as alcohol, salicylates, sulfa medications, haloperidol, pentamidine, and quinine. It may also be factitious, caused by accidental or intentional ingestion of hypoglycemic agents such as insulin, or a side effect of certain medications. Insulinomas are rare tumors that produce excessive amounts of the hormone insulin, which leads to hypoglycemia.

Hypoglycemic disorders can be categorized as fasting or postprandial/reactive, or insulin mediated or noninsulin mediated. However, it is more useful to classify the patient according to symptoms and differentiate the sick from not sick. The patient may have hypoglycemia alone or it may be part of a disorder. A detailed evaluation is key with a thorough review of the patient's past medical history and medication history. The differential diagnosis is different for different age groups.

For example, hypoglycemia is rare in the pediatric population. The most common cause of hypoglycemia in noninsulin-dependent children over the age of 1 year is idiopathic ketotic hypoglycemia. This is a syndrome that occurs after periods of fasting or during times of illness; it resolves with glucose administration. In neonates, infants, and children, hypoglycemia may be caused by inborn errors of metabolism. Common etiologies among adults include diabetic medication, ethanol (alcohol) use, and sepsis. In diabetic patients, hypoglycemic medications, inadequate food intake, increased physical exertion, illness, and drug interactions can all lead to hypoglycemia. Treatment depends upon the etiology, but usually involves the administration of dextrose orally or intravenously.

SEE ALSO: Diabetes; Endocrinology.

BIBLIOGRAPHY. W.J. Brady, and A.H. Richard, "Section 17—Endocrine Emergencies," in *Emergency Medicine: A Comprehensive Study Guide*, http://statref.com (cited September 2006); F. J. Service, *IX Hypoglycemia*, ACP Medicine, http://statref.com (cited September 2006).

Christina Murray
Angela J. Garner, M.D.
University of Missouri–Kansas City
School of Medicine

Hypothermia

Hypothermia refers to when the body's temperature falls below a temperature necessary to maintain normal metabolic functions. The normal body temperature is 37 degrees C and hypothermia occurs when the body drops to below 35 degrees C. Nearly 700 people die each year from hypothermia in the United States.

There are many causes of hypothermia such as decreased heat production. This can be because of endocrine abnormalities such as hypopituitarism or hypothyrodism. Decreased heat production can also be due to hypoglycemia or malnutrition. It is important to consider these causes of hypothermia when a person's normal body temperature does not rise through treatment, such as blankets and warming. Another cause of hypothermia can be due to increased heat loss. There are many factors that can lead to this cause, such as immersion in a cold body of water, or being in cold weather without sufficient clothing. Another common cause of increased heat loss is due

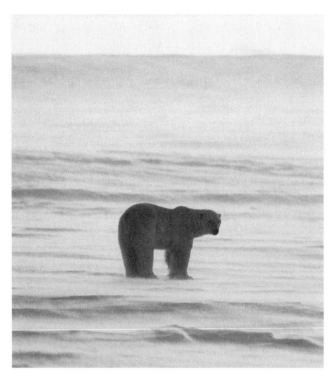

Hypothermia occurs when the body drops to below 35 degrees Celsius and kills nearly 700 people per year in the United States.

to alcoholic intoxication. Alcohol causes cutaneous vasodilation of arteries which warms the skin. Core body temperature decreases due to shunting of blood to the periphery and leads to hypothermia. Finally, another cause of hypothermia is impaired thermoregulation which is caused by failure of the hypothalamus to regulate body temperature. At-risk populations for hypothermia are elderly adults, children, and mentally impaired individuals.

Different publications have different criteria to determine mild, moderate, and severe hypothermia. In general, mild hypothermia begins when the temperature of the body falls below 35 degrees C but is still above 32 degrees C. The person will show signs of shivering, pale blue skin, slurring speech, confusion, and respiratory rate may increase. Moderate hypothermia occurs when body temperature is between 28 to 32 degrees C. Patients present in a stupor, they usually are not shivering anymore, body becomes rigid, and breathing becomes shallower. Severe hypothermia occurs when the body temperature is below 28 degrees C. Symptoms of severe hypothermia include difficulty breathing, unconsciousness, no pulse, and extreme rigidity. Patients with severe hy-

pothermia also have an increased risk for ventricular arrhythmias, which can be life threatening.

There are many tests and observations that can be done that will tell if a person is hypothermic. If the person can voluntarily stop his or her shivering then he or she most likely has mildly hypothermic. Another test is to ask the patient to count backward from 100 by a certain multiple, such as six. This requires higher reasoning by the brain and if the person is hypothermic they will not be able to accomplish this task. Another test is to check the radial pulses. If the person has a very faint or no radial pulse, then they are most likely severely hypothermic.

Treatment for patients with hypothermia is to slowly warm the body back to normal body temperature. Remove the person from the external stimulus that may be causing the hypothermia, such as cold water. Also provide warm beverages for the person to drink and monitor his or her breathing. Do not apply direct heat to a person that is hypothermic, such as a heating pad or warm water. If a heating pad is placed on the arm or legs, then cold blood will get shunted to the core and can lead to complications. Also do not massage the body of the person who is hypothermic. Individuals who are hypothermic are at an increased risk for cardiac complications and so massaging the body can exacerbate this risk. In the hospital, doctors will treat hypothermia differently based on the severity and cause. In general, doctors will use blankets and external actions to warm the body. If the patient is severely hypothermic, the doctor may infuse warm fluids into the person or have the person placed on hemodialysis. Most people with hypothermia recover without any long-term complications.

SEE ALSO: Alcoholism; Alcohol Consumption; Alzheimer's Disease; Parkinson's Disease; Hypopituitarism; Hypothyroidism.

BIBLIOGRAPHY. Rick Curtis, "Outdoor Action Guide to Hypothermia and Cold Weather Injuries," www.princeton.edu (cited November 2007); "Hypothermia," www.mayoclinic.com (cited December 2006); "Hypothermia," www.webmd.com (cited January 2007); Vinay Kumar, et al., *Pathologic Basis of Disease* (Elsevier Saunders, 2005).

PAVAN BHATRAJU
UNIVERSITY OF LOUISVILLE

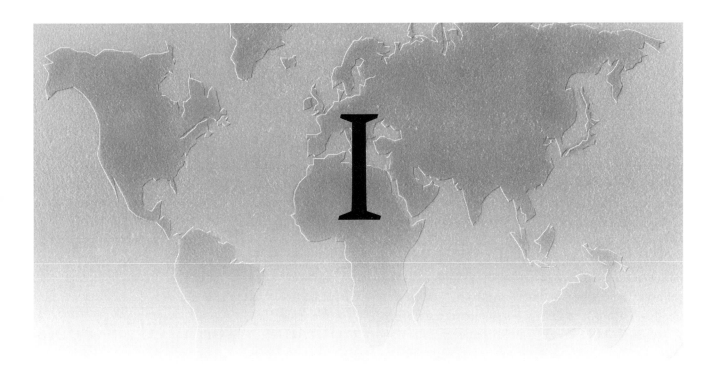

Iceland

Located in northern Europe between the Greenland Sea and the North Atlantic, the island of Iceland has the second highest living standard in the world according to the United Nations Development Programme's (UNDP) Human Development Report and is outranked only by Norway. With a per capita income of $35,700, Iceland ranks as the 12th richest nation. Although the fishing industry employs only four percent of the labor force, it generates 70 percent of export earnings. The standard of living is high, and Iceland scores particularly high on literacy, longevity, income, and social cohesion. Income is fairly evenly distributed, and unemployment is extremely low (2.1 percent). The government provides a broad safety net that includes universal access to healthcare and a generous housing subsidy.

Government spending on healthcare is extremely high in Iceland, and the government allocates an average of 26 percent of the total budget to health. In international dollars, Iceland spends $3,110 per capita, with 10.5 percent of the Gross Domestic Product (GDP) earmarked for health programs. Due to the national plan, approximately 85 percent of healthcare spending is generated by the government, and 36.5 of that spending is used to finance social security, which

is mandatory. The only private funding of healthcare in Iceland is derived form the 15 percent service fee required of all Icelanders. There are 3.62 physicians, 13.63 nurses, 0.60 midwives, 1.00 dentists, and 1.30 pharmacists per 1,000 population in Iceland.

In 1990, Parliament passed Health Services Act No. 97, which guarantees universal healthcare access to Icelanders to protect their mental, social, and physical health. The national health plan is financed through taxes (85 percent) and user fees (15 percent). Iceland is divided into healthcare regions, and primary health centers are located throughout each region. These centers provide routine healthcare, disease prevention, and home care. The centers also have responsibility for family planning, school health, and mother and child healthcare.

Iceland's population of 299,388 enjoys a life expectancy of 80.31 years, the 11th highest life expectancy rate in the world. Females outlive males an average of four years. Access to education at both the primary and secondary levels is universal, and 99 percent of the population over the age of 15 is literate. All Icelanders have access to safe drinking water and improved sanitation. Women give birth to an average of 1.92 children.

Between 1990 and 2004, infant mortality was slashed by two-thirds in Iceland, falling from six to two deaths per 1,000 live births. The current infant mortality rate of 3.29 deaths per 1,000 live births is the fifth lowest in the world. During that same period, under-5 mortality fell from seven to three deaths per 1,000 live births. Icelandic children are remarkably healthy, but four percent of infants are underweight at birth. All infant immunization rates are in the 90s: 99 percent of infants are immunized against diphtheria, pertussis, and tetanus (DPT1 and DPT3), polio, and *Haemophilus influenzae* type B, and 93 percent are immunized against measles.

Periodic earthquakes threaten the general wellbeing in Iceland. Environmental threats include water pollution caused by the runoff from fertilizer and the government's inability to sufficiently treat wastewater. HIV/AIDS is not a major concern in Iceland. With a 0.2 percent adult relevancy rate, only 220 Icelanders are living with the disease. HIV/AIDS has proved fatal to around 100 people.

When the Askja volcano erupted in 1873, it was a major economic and social catastrophe for Iceland. One in every five Icelanders died, and the country lost a fifth of its remaining population to Canada and the United States. Some scientists predict that Iceland will at some indefinite time be devastated by another volcanic eruption. Excavations of the graves of some of the 10,000 Icelanders who died in the 1873 eruption have provided scientists with new information on causes of death. Scores of Icelanders died from poisonous hydrofluoric acid that contaminated food and water sources or from illness brought on by extreme weather conditions that resulted from the eruption; the weather spread over parts of Europe. In an article published in the *Journal of Geophysical Research* in October 2004, two volcanologists predicted that a similar eruption is on its way and surmised that the aftermath would affect much of the Northern Hemisphere for months. Other volcanologists insist that the chance of a modern eruption that would threaten the health and well-being of Iceland and the surrounding area is low.

SEE ALSO: Healthcare, Europe.

BIBLIOGRAPHY. Spencer Di Scala, *Twentieth Century Europe: Politics, Society, Culture* (McGraw-Hill, 2004); Sandra Halperin, *War and Social Change in Modern Europe: The Great Transformation Revisited* (Cambridge University Press, 2004); Martin A. Levin and Martin Shapiro, eds., *Transatlantic Policymaking in an Age of Austerity: Diversity and Drift* (Georgetown University Press, 2004); Jeremy Rifkin, *The European Dream: How Europe's Vision of the Future Is Quietly Eclipsing the American Dream* (Jeremy P. Tarcher/Penguin, 2004); Richard Stone, "Iceland's Doomsday Scenario?" *Science* (v.306/5700, 2004); Peter Taylor-Gooby, *New Risks, New Welfare: The Transformation of the European Welfare State* (Oxford University Press, 2004).

ELIZABETH R. PURDY, PH.D.
INDEPENDENT SCHOLAR

Immune System and Disorders

The immune system protects the body from invasion by nonself organisms with an array of tissues, cells and organs working together through primary and secondary mechanisms. The primary line of defense is physical and chemical barriers to keep out invaders. The skin forms a tough physical barrier and secretes oil and sweat as chemical defenses. Other chemical defenses are the acid secretions in the stomach and vagina, mucous secretions in the respiratory tract and lysozymes (antibacterial enzymes) in tears. Colonies of friendly bacteria live in the intestines to use up nutrients invaders could thrive on. The flushing action of urine removes invaders from the urinary tract.

If an invader makes it past the first line of defense, a two-pronged secondary attack with nonspecific and specific responses is triggered into action. The nonspecific response is direct and immediate with chemical and cellular agents. The specific response is complex, specific to the invader and takes longer to prepare. The immune system recognizes the body's cells because they carry specific markers for recognition under normal conditions as cells that belong. When the immune system agents encounter an unrecognized invader it triggers the immune response.

To carry out the function of the immune system, organs throughout the body deploy lymphocytes (specialized white blood cells). The organs are often referred to as lymphoid organs and include the bone marrow, thymus, lymph nodes, spleen, tonsils, adenoids, appendix, lymphatic vessels to carry lymphocytes and Peyer's patches clumps of lymphoid tissue in the small intestine. Lymphocytes (B cells and T cells) and phagocytes, the cells which will become immune cells grow in the bone marrow. B cells mature in the bone marrow and T cells migrate to the thymus where they learn to distinguish self-cells from non-self invaders. Mature lymphocytes either collect in the immune tissue and organs or travel in lymphatic vessels throughout the body.

NON-SPECIFIC SECONDARY RESPONSE

Chemical nonspecific secondary response includes the release of histamine at the site of invasion to increase blood flow to the area and to increase the permeability of capillaries to allow other defense agents to enter. Kinins are released in the invaded area to increase inflammation and sensitivity and attract phagocytic white blood cells. Complement (plasma proteins) attacks the invader, penetrates the outer barrier and causes it to burst. Complement also may coat the surface of the invader to make it susceptible to phagocytic action. Interferon stimulates the inflammatory response and is antiviral by blocking synthesis of viral coat protein and halting viral cell growth.

Cellular nonspecific secondary response includes the release of phagocytes (eosinophils, neutrophils, and monocytes which grow to macrophages at the site). The invader is trapped inside a vacuole and digested with powerful enzymes. Phagocytes are also destroyed and form pus at the site of infection. Natural killer cells are totally non-specific; they contain chemicals and kill invaders (tumor cells, pathogens, viruses and even the body's own diseased cells) on contact by binding and then releasing the chemicals to make the cell membrane of the invader permeable causing it to burst.

SPECIFIC SECONDARY RESPONSE

Chemical specific secondary response includes the humoral response with the creation of specific antibodies. B-Lymphocytes (B-cells) make and secrete antibodies with a few acting as memory cells to ensure lasting immunity are produced in the bone marrow and in the fetal liver. Each lymphocyte is programmed to recognize only one specific antigen and yet B-lymphocytes can respond to millions of different antigens both naturally occurring and artificially created. T-lymphocytes are produced in the thymus and directly attack and destroy infected cells.

When the body is exposed to an invading agent, helper T-cells (also known as CD4 cells) send a signal to the B-cells to initiate the humoral response and begin antibody production. The immune system utilizes B-cells to recognize and identify the invading agent. The B-cells produce and release antibodies through the humoral response and some B-cells commonly called memory-cells record and retain the information specific to the antigen to provide long-lasting protection against each specific invading agents.

The Y-shaped antibodies have receptor binding sites that attach to the antigen or invading agent. Antibodies work in three similar though different ways; by binding to several antigens to form a clump to be devoured by phagocytes, by the complement system brings water into the cells causing the cells to burst and by opsonization coating the invading cells with antibodies with a constant region providing a receptor site matching a receptor on the phagocyte allowing the phagocyte to engulf and destroy the invading agent.

Cellular specific secondary response is mediated by T-cells. Helper T-cells activate B cells, other T cells, natural killer cells and macrophages. Cytotoxic T-cells kill cells infected by viruses, cancer and are responsible for the rejection of tranplanted organs or tissues. Suppressor T-cells slow down and turn off the immune response. Memory T-cells record information to immediately recognize an invading agent if it shows up again in the body and trigger antibody production.

DISORDERS OF THE IMMUNE SYSTEM

When the body's immune system fails to work properly, attacks the body's own cells, is compromised by a chronic or acute disease state, the body is unable to keep up with the progression of the disease. Several disorders may result.

Allergy is a hypersensitivity reaction to an invader with tissue inflammation and organ dysfunction. Because the allergen is foreign to the body, it often effects the organs with the first line of defense, the respiratory and digestive tracts. The allergic reaction may be atopic localized to a susceptible target, inherited development antigen-specific immunoglobulin to environmental or food allergens or it may be anaphylactic causing a general release of immune system mediators to certain allergens (drugs, foods, insect venoms) resulting in wide-spread immune response with vaso-dilation, itching, swelling, bronchospasm, and digestive tract or uterine muscle contractions. Cytotoxic reactions activate complement to destroy cells bound to antigens. Antigen-antibody complexes may deposit in tissues and are destroyed by the immune system causing tissue damage commonly affected organs are the skin, joints, and kidneys. Delayed hypersensitivity results from the deposit of antigen in tissues and when the immune system attacks the antigen, a later, localized inflammation occurs.

Autoimmune disease occurs when the immune system attacks the body's own tissues and create antibodies against its own cells. Common known or suspected diseases resulting from autoimmunity include arthritis, rheumatic fever, scleroderma, systemic lupus erythematosus, hormone disorders, and insulin-dependent diabetes mellitus. Nearly every tissue and organ in the body is susceptible to autoimmune attack. Autoimmunity may also occur after an infection with a disease organism with similar surface antigens to the body's. The antigen may circulate in the body until the immune system recognizes the antigen as foreign. The specific antibodies then developed for these similar organisms may then in turn react with the body's cells.

Immunodeficiency diseases result from abnormalities in the immune system leading to increase susceptibility to infection, longer-lasting infection, or more severe infection. The immunodeficiency may be genentic or caused by external factors. Individuals with immunodeficiencies often succumb to infections. Genetically caused immunodeficiency diseases include X-linked agammaglobulinema (affects males where B-cells fail to mature into antibody producing cells), DiGeorge's syndrome (thymus fails to develop resulting in suppressed T-cell response), and adenosine deaminase deficiency (absence of enzyme leads to death of B-cells and T-cells). A suppressed immune system caused by an external factor is AIDS. AIDS is caused by a retrovirus that attacks helper T-cells leading to a decrease in B-cell activity. The body is unable to form antibodies and becomes susceptible to attack from numerous rare diseases and opportunistic infections.

Cancers of the immune system, as in other organs and cells of the body, result from the proliferation of cells in the organ. Cancers of the immune system include leukemia (malignancy of the white blood cells replacing normal bone marrow elements), multiple myeloma (malignancy of plasma cells with replacement of the bone marrow leading to anemia and bone marrow and bone destruction) and non-Hodgkin's lymphomas (malignancy of T-cells and B-cells within the lymph nodes) and Hodgkin's disease (Reed-Sternberg cells, arises in one lymph node and spreads to others).

SPECIAL IMMUNE SYSTEM CONSIDERATIONS

The recognition of self versus non-self invaders can cause difficulties with organ and tissue transplants (the immune system will recognize the transplant as foreign and attempt to reject it), bone marrow transplants (graft vs. host disease where the T-cells from the donor attack and destroy the tissues of the recipient) and Rhesus antigen (a red blood cell surface antigen may cause hemolytic disease the second positive Rh factor fetus for a negative Rh factor mother).

Immunosuppressive drugs are used to prevent rejection of transplants. Corticosteroids result in reduced inflammation. Cytotoxic drugs can inhibit T-cell and B-cell immunity and inflammation. Antimetabolites inhibit the proliferation of T-cells and B-cells and some prevent T-cell activation. Cyclosporine and tacrolimus inhibit T-cell response.

Bone marrow can be cleansed of mature T-cells to prevent graft versus host disease with chemicals or monoclonal antibodies.

Passive immunity for protecting fetuses from hemolytic disease caused by Rhesus factor by administering Rh immune globulin to Rh-negative mothers within 72 hours of birth of the first Rh-positive child to destroy Rh positive cells so the mother will not produce antibodies to the Rh-positive cells.

CURRENT RESEARCH AND GLOBAL IMPLICATIONS

Stimulating or suppressing the immune response to treat disease either by increasing the body's own defense mechanisms, injecting specific immunologic proteins, creating abundant T-lymphocytes to destroy infected cells or genetically altering T-lymphocytes to recognize and destroy cancer cells when reinjected into the body has the potential to improve quality of life.

Continued research on the function, stimulation and suppression of the immune system could decrease the disease states caused by immune system disorders, the development of new vaccines. The potential may exist to treat immune system disorders with immune-system components to fight diseases such as cancer, AIDS, allergies, and autoimmune diseases.

SEE ALSO: Acquired Immunity; Active Immunity; AIDS; Autoimmune Diseases (General); Chronic Fatigue Syndrome; Diabetes Type I (Juvenile Diabetes); Guillian-Barr Syndrome; Immunization/Vaccination; Infectious Diseases (General); Lupus; Lymphatic Diseases; Multiple Sclerosis; Myasthenia Gravis; Passive Immunity; Rheumatoid Arthritis; Scleroderma.

BIBLIOGRAPHY. Allan R. Cook, ed., *Immune System Disorders Sourcebook* (Omnigraphics, 1997); Jeffrey L. Kishiyama, and Daniel C. Adelman, "Allergic and Immunologic Disorders," in *Basic and Clinical Pharmacology* (Appleton & Lange, 1998); Maya Pines, *Arousing the Fury of the Immune System: New Ways to Boost the Body's Defenses* (Howard Hughes Medical Institute, 1998).

LYN MICHAUD
INDEPENDENT SCHOLAR

Immunization/Vaccination

Human beings are frequently infected with a variety of pathogens, including bacteria, viruses, fungi, and parasites. A vaccine is a preparation that, when administered, can provide protection against a particular infectious agent. The idea for a vaccine was borne of observations that once an individual had suffered a particular infectious ailment, that person was unlikely to contract that disease again. There are reports dating to 200 B.C. of individuals in India and China inoculating themselves and others with infected matter from those suffering with mild cases of smallpox. Much later, Edward Jenner observed that milkmaids who had come into contact with cowpox did not develop smallpox when exposed. He subsequently tested this observation by directly exposing individuals to the fluid from cowpox lesions and then challenging them with a controlled infectious exposure, or inocu-

lation, of smallpox. His test subjects did not become ill with smallpox, providing preliminary validation of the concept of vaccination.

Ultimately, vaccination seeks to expose the immune system to a weakened, killed, or fragment of a pathogen in a way that generates an immune response so that upon exposure to that actual pathogen there is a rapid removal of the pathogen. This rapid response ultimately will prevent spread of the invading organism from the portal of entry and would also prevent subsequent replication and disease manifestations.

THE IMMUNE SYSTEM

A basic understanding of the immune system helps to clarify the importance and problems inherent in vaccinations. When the body is exposed to a pathogen the body responds in several ways. There are components of the innate immune system that react to whatever pathogen gains entry into the body. The innate immune system reaction is rapid, but is nonspecific and confers no "memory" meaning that if the body is exposed to the same pathogen again the response is not faster nor stronger the second time. There are several cell types that are involved in the innate immune response including mast cells, neutrophils, basophils, eosinophils, dendritic cells, and neutrophils. While these cells all have specific functions, they have the capacity to kill a broad range of infecting organisms. Innate immunity is a more primitive response, and there are similar defense mechanisms in not only humans, but all plant and animal life.

In contrast, the adaptive immune system is composed of several different cell types, including B cells which are responsible for making antibodies. Antibodies recognize specific features of an infectious organism, and by binding, can promote the sequestration, removal or engulfment of that pathogen. T-cells can help direct the immune system and can also directly kill cells of the body that are infected with a pathogen. It takes longer for the adaptive immune system to respond to an infectious agent. However, upon exposure to a bacteria or virus there is concurrently the process of eliminating the offending agent and also the development of "memory" cells. These memory cells, both B and T-cells, have been exposed to a particular infectious agent so that upon a second exposure there is a more rapid and specific response that can clear the body of that particular infection

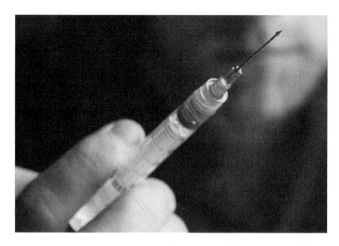

A vaccine is a preparation that, when administered, can provide protection against a particular infectious agent.

before it has a chance to cause disease. Oftentimes there is a cumulative response, in that a single exposure does provide some level of memory and protection, but multiple exposures are needed to develop a high level of immunity. The process of immunization takes advantage of the ability of the immune system to remember an infection and become more prepared to clear a subsequent infection.

ACTIVE IMMUNIZATION

Immunizations are frequently divided into two types: active and passive immunization. Active immunization takes into account the properties of the adaptive immune system described above. The goal of an active immunization is to stimulate a response in the immune system by exposing the body to a particular infectious agent. There are several different vaccine preparations that exist.

For both bacteria and viruses, often the whole organism that has been killed will be used as the vaccine. Other times, an attenuated, or weakened, form of a bacteria or virus can be used. These attenuated vaccines are recognized by the immune system as foreign and the immune system generates a response against them, but the pathogens themselves are not capable of causing disease. Other times, the vaccine will contain only a fragment, subunit, or protein component of a particular bacteria or virus. Lastly, some pathogens do not cause damage to humans themselves, but rather they secrete toxins that can cause disease. Some vaccines use modified versions of those toxins to stimulate an immune response. Alternatively, vaccination can be accomplished by exposing an individual to a similar and related infectious organism that does not cause disease but can generate cross-immunity.

PASSIVE IMMUNIZATION

Passive immunization is used when there is a need to provide short-term and rapid protection against a particular infection and there is not time to administer an immunization and await the development of the stronger, memory immune response or in an individual that is immunocompromised and unable to mount a sufficient response on his or her own. Passive immunity involves administration of antibodies taken from human serum and transfusing it into the individual who has been exposed to the specific pathogen. This method of vaccination is not part of routine disease prevention.

VACCINE AVAILABILITY

There are several factors that influence whether or not a vaccine is available for a particular bacteria or virus. For some organisms, the lifecycle and the components of a successful immune response are not known, precluding the successful development of a vaccine. In other cases, the pathogen has developed mechanisms to evade the immune system and may mutate rapidly, may change the surface proteins, or use other techniques such that each time the immune system encounters it, the appearance is different and memory cells are not able to respond appropriately. For example, while HIV is very well studied, it mutates rapidly making it difficult to develop a successful vaccine.

There are other factors that influence whether a particular vaccine is available on a global market, including storage requirements, such as need for refrigeration or a need for sterile syringes. In addition, the cost of some vaccines makes wide distribution unrealistic. For example, a vaccine against human papillomavirus was recently developed; however, the price is sufficiently prohibitive, and it is not widely available.

There are a number of infectious agents for which vaccines are available, including hepatitis A, hepatitis B, Poliovirus, yellow fever, influenza virus, diphtheria, *haemophilus influenzae*, measles, mumps, pertussis, rubella, tetanus, varicella, smallpox, tuberculosis, human papillomavirus, meningococcus, rotavirus and others.

Many countries have mandated certain vaccines for entry into the school system or travel into the country. Mass vaccinations have led to the elimination of smallpox worldwide, and the near-eradication of polio. In addition, in areas with a large percentage of the population receiving vaccinations (herd immunity) there have been significant decreases in infections such as measles, mumps, rubella, *haemophilus influenzae* and others. Increased global access to vaccination and primary health services will further reduce the global burden of infectious disease.

SEE ALSO: Acquired Immunity; Active Immunity; Immunology; Infectious Diseases (General); Innate Immunity.

BIBLIOGRAPHY. Allan R. Cook, ed., *Immune System Disorders Sourcebook* (Omnigraphics Inc, 1997); Catherine J.M. Diodati, *Immunization: History, Ethics, Law and Health* (Integral Aspects, 1999).

CHRISTINE CURRY
INDEPENDENT SCHOLAR

Immunologist

Immunologists are people working in the biomedical field of immunology studying the immune systems of biological organisms from a variety of perspectives including the investigation of molecular structure and function, and evolutionary, clinical, diagnostic, and therapeutic angles. They examine the relationships between pathogens, immune responses, and the environment in the field of host defense. Immunologists may be medical specialists trained in the field of immunology, physician-scientists, or research scientists. The work of immunologists intersects with professionals in many other fields such as rheumatology, infectious disease, hematology, and organ transplantation. At the nexus of the study and practice of immunology lies the study of epidemiology, which informs the transmission course of and adaptation to disease.

The historical origins of immunology can be traced back to at least 430 B.C.E. when Thucydides recorded the plague in Athens. In many ways, he became a fore-runner for future immunologists. He described in his writings that many people who recovered from the illness could care for the sick without contracting the plague for a second time. The next pivotal moment in the history of immunologists occurred centuries later. In 1796, Edward Jenner, a doctor in England, introduced the concept of vaccination immunity using cowpox to provide cross-immunity for smallpox in humans.

A scientific approach to the study of immunology developed later in the 19th and 20th centuries. Louis Pasteur furthered concepts used by Jenner and contributed to the fields of bacteriology and immunity through studies of cholera, rabies, and anthrax. The experimental work of Pasteur and Robert Koch in the 19th century cemented the foundation of germ theory (i.e., the notion that diseases are caused by pathogens) intricate to the understanding of immunology. Shibasaburo Kitasato and Emil von Behring provided the ground for understanding antibodies and immunity in the late 1890s through their studies of animals immune to tetanus and diphtheria, diseases caused by organisms that produce toxins harmful to their host.

Many Nobel laureates and scientists of the 20th century have made seminal contributions to the evolution of field of immunology. For example, Jules Bordet provided evidence about the existence and role of the complement system in the immune response. Karl Landsteiner developed a classification system for blood groups intricate to the understanding of blood transfusion science. Gerald Edelman and Rodney Porter discovered the exact chemical structure of an antibody protein and were awarded a Nobel Prize in 1972 for their work. Edward Thomas and Joseph Murray received a Nobel Prize in 1990 for their important contributions to cell and organ transplantation in treating human disease, notably leukemia.

Increasing scientific knowledge and rapid technological growth in the 21st century increasingly provides immunologists an opportunity for a deeper understanding of the function, adaptation, and behavior of the immune system. Advances in the characterization and treatment of autoimmune disorders and inflammatory processes, better donor–recipient matching and rejection prevention in allograft cell and organ transplantation, and new developments in genomic medicine for individualized patient treatment for a variety of autoimmune and pathogenic diseases are current areas of exciting growth in the field of immunology. Gene therapies remain in their infancy in the treatment of a variety of immune disorders, but they hold an amazing therapeutic potential. An increasing understanding of the complexities in immune signaling pathways is allowing immunologists to create a rapidly evolving landscape of options in the diagnosis and treatment of acquired infections, cancers, autoimmune diseases, and organ transplantations.

SEE ALSO: Allergy; Bacteriology; Bone Marrow Diseases; Immune System and Disorders; Immunization/Vaccination; Immunology; Immunosuppression; Immunotherapy; Organ Transplantation; Pasteur, Louis; Psychoimmunology; Psychoneuroimmunology; Virology.

BIBLIOGRAPHY. Charles Janeway, *Immunobiology: The Immune System in Health and Disease* (Garland, 2005); Arthur Silverstein, *A History of Immunology* (Academic Press, 1989).

JUSTIN M. LIST, M.A.R.
STRITCH SCHOOL OF MEDICINE
LOYOLA UNIVERSITY CHICAGO

Immunology

In the late 18th century Dr. Edward Jenner stumbled upon the notion of the immune system following his discovery that cowpox protected him against a human pathogen known as smallpox. This process of immunity by introduction of more mild strains of a disease became known as vaccination. Unfortunately, very little was understood about the etiology of infection and the subsequent induction of the host immune response. Dr. Robert Koch, over 100 years later, established the first relationship between cause and effect as it relates to infection. Out of his work came specific postulates used to understand which pathogens are fundamentally responsible for specific diseases and what components of those pathogens contribute to disease progression. The concept of immunology was born.

Immunology is the study of the immune system, the primary defense mechanism of the body. In humans, the immune system is composed of specific immune cells and produces and utilizes numerous unique, chemical signals. Each component of the immune system works collectively to prevent invasion by foreign substances, or pathogens. Examples of such pathogens include bacteria, viruses, fungi, and parasites. Each utilizes a specific method of transmission such as fecal-oral, airborne, direct inoculation, direct contact, and congenital. To elicit an immune response, these pathogens must not only be foreign to the body, but they must be large enough molecules, chemically complex, and degradable. Still heavily studied area, the human immune system consists of both innate and acquired responses to pathogenic invasion with both types of responses interacting on many complex, biological levels.

Typical components of the innate immune system include normal physiologic and chemical barriers such as the skin, saliva, the pH of the stomach, tears, enzymes, and mucous. During the innate response, the human body utilizes immune cells such as neutrophils, monocytes, NK cells, and tissue macrophages. These cells respond to specific foreign patterns through preexisting pattern recognition receptors. Each type of cell has the ability to kill the invading organism through a nonspecific process known as phagocytosis, a mechanism first discovered by the Russian immunologist Dr. Elie Metchnikoff. This process includes engulfment of the pathogen and fusion with acidic enzymes within the host cell. Innate immune cells can also kill through the complement cascade as well as extracellular mechanisms involving soluble mediators. Complement activation includes first lysing the pathogens, and then coating them with a material targeting them for phagocytosis. Complement involves the following three pathways: classical, alternative, and lectin binding. All converge on a common pathway where a pore is created within the target cell membrane leading to lysis of that cell. In innate immunity, the characteristic immune response includes chemical messages in the form of cytokines, pyrogens (fever producers), interferon, and complement. While innate immunity is an effective means of fighting off foreign bodies, it is sometimes not enough. Thankfully, our bodies possess another type of immunity known as acquired immunity.

Acquired, or adaptive immunity, can be divided into humoral and cell mediated immunity. The response time is much slower when compared with innate immunity. Both humoral and cell-mediated responses depend on specific cells known as B and T cells which develop and mature in the primary lymphoid organs of the bone marrow and thymus gland, respectively. Following maturation, these cells leave the primary lymphoid organs and move to secondary lymphoid organs, which include the spleen, lymph nodes, and tonsils. B cells recognize intact pathogen, whereas T cells only recognize pathogen that has been broken down into protein components and presented on the cell surface of another immune cell. B cells communicate with other cells through a specific receptor, whereas T cells must bind using a receptor and an additional cell surface molecule known as the MHC. There are two important types of T cells, CD8 and CD4, and each binds to a specific set of cell surface molecules.

Already armed with a set level of specificity for an invading pathogen, B and T cells are induced to proliferate once they encounter pathogen so that the population of immune cells with identical specificity for a pathogen increases. This increases the potential for specific destruction and containment of the foreign organism. This proliferation, or clonal expansion of cells, in response to the first encounter with pathogen is considered the primary response, and it is soon followed by a more rapid and larger secondary response when the immune system encounters the same pathogen again. This secondary response includes memory B and T cells which contribute to the faster nature of this response.

It is during this secondary response that the different functional capacities of B and T cells are revealed. B cells will differentiate into plasma cells, which will secrete antibodies, or immunoglobulins. There are five different groups of immunoglobulins each with distinct functions and biologic properties: IgG, IgM, IgE, IgD, and IgA. These antibodies are specific for antigens found on the pathogens. Antigens, or any foreign substance recognized by a specific receptor, can include the following: proteins, carbohydrates, lipids, or nucleic acids considered foreign to the body. Once T cells encounter pathogen a second time they also possess the capacity to become memory cells. They function as either helper T cells or cytotoxic T cells both of which play integral roles in pathogenic destruction and induction of the host immune response.

Immunology utilizes many tests to determine the presence or absence or antibodies or antigens. These include radioimmunoassay (RIA), enzyme-linked immunosorbent assay (ELISA), direct immunofluoresence, monoclonal antibody production, and Western blotting.

Our understanding of the process of immunology is crucial, for it allows further exploration into disease prevention, leads to the discovery of vaccines, offers insight into effective and successful methods to fight infection, and uncovers the intricate mechanisms involved in the immune response to pathogenic invasion. Maybe the most important of all of the benefits to our understanding of immunology lies in the ability to improve quality of life and to evade death.

SEE ALSO: Acquired Immunity; Immunologist; Innate Immunity.

BIBLIOGRAPHY. Charles Janeway, Paul Travers, and Mark Walport, *Immunobiology, the Immune System in Health and Disease* (Elsevier Science Ltd./Garland Publishing 1999); Ian Todd, and Gavin Spickett, *Immunology* (Blackwell Publishing, 2005).

Melissa K. Wolinski
Michigan State University

Immunosuppression

Immunosuppression is a natural act or medical treatment that reduces the activation or efficacy of the natural immune system in humans and animals. Generally, immunosuppression is a result of viral activity (such as human immunodeficiency virus [HIV]) or other natural causes. In some cases, immunosuppression is an unwanted side effect of treatment for particular diseases or conditions. In recent years, this process been very important in allowing people to accept transplants such as kidneys which might otherwise be rejected by the natural immunities of the patient.

There have long been particular conditions that lower the response of the human immune system, with the most wellknown in recent years being HIV. In fact, suffering from many illnesses and medical conditions may weaken a person, and as a result, lower the activation of their immune system, making them more susceptible to other illnesses or diseases. This phenomenon has been observed since ancient times. Often, when someone is suffering from a particular condition, others with any type of potentially infectious disease—even the common cold—are prevented from visiting to help ensure that the patient avoids additional illnesses, an even made more possible due to the patient's compromised immune system.

Additionally, some diseases and conditions are best treated by methods that can further reduce or compromise the patient's immune system. For this reason, people who are having or have recently had treatment by chemotherapy are often advised not to visit friends or relatives in hospitals; as their immune system has been suppressed by treatment, exposure to other conditions may result in infection or additional serious complications.

The immune system often reacts to the transplantation of new organs by attempting to reject the organ as if it were an infection or disease. For this reason, the recipient is often treated with immunosuppressive drugs. The first of these to be identified was cortisone, but it had many side effects that limited its use. In 1959, azathiprine was produced and found to be far more specific in its treatment of organ donor recipients. The discovery of cyclosporine in 1970 as an effective immunosuppressive drug changed the nature of kidney transplantation, allowing it to become a far more common practice for using organs from donors who did not perfectly matched those of recipients. Since then, this drug has been used successfully for liver transplants, lung transplants, pancreas transplants, and heart transplants.

Some of the pioneering research in the field of immunosuppression was conducted by Dr. Joseph E. Murray, professor of surgery at Harvard Medical School since 1970, who was the chief plastic surgeon at the Children's Hospital, Boston, from 1972 until 1985. In 1990, he was awarded the Nobel Prize in Physiology or Medicine for his work; Dr. Murray and his team were credited with the first successful kidney transplant, which took place at Peter Bent Brigham Hospital in Boston on December 23, 1954. Eight years later, he conducted the first kidney transplant with a kidney from a donor unrelated to the patient; immunosuppressive drugs were key to the success of the operation.

SEE ALSO: Organ Transplantation.

BIBLIOGRAPHY. Steven A. Frank, *Immunology and Evolution of Infectious Disease* (Princeton University Press, 2002); Janis Kuby, *Immunology* (W. H. Freeman, 2003).

JUSTIN CORFIELD
GEELONG GRAMMAR SCHOOL, AUSTRALIA

Immunotherapy

The immune system, through a variety of responses working together, protects the body from invading pathogens and eliminates disease. When the body's immune system fails to work properly or is compromised by a chronic or acute disease, the body is unable to keep up with the progression of the disease and needs additional help to fight off debilitating effects.

Providing passive immunity is one of the most widely recognized and used forms of immunotherapy. This process transfers immunity by direct injection of antibodies or antiserum to prevent infectious disease. This provides immediate—though temporary—protection from a specific disease-causing bacteria, virus, or toxin and can also protect persons unable to produce antibodies themselves. These injected antibodies have a short lifespan. No memory cells are created leaving the individual is left susceptible to infection by the same antigen.

Any immunotherapy, whether classified as investigational or approved for use, relies on stimulating the immune response to treat a disease either by increasing the body's own defense mechanisms, injecting specific immunologic proteins, creating abundant T-lymphocytes to destroy infected cells, or genetically altering T-lymphocytes to recognize and destroy cancer cells when reinjected into the body. According to the American Cancer Society, immunotherapy is used to enhance the primary treatment. Immunotherapy relies on activating a portion of the immune system through the use of proteins or medications to improve immune function. An approved use of BCG (an extract of weakened tuberculosis) has been effective in treating bladder cancer by increasing production of T-lymphocytes. Levamisole is approved as an adjunct to fluorouracil for colon cancer to increase macrophage activity.

The discovery of cytokines, a large diverse group of proteins functioning and released by various cells of the immune system has led to numerous uses of specific cytokines for treating infections, inflammations, autoimmune disorders, and neoplasms. The approved uses of cytokines include interferon–alpha for the treatment of two forms of leukemia, malignant melanoma, and Kaposi's sarcoma; interferon–beta for treating relapsing multiple sclerosis; interferon–gamma for treating chronic granulomatous disease; and interleukin–2 for treating metastatic renal cell carcinoma. Research continues into numerous uses of cytokines for immunotherapy.

Other forms of immunotherapy are still being investigated. Gene therapy is being tested as a way to remove melanoma tumors throughout the body. Researchers are experimenting with isolating white blood cells and inserting T-lymphocyte receptors to recognize and destroy cancer. When reinjected into the body, these altered cells seek out and destroy specific cancer cells throughout the body.

Another possible use for immunotherapy is in HIV infection. The HIV virus destroys helper T-lymphocytes. These cells are important to modulating the immune response. When these cells are destroyed, the entire immune system becomes compromised. T-lymphocytes, the so-called natural killer cells exist in the blood; some have the specificity to seek out and destroy HIV. Theoretically, a patient could have blood drawn, and, in a laboratory environment, have the number of these HIV-specific T-lymphocytes created using a polymerase chain reaction (PCR). These could then be injected back into the patient to assist in fighting disease.

In theory, the purpose of treating the immune system with immune-system components increases the body's ability to fight diseases such as cancer, AIDS, allergies, and autoimmune diseases. In these conditions, the body fails to recognize its own cells and the immune system begins to automatically destroy those cells.

With some success, immunotherapy has attracted attention from governments and academic researchers. While currently being used effectively for some forms of cancer and allergies, failures have occurred as well. There is hope that immunotherapy can be used for other diseases and to prevent rejection of transplanted organs.

SEE ALSO: Acquired Immunity; Active Immunity; Allergy; Cancer Alternative Therapy; Immune System and Disorders; Passive Immunity.

BIBLIOGRAPHY. Jose Alexandre M. Barbuto, Emmanuel T. Akporiaye, and Evean M. Hersch, "Immunopharmacology," in *Basic and Clinical Pharmacology* (Appleton & Lange, 1998); *Merck Manual of Medical Information*, 2nd home ed. (Merck Research Laboratories, 2003); *New Ways to Boost the Body's Defenses Arousing the Fury of the Immune System* (Howard Hughes Medical Institute, 1998); "What Is Immunotherapy?" www.cancer.org (cited April 2005).

LYN MICHAUD
INDEPENDENT SCHOLAR

Impetigo

Impetigo is a superficial skin disease that is usually found in children between 2 and 6 years old as well as older people who play close contact sports such as American football, rugby, and wrestling. The name *impetigo* derives from the Latin *impetere* ("assail") because it often results from these contact sports. It is sometimes commonly known as "school sores."

The most common form of impetigo starts as an inflamed region of skin about half an inch in diameter. The incubation period of the infection is between one and three days and is indicated by the appearance of pimple-like lesions with the skin around these lesions turning red. The lesions then fill with pus that breaks down over the next four to six days and forms a thick crust.

The main cause of impetigo is from the streptoccocus strain known as *Streptoccocus pyogenes*, which also causes strep throat; impetigo can also be caused by *Staphylococcus aureus*. The infection is initially spread by lesions or with nasal carriers and cannot be carried by dead streptococci in the air.

Impetigo often occurs alongside other injuries to the skin such as insect bites and cuts, which can make it difficult to diagnose correctly. Aside from examination, the most common method of discovery of impetigo is in the form of itchy skin. Patients with a history of cold sores are statistically more likely to have infections of impetigo.

Treatment of impetigo depends on the type of skin lesion that appears and the age of the infected person. At its simplest, treatment can involve washing the affected areas with soap and water or using diluted tea tree oil with an inert carrier oil. Many general practitioners recommend the use of bactericidal ointment and, in more severe cases, the use of oral antibiotics. In all cases, it is important to dissolve the skin scabs with ointment, as the bacteria that causes impetigo lives underneath the scabs. The tea tree oil solution is an exception to this rule, as this solution is generally capable of penetrating the scab. Once treated, impetigo usually clears up in three to five days.

SEE ALSO: Skin Diseases; Staphlococcal Infections; Streptococcal Infections.

BIBLIOGRAPHY. Wayne Biddle, *Field Guide to Germs* (Henry Holt, 2002); Prisca Middlemiss, *What's that Rash? How to Identify and Treat Childhood Rashes* (Hamlyn, 2002); Carol Turkington, *Encyclopedia of Skin and Skin Disorders* (Facts on File, 2002); David Weeden, *Skin Pathology* (Harcourt, 2002).

JUSTIN CORFIELD
GEELONG GRAMMAR SCHOOL, AUSTRALIA

Impotence

Impotence, often called erectile dysfunction (ED) when discussed in a biomedical context, is the inability to sustain a penile erection sufficient for satisfactory sexual intercourse. An estimated 15 to 30 million men worldwide suffer from some degree of this condition; more prevalent among older men, younger men are also vulnerable to ED. While biomedical treatments for ED, like Viagra®, have become popular worldwide, the causes of this condition can be physical and psychological, and are often a mixture of both. Although the majority of cases of ED can be treated pharmacologically, the causes of each case are unique to the individual sufferer. Further, the practical understanding of what kind of sexual performance constitutes ED or impotence varies according to culture and location, since individual ideas about what constitutes "satisfactory" sex vary according to these factors. Ideas about the causes of ED or impotence vary similarly; depending on the particular healing systems to which individual men subscribe, elements as diverse as poor blood flow and witchcraft may be viewed as etiological factors. In the biomedical view, ED is caused by physical factors that impede blood flow to the penis; these include noncommunicable diseases (NCDs) like type 2 diabetes and heart disease, and nerve damage, often caused by spinal cord injury, prostate surgery, or degenerative nerve disease. ED is compounded, and in some cases caused, by emotional factors including stress, depression, and interpersonal disharmony.

IMPOTENCE IN NON-WESTERN CULTURES

Less-than-ideal erections have long been seen as a concern worldwide, although different cultures hold different ideals of sexual performance and understand erectile difficulty to be caused and cured by different factors. In China, for instance, traditional medicine has dealt with impotence for over 2,000 years. Chinese traditional medicine understands impotence as a problem resulting from a bodily energy blockage located in the liver or kidney; this condition is treated with herbal medicine and acupuncture. In many cultures, such as that of the Azande of north central Africa, illness is believed to be caused by the intervention of malevolent spirits; the cause of impotence is thought to be witchcraft, and the condition is treated by counteracting the witch. The herbal treatment of impotence, as well as ideas of erectile difficulty caused by spirit intervention, coexist in many areas with the use of pharmaceutical treatments for ED.

RECENT HISTORY OF IMPOTENCE IN THE WEST

Ideas about the causes and nature of impotence have changed dramatically in western societies over the past century. At the turn of the 19th century, persistent impotence was understood as a medical problem, but one with behavioral roots. Too much sex, masturbation, or "perverse"(other than heterosexual, procreative) sex were thought to physically damage the penis and deplete what was thought to be a limited supply of energy-giving sperm. Impotence was treated with behavioral change, specifically warnings to reduce sexual activity and perform only heterosexual, traditional sexual acts. Behavioral treatment was often accompanied with medical treatment, such as surgical treatment for urethral strictures to address the physical damage that doctors thought was caused by excessive sex.

As psychoanalysis, Sigmund Freud's theory of the unconscious and the treatment of neuroses, became popular in the first half of the 20th century, impotence came to be seen as a symptom of underlying psychological problems. With the popularity of psychoanalysis, sexuality became to be commonly seen as a natural drive, albeit one that could be expressed incorrectly in individuals suffering from childhood trauma. Thus, the treatment for impotence was no longer behavioral change but participation in a psychoanalytic talking cure designed to uncover trauma and set sexual development on a healthy path.

Psychoanalysis fell out of favor in the latter half of the 20th century, and biomedical explanations for physical conditions previously thought to be caused by psychological problems have since been adopted. Sexual response has come to be understood as a largely biological issue, although one that could be affected by emotions. From this, impotence came to be understood as a largely biological pathology. The development of biomedical treatments for impotence, beginning with sale of the penile implant in 1973, cemented this view. The penile vacuum pump, introduced in 1983, and the pharmacological remedies of injectible papaverine (1995) and similarly acting urethral suppositories (1997) followed. While these biomedical interventions never became widely popular due to the difficulty and discomfort of their use, their existence helped to support and spread the idea that nonnormative erections are a biomedically treatable problem.

FROM IMPOTENCE TO ERECTILE DYSFUNCTION

The current popularity of thinking about, and treating, less-than-ideal erections as a biomedical problem is largely due to two factors: the clear redefinition of impotence as a medical issue and the introduction of noninvasive pharmaceutical interventions for impotence. Because the concept of "impotence" connoted weak masculinity, in the early 1990s health professionals and pharmaceutical companies sought to destigmatize less-than-ideal erections by clearly redefining them as a disease condition; they accomplished this by terming impotence "erectile dysfunction." This reconceptualization went hand-in-hand

with a new and more appealing treatment option: Viagra. While earlier medical treatments were cumbersome and uncomfortable, Viagra (sildenafil) is a pill. The drug was introduced by Pfizer in 1998, and it revolutionized the medical treatment of ED. Viagra was introduced simultaneously in multiple countries, and was soon available (if sometimes via smuggling, internet pharmacy, or "Viagra tourism") worldwide. Viagra, a vasodilator, works by enlarging penile blood vessels to increase blood flow, which in turn causes an erection. This drug was followed in 2003 by Eli Lilly Icos' Cialis® (tadalafil) and in 2005 by Bayer's Levitra® (vardenafil), which work in essentially the same way as Viagra.

With the advent and global sale of these medications, the idea of nonnormative erections as a biomedical problem has spread worldwide. The popularization of the ED model for understanding nonnormative erections has helped to destigmatize and provide medical assistance for the condition, bringing relief to millions of men. However, the global spread of this sort of understanding has also been critiqued. Studies of couples in which men have begun to use Viagra have revealed that women are often unhappy with the new focus on penetrative sexuality that Viagra may induce, and sexologists have argued that the focus on restoring normative erectile function limits human sexuality and enforces traditional gender roles. Critics of medicalization have voiced the concern that the medicalization of aging, including age-related changes in erectile function, makes individuals unhappy with their natural bodies and dependent on costly and unnecessary drugs.

IMPOTENCE AND CHRONIC DISEASE

Medical studies report that ED is increasing at epidemic rates across the globe. While this is due in part to growing understandings of nonnormative erections as cases of ED, problems with erectile function are also increasing as a symptom of the global epidemic of NCD. Developed nations have gone through an "epidemiologic transition" in which the leading causes of morbidity shift from infectious disease and injury to chronic NCDs like cancer, diabetes, and heart disease. As people in developing nations adopt processed-food, heavy Western diets, and sedentary lifestyles, NCDs have become a global epidemic and significant cause of global morbidity. ED is a symptom of many NCDs, like type 2 diabetes and heart disease, which impede blood flow. Thus, as NCDs have increased, so has the occurrence of ED.

Public health campaigns, as well as pharmaceutical marketing, have begun to make use of the link between ED and NCDs to encourage men to seek medical help and make healthful lifestyle changes. Men who do not see their doctors for treatment of NCDs may be encouraged to do so by the fear or experience of ED. Thus, a growing number of public health interventions aimed at preventing or treating NCDs make use of ED treatment as a way to draw men to healthcare providers.

SEE ALSO: American Urological Association (AUA); Diabetes Type II; Heart Diseases (General); Male Genital Disorders; Prostate Cancer; Reproductive Health (General).

BIBLIOGRAPHY. Andrew S. Crimmel, Chad S. Conner, and Manoj Monga, "Withered Yang: A Review of Traditional Chinese Medical Treatment of Male Infertility and Erectile Dysfunction," *Journal of Andrology* (v.22/2, 2001); Ian Eardley and Sethia Krishna, *Erectile Dysfunction: Current Investigation and Management* (Mosby, 2003); Maud Kamatenesi-Mugisha and Hannington Oryem-Origa, "Traditional Herbal Remedies Used in the Management of Sexual Impotence and Erectile Dysfunction in Western Uganda," *African Health Sciences* (v.5/1, 2005); Annie Potts, et al., "'Viagra Stories': Challenging "Erectile Dysfunction," *Social Science & Medicine* (v.59, 2003); Leonore Tiefer, "The Medicalization of Impotence: Normalizing Phallocentrism," *Gender & Society* (v.8/3, 1994).

EMILY WENTZELL
UNIVERSITY OF MICHIGAN

In Situ

The term *in situ* comes from the Latin and means "in the/its place." In biology, the term usually refers to the study of an organism where it naturally occurs, such as in arid and desert conditions or at the bottom of deep ocean troughs, rather than how the organism reacts in a laboratory. In medical research, in situ research means studying the way people interact with their normal work or home environment to discover the potential sources of the various problems or disorders that may and do occur. This is particularly important when working out causes of problems based on occupational or residential factors, such as working in a place with regular exposure to radiation or living in a house that has major environmental problems such as dampness or pollution.

The study of problems in workplace environments has led to medical researchers developing the concept of occupational cancer, first developed by the British surgeon Sir Percivall Pott who, in 1775, made the discovery of the link between scrotal cancer in chimney sweeps with their regular exposure to soot.

The term *in situ* when used by oncologists usually refers to the study of malignant cancer cells in their location within a person rather than isolated on a petri dish or in a test tube. It can also be used to describe a carcinoma to refer to malignant cells that are present in the epithelium which have not been invaded beyond the basal lamina into deeper tissues. This is particularly important for developing techniques, including laser surgery. Bladder cancer at stage 0 is called a carcinoma in situ while it remains localized in the inner layer of the urinary bladder; however, as soon as it spreads, it is said to be no longer in situ. Similarly, while a stomach cancer carcinoma is only affecting the stomach, it is known as being in situ.

Geneticists have used the term *in situ* meaning "in the chromosome." An example of this is "fluorescent in situ hybridization," abbreviated as "FISH," which can happen to chromosomes in cells when a target sequence is being observed.

SEE ALSO: Oncology.

BIBLIOGRAPHY. K. H. Choo, ed., *In Situ Hybridization Protocols, Vol. 33* (Springer-Verlag, 1994); Bruce E. Rittmann, et al., *In Situ Bioremediation* (Noyes Publications, 1994).

JUSTIN CORFIELD
GEELONG GRAMMAR SCHOOL, AUSTRALIA

In Vitro

The strict translation of *in vitro* from Latin is "in glass." Historically, in vitro studies were carried out in glass containers (test tubes, beakers). Now, in vitro research refers to research performed in an artificial environment and refers to experiments in culture media, petri dishes, or other controlled environments outside of living organisms.

In vitro research is common to formal laboratory settings. Because of the controlled environment, there are typically fewer variables and results are easier to distinguish. An advantage of this type of research is the ability to focus on specific component parts of organisms and how they function. Often, in vitro research is centered on one modification and the subsequent reaction upon the specific cellular component being tested. For example, in vitro studies could be used to discern function of specific enzymes and receptors. In addition, in vitro research is typically less expensive to perform and yields results that can be extended into different fields of technology. Initial pharmaceutical research is typically done in vitro, as metabolic pathways are better defined and the mechanism of action delineated. This background is necessary prior to the creation of new medications.

One current use of in vitro technology is in vitro fertilization (IVF). Infertility is typically defined as inability to conceive within 12 months of unprotected intercourse. Couples with certain types of infertility have achieved pregnancy using this technique. Specifically, a patient's ovaries are stimulated with a particular hormone to cause ovulation and maturation of eggs. Then, the eggs are surgically retrieved and fertilized with sperm in an in vitro laboratory setting, typically in petri dishes. The fertilized eggs become zygotes and typically, when they develop into six- to eight-cell embryos (approximately two to three days later), they are then transferred to the patient's uterus with the intent to progress to a successful pregnancy. Potential risks of IVF may include difficulties with the medication to initially stimulate the ovaries (resulting in either lack of ovulation or ovarian hyperstimulation syndrome), operative risks in obtaining the eggs or transferring the embryos, lack of adequate fertilization or progression to viable embryos, multiple gestations, other complications of pregnancy, and psychological stress. Additionally, the several-step procedure of IVF is expensive, and may be cost prohibitive to some couples, as insurance coverage for the management of infertility varies between different carriers and different states.

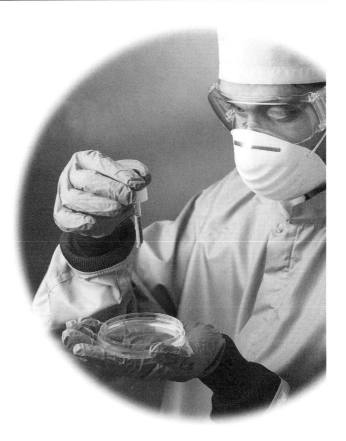

In vitro fertilization (IVF) has enabled couples with certain types of infertility to achieve pregnancy through this method.

The controlled environment of in vitro studies is sometimes a disadvantage when drawing conclusions as to how living organisms will respond with the same modification. Because living organisms may have multiple other adaptations related to the experimental change, sometimes results of in vitro studies are not only inaccurate, but they can be completely unpredictable. In fact, over time, uses of pharmaceuticals tested in vitro can change dramatically over time. A recent prominent example of this is aspirin. Initially, the synthetic drug was used as an analgesic. For the 100 years following its discovery, its uses increased and in the last 30 years aspirin has been recognized to reduce the risk of all vascular events (myocardial infarction, stroke, and deep vein thromboses) by about one-third. Therefore, results from studies performed in vitro do not always show precisely how living organisms will respond; because of this it may be difficult to draw conclusions from in vitro studies directly to living organisms and to how they actually respond internally.

SEE ALSO: Hormones; In Vivo; Infertility.

BIBLIOGRAPHY. Peter Elwood and Michael Stillings, "Aspirin—The First Miracle Drug," *The Pharmaceutical Journal* (v.266/7138, 2001); Emily C. Harrison and Julie Scott Taylor, "IVF Therapy for Unexplained Infertility," *American Family Physician* (v.73/1, 2006); *Illustrated Stedman's Medical Dictionary*, 24th ed. (Williams & Wilkins, 1982); Wikipedia, "In Vitro," http://en.wikipedia.org/wiki/In_vitro (cited February 22, 2007); Wikipedia, "In Vitro Fertilisation," http://en.wikipedia.org/wiki/In_vitro_fertilization (cited February 22, 2007).

ANN M. KARTY, M.D.
KANSAS CITY UNIVERSITY OF MEDICINE
AND BIOSCIENCES

In Vivo

The literal translation of *in vivo* from Latin is "in the living being." This phrase refers to those things occurring inside of a living entity. In vivo research refers to research performed within the tissue of a living being as opposed to research performed on dead materials or on specific metabolic components.

In vivo research is commonly used to observe the overall effects on the living organism being studied rather than one specific outcome. Accordingly, there are more external variables with in vivo research. Although optimal studies attempt to limit outside factors potentially confounding the project, results of studies are sometimes difficult to determine because there may be factors (both predicted and not predicted) that alter results or factors that alter the specific interpretation of results.

In vivo research, by definition, must be performed within the system in which it is meant to be used. New pharmaceuticals and compounds created in laboratories may prove worthless or even harmful to living tissue, and thus must be tested on live subjects. Live organisms used for these tests can vary from plants to mice to human subjects.

The value of in vivo testing is revealed in cases where, for instance, a substance that has been found to be active and effective in laboratory, in vitro tests virtually disappear when tested in vivo; this can happen because of the interaction of another in vivo factor that interacts negatively with the substance being tested.

In vivo research is generally conducted by pharmaceutical companies when testing new drugs; often, these in vivo trials involve human subjects. Typically, background research on the potential pharmaceutical being tested has already been conducted on individual metabolic components, and an intervention has been created to treat a medical condition.

In the United States and several other countries, clinical trials must be performed to evaluate new drugs/biologics, medical devices, and other interventions used on patients under scientifically controlled settings. Before the intervention can be released to the public, clinical research trials must be performed to determine safety and efficacy of the drug. The Food and Drug Administration (FDA) has published specific guidelines to be used during the in vivo clinical trials on human subjects.

Pharmaceutical trials are commonly described in four phases that occur over several years. If the studies demonstrate continued safety and efficacy during this time period, the drug development process typically proceeds. The initial phase involves the first testing in human subjects to observe the in vivo results and delineate safety, tolerability, pharmacokinetics, and pharmacodynamics upon a small group of healthy individuals. The second phase is designed to assess the in vivo results on a larger group of human subjects assessing clinical efficacy. The third phase is typically designed to delineate assessment of the efficacy compared to current standard of care therapies; larger groups of subjects are used for this phase. The final phase of pharmaceutical trials involves the postlaunch safety surveillance. Sometimes long-term or unexpected and rare adverse effects are discovered once larger groups of patient populations are using the treatment and undergoing the in vivo human subject exposure.

The use of human subjects raises ethical issues for in vivo research. Consequently, institutional review boards (IRBs), also commonly known as an ethical review boards, exist to formally review and monitor research involving human subjects. The mission of these boards is to protect the rights and welfare of research subjects. IRB approval is required to conduct research funded by both the FDA and the Department of Health and Human Services.

SEE ALSO: Food and Drug Administration (FDA); In Vitro; Institutional Review Board (IRB); Medical Jurisprudence.

BIBLIOGRAPHY. Robert Amdur, *Institutional Review Board Member Handbook* (Jones and Bartlett, 2002); *Illustrated Stedman's Medical Dictionary*, 24th ed. (Williams & Wilkins, 1982); Bruce R. Neibuhr, *Handbook of Clinical Trial and Epidemiological Research Designs January 2000*, http://www.sahs.utmb.edu/Pellinore/intro_to_research/clinirls.htm (cited February 22, 2007); Wikipedia, "In Vivo," http://en.wikipedia.org/wiki/In_vivo (cited February 22, 2007);

ANN M. KARTY, M.D.
KANSAS CITY UNIVERSITY OF MEDICINE
AND BIOSCIENCES

Inbreeding

Inbreeding is the mating of closely related individuals, yielding offspring characterized as inbred. The principle biological consequence of inbreeding is decreased genetic variation in inbred individuals as compared to non-inbred individuals. This can manifest a higher incidence of diseases with a recessive genetic basis and other abnormal pregnancy outcomes (stillbirth, etc.). Because individuals in different societies (as well as different individuals within the same society) may have different definitions of "closely related," some prefer the use of the term *consanguinity*, which refers to the existence of any common ancestor among a subject's parents (although in practice, such analysis rarely looks at relationships more distant than the second or third cousin or equivalent). It is also worth noting that distinctions between "inbreeding" and "consanguinity" are not uniformly agreed upon and that sources often use the two interchangeably.

BIOLOGICAL SIGNIFICANCE

The relative importance of inbreeding in contributing to the incidence of disease depends largely on the prevalence of the recessive allele in the population at large. If the recessive allele in question is relatively common, then the impact of inbreeding or consanguinity will not be significant unless the frequency of inbreeding is such that it is the rule rather than the exception. A good example of this is Tay-Sachs disease and a population of Ashkenazi Jews in the United States. Carrier frequency in this population is thought to be as high as one in 30. If this population mated randomly, the incidence of Tay-Sachs would be sufficiently high that the increased incidence from sporadic inbreeding would be negligible. This incidence can be contrasted with that of the general public, which is one in 300. Because the background rate of Tay-Sachs in such a population is much lower, the influence of any inbreeding is necessarily greater.

It should be cautioned, however, that the risks of inbreeding are not so great as is popularly imagined. While the risk for particular (rare) conditions may be markedly increased when inbreeding is present, it should be remembered that the average, non-inbred individual contains 8 to 10 mutations for autosomal recessive disorders. Thus, while it has been estimated that three to five percent of pregnancies arising from the mating of first cousins produces an abnormality (stillbirth, neonatal death, or congenital malformation), the overall rate of birth abnormalities for the general population stands at two to three percent.

INBREEDING AROUND THE WORLD

The risk of inbreeding is only half the picture when considering the overall impact of inbreeding. Consideration must also be given to the prevalence of inbreeding. Unfortunately, there is a paucity of population-level data on inbreeding prior to the end of World War II. While anecdotal evidence and sporadic studies on the phenomenon exist from before this time, there was not much serious outside scholarship looking at the issue, a key when considering a social practice considered unremarkable by those who practice it. What is known is that currently, rates of inbreeding vary significantly between countries and that those countries with high rates of inbreeding are concentrated in a region stretching from Morocco to southern India or China and east Asia depending on the definitions and survey methods used. Furthermore, immigrants from these countries continue the marriage practices of their home countries even in countries where such practices are not the norm.

RELIGION AND INBREEDING

There appears to be no consistent reason given by the world's major religions for the various forms of marriage preference, and even within the major religions there are marked differences in attitude to varying forms of inbreeding. Within Christianity, the Orthodox churches prohibit consanguineous marriage; the Roman Catholic Church currently requires diocesan permission for marriages between first cousins (and discourages several other forms of inbreeding), and many Protestant denominations permit marriages up to and including first-cousin marriages.

A similar degree of nonuniformity exists in Hinduism, both as a matter of theology and in practice. Hindus from the northern region of India typically frown upon marriage between biological kin for several generations (far in excess of the Western first-cousin taboo). By comparison, Hindus in south India strongly favor marriage between a son and the mother's brother's daughter; uncle–niece marriages also are seen.

In general, Muslim regulations on marriage parallel the Judaic pattern detailed in *Leviticus* 18. However, uncle–niece marriages are permitted in Judaism. They are forbidden by the Koran, even though double first-cousin marriages, which have the same coefficient of inbreeding, are recognized within Islam.

Buddhism sanctions marriage between first cousins, as does the Zoroastrian tradition. The Sikh religion forbids consanguineous marriage, although some minority Sikh groups appear to honor this commandment in the breach, particularly with more-distant relations.

It has also been claimed that diaspora groups engage in higher rates of inbreeding than their nonmigratory companions because such groups tend to immigrate as families and because immigration law in the Western countries they immigrate to (Canada, the United Kingdom, and the United States) tend to favor the granting of visas to spouses over cousins and uncles. Research in this area is ongoing; it is not yet clear if other sociodemographic factors explain this differential rate of inbreeding.

LEGISLATION

Just as different religions have different perspectives on what level of inbreeding is unacceptable, so do various legal jurisdictions. Whereas first-cousin marriages are legal in the United Kingdom and Australia, they are illegal in many U.S. states (although exceptions can be incorporated into state laws, particularly for the practices of particular religious and ethnic groups). Legal analysis in this area should be considered carefully as not all legislation is enforced in practice. For example, in India, the 1955 Hindu Marriage Act bans uncle–niece marriage, but a study conducted between 1980 and 1989 in two large cities in southern India concluded that 21.3 percent of Hindu marriages there were uncle–niece marriages.

SOCIODEMOGRAPHIC FORCES AND INBREEDING

Just as there is variation in religious and legal guidance on an institutional level, there is also variation in social forces felt at a local level, influencing inbreeding practices in communities around the world. The reasons most commonly given for the popularity of inbred marriage can be summarized as tradition, social cohesion, maintenance of scarce resources (particularly in societies where dowries are common), domestic harmony, and greater stability of marriage. The degree of social similarity and the reduction in the number of in-laws may explain the greater stability that has been claimed for inbred unions (which do have lower divorce rates and a higher degree of female autonomy than non-inbred marriages from the same social group).

Incidence of inbred marriage has been associated with low socioeconomic status, illiteracy, and rural residence, although counterexamples are rife. The most prominent example of this is the ruling aristocracy of Europe: the imperative to marry other members of the same ruling class and the use of marriage as a method to seal alliances created significantly inbred family trees with well-known consequences, the most commonly known being the hemophilia of the Romanov Dynasty in Russia.

Despite the prominent counterexample of inbred royalty, the vast majority of inbred marriages occur in the region from Morocco to south India, one that has historically been relatively poor and rural. Although such practices in this region are centuries old, trends may soon change. Whereas as many abnormal pregnancies previously ended in stillbirth and infant mortality was high, modern advances in medical care are creating a growing population of offspring dependent on the state for expensive support services. This may eventually prompt efforts to lower the rate of inbred marriage in this region to levels seen in the West. While tradition cannot be readily overturned, it is likely that as the correlates for inbred marriage are eradicated by improving economic conditions, improved educational infrastructure and increasing urbanization, societies will be increasingly unwilling to tolerate traditions that impose such consequences.

SEE ALSO: Birth Defects; Coefficient of Inbreeding.

BIBLIOGRAPHY. A.H. Bittles, A. Shami, and N. Appaji Rao, "Consanguineous Marriage in Southern Asia: Incidence, Causes and Effects," *Minority Populations: Genetics, Demography and Health*, eds. A.H. Bittles and D.F. Roberts (Macmillan, 1992); R.L. Nussbaum, et al., *Thompson & Thompson: Genetics in Medicine*, 6th ed., revised reprint (Saunders, 2004); S. Sailer, "Cousin Marriage Conundrum," *The American Conservative* (January 13, 2003).

BIMAL P. CHAUDHARI
BOSTON UNIVERSITY

Incidence

Incidence is a measure of disease occurrence used in the field of epidemiology. Incidence describes the number of new cases of a disease or condition that occur in a population at risk. There are three primary components needed to calculate incidence: the population at risk, the length of time that the population is at risk, and the number of new cases that arise. Two types of measures are used to describe incidence: *cumulative incidence* (also called incidence proportion) and *incidence rate* (also called incidence density).

Cumulative incidence describes the number of new cases among the population at risk observed over the observation period of interest. Conceptually, this describes the probability that an individual in the observed population at risk will contract the disease or condition. It is best used in studying a closed cohort, which includes an identifiable population at a given point of time, allowing only loss to follow-up. The formula used to determine cumulative incidence is:

cumulative incidence = (# new cases)/
(*n* of population at risk during observation period)

Incidence rate describes the number of new cases over person-time, or the sum of the time that individuals in the population at risk are observed. Conceptually, this describes the change in the number of cases in relation to change in a unit of person-time. This is best used for an open cohort, where individuals join and leave, thus contributing varying amounts of observed time to the analysis. It is described by the following formula:

incidence rate = (# new cases)/(person-time)

Calculating appropriate incidence requires properly determining the population at risk, which is impacted by additions through birth, or loss through death, migration, and other similar events. Individuals also typically cease to be included in the population at risk once they have developed the disease or condition under study. Incidence is also affected by determination of new cases. If the condition of interest can occur within a given subject more than once, the determination to count each episode or only the first or last episode of the disease or condition changes the calculation.

SEE ALSO: Cohort Study; Epidemiology; Prevalence.

BIBLIOGRAPHY. Donna Crowley, *Handbook of Statistics in Clinical Oncology* (Marcel Dekker, 2005); Jose Granados, "On the Terminology and Dimensions of Incidence," *Journal of Clinical Epidemiology* (v.50, 1997).

CONSTANCE W. LIU, M.D.
CASE WESTERN RESERVE UNIVERSITY

Incontinence

Incontinence is defined as the inability to control excretory functions, generally the inability to control urine and fecal excretion. Incontinence is a common medical problem in both children and adults, generally affecting the earliest and latest years of life. Urinary incontinence alone, for example, affects an estimated five to 15 percent of community-dwelling older adults.

Normal urination and defecation are controlled by the autonomic nervous system of the body, which is composed of the parasympathetic and sympathetic nervous system. In general, the sympathetic nervous system promotes retention of feces and urine, while the parasympathetic nervous system promotes elimination. The balance of these systems occurs in the levels of the organs involved, spinal cord, brainstem, and cerebral cortex. Voluntary control over elimination occurs in the cerebral cortex.

ADULTS—URINARY INCONTINENCE

More than 50 percent of adult residents in long-term care facilities are estimated to have either urinary or fecal incontinence. Incontinence can dramatically influence quality-of-life issues, often leading to social isolation, depression, and institutionalization (in the case of older adults). Nevertheless, it is largely unrecognized and underaddressed in the healthcare setting. Neurologic impairment, immobility, and gender—females are more likely to suffer urinary incontinence than males—are major independent risk factors in adults.

Urinary incontinence in adults can be originate from wide range of medical and psychological causes. In many cases, incontinence is only transient. Common causes of transient incontinence include medication side effects, delirium, fecal impaction (often from constipation), urinary tract infections or other infections, irritation of the vagina or urethra, psychological factors such as depression, or physical mobility limitations. There are several forms of more chronic incontinence commonly experienced by individuals.

Urge Incontinence—This form of incontinence results from overactivity of the detrusor muscle, a muscle in the bladder wall that promotes elimination. Urge incontinence is generally believed to be the most common form of chronic incontinence. Individuals with this form of incontinence commonly describe a sudden feeling of needing to void before involuntary voiding. Treatments include behavioral management, such as timed voiding schedules and visualization techniques, as well as pharmacologic treatment through medications that decrease contractions of the detrusor muscle.

Stress Incontinence—This form of incontinence results from impaired urethral closure. Individuals with this type of incontinence often describe involuntary loss of urine associated with sneezing, coughing, laughing, or lifting objects. Treatment options include pelvic muscle exercises, weight loss in obese patients, use of estrogen, pharmacologic treatments, and surgical procedures, which are generally used for those who fail medical management.

Overflow Incontinence—This form of incontinence results from incomplete emptying of the bladder and abnormally high bladder volumes. This often results from mechanical obstruction of outflow, such as by an enlarged prostate, or from decreased contraction of the detrusor muscle. Individuals generally complain of frequent dribbling of urine, which can be constant, and a feeling of incomplete emptying of the bladder. They often also complain of a decreased force of urinary stream. Treatment options include intermittent catheterization, pharmacologic therapy, and surgery.

Functional Incontinence—This form of incontinence results from the inability of an individual to transport in a timely manner to a location to void. Examples include individuals with severe mobility limitations or with dementia.

Mixed Incontinence—Many individuals with incontinence often have a combination of the various above types.

ADULTS—FECAL INCONTINENCE

Fecal incontinence is common, affecting three to 21 percent of community-dwelling elderly individuals over age 65. Fecal incontinence is also referred to as encopresis, although this term is more commonly used in children. Like urinary incontinence, fecal incontinence can have enormous impact on the lifestyle of an individual. Fecal incontinence can occur transiently in healthy adults in cases such as diarrhea. Fecal incontinence, similar to urinary incontinence, can result from functional difficulties, such as arthritis or other gait difficulties, or poor access to toileting facilities. It can also result from neurological disease, such as spinal cord damage, or damage to the nerves in the intestinal tract or rectum. Other causes include dementia, severe depression, fecal impaction (constipation), neoplasm, and cerebral vascular disease.

CHILDREN—URINARY INCONTINENCE

Girls typically gain bladder control before boys. Toilet training usually begins between ages 2–4. By the age of 5, 90 to 95 percent of children are nearly completely continent during the day, and 80 to 85 percent are continent at night.

Diurnal (Daytime) Incontinence—The most common pediatric cause of this form of incontinence is unstable (overactive) bladder. This form is associated with a smaller-than-normal bladder, which has strong, uninhibited contractions. Other causes can include urinary tract infections, neurological disease, infrequent voiding, giggle incontinence, sphincter abnormalities, anatomical abnormalities of the urinary tract, overflow incontinence, sexual abuse, and behavioral causes. Treatment of daytime incontinence varies depending on the etiology. Most children outgrow this problem; however, pelvic floor exercises, behavioral training, and pharmacologic therapy may be helpful.

Nocturnal Enuresis—Children often deal with nocturnal enuresis, the occurrence of involuntary voiding at night at 5 years old and older. This problem is more common in boys and it seems to occur more often in children with a family history of the problem. Nocturnal enuresis without overt daytime symptoms affects up to 20 percent of children at the age of 5. Causes may include sleep disorders, psychological factors, urinary tract infections, urinary tract obstruction, sleep apnea, genetic factors, and delayed neurological development allowing voluntary control of voiding.

In the majority of cases, the problem ceases spontaneously. Treatment depends on the cause but may include nighttime fluid restriction, motivational measures (reward systems), conditioning therapy (such as use of alarms), psychological therapy, and pharmacologic therapy.

CHILDREN—FECAL INCONTINENCE

In children, more than 90 percent of fecal incontinence, or encopresis, is associated with constipation. Other problems include neurological disease, poor toilet training, psychosocial problems, and other digestive tract disease. Treatment generally involves treating the constipation. More than half of cases resolve spontaneously in two years.

SEE ALSO: Constipation; Urinary Tract Infection.

BIBLIOGRAPHY. John Noble, *Textbook of Primary Care Medicine*, 3rd ed. (Mosby, 2000); S. H. Tariq, "Geriatric Fecal Incontinence," *Clinics in Geriatric Medicine* (v.20/3, 2004); Richard E. Behrman, "Voiding Dysfunction," in *Nelson Textbook of Pediatrics*, 17th ed. (Saunders, 2004).

ELIZABETH VAN OPSTAL
MICHIGAN STATE UNIVERSITY

India

The Republic of India, commonly known as India, is a country in south Asia. With a total population of 1,103,371,000 people (67 percent living in rural areas and 33 percent in urban areas), India is the world's second most populous country, and the most populous liberal democracy in the world. It is the seventh largest country by geographical area and has a coastline of over 7,000 kilometers. India is bounded by the Indian Ocean on the south, the Arabian Sea on the west, and the Bay of Bengal on the east. India borders Pakistan to the west; the People's Republic of China, Nepal, and Bhutan to the northeast; and Bangladesh and Myanmar to the east. The country's 26 states are bordered to the north by the world's highest mountain chain, the Himalayas. To the south, India is in the vicinity of Sri Lanka, the Maldives, and Indonesia.

With the world's fourth largest economy in purchasing power and the second fastest growing large economy, India has made rapid progress in the last decade, especially in information technology. Today, India has a Gross Domestic Product (GDP) per capita of $1,830. Total health expenditure per capita is $82 (2003 international dollars). Total health expenditure as a percentage of GDP (2003) is 4.8 percent. Although India's standard of living is projected to continue to rise sharply in the next half-century, the country currently battles high levels of poverty, persistent malnutrition, and environmental degradation. Literacy, defined as the population over age 15 that can read and write, is 59.5 percent. This percentage is highly segregated by gender, as 70.2 percent of males were literate, while only 48.3 percent of females were literate in 2003. The current life expectancy at birth is 61.0 years for males and 63.0 years for females. Child mortality per 1,000 is 81 for boys and 89 for girls. Adult mortality per 1,000 is 275 for males and 202 for females. In India, the risk for major infectious diseases is high. The food- and waterborne disease that are prevalent include bacterial diarrhea, hepatitis A and E, and typhoid fever. Vectorborne diseases that are prevalent and are at high risks in some locations include dengue fever, malaria, and Japanese encephalitis.

Indigenous or traditional medical practitioners continue to practice throughout the country. The two main forms of traditional medicine practiced are the ayurvedic ("science of life") system, which deals with

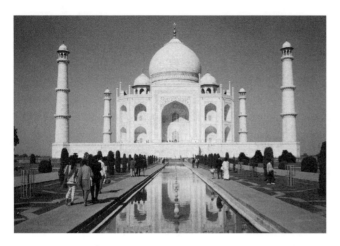

There are two main forms of traditional medicine practiced in India, the ayurvedic system, and the unani system.

causes, symptoms, diagnoses, and treatment based on all aspects of well-being (mental, physical, and spiritual), and the unani (so-called Galenic medicine) herbal medical practice. A vaidya is a practitioner of the ayurvedic tradition, and a hakim (Arabic for a Muslim physician) is a practitioner of the unani tradition. These professions are frequently hereditary. A variety of institutions offer training in indigenous medical practice. It was not until the late 1970s that health policy referred to any form of integration between Western-oriented medical personnel and indigenous medical practitioners. In the early 1990s, there were 98 ayurvedic colleges and 17 unani colleges operating in both the governmental and nongovernmental sectors.

Despite the centuries of traditional medicine, primary health centers remain the cornerstone of the rural healthcare system. By 1991, India had approximately 22,400 primary health centers, 11,200 hospitals, and 27,400 dispensaries. These facilities are part of a tiered healthcare system that funnels more difficult cases into urban hospitals while attempting to provide routine medical care to the vast majority in the countryside. Primary health centers and subcenters rely on trained paramedics to meet most of their needs.

The main problems affecting the success of primary health centers are the predominance of clinical and curative concerns over the intended emphasis on preventive work and the reluctance of staff to work in rural areas. Healthcare facilities and personnel increased substantially between the early 1950s and early 1980s, but because of fast population growth,

the number of licensed medical practitioners per 10,000 individuals had fallen by the late 1980s to 3 per 10,000 from the 1981 level of 4 per 10,000. In 1991, there were approximately 10 hospital beds per 10,000 individuals. In addition, the integration of health services with family planning programs often causes the local population to perceive the primary health centers as hostile to their traditional preference for large families. Therefore, primary health centers often play an adversarial role in local efforts to implement national health policies.

INDIA AND HIV/AIDS

India is estimated to have the second largest population of people living with human immunodeficiency virus (HIV)/AIDS, next to South Africa. The National AIDS Control Organization (NACO) estimated that the number of people infected with HIV in India increased from 3.86 million in 2000 to 5.13 million in 2004. In areas that are more severely affected, the epidemic has started to challenge recent development achievements and to raise fundamental issues of human rights concerning people living with HIV/AIDS. The HIV/AIDS epidemic in India is heterogeneous; it seems to be following the type 4 pattern, where the epidemic shifts from the most vulnerable populations (such as sex workers, injecting drug users, and men who have sex with men) to bridge populations (clients of sex workers, people with sexually transmitted infection, and partners of drug users) and then to the general population. The shift usually occurs when the prevalence in the first group exceeds five percent, with a two- to three-year time lag between shifts from one group to another. As of 2004, about 39 percent of people living with HIV/AIDS were women and about 58 percent lived in rural areas where HIV/AIDS services are poor. By the end of November 2005, the total number of reported AIDS cases in India was 116,905, of which 34,177 were women. These data also indicate that about one-third of reported AIDS cases are among people younger than 30 years old.

However, many more AIDS cases go unreported. Only 8,097 total AIDS deaths have been reported as of December 2005. This is because many deaths due to AIDS-related causes go unreported because of stigma, discrimination, and problems in claiming life insurance coverage. The spread of HIV is as diverse as the societal patterns between India's different regions, states, and metropolitan areas. A total of 111 districts in 18 states are currently considered high-prevalence districts. Another growing problem is that of orphans and vulnerable children and, although official figures are not available, the Joint United Nations Programme on HIV/AIDS (UNAIDS) estimates that more than 170,000 children under 15 years are living with HIV/AIDS.

INDIA AND TUBERCULOSIS

India has more new tuberculosis (TB) cases annually than any other country. Following the sharp growth in spending on TB control and the rapid implementation of directly observed treatment, short course (DOTS), India reached 57 percent case detection countrywide in 2004, and 70 percent within DOTS areas. However, there is not yet sufficient evidence from surveillance and survey data to demonstrate that the TB epidemic is nationally in decline. India's challenge is to sustain and improve the quality of DOTS, to expand services to manage multidrug-resistant TB and TB linked to HIV, to involve all care providers, and to demonstrate that DOTS is having an impact.

MEDICAL TOURISM

Medical tourism is on the rise worldwide; now multibillion-dollar industry, medical tourism involves patients traveling to different countries for either urgent or elective medical procedures. The reasons patients travel for treatment vary. Many medical tourists from the United States are seeking treatment at substantially reduced costs. Medical tourists from Canada are often people who are frustrated by long waiting times. Patients in Great Britain often feel they cannot wait for treatment by the National Health Service and are unable to afford to see a physician in private practice. For others, becoming a medical tourist is a chance to combine a tropical vacation with elective or plastic surgery. Now more than ever, patients are coming from poorer countries such as Bangladesh where treatment may not be available.

India is considered the leading country promoting medical tourism, and now it is moving into a new area of "medical outsourcing," where subcontractors provide services to the overburdened medical care systems in Western countries. India's National Health Policy declares that treatment of foreign patients is legally an "export" and deemed "eligible for all fiscal incentives extended to export earnings." Government

and private sector studies in India estimate that medical tourism could bring between $1 billion and $2 billion into the country by 2012. The reports estimate that medical tourism to India is growing by 30 percent a year. In fact, India's top-rated education system is not only churning out computer programmers and engineers, but also an estimated 20,000 to 30,000 doctors and nurses each year.

SEE ALSO: HIV/AIDS; Healthcare, Asia and Oceania; National Center for Infectious Diseases (NCID); Malaria; National Center for Injury Prevention and Control (NCIPC); Tuberculosis.

BIBLIOGRAPHY. J.G. Lipson, S.L. Dibble, & P.A. Minarik, eds., *Culture & Nursing Care: A Pocket Guide* (University of California San Francisco Nursing Press, 1996); B.J. Paulanka and L.D. Purnell, eds., *Transcultural Healthcare: A Culturally Competent Approach* (CD-ROM) (F.A. Davis, 1998).

BARKHA GURBANI
UNIVERSITY OF CALIFORNIA, LOS ANGELES

Indian Health Service (IHS)

The Indian Health Service (IHS), an agency within the Department of Health and Human Services, is responsible for providing federal health services to American Indians and Alaska Natives. The provision of health services to members of federally recognized tribes grew out of the special government-to-government relationship between the federal government and Indian tribes. This relationship, established in 1787, is based on Article I, Section 8 of the Constitution, and has been given form and substance by numerous treaties, laws, Supreme Court decisions, and Executive Orders.

The IHS is the principal federal healthcare provider and health advocate for American Indians and Alaska Natives. Its goal is to raise the health status of these people to the highest possible level. The agency employs approximately 15,500 people, with examples from nearly every medical discipline providing healthcare, social, and environmental health services. The clinical staff consists of more than 5,000 nurses, physicians, pharmacists, dentists, sanitarians engineers, and various allied health professionals, such as nutritionists, health administrators, and medical records administrators. Individuals who have health-related degrees have the option of joining the IHS as civil servants or as commissioned officers in the Public Health Service (PHS).

The IHS currently provides health services to approximately 1.5 million American Indians and Alaska Natives who belong to more than 557 federally recognized tribes in 35 states. The IHS provides a comprehensive health services delivery system for American Indians and Alaska Natives with opportunity for maximum Tribal involvement in developing and managing programs to meet their health needs. The IHS goal is to ensure that comprehensive, culturally acceptable personal and public health services are available and accessible to all American Indians and Alaska Natives.

The IHS assists tribes in developing their health programs through activities such as health management training, technical assistance, and human resource development, coordinating health planning, obtaining and using health resources available through a number of government programs, operating comprehensive healthcare services and health programs, providing comprehensive healthcare services including both hospital and ambulatory medical care and preventive/rehabilitative services, and developing community sanitation facilities. The IHS also serves as the principal federal advocate in the health field for Indians to ensure comprehensive health services for Indian people.

Many IHS programs center on preventive measures involving environmental, educational, and outreach activities are combined with therapeutic measures into a single national health system. Within these broad categories are special initiatives in traditional medicine, elder care, women's health, children and adolescents, injury prevention, domestic violence and child abuse, healthcare financing, state healthcare, sanitation facilities, and oral health. Most IHS funds are appropriated for American Indians who live on or near reservations. Congress also has authorized programs that provide some access to care for Indians who live in urban areas.

SEE ALSO: Department of Health and Human Services (DHHS).

BIBLIOGRAPHY. Indian Health Services, www.ihs.gov/index.asp (cited September 2006); Everett R. Rhodes, *American Indian Health: Innovations in Health Care, Promotion, and Policy* (Johns Hopkins University Press, 2002); United States Department of Health and Human Services, www.hhs.gov/ (cited September 2006).

BEN WYNNE, PH.D
GAINESVILLE STATE COLLEGE

Indonesia

The Republic of Indonesia covers a large archipelago of islands in southeast Asia and was the Dutch colony known as the Netherlands East Indies until World War II. During the war, it was occupied by the Japanese, and after the war, there was another conflict which saw the Indonesian nationalists defeating the Dutch, achieving independence. Indonesia has a population of 238,453,000 (2004) and has 16 doctors and 50 nurses per 100,000 people.

The provision of healthcare in Indonesia varies considerably with the capital, Jakarta, having the best facilities, and also good facilities in many other major cities, and on the island of Bali which is visited by many tourists. The Dutch did not invest much in healthcare, with hospitals catering for Europeans and the Indonesian elite. Indeed, the life expectancy was so low, with Europeans often only lasting one year in Batavia, the administrative capital (modern-day Jakarta), that when Willem Daendels was appointed governor of the Netherlands East Indies in 1807, he did try to improve the terrible levels of sanitation in Batavia. This involved moving the city's cemetery, and clearing the canals to allow for sewage to flow out of the city into the sea.

From 1910, the Dutch started to improve the provision of public healthcare, giving injections for smallpox to many people throughout the archipelago. During the 1930s as advances were made in tropical medicine, the provision of healthcare improved considerably in the country, and by 1936, there were 500 hospitals throughout the Netherlands East Indies, some of which were really clinics, 15 asylums for the insane, 42 leper colonies, and 970 dispensaries. Most of these were run by the Government Medical Service, but there was also a considerable private input. The Dutch also ran a model program which was established at Purwokerto in Jawa Tengah province (West Java). With the Japanese invasion of the Netherlands East Indies, the health services collapsed with the Dutch medical personnel either being killed, fleeing, or being interned by the Japanese. After World War II, the Dutch-Indonesian War saw little new investment in hospitals, but the situation changed in the 1950s.

The major health problems that faced Indonesia were to do with diet, and also malaria, dysentery, typhoid, and cholera. There has also been a problem with venereal disease, rabies, hepatitis, and, in more recent years HIV/AIDS, and also strains of influenza. In some places there has also been the need to treat people suffering from snake or jellyfish bites. To combat these problems, President Sukarno, who controlled the country until 1965, invested heavily in building up the healthcare system, with hospitals, clinics, and pharmacies opening throughout the country. President Suharto, who followed him, and ruled until 1998, presided over a period of great prosperity which saw more hospitals and medical care facilities being built. However, unlike most other countries in southeast Asia, the provision of healthcare has, since 1965, received little government subsidy, although it is overseen by the Ministry of Health and Social Welfare.

The Ikatan Dokter Indonesia (Indonesian Medical Association) was founded in 1950 and has 45,000 members. It publishes *BIDI* each fortnight, and the *Majalah Kedokteran Indonesia*. There are also a number of research institutes in the country catering for particular disease, including the Lembaga Malaria (Malaria Institute), founded in 1920; the Clinical Institute for Leprosy Research, founded in 1935; and the Unit Diponegoro, catering for nutrition, founded in 1937. A Research Center for Cancer and Radiology was established in 1974, under the direction of the National Health Research Institute; and three years later, the Indonesian Cancer Society was founded in Jakarta. Mention should also be made of the Indonesian Index of Medical Specialties (IIMS) which provides a list of pharmaceutical preparations which can be prepared in the country.

The hospitals in Jakarta include Pondok Indah in the southern part of the city, and St. Carolus Hospital, a Roman Catholic hospital which provides emergency care. For the island of Bali, with large numbers of tourists, the healthcare system has been much better than many other parts of the country. However, in spite of that, during the Bali bombings in 2002, many of the injured were evacuated to Darwin in Australia for treatment for burns. Elsewhere in Indonesia, most cities and towns have hospitals and clinics, with serious illnesses either being treated in regional capitals, and some foreigners in the country preferring treatment either in Jakarta or overseas in Singapore.

SEE ALSO: Healthcare, Asia and Oceania; Malaysia.

BIBLIOGRAPHY. *Indonesia: Health Planning and Budgeting* (The World Bank, 1991); Ann Pembrooke McCauley, *The Cultural Construction of Illness in Bali*, (Ph.D. thesis, University of California, Berkeley, 1984); David Mitchell, et al., eds., *Indonesian Medical Tradition: Bringing Together the Old and the New* (Australian Indonesian Association, 1982); Charles Robert Snyder, *Indonesian Civil Service Physicians and Private Medical Practice: Incentives and Disincentives for Physician-Delivered Health Service in the Public Sector* (PhD thesis, University of Michigan, Ann Arbor, 1990).

Justin Corfield
Geelong Grammar School, Australia

Indoor Air Pollution

The presence of polluted air inside livable spaces is as old as civilization itself. In earlier societies, the primary causes of pollution came from burning wood, peat, and fossil fuels in conjunction with poor ventilation. However, present-day sources of indoor air pollution are more varied and have wide-ranging health consequences. Sources of indoor pollution include ambient air pollutants, bioaerosols, and physical pollutants such as radon, asbestos, heavy metals and particulates; volatile organic compounds such as formaldehyde, polynuclear aromatic compounds, polychlorinated biphenyls; pesticides; and noise.

Many people assume the air inside their homes or offices are cleaner than the air outside. This, however, is not necessarily true. While indoor air does not have automobile or factory emissions to contend with, there are many other pollutants that are found indoors. In most cases, there are multiple pollutants that can be found in the home. While pollutant levels from individual sources may not pose a significant health risk by themselves, most homes have more than one source that contributes to indoor air pollution. Alone, these pollutants are not significant but their cumulative effect poses a serious health risk.

Asbestos is a major source of indoor air pollution and can be found mostly in older homes within pipe and furnace insulation materials and floor tiles. Each of these presents a significant health risk indoors. Smoking is one of the largest sources of indoor air pollution and is a significant cause of lung cancer. Tobacco smoke contains many different chemicals that cannot be completely eliminated with ventilation and air filters. Carbon monoxide and nitrogen dioxide are emitted by combustion products like stoves, fireplaces, and heaters. These gases comprise a large health risk and at high concentrations can lead to death. Outside, the health risk presented by these pollutants is much smaller and not of much concern.

Asbestos, a fibrous mineral, is most often too small to be seen by the naked eye and is found mostly in building material; when asbestos fibers become damaged, they can become airborne and are a serious health risk. Asbestos is common on surfaces in older buildings; the exposure of these materials to wear and damage makes the asbestos likely to fray. Because of the small size of asbestos fibers, once they are inhaled, they accumulate in the lungs. The symptoms of diseases caused by continual exposure may not be noticed until years later. Asbestos can cause lung cancer, mesothelioma (a cancer of the chest and abdominal linings), and asbestosis (irreversible lung scarring that can be fatal). In removing asbestos, it is possible that it could become airborne, so as long as it is in good condition, there is no health risk.

Tobacco smoke contains many different compounds, some of which can lead to cancer and other respiratory diseases. Tobacco smoke contains approximately 4,700 different types of chemicals. There is an obvious health risk among people who smoke; however, because of secondhand smoke, there is a significant health risk among people who do not smoke. Indoors, tobacco smoke tends to become concentrated, even with ventilation and air filters, which cannot eliminate it completely, mainly because of the large number of pollutants such smoke contains. Tobacco smoke is the

leading cause of lung cancer; the best defense against it is to eliminate it from indoor settings.

Carbon monoxide, another common indoor air pollutant, is an odorless gas that comes from many different sources including tobacco smoke, automobiles, and improperly adjusted gas appliances. Extreme exposure can result in death. Health effects, at low concentrations, include fatigue in healthy people and chest pain in people with heart disease. At higher concentrations, effects include impaired vision and coordination, headaches, dizziness, confusion, and nausea. Many of these symptoms are misdiagnosed as symptoms of the flu and are overlooked. Many people are asleep when overcome by carbon monoxide gas or fall asleep as a result of the poisoning and never wake up.

When a series of symptoms and ailments that impact humans is connected with a building, the building becomes known as a sick building. The sick-building syndrome and building-related illnesses such as Pontiac fever, *Legionella pneumophila* fever, rhinitis, humidifier fever and hypersensitivity pneumonitis or lung infections, cancer, bronchide asthma, headache, dizziness, fatigue, and difficulty concentrating are caused by a variety of contaminants. Identifying and controlling these contaminants helps to eliminate sickness related to indoor air pollution.

The best way to eliminate indoor air pollution is to eliminate its source. For pollutants such as tobacco smoke, elimination of its presence indoors is the only way to eliminate the pollution it creates. However, this strategy will not work for every type of indoor air pollution simply because some of the sources of pollution are within the building itself or emitted from important appliances. The next best solution would be to regulate the pollution with proper ventilation. Ventilation, coupled with air filters, helps regulate pollution; however, the only way to completely eliminate any type of indoor air pollution is to eliminate the source.

SEE ALSO: Asbestos/Asbestosis; Asthma; Asthma in Children; Legionnaire's Disease.

BIBLIOGRAPHY. H.E. Burroughs and Shirley J. Hansen, *Managing Indoor Air Quality*, 3rd ed. (Fairmont Press, 2004); Consumer Product Safety Commission (CPSC) and Environmental Protection Agency (EPA), *The Inside Story: A Guide to Indoor Air Quality*, CPSC Document

#450 (CPSC and EPA, 1993); E. Willard Miller and Ruby M. Miller, *Indoor Pollution* (ABC-CLIO, 1998).

DeMond Shondell Miller
Joel Yelin
Rowan University

Infant and Newborn Care

The goal of routine care for newborns and infants is to promote healthy development through proper nutrition, routine vaccinations, and early detection and prevention of disease.

NEONATAL PERIOD

Directly after delivery, neonates should be assessed using the APGAR score. The APGAR score is a method of assessment using five areas, scored on a scale of 0–2, to evaluate neonates after birth. The areas assessed include appearance (skin coloration), pulse (heart rate), grimace (reflex irritability), activity, and respirations (breathing rate and effort). Generally, an APGAR score above 7 is considered normal. The APGAR score determines the need for immediate medical care and is not a predictor of long-term development.

Within the neonatal period, preventative measures should be taken to guard against commonly acquired infections and conditions. This includes the administration of an antimicrobial agent such as erythromycin to both eyes and vitamin K given intramuscularly to prevent conjunctivitis of the newborn and hemorrhagic disease of the newborn, respectively. Neonates should be monitored for jaundice (elevated bilirubin levels in the blood) and screened for specific disease states and inherited conditions. Screening recommendations vary from state to state; however, at minimum, all states must screen for phenylketonuria (PKU) and congenital hypothyroidism. Most states also screen for additional inherited diseases such as sickle cell disease and congenital adrenal hyperplasia (CAH). Certain states participate in an expanded newborn screening. Human immunodeficiency virus (HIV) testing, while not routinely done, should be conducted if the mother is HIV positive or engaging in high-risk behaviors. Blood typing is done if the mother has type O blood or is Rh (Rhesus factor) positive to monitor the neonate for erythroblastosis fetalis which consists of anemia, jaundice, respiratory difficulties, and enlargement of the liver and spleen. Many, but not all, states require a hearing screen before the baby is discharged. The umbilical cord should be exposed to air and swabbed daily with rubbing alcohol to prevent infection. The umbilical cord stump detaches spontaneously in approximately one to three weeks. Circumcision of male neonates should be offered and, if desired, should be done within the first few days of life. The American Academy of Pediatrics' policy regarding circumcision is that while newborn male circumcision has potential medical benefits, it also has disadvantages and risks; thus, parents should determine what is in the best interest of their child. Healthy neonates are usually discharged at 48 hours of life and should be followed up in approximately three days by a healthcare professional.

NUTRITION

Both the World Health Organization and the American Academy of Pediatrics endorse breastfeeding as the optimal form of nutrition for infants and recommend exclusive breastfeeding for a minimum of six months. In addition to nutritional completeness, breastfeeding provides psychosocial and immunological benefits. Human milk supplies all of the fluid and nutrition an infant needs. However, iron-fortified rice cereals should be encouraged at the age of 6 months. Infants should not be given additional water for drinking due to the risk of hyponatremia (low sodium in the blood). Infants less than 1 year should not be given cow's milk. The only acceptable replacement for breast milk in the first year of life is commercially manufactured infant formula. Types of infant formulas include cow's milk-based, soy protein-derived, and specialized infant formulas, such as those for premature infants. Both breast milk and the typical infant formula contain 20 kcal/oz. Depending on age, infants should gain between three to eight ounces per week. Breastfed infants should be fed on demand or approximately every two hours, with a decreasing frequency as the infant ages. Bottle-fed infants can go approximately three to four hours between feedings, as formula is digested more slowly than human milk. At 1 year of age, whole cow's milk may be substituted for breast milk or formula.

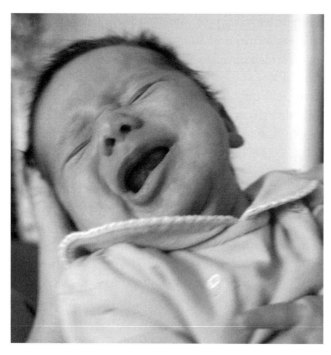

Routine healthcare is important for newborns and infants to promote healthy development.

VACCINATION

Immunizations help to prevent communicable diseases. Childhood immunizations are responsible of the control of once prevalent infections such a polio, measles, mumps, and tetanus. The Centers for Disease Control and Prevention (CDC) publishes a recommended vaccination schedule for infants, children, and adults.

SAFETY

Infants should be placed on their back to sleep to reduce the risk of sudden infant death syndrome (SIDS). Infants should ride in rear-facing car seats until they reach nine kilograms (20 lb) and 1 year of age. To prevent falls, the use of baby walkers should be avoided and infants should never be left alone on changing tables or other elevated areas.

SEE ALSO: Child Safety; Childhood Immunization; Infant and Toddler Health; Neonatology; Nutrition; Pediatrics.

BIBLIOGRAPHY. Mark Beers, et al., eds., "Approach to the Care of Normal Infants and Children," in *Merck Manual of Diagnosis and Therapy,* 18th ed. (Merck Research Laboratories, 2006); Abraham M. Rudolph, et al., eds., "Routine Postnatal Care and Observation," in *Rudolph's Pediatrics,* 21st ed. (McGraw-Hill, 2002); World Health Organization, "WHO Child Growth Standards," www.who.int/childgrowth/en/ (cited April 2007).

ANGELA J. GARNER, M.D.
DANIELLE WEBSTER
UNIVERSITY OF MISSOURI–KANSAS CITY
SCHOOL OF MEDICINE

Infant and Toddler Development

In order to provide the optimum environment for healthy infant and toddler growth and development, it is essential to understand markers that characterize each stage of growth. If a number of these markers are absent or delayed, there may be an underlying physical or mental condition that needs to be addressed. Early identification of problems is vital to children's health. Teachers and child care workers may spot problems that parents have not noticed or have been afraid to acknowledge. They may also be able to identify abused or neglected children who exhibit abnormal development. Child development may vary according to culture and environment. Socioeconomic status also plays a major role in development. A child growing up in poverty may develop more slowly in response to nutritional deficiencies and a lack of social stimuli. Limited access to safe food and water and proper healthcare may also delay development.

Early in the 20th century, child development scholars in industrialized nations began to understand that children were not just "small adults" but were individuals with unique personalities and distinct needs. In 1933 during the Great Depression, the Society of Research in Child Development (SRCD) was established to apply this concept to improving the lives of America's children. The focus was on understanding how poverty and social deprivation affected development and on using that knowledge to design policies and programs to alleviate negative effects of poverty. In 1965, President Lyndon Johnson (1908–73) launched his War on Poverty, and Congress established the Head Start Program, which teaches reading and math skills to qualifying children from birth to three years to promote school readiness. Working under the auspices of the Department of Health and

Human Services, the program also offers health, nutritional, and social support to children and families enrolled in the program.

INFANCY

Within hours of a normal birth, most infants are alert and beginning to react to their surroundings. Although immature, all body systems are operating. Infants have the ability to swallow, suck, gag, cough, yawn, blink, and eliminate waste.

Hearing is well developed, but it takes several years for vision to reach adult levels. Studies conducted on newborns demonstrate that newborns can already discriminate face-like shapes from straight lines. The startle reflex is also apparent, and newborns react to sudden, unexpected movements and load noises. The grasping reflex allows even the tiniest infants to hold onto someone's finger. The sense of smell and taste are also evident, and infants will turn away from unpleasant smells and express preferences for sweet tastes over bitter.

Physically, heads are large in proportion to the rest of the body. Average birth weight varies from 6.5 to 9 pounds (3 to 4.1 kg) and length varies from 18 to 21 inches (45.7 to 53.3 cm). After losing five to seven percent of birth weigh, infants begin to gain an average of five to six ounces a week. Over the next few days, infants develop their own patterns, alternating from sleep to crying to alertness and returning to sleep. Young infants sleep in the fetal position and should be placed on their backs to offset the chance of sudden infant death syndrome (SIDS). Many infants sleep from three to four hours between feedings, initially requiring from six to 10 feedings per day.

Crying and fussing are the major forms of communication for infants. Research reveals that babies respond well to "baby talk," which is considered essential to language development. Infants react to touch and will turn toward a voice, particularly that of the mother, and will seek out the breast or bottle. They like to be held close over the heart, and wrapping them firmly in blankets (swaddling) is often soothing. A distressed infant may also be quieted by shushing sounds, which remind them of noises heard in the womb.

Between two and three months, newborn reflexes begin to disappear. If this does not occur, it may be an indication of neurological problems. At this stage, infants cry less and begin to engage in social smiling. They entertain themselves as they discover their own fingers and toes. Favorite toys are mobiles and rattles, and babies enjoy games such as bye-bye and pat-a-cake. Attachment to parents and primary caregivers is normal. Around 8 or 9 months, separation anxiety surfaces, and babies object to being away from parents or caregivers.

By four months of age as vision improves, and infants pay attention to bright objects, preferring primary colors, particularly red. In one study, infants who were shown both symmetrical and asymmetrical faces expressed a preference for the symmetry of faces that had been identified as "attractive" by adults. Between the ages of five and eight months, however, infant preference was for asymmetry. Young infants who tended to prefer consonant musical tones reacted to variations in rhythm by eight months. Children learn by imitation, and how well infants and toddlers learn to mimic others is a vital key in tracking healthy development. One of the first signs of infant imitation is responding to a smile with a smile. Later, infants learn to mimic other facial expressions and sounds.

As normal infants grow, the head and chest circumference become relatively equal. Infants learn to flip from one side to the other in a prone position. They progress to sitting alone and to crawling. Pulling up on someone's hands or furniture is followed by standing alone. By the end of the first year, many babies have taken their first steps. Following the cooing of early infancy, older infants vocalize simple sounds and begin to say words such as "dada," "mama," and "bye-bye." The infant can now pick up small pieces of food and manipulate a spoon and baby cup. Infants try to brush their own hair and turn the pages of books. They enjoy songs and rhymes and may try to dance and sing. Babies are highly social at this stage and like to be included in family life. They understand approval and will join in clapping. Some infants also exhibit independence by resisting, kicking, or screaming. In some cultures, this independence is strictly discouraged, while others see it as normal.

TODDLER YEARS

At the end of the first year of life, infants become toddlers. Between the ages of 1 and 3, physical growth slows as toddlers learn to master motor and communication skills. Imitation continues to be a major element in normal development, often taking the shape of playing house or school or pretending to be princesses or superheroes. Normal toddlers have seemingly unlimited energy, enthusiasm, and curiosity, and they develop more complex thinking and learning abilities. Emotional communication ranges from freely bestowed hugs and kisses to crying and tantrums. Older toddlers understand the concepts of guilt, pride, and shame and display them at appropriate times. Toddlers tend to believe they are the center of the universe. They understand the concept of ownership but may be unwilling to share or take turns.

The circumference of the head, which indicates healthy brain development, continues to grow at a rate of one-half inch (1.3 cm) every six months. By the age of 3, most toddlers will have quadrupled their birthweight and doubled their birth height. The toddler body begins to develop an adult-like appearance, although the abdomen protrudes and the back appears swayed until age 3. Even toddlers who walk well may fall when hurrying. Push and pull toys and large balls are ideal for toddlers and help them to develop motor skills and coordination. The toddler can climb into a large chair or sit in a small chair unaided.

At the age of one, a toddler draws using whole-arm movement. By the age of the 3, these skills have progressed to finger/thumb manipulation. By the end of the third year, most toddlers are potty trained, but may continue to have accidents when they are engrossed in an activity or while sleeping. By the age of 2, many toddlers learn to manipulate doorknobs. If no child-safety measures are in place, the toddler may leave a room or dwelling without adults being aware. This ability combined with an inherent curiosity makes toddlers prone to wander. Thus, they requires constant adult attention, particularly in public and unfamiliar places.

Because the toddler now understands the concept of object permanence, he/she enjoys hiding objects and playing hide and seek. Although toddlers like to play with other children, they may not cooperate or follow established rules. The ability to hold toys or objects in both hands at one time is a key indicator in normal neural development. The toddler should be able to identify body parts and objects, place one object inside another, and make mechanical objects perform their intended functions. The toddler is able to follow simple directions. Language skills progress

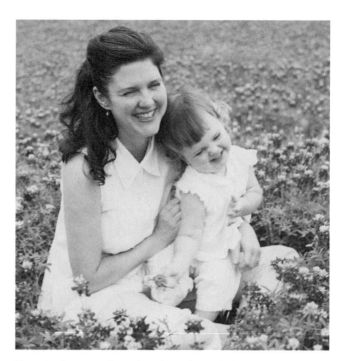

Between the ages of 1 and 3, physical growth slows as toddlers learn to master motor and communication skills.

rapidly, and the toddler advances from simple words to whole sentences. By the age of 3, the toddler is able to carry on conversations with others, although some words may not be intelligible. Toddlers begin to understand the concept of cause and effect, but are not always able to identify situations that may pose danger. Appetite begins to decline, and toddlers frequently insist on eating only one or two preferred foods. They can undress themselves and assist in getting dressed, manipulating large buttons, zippers, and Velcro fastenings. The toddler is able to wash his/her hands and imperfectly brush his/her own teeth. Toddlers may sleep 10 to 12 hours a night, but they may try to put off bedtime.

By age 3, most toddlers have progressed beyond the "terrible twos" to become friendlier and more cooperative. Females have reached 57 percent of their adult height, and males have reached 53 percent. The average 3-year-old weighs from 30 to 38 pounds (13.6 to 17.2 kg). The head now appears in proportion to the rest of the body, and the body is more erect. Most 3-year-olds have all of their baby teeth, and vision has improved to 20/40. Jumping and hopping are favorite means of locomotion. The child is able to manipulate the pedals of small riding toys, and hand dominance is apparent. Many toddlers are able to identify primary colors, identify common shapes, and count from one to 10 or 20. The 3-year-old vocabulary generally contains between 300 and 1,000 words, and the child may memorize favorite songs, stories, and nursery rhymes. In rare cases, 3-years-old have mastered the ability to read.

In 2007, research into the development of toddlers took a new direction with the introduction of a Japanese humanoid known as Child-Robot with Biominetic Body (CB2). The focus of the Osaka University project is to amass knowledge of how toddlers learn language and develop object recognition and communication skills. The robot is designed to mirror the motions of a human child, responding to both touch and sound. The 4-foot tall robot weighs 56 pounds and has 56 actuators, 197 touch sensors, and one audio sensor. Cameras serve as eyes, and an artificial vocal cord allows the robot to mimic human speech. When in motion, the robot "toddles."

SEE ALSO: Birth Defects, Child Abuse, Child Development, Child Safety, Infant and Newborn Care, Infant and Toddler Health, Neurology, Sudden Infant Death Syndrome (SIDS).

BIBLIOGRAPHY. J. Lawrence Aber, et al., *Child Development and Social Policy* (American Psychological Association, 2007); Administration for Children and Families, "About Head Start" http://www.acf.hhs.gov/programs/hsb/about/index.htm (cited June 2007); K. Eileen Allen and Lynn R. Marotz, *Developmental Profiles: Pre-Birth through Twelve* (Thomson, 2007); Leslie J. Carver and Brenda G. Vaccaro, "Twelve-Month-Old Infants Allocate Increased Neural Resources to Stimuli: Associated Negative Adult Emotion," *Developmental Psychology* (v.43/1, 2007); Ann E. Ellis and Lisa M. Oakos, "Infants Flexibility Use Different Dimensions to Categorize Objects," *Developmental Psychology* (v.42/6, 2006); "Humanoid Toddler Reacts to Touch, Sound: Robot Designed to Move Just Like A Real Child between One and Three Years Old," http://www.msnbc.msn.com/id/19112210/ (cited June 2007); Jerome Kagan Norbert and Herschkowitz A. Young, *A Young Mind in a Growing Brain* (Lawrence Erlbaum, 2005); Alice Park, "Baby Faces," *Time*, (v.169/24).

ELIZABETH R. PURDY, PH.D.
INDEPENDENT SCHOLAR

Infant and Toddler Health

Access to medical care and proper nutrition are essential to the normal growth and development of infants and toddlers. Infant mortality is one of the most significant indicators of the level of social development within each country. Consequently, mortality rates tend to be lowest in the most industrialized nations and highest in the poorest developing countries. The countries with the highest infant mortality rates are Angola (184.44 deaths per 1,000 live births), Sierra Leone (158.27), and Afghanistan (157.43). Singapore (2.30), Sweden (2.76), and Japan (2.80) have the lowest infant mortality rates. Since the 1950s, infant morality rates have declined in the United States. However, cuts to programs that fund immunization, nutrition, and health initiatives for infants and toddlers, particularly those of the Reagan administration of the 1980s, have meant that the United States trails most other industrialized nations in infant mortality (6.37 deaths per 1,000 live births). In response to improved medical knowledge and technology and the increased attention paid to the correlation between prenatal care and infant and toddler health, the perinatal (within the first month of life) mortality rate has also dropped, and fewer incidences of low birthweight newborns and short gestational births are occurring, thereby improving the overall health of surviving infants and toddlers

One of the most important factors in promoting infant health is breastfeeding, which provides strong health protections for infants and has the advantage of being more convenient than bottle feeding. In developing countries, young children are often breastfed for extended periods because breast milk is their primary source of nutrition. Both the World Health Organization (WHO) and the United Nations Children's Fund (UNICEF) encourage breast feeding for at least two years. In industrialized nations, most infants are weaned by the end of the first year of life, if not sooner. Breastfeeding rates are as high as 98 percent in countries such as Sweden and Norway where government policies encourage the practice. In the United States, 70.0 percent of women breastfeed newborns, but only 36.2 percent continue breastfeeding until the baby is 6 months old. Working mothers who choose to can use a breast pump to express breast milk to be fed to infants by other caregivers. Solid foods are introduced as instructed by pediatricians, beginning with cereals and progressing to vegetables, fruit, and meats. Only one new food should be introduced at a time to make it easier to identify allergies that may develop and to determine whether certain foods can be tolerated by individual infants. By 8 to 12 months, infants may eat soft or pureed table food. Nuts, popcorn, whole grapes, and hot dogs should never be fed to infants or toddlers because of the high risk of choking.

Infants and toddlers need to visit medical care providers at designated intervals to chart growth and development, have hearing and vision checked, and identify potential problems. UNICEF estimates that of the 10.6 million children under the age of 5 who die each year, two-thirds die from vaccine-preventable diseases. Immunizations that protect children from a variety of preventable infectious diseases are available at physician's offices and at health clinics around the world. Required vaccinations generally include diphtheria, pertussis (whooping cough), tetanus, polio, measles, mumps, rubella (German measles), *Haemophilus influenza* type B (Hib), hepatitis B, and chicken pox. Some of these vaccinations are controversial because of suspected links to conditions such as autism and seizures. However, schools may refuse to enroll any child who has not received required inoculations. In developing countries, international organizations such as UNICEF and WHO often work with local governments to promote immunization programs.

Immunizations do not protect children from accidental injury, nor do they act as barriers to frequent ear, respiratory, and gastrointestinal infections. Normally, these infections respond well to treatment; however, ear infections have become so common that there is concern that they may become resistant to common antibiotics. When ailing infants and toddlers have diarrhea, they are susceptible to dehydration, which if left untreated, could lead to death. Rehydration formulas are widely available to restore fluid and electrolytes. Even in industrialized nations, poor and immigrant children tend to be in poorer health than those in the general population. Rates of lead and pesticide poisonings are also considerably higher among those segments of the population. Infants and toddlers in developing countries, where access to safe water and food and improved sanitation is limited, are highly susceptible to a host of water, and foodborne diseases

such as hepatitis A and typhoid and to vectorborne diseases such as malaria and dengue fever.

Either at birth or shortly thereafter, infants may show the first sign of transmitted or inherited abnormalities. For instance, in developing countries of Africa and Asia, large numbers of infants are exposed to HIV/AIDS. In 1996, the United Nations and the World Health Organization (WHO) estimated that 2.6 million children had HIV/AIDS. Within four years, that number had risen to between five and 10 million. In the absence of intervention, the virus may be transmitted from mother to child. Within the first three or four months of life, recurrent infections and fluid in the ears of exposed infants may be the first indications of AIDS. Three-fourth of all infants with AIDS experience neurological damage. These infants may also experience lung damage, growth failure, craniofacial abnormalities, weakness and apathy, warts on hands, swollen lymph nodes, and thrush. If the new mother is a drug user, newborns may show signs of drug withdrawal and have a number of birth defects.

Sudden infant death syndrome (SIDS) has been one of the most mystifying causes of death among infants. SIDS is diagnosed in cases where no other explanation is feasible following an investigation and autopsy. In the past, apparently healthy infant sometimes died while sleeping. The campaign to place sleeping infants on their backs has slashed the rate of SIDS. Today, the leading causes of SIDS deaths are congenital malformations and low birth weights. At-risk infants often wear monitors to alert parents and caregivers to changes in breathing patterns and heart rates. Mortality rates from SIDS are still higher than normal in inner cities and in some southern states. Some researchers believe there are environmental factors involved in SIDS.

In the United States, the Healthy People 2010 initiative has targeted infant and toddler health as part of the effort to improve overall health. Specific goals include reducing iron deficiency by five percent, slashing nonfatal poisonings to no more than 292 per 100,000, reducing growth retardation in under-5, low-income children to less than five percent, decreasing infant deaths to no more than 4.5 per 1,000 live births, cutting SIDS rates to 0.30 per 1,000 (in part by increasing the number of infants sleeping on their backs to 70 percent), and improving accessibility to vaccinations and rehydration therapies. As infants and toddlers become mobile, health risks increase. Therefore, Healthy People 2010 is also working to reduce the risk of drowning deaths among children under the age of 4 to no more than 0.9 per 100,000, increase the use of automobile child restraints for this age group to 100 percent, reduce antibiotic courses for ear infections to 88 courses per 100 children under the age of 5, and reduce lead blood levels in all children under the age of 5.

SEE ALSO: AIDS; Autism; Birth Defects; Disease Prevention; Gastroenterology; Infant and Toddler Development; Otology; Pregnancy; Preventive Care; Respiratory Diseases (General); Sudden Infant Death Syndrome (SIDS); United Nations Children's Fund (UNICEF); World Health Organization (WHO).

BIBLIOGRAPHY. Michael S. Clement, *Children at Health Risk* (Blackwell, 2003); Andrew Curtis and Michael Leitner, *Geographic Information Systems and Public Health: Eliminating Perinatal Disparity* (IRM Press, 2006); Carole Lium Edelman and Carol Lynn Mandle, *Health Promotion throughout the Life Span* (Elsevier Mosby, 2006); Healthy People, http://www.healthypeople.gov/ (cited July 2007); Jenifer, Swanson, *Infant and Toddler Health Source Book: Basic Consumer Health Information* (Omnigraphics, 2000); H.,B. Valman and R.M. Thomas, *ABC of the First Year* (BMJ Books, 2002); UNICEF, "One in Four Infants Still at Risk from Vaccine Preventable Diseases" http://www.unicef.org/media/media_28400.html (cited cited July 2007); James Wynbrandt and Mark D. Ludman, *The Encyclopedia of Genetic Disorders and Birth Defects* (Facts on File, 2000).

ELIZABETH R. PURDY, PH.D.
INDEPENDENT SCHOLAR

Infectious Diseases (General)

By definition, those diseases that are transmitted from one person to another or between animals and humans (animal to animal, animal to human, human to human, human to animal), implying the transfer of a microorganisms or/and an infectious pathogen agent, are infectious diseases. Infectious agents are living (or at least nucleic acid encoding or proteins) units that must invade the insect host in order to initiate an infection.

Infectious diseases could be caused by bacteria, fungi, viruses, parasites (protozoan and helminthes) and prions. Ectoparasites produce infestation, a different term to express the presence of a pathogen agent on the external region of the body of the host.

Pathogens can be spread by many routes other than direct contact, including through water, food, air, and bodily fluids—blood, semen, saliva, and so on. Many diseases may be transferred by vectors—animals (usually insects) that carry microorganisms (mostly viruses and parasites). Vectors may spread a disease either by mechanical or by biological means (the organisms require a vector to reach specific stages of its life cycle, particularly the infectious stage for the intermediary, accidental and definitive hosts). Mechanical transmission occurs, when flies transfer the germs for typhoid fever from the feces (stool) of infected people to food eaten by healthy people. Biological transmission takes place when an insect bites a person and takes infected blood into its own system. Once inside the insect's gut, the disease-causing organisms may reproduce, increasing the number of microorganisms that can be transmitted to the next victim. This is how the *Anopheles* spp. or *Aedes spp.* mosquito vector, for instance, transfers malaria or dengue, respectively. Additionally, the advance in new areas of activity has let the emergence of new infectious diseases as well new pathogens behavior, and the modification of established methods of transmission. In the medical management of patients, particularly in hospitals, healthcare-associated infections are also a raising concern worldwide (nosocomial infections).

Historically, the record of human suffering and death caused by smallpox, cholera, typhus, dysentery, malaria, and so forth establishes the eminence of the infectious diseases. Despite the outstanding successes in control afforded by improved sanitation, immunization, and antimicrobial therapy, the infectious diseases continue to be a common and significant problem of modern medicine. The most common disease of humankind, the common cold, is an infectious disease, as is the feared modern disease AIDS. Some chronic neurological diseases that were thought formerly to be degenerative diseases have proven to be infectious. Day by day, news scientific findings have revealed the role of the infectious agents in chronic diseases such as asthma, multiple sclerosis, some chronic cardiovascular diseases, Whipple disease, gastric diseases, diabetes, and many types of cancer, among others. There is little doubt that the future will continue to reveal the infectious diseases as major medical problems.

The infectious agent is carried by healthy hosts called reservoirs (e.g., water birds for the flu virus). It is transmitted to the target organism either directly or through carrier organisms. For example, the protozoa responsible for malaria live in mosquitoes, carriers that transmit them through their bites to humans, who develop the disease. The worldwide emergence of diseases once restricted to a particular region is caused by changes in lifestyle and human modification of the environment due to high demographic growth (clearing and deforestation, contact with wild fauna, overcrowding in megalopolises, tourism, immigration, etc.).

Since an epidemiological point of view, worldwide, bacterial and viral infectious diseases represent and call the major attention of healthcare systems, in part due to the economical burden for them, related to the medical management of such infections, such antibiotics for bacterial infections. Treating viral illnesses or noninfective causes of inflammation with antibiotics is ineffective, however, and contributes to the development of antibiotic resistance, toxicity and allergic reactions, leading to increasing medical costs.

For these reasons in the field of infectious diseases different markers related to distinguish the general etiology of the disease have been aimed and developed. Markers such as the leukocyte and neutrophil counts, serum C-reactive protein (CRP) level and erythrocyte sedimentation rate (ESR), which have relatively poor sensitivity and specificity. But other news, such as procalcitonin, inflammatory mediators such as G-CSF, TNF-a, IL-1b, IL-6, and IL-8, the triggering receptors expressed on myeloid cells (TREM), the neutrophil FcgRI (CD64), the phagocyte complement receptors and the product of platelet and neutrophil counts (PN product), among others, which have been showing relatively good sensitivity and specificity.

There are a shifting pattern in the profile of infectious diseases among the countries, developed and developing countries. The majority of developed countries have undergone a prototypical epidemiologic and demographic transition. Host–infectious agent relations have evolved over centuries, but these transitions are largely attributed to a decrease in the burden and mortality from infectious diseases. As a result, life expectancy has radically changed over the past century

with a significant increase in longevity. Although we welcome these improvements in health status, we never imagined that prolongation of life due to fewer infectious diseases would have disadvantages in future generations. It has become evident that inflammatory disorders, including both autoimmune and allergic diseases, are increasing in prevalence to epidemic proportions, particularly in more affluent, industrialized countries over the past 40 years. At the same time, the rate of allergic diseases in the developing world has not changed over the same period of time. There is current scientific evidence that a major player in explaining this tendency could be partially explained by decreased incidence of infectious diseases. In the case of developing countries the situation is different. The world is marked by extremes of economic inequality, across and within countries in which poverty is a common denominator. With incomes in resource-rich countries exceeding thousands of dollars, 20 percent of the world's population nonetheless survives on less than $1 a day. Inevitably, the economic health of a country both affects and is affected by its people's health and life expectancy. It has been argued that the health effects of inequalities with respect to income and assets impose a major burden on the poor, which reduces the competitiveness of societies and has an effect on the global marketplace. Therefore, it is in the world's best interest to ensure the health of all its people, because human health is the foundation of economic growth and development.

Many infectious diseases previously seen only in resource-constrained settings can be currently diagnosed anywhere in the globe due to increased travel, immunosuppression, HIV/AIDS; organ transplantation and blood transfusion.

SEE ALSO: Environmental Health; Epidemiology; Immunology; Medical Entomology.

BIBLIOGRAPHY. Gordon Cook and Alimuddin Zulma, *Manson's Tropical Diseases* (Saunders, 2003); Paulo Sergio Lucas Da Silva, et al., "The Product of Platelet and Neutrophil Counts (PN Product) at Presentation as a Predictor of Outcome in Children with Meningococcal Disease," *Annals of Tropical Paediatrics* (v.27/1, 2007); Erick Folch, et al., "Infectious Diseases, Non-Zero-Sum Thinking, and the Developing World," *American Journal of Medical Sciences* (v.326/2, 2003); Carlos Franco-Paredes, Ildefonso

Tellez, and Carlos del Rio, "Inverse Relationship between Decreased Infectious Diseases and Increased Inflammatory Disorder Occurrence: the Price to Pay," *Archives of Medical Research* (v.35/3, 2004); Carlos Franco-Paredes, et al., "Cardiac Manifestations of Parasitic Infections Part 3: Pericardial and Miscellaneous Cardiopulmonary Manifestations," *Clinical Cardiology* (v.30/6, 2007); Jari Nuutila, and Esa-Matti Lilius, "Distinction between Bacterial and Viral Infections," *Current Opinion in Infectious Diseases* (v.20/3, 2007).

Alfonso J. Rodriguez-Morales, M.D., M.Sc.
Universidad de Los Andes, Venezuela
Carlos Franco-Paredes, M.D., M.P.H.
Emory University

Infertility

The clinical definition of infertility is one year of having normal sexual activity without pregnancy, without using contraceptive methods. According to the World Health Organization, infertility affects one out of 10 couples at some point in their lives, with 80 million people affected worldwide. Males contribute to between 40 to 50 percent of infertility cases. While normal male spermatogenesis means men are potentially fertile all the time and throughout their lives, women have a small window each month of approximately six days, ending with ovulation when they are fertile and a limited fertile time between the onset of menses and the cessation of menstruation at menopause. To maximize the chance of getting pregnant, both women and men should understand how the reproductive system works to ensure they are timing sexual activity during a fertile time.

The causes of infertility can be on the part of either the man or the woman and vary from blockage in the sexual organs, to being secondary from other illnesses or biologic indicators, to having psychological characteristics, or being caused by environmental exposure to toxic substances.

Similarities of infertility issues can be analogous between the genders in the case of hormonal considerations. Not producing or releasing enough sex hormones can lead to anovulation or lack of spermogenesis. The hypothalamus releases gonadotropin releasing hormone (GnRH), to signal the pituitary to release luteinizing hormone (LH) and follicle stimulating hormone (FSH), which in turn regulates the gonads. A feedback loop of steroid hormones in the circulating blood turns off or stimulates hypothalamic activity.

MALE CONTRIBUTING FACTORS

A reproductive health exam with a specialist will take into account common general factors affecting male fertility, including stress, obesity (estrogen production by adipose tissue blocks GnRH release), genetic disorders, cancer, and tobacco, drug, or anabolic steroid use. Specific factors affecting male fertility include undescended testicles, erectile dysfunction, premature ejaculation, excessive heat (increased temperature impede sperm production), blockage in spermatic cord, and viability of sperm.

Average seminal fluid has a neutral pH (approximately 7.2) and contains nutrients for the sperm to use for energy. On average, 100 to 300 million sperm are produced each day. Fertile ejaculate contains adequate volume and concentration of sperm (100 to 400 million sperm) with enough sperm of normal morphology or shape, and the motility or ability to move from the vagina to the fallopian tubes. Problems with morphology or motility are apparent with the occurrence of sperm with pinpointed head, tapered heads, crooked heads, two heads, and coiled or kinked tails.

Primary hypogonadism is defined as testicular failure, and secondary hypogonadism is defined as defective secretion of gonadotropins from the hypothalamus and/or pituitary. These hormones target three specialized cells for reproduction—the spermatogonia in the seminiferous tubules, the Leydig cells in the connecting tissue between the coiled seminiferous tubules, and the Sertoli cells forming the basement member of the seminiferous tubules. They provide the environment necessary for germ cell differentiation and maturation.

FEMALE CONTRIBUTING FACTORS

As with male reproductive health, general factors affect female fertility, including age (women in their late 30s are less fertile than those in their 20s), excessive exercise, stress, weight (either loss or gain), chronic diseases (lupus, polycystic ovary syndrome, arthritis, hypertension, asthma, cancer), and tobacco or drug use. Specific factors affecting female fertility include sexually-transmitted disease resulting in tubal blockage, cervical narrowing from infection, cervical fluid inhibiting sperm motility, immune system antibodies attacking sperm, uterine fibroids, and production of viable eggs. Scientists have in the past stated that women are born with all of the eggs they will produce in their lifetime, but new research indicates stem cells may allow women to produce more eggs and extend reproductive ability.

Cervical fluid must be conducive to assisting the sperm. During nonfertile times, the cervical fluid is either dry or sticky. During fertile times the cervical fluid assists the sperm into the cervix, and provides additional nourishment to keep the sperm alive. In this type of fluid, the sperm can survive up to five days. In nonconducive or "unfriendly" cervical fluid, the sperm may only live a couple hours, or up to a day or two. Precise timing in regards to sexual activity and ovulation are essential. Endometriosis is the growth of the endometrium outside the uterus, increasing the risk of infertility. Pelvic inflammatory disease (PID) increases risk of infertility with repeated episodes of salpingitis.

In addition to physical barriers to fertility, a woman's reproductive cycle, with involvement by the hypothalamus, pituitary, and ovaries, creates a variety of infertility causes, including timing sexual activity with the short fertile window each month and hormonal adequacy for control and regulation of ovulation and hormonal preparation of the uterus for implantation.

The follicular phase is the growth and release of the oocyte. Under the stimulation of FSH, one follicle or more enlarges. The progesterone levels remain low, and estradiol begins a slow rise progressively to its maximum level, 24 hours before the LH/FSH peak and ovulation. The LH peak signals the end of the follicular phase and ovulation commences within 16 to 18 hours of this peak. High doses of estrogen suppress LH and FSH by inhibiting GnRH.

Primary hypogonadism is defined as ovarian deficiency either by decreased ovulation or decreased hormone production, and secondary hypogonadism is defined as defective secretion of gonadotropins from the hypothalamus and/or pituitary.

Ovarian hormones are necessary for maturing the primordial germ cells into oocytes, developing tissues for implantation of the fertilized oocyte (blastocyst), and for hormonal timing for ovulation. Estrogen stimulates vaginal and uterine epithelium. Progestins decrease the action of estrogen and begin the secretory process. This decreases peripheral blood flow and heat loss, resulting in increased body temperature during the luteal phase, and indicates ovulation. Persistent anovulation, as in the case of polycystic ovary syndrome, medications can be given to stimulate the ovaries.

TESTING

An initial consultation for fertility includes medical and psychosexual history, followed by physical and genital examinations, and blood testing. Sperm analysis is preformed after three days of sexual abstinence to check for appropriate volume, concentration of sperm, motility and morphology, to determine male contribution to infertility. Abnormal results will require further evaluation for cause (environmental or workplace toxins, drug or alcohol abuse and hypogonadism).

Some controversy exists about the cervical factors affecting fertility, even so most gynecologists include a postcoital test. Timing the test just before ovulation and within six hours of sexual activity, and a small drop of cervical fluid is obtained from within the cervical os (the opening in the cervix) is examined under the microscope. The presence of five or more active sperm per field is a satisfactory reading. The presence of three or more white blood cells in the test indicates either female cervicitis or male prostatitis.

After the next menstrual period, an X-ray can determine uterine abnormalities and tubal obstruction.

Additional testing may include testing of LH and FSH levels, an ultrasound examination of the ovaries for maturing and unruptured follicles, and an endometrial biopsy during the luteal phase, to rule out luteal phase deficiency.

TREATMENT OPTIONS

While maintaining a healthy lifestyle is necessary, physicians will provide options for treatment, including counseling to find fertile times, using ovulation predicting kits, and following basal body temperature changes. Surgery and medication to correct reproductive problems may be necessary.

Agonists 17 α-ethinyl estradiol and mestranol are oral contraceptives used to regulate the reproductive cycle, in preparation for additional medication therapy, to promote fertility as soon as the contraceptive is discontinued. Antagonists compete with estradiol for intracellular receptor. Clomiphene competes with estradiol for hypothalamic receptor sites. GnRH is not restrained, and increasing amounts of LH and FSH are released by the pituitary to make multiple follicles mature simultaneously with the potential for multiple pregnancies.

For cases of inadequate transport of sperm, intrauterine insemination is an option, where sperm with seminal fluid, debris, mucus, and fat globules are removed is injected into the uterus with a catheter.

Assistive reproductive technology includes three different technologies—invitro fertilization (eggs and sperm are collected, fertilized, and transferred into the uterus), zygote intrafallopian transfer, and gamete intrafallopian transfer. Of these, invitro fertilization is most common and more universally offered.

Artificial insemination is available for those who are unable to have a biologically shared child. Sperm donation allows the woman to have a biological child with donated sperm; egg donation can combine the man's sperm with a donated egg followed by invitro fertilization, or embryo donation with donated sperm and egg can be used for women healthy enough to give birth.

The prognosis is positive for minor, including multiple, causes of infertility, with treatment. Severe infertility is untreatable and of prolonged duration. Regardless of the cause of infertility, couples may experience feelings of inadequacy and additional stress and strain on the relationship. As important as the physical treatment, counseling and therapy may be needed to deal with the psychological aspects of difficulty or absence of reproduction. If treatment does not work, couples additionally have the option of adoption, foster parenting, and birth by surrogate.

SEE ALSO: Gynecology; Impotence; Menstruation and Premenstrual Syndrome; Reproductive Health (General).

BIBLIOGRAPHY. H. Trent MacKay, "Gynecology," in *Current Medical Diagnosis & Treatment 2004* (Lange, 2004); Daniel A. Potter, and Jennifer S. Hanin, *What to Do When You Can't Get Pregnant* (Marlowe, 2005); World Health Organization, "Infertility," www.who.int/reproductive-health/infertility/ (cited April 2007).

LYN MICHAUD
INDEPENDENT SCHOLAR

Inflammatory Bowel Disease

Inflammatory bowel disease consists of two disorders: Crohn's disease and ulcerative colitis. Both conditions result from abnormal activation of the body's immune system, resulting in an inflamed bowel and concurrent systemic symptoms. These are chronic, idiopathic, and relapsing and remitting disorders, more common in the developed world. Crohn's disease is autoimmune and involves widespread inflammation throughout the gastrointestinal tract, while ulcerative colitis is limited to the colon.

The luminal layer of the gastrointestinal tract (called the mucosa) is colonized normally with microflora. This flora is of functional significance. The human body does not consider the flora as an antigenic or pathogenic entity. In inflammatory bowel disease, the tables turn, and the host's immune system gets activated against its own flora, causing an inflammation against the normal mucosa, resulting in defective function. Because the immune response is directed against the body's own tissues, this is an autoimmune disorder, involving abnormal immune responses, genetic predisposition, and environmental triggers.

The development of this disease strongly depends on genetic predisposition. Fifteen percent of inflammatory bowel disease patients have first-degree relatives who also have the disease, and the lifetime risk of either a parent or a sibling being affected is 9 percent. However, the disease is a multigenic trait. This means that several genes will control the eventual clinical presentation of the disease, thus resulting in variable symptoms.

Animal studies have elucidated the importance of gut flora in the development of inflammatory bowel disease. It is thought that defects in the barrier of the gut wall could cause the lymph tissue to be exposed to the microflora resting on the mucosal surface. This causes an immediate immune response against the normal gut flora, causing the inflammation. Environmental triggers, such as irritants in the diet, can also trigger a relapse by acting as a microbe against which an immune response is launched by the body.

The specific nature of the type of immune response is another aspect of inflammatory bowel disease research. T cells of the immune system are involved in autoimmune responses against self-antigenic in the body. These cells are cytotoxic and kill the cells of the body if they exhibit certain apoptotic (suicidal) proteins, or abnormal antigens (such as viral proteins exhibited on the surface of the cell that is infected with the virus). Such cells attack the normal cells in cases of autoimmune disease, and in inflammatory bowel disease, they target the intestinal mucosal cells.

Crohn's disease is a type of delayed hypersensitivity response that is chronic and induced by interferon gamma–producing T helper cells 1. Ulcerative colitis is cause by T helper cells 2. Diagnosis of inflammatory bowel disease is largely dependant on clinical history, radiographic examination, laboratory findings, and pathological examination of tissue. Microscopic histological assessment defines the diseases.

Crohn's disease is also called regional enteritis. The disease consists of patchy areas of affected mucosa alternated by areas of normal mucosa. The region of inflammation could be anywhere throughout the length of the gastrointestinal tract, that is, from the mouth, esophagus, stomach, small intestine, large intestine, rectum to the anus. As a consequence of repeated inflammation, the intestinal wall becomes rubbery and thick due to edema. The tissue undergoes fibrosis and scar formation and the muscular layer of the intestinal wall hypertrophies, causing the lumen itself to reduce. The narrow lumen causes the classic presentation of "stringy sign" in a barium meal's X-ray. Despite the severity of the disease in some areas, other parts of the gastrointestinal tracts may be very much unaffected. Early features of the disease show point sores that progress to ulceration. Ulcerated areas coalesce causing serpentine ulcers along the long axis of the bowel. The normal smoothness of the mucosal surface is lost and fistulas and fissures commonly develop.

Clinical symptoms of the patient include mild diarrhea, fever, and abdominal pain. The episode is followed by an asymptomatic period, which can vary in duration. Fecal blood loss can be present but is usually not as severe as that in ulcerative colitis. Acute flare-ups can also present themselves as an appendicitis episode, with pain in the lower right quadrant of the abdomen. Repeated bouts of diarrhea cause fluid loss and electrolyte imbalances. Furthermore, fibroses and fistulas can be common complications; because the normal functional capacity of the mucosa is lost, there can be substantial loss of protein and fat and considerable malabsorption.

Systemic symptoms include arthritis, sacroiliatis, ankylosing spondylitis, and migraines. Such patients have an increased risk to develop cancer over the years of their illness; however, the risk is not as high as that in ulcerative colitis.

Ulcerative colitis is a type of inflammatory bowel disease that is limited to the colon. It involves mucosal and submucosal damage. Unlike Crohn's disease, this disease spreads proximally from the anus and rectum toward the descending colon, transverse colon, and ascending colon. Aside from the normal symptoms of diarrhea, fever, and fecal blood loss, there are several systemic symptoms such as ankylosing spondylitis, migratory polyarthritis, hepatitis problems, and uveitis.

The incidence of ulcerative colitis is higher than that for Crohn's disease and is more widely distributed. It is thought that the inflammation of the colon is probably caused by regurgitation of iliac contents into the colon by the presence of an abnormal and incompetent ileocaecal valve. The vale links the cecum to the ileum. These conditions can also result in a clinical presentation of appendicitis, because the cecum is close to the appendix.

The mucosal involvement is of such a nature that the mucosa bleeds easily, and overt fecal blood loss can lead to dire consequences. Inflammation progressively worsens the condition and the mucosa has a patchy appearance of ulcers alternating with segments of regenerating mucosa that looks like a polyp. Ulcers are rarely serpentine, but damage spreads to the underlying neural plexus of nerves that gets damaged cause a toxic megacolon. This condition could be lethal as loss of the nerves supplying the colon causes cessation of bowel functioning.

It cannot be overemphasized that ulcerative colitis leads to epithelial damage that causes epithelial dysplasia and significantly increases the chance of colonic cancer. Clinical symptoms include mucoid bloody diarrhea that may persist invariably. Spasmodic pain generating from the lower left quadrant, spreading throughout the abdomen, is characteristic. The first attack may be the last in lucky patients. Attacks may be triggered by emotional or physical stress.

The treatment of inflammatory bowel disease can involve immunosuppressive drugs such as azothiaprine and corticosteroids. Maintenance therapy is done by using antiinflammatory drugs. Such patients are very vulnerable to depression and, therefore, should be encouraged not to be stressed or exert themselves emotionally or physically. In case of a toxic megacolon, surgery is the only option, sealing the rectum and attaching a synthetic colostomy bag for collection of fecal matter.

SEE ALSO: Diarrhea; Immunosuppressive Drugs; Inflammation; Psychosomatic Disorders.

BIBLIOGRAPHY. Fred Saibil, *Crohn's Disease and Ulcerative Colitis: Everything You Need to Know* (Firefly Books, 2003); Ramzi S. Cotran, et al., *Robbins Pathological Basis of Disease*, 6th ed. (Saunders, 1999).

QURATULAIN FATIMA
INDEPENDENT SCHOLAR

Influenza

Influenza, or "flu" for short, is a contagious viral disease that affects the respiratory system. The influenza virus is contracted through airborne exposure. It has also been called the grippe, the "sweating sickness" and in the great pandemic of 1918, Spanish fever.

Laypeople sometimes confuse influenza with other respiratory infections that are have flu-like symptoms but different causes. Influenza can be contracted by anyone at any age. Influenza viruses are RNA viruses of the family Orthomyxoviridatge. The viruses affect birds and mammals including humans. The disease is usually spread by sneezes and coughs which create an aerosol containing the virus. It can also be spread through blood, feces, nasal secretions, and saliva. Birds infected with influenza virus spread the disease via their droppings. The disease can remain infectious for sometime. In the human body, it is infectious for about a week. However, birds that carry the disease to the Artic regions can leave infectious droppings that are contagious for a month or more at near-freezing temperatures.

Common disinfectants and detergents can be used to kill influenza viruses. There are some few strains that resist this type of prophylactic activity.

Influenza can cause illness that ranges from mild to very serious. Specific symptoms are often called "flu-like" symptoms. They include fever, chills, headaches, runny or stuffy nose (rhinitis), dry cough (unproductive cough), sore throat, muscle aches (myalgia) that are nonspecific, and general weakness (malaise).

Stomach symptoms are more common in children than in adults. Symptoms in children can include ear infection (otitis media), nausea, diarrhea, and vomiting. The stomach symptoms are not caused by "stomach flu" which does not exist. The stomach upset is caused by different viruses or by secondary reactions.

Generally, people infected with a case of uncomplicated influenza recover in a few days to two weeks. However, the virus may weaken the immune system so that it creates opportunistic infections from bacteria. Pneumonia is a common secondary infection. It may be a secondary infection or caused by a primary influenza viral pneumonia. Other secondary infections are bronchitis and ear infections.

Most deaths associated with influenza are due to secondary infections. Annually, between five to twenty percent of the American population catch the flu every year. This number is in the millions with most recovering soon. However, around 200,000 people have to be hospitalized every year and about 35,000 people die from influenza complications every year.

The population groups most threatened by influenza are children, those over 65 years of age, and those with chronic health problems. The influenza virus exacerbates their underlying medical condition. Asthmatics and people with cardiac disease such as chronic heart failure are vulnerable because their condition is worsened by the disease.

Treatment for the flu includes rest, drinking plenty of fluids, and avoiding the use of tobacco and alcohol. Medications may also be taken. Some such as aspirin seek to control fever. Other medications control aches and pains. Physicians may prescribe antibiotics to combat secondary infections. Antiviral medications may be prescribed to combat the influenza virus.

Aspirin can be given to adults as part of the treatment for flu, but it should never be given to children or teenagers unless ordered by a licensed physician. Medicine for relieving symptoms are readily available for children or teens. For them to take aspirin when flu-like symptoms are present is to risk contracting Reye syndrome. This is a rare but very serious illness.

Influenza can be spread by physical contact, but is usually contracted from breathing the virus. It spreads from person to person through respiratory droplets ("droplet spread") beginning one day prior to the development of symptoms to five days after infection. Children can be contagious for seven days or longer.

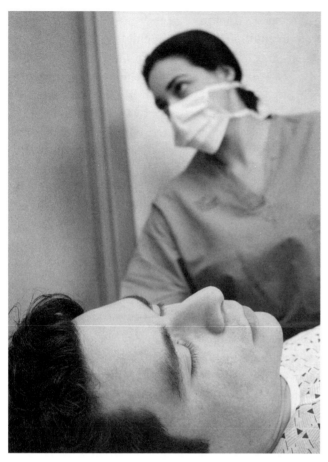

Influenza, or "flu" for short, is a contagious viral disease that affects the respiratory system. It can be contracted by people of all ages.

The influenza virus can also be spread if respiratory droplets touch the hands of uninfected people before they wash their hands. They may then transmit the disease to their respiratory system through contact.

When the virus is inhaled, it comes into contact with the cells lining the upper air passages. The virus is able to penetrate the cells and to begin its replications. As it reproduces, it spreads to other cells and then to the whole respiratory tract. As breathing occurs, the virus penetrates deep into the lungs and is also expelled into the air where it awaits an opportunity to infect others. Symptoms usually begin from one to four days after infection.

Most of the time, the human body develops enough antibodies to defeat the virus. It also develops an immunity against further influenza infections. The body develops cytotoxic T lymphocytes that have the genetic structure necessary to identify and to destroy the influenza virus. However, the influenza virus undergoes constant changes in its genetic code so that its chemical composition constantly changes. As a consequence, the body may have developed an immunity to an old strain of the virus but not to its new versions.

Because deaths from influenza are common especially in the very young, the elderly, and those with weakened immunes systems, vaccinations are promoted by health authorities. The influenza vaccine is made about six months in advance of the oncoming flu season. Vaccines against influenza have been made from either killed or live viruses.

Vaccines made from killed influenza viruses have been the most common. However, this type of vaccine has only a limited effectiveness. Research in the 1970s led to the development of live influenza vaccines. These have been more effective in combating the disease. Annual vaccination against flu is the best preventative strategy; however, some antiviral drugs have also been developed. These drugs can also be used to fight the influenza virus because they have a chemoprophylaxis effect. Amantadine, oseltamivir, rimantadine, and zanamivir are the only antiviral agents licensed in the United States. Other antiviral drugs are used in other countries. Like most drugs, all of them carry the possibility of negative side effects.

Antiviral drugs used to fight influenza viruses have encountered the development of resistance. Influenza A can quickly develop resistance; however, as the A strain mutates, it can redevelop susceptibility to antiviral drugs. During the 2006–07 flu season, American and Canadian studies indicated that Influenza A had developed resistance to amantadine and rimantadine during treatment. These two antiviral drugs were not recommended by the Centers for Disease Control and Prevention (CDC) until susceptibility was reestablished.

Oseltamivir and zanamivir are effective in treating influenza. Oseltamivir can be prescribed to infants and zanamivir can be approved for people 7 years old and older. Oseltamivir is made by Roche Laboratories and marketed as Tamiflu® (Oseltamivir Phosphate). In November 2006, the Food and Drug Administration approved a supplement to the possible side effects of the drug. Children taking the drug in Japan were reported as presenting psychiatric behaviors that caused self-injury. Administration of the drug in children now requires several minutes supervision to check for unusual behavioral signs.

Most cases of influenza occur in the winter months in both hemispheres. Beginning in November rising during December and January, the disease usually peaks in February and then begins to recede in March and ends in May. However, it may peak in any of the flu season months.

The flu season is not caused by the onset of cold weather as a direct cause. Rather, as the cold weather pushes people to get out of the cold in warm places, they congregate more which allows more opportunities for influenza viruses to spread. The best preventative against influenza is vaccination in the fall prior to the onset of flu season. Vaccines are prepared influenza virus strains that are most likely to be the prevalent strain during the oncoming flu season. In addition to vaccination, good health habits are very useful in preventing flu. These include avoiding contact, good hygiene, and healthy physical activity.

The influenza virus constantly mutates. As a result, its potency varies from year to year. Scientists have categorized influenza viruses into three main types. These are type A, type B, and type C. Types A and C affect many species including humans. Type B seems to affect only human beings.

Type A influenza is the most virulent of the three strains. It has been subdivided into categories based upon its responses to different antibodies and it pandemic potential. Type A strain, H1N1 (Spanish flu), H2N2 (Asian flu), H3N2 (Hong Kong flu), H5N1 (potential pandemic in 2007), H7N7, H1N2 endemic in humans and pigs, and H9N2, H7N2 H7N3 and H10N7.

The type A influenza viron is not a single genetic string of nucleic acid. It has eight segments that can perform different chemical reactions.

Type B influenza affects only humans and possibly seals. Most people are exposed to the strain at an early age and develop a limited immunity. Type C influenza is less common than the other two types. However, it causes local epidemics.

Swine and birds are carriers of influenza viruses. Birds may be the main reservoir of influenza stains. They can in some cases transmit the virus to each other where it undergoes genetic modification. In some cases, the genetic modifications allow the virus to infect human beings. Strains of flu are usually named for the location in which they are first identified. Or they may be named after the species in which a new strain was first found such as bird flu, swine flu, human flu, horse flu.

Influenza is a global disease that travels rapidly. It may be carried by migrating birds that then communicate it to other species and then to humans. Outbreaks occur annually, spreading around the world through contact with travelers. Great number of people are sickened every year with a large annual death toll. Economic losses from lost wages and healthcare costs are very large.

As influenza strains mutate, they can cause pandemic outbreaks in which there are great losses of life. The Spanish flu or the Great Influenza outbreak occurred in winter of 1918–19. Over 500,000 Americans died. Deaths globally were over 20 million people. Global deaths may have been much higher.

There were two other influenza pandemics in the twentieth century. Each killed millions of people. In 1956–57, the Hong Kong flu caused a great many deaths.

Pandemics are difficult to predict nor is it possible to predict how severe they may be. However, if one starts, the whole world is at risk. Countries that close their borders are simply delaying the inevitable. In a human pandemic, millions will die and the economic losses will be enormous.

In the 1990s, a new strain of flu appeared in Asia, the deadly avian strain called H5N1. So far, very few humans have been infected, but the number is growing. Of those infected, half died. Exposure to infected poultry is the suspected as the source of contraction of the disease.

The H5N1 strain has spread throughout Asia and Africa as birds migrate annually. Its appearance in the Americas is expected because of contact between birds around the Artic Circle between Asian and American bird flocks. The concern of health officials is that bird flu will interact with swine flu and then be genetically modified so that it become contagious to humans. Human-to-human contagion will then become a pandemic.

SEE ALSO: Epidemic; Infectious Diseases (General); Respiratory Diseases (General).

BIBLIOGRAPHY. John M. Barry, *The Great Influenza: The Epic Story of the Deadliest Plague in History* (Viking Penguin, 2005); Alfred W. Crosby, *America's Forgotten Pandemic: The Influenza of 1918* (Cambridge University Press, 2003); Michael Greger, *Bird Flu: A Virus of Our Own Hatching* (Lantern Books, 2006); *Influenza—*

a Medical Dictionary, Bibliography, and Annotated Research Guide to Internet References (ICON, 2004); Roy Jennings and Robert C. Read, *Influenza* (Royal Society of Medicine Press, 2000); Daniel Kalla, *Pandemic* (Tor Books, 2005); Y. Kawaoka, *Influenza Virology: Current Topics* (Caister Academic Press, 2006); Gina Bari Kolata, *Flu: The Story of the Great Influenza Pandemic of 1918 and the Search for the Virus that Caused It* (Simon & Schuster, 2001); Robert M. Krug, *Influenza Viruses* (Springer-Verlag, 1989).

ANDREW J. WASKEY
DALTON STATE COLLEGE

Inhalants

Inhalants are toxic substances found in common household products such as spray paint, glue, nail polish remover, and cleaning fluids. These substances produce breathable chemical vapors, which are inhaled to produce mind-altering effects. Inhalants are often used as a substitute for alcohol with effects that mimic acute alcohol intoxication. Most inhalant abusers are younger than 25 and are often unaware of the dangers associated with inhalant use, which include organ damage and possible death. Education, early identification, and intervention are necessary to stop inhalant abuse before it causes serious consequences.

Inhalants are easily available, inexpensive, and difficult to detect, resulting in widespread potential for abuse among children and teenagers in both urban and rural areas. Inhalant abuse is most common in the south and southwestern United States and among Native American children. Poverty, a history of sexual or physical abuse, and poor grades have all been associated with an increased risk of inhalant abuse. Government surveys have shown that inhalant abuse typically peaks between the seventh and ninth grades and results from the 2006 Monitoring the Future study indicate that 29.2 percent of eighth graders report lifetime use of inhalants.

Inhalants include large variety of substances such as solvents (e.g., gasoline, paint thinner, glue, felt-tip marker, correction fluid), aerosols (e.g., spray paint and hair spray), and gases (e.g., butane light-ers, ether, halothane, nitrous oxide) that have varying pharmacological effects. Inhalants can be abused in many different ways including inhaling nitrous oxide from balloons, spraying aerosols directly into the mouth, "sniffing" which describes direct inhalation of fumes from containers, "bagging" which involves inhalation of solvents from a plastic or paper bag, and "huffing" which describes inhaling vapors from a cloth soaked in solvent that is held close to, or stuffed inside of, the mouth. Most inhalants produce rapid euphoria and central nervous system depression. This resembles acute alcohol intoxication, with drunken appearance, slurred speech, disorientation, nausea, and vomiting. Inhalant abusers are also likely to have chemical odors or paint stains on their face, hands, or clothing.

Research from animals and humans show that inhalants are extremely toxic and hazardous to health. High concentrations of certain inhalants, such as butane, can induce rapid and irregular heart rhythms that may progress to heart failure and death within minutes, a syndrome described as "sudden sniffing death." Inhalants can also lead to death through suffocation and asphyxiation. Chronic use of inhalants can cause organ damage to many structures including the brain, heart, liver, lungs, and kidneys.

Although inhalants are not regulated under the Controlled Substances Act, they have a high potential for abuse and many state legislatures have passed laws restricting the sale of products such as spray paint and glue to minors. Adults should be aware of the temptations that inhalants pose to children and store household products carefully to avoid accidental ingestion or intentional abuse.

SEE ALSO: Adolescent Health; National Institute on Drug Abuse (NIDA).

BIBLIOGRAPHY. Jerrold S. Meyer and Linda F. Quenzer, *Psychopharmacology: Drugs, the Brain, and Behavior* (Sinauer, 2004); National Institute on Drug Abuse, "Info Facts: Inhalants," www.drugabuse.gov (cited January 2007); National Institute on Drug Abuse, "NIDA Community Drug Alert Bulletin: Inhalants," www.drugabuse.gov (cited January 2007).

BERNADETTE MIETUS STEVENSON, M.D., PH.D.
UNIVERSITY OF NORTH CAROLINA

Innate Immunity

An inflammatory response is the body's reaction to tissue damage or infection by foreign substances. It is a complex phenomenon composed of two very distinct types of immunity: innate and acquired. In innate immunity, the body utilizes natural and physiologic barriers to initiate cellular repair, to protect itself from invasion, and to attempt to limit the spread of pathogen through activation of a complex inflammatory cascade.

The natural barriers of innate immunity include the skin, mucous membranes, hair, and the acidic environments of the stomach and sweat. Examples of the physiologic responses include the coughing reflex, the release of antifungal and antibacterial secretions from skin glands, the beating of respiratory cilia, the production of hydrolytic enzymes in tears and saliva, the production of chemical signals known as cytokines, and the stimulation of specific innate cellular components which aid in the fight against infection. Effective innate immunity does not rely on previous interaction with the pathogen and is therefore a non-specific cellular immunity.

Phagocytosis, characterized by host cell migration, recognition, attachment, engulfment, and processing of pathogens, is the main mechanism of innate immunity. In this process, host cells are protected from invasion and attempt to control the spread of a pathogen. The primary cells involved are neutrophils and macrophages. Neutrophils are considered the first responders during inflammation and are often replaced by macrophages arriving at the exposure site within 48 hours. Activation of this process often follows exposure of the body to specific bacterial components, like lipopolysaccharide (LPS), a polysaccharide on certain bacterial cell membranes.

The body also responds to bacterial peptides, membrane components like peptidoglycan and techoic acid, and foreign nucleic acids. Each of these substances contains unique sequences known as pathogen-associated molecular patterns, or PAMPs, that the body recognizes as foreign. The body possesses its own recognition machinery in the form of toll-like receptors, or TLRs, found on host innate immune cells, and these are used to recognize and bind these PAMPS. Initiation of downstream cellular responses then occurs and leads to the production of exudate and specific chemical messages such as interferon, interleukins 1 and 6, and tumor necrosis factor.

Another process by which host cells are protected from invasion and attempt to control the spread of a pathogen is via complement activation. A complement is an immune complex comprised of three activating pathways: the leptin pathway, the alternative pathway, and the classical pathway, all of which allow for the destruction of the invading pathogen.

The typical signs and characteristics of the innate immune response include heat, redness, swelling, pain, and loss of function. The heat and redness accompany vascular dilatation while swelling is the result of the escape of fluid, plasma protein, and cellular accumulation within the area of exposure. Pain results from released chemical mediators and nerve compression. The severity of the pathogen, the immune status of the host, and the site of exposure determine the intensity of each symptom. Without such a complex response, the body would be unable to effectively fight off infection and disease.

SEE ALSO: Acquired Immunity; Immunology.

BIBLIOGRAPHY. Stefan H.E. Kaufmann, Ruslan Medzhitov, and Siamon Gordon, eds., *The Innate Immune Response to Infection* (ASM Press, 2004).

MELISSA K. WOLINSKI
MICHIGAN STATE UNIVERSITY

Inpatient

An inpatient is someone staying at a hospital for one or more nights while undergoing medical treatment. The word comes from the term *patient* which is derived from the Latin word *patiens*, which refers to enduring or suffering. The adjective *patient* from the word *patience* comes from the same origin, but obviously, has a different meaning.

A hospital is the medical facility where patients can be treated overnight, as opposed to a clinic or medical center, where this is generally not possible. As a result, an inpatient is officially defined as someone who goes to the hospital with a serious ailment or condition, and needs to stay overnight or until he or she recovers. This may be for several days or weeks; in extreme cases, such as with coma patients, stays can last decades.

In emergencies, patients are admitted immediately. Visitors to emergency rooms are generally seen quickly, with an immediate report of the patient's condition made. Staff in the emergency room determines the urgency of the patient's need for medical treatment. Depending on these decisions and the number of patients waiting for emergency treatment, there can be a wait before a given patient is formally admitted. At this point, medical professionals determine whether or not the patient can be treated and released or will need a more prolonged stay for treatment, rest and recovery, or because of the patient's home situation; in some cases, a patient may be admitted because of the inability to return home or the need to notify family members.

If it is determined that the patient will be staying at the hospital for at least one night, the patient's status becomes "inpatient." Hospital staff must then find an available bed, either at their hospital or at another nearby facility. Patients awaiting an operation, those recovering from a fall or accident, and those recovering from medical procedures are classified as inpatient until they have recovered sufficiently to allow a return home. Patients who arrive at the hospital for a planned medical procedure are generally classified as inpatient as well.

Upon discharge from a hospital, a person ceases to be an inpatient.

SEE ALSO: Outpatient.

BIBLIOGRAPHY. Sanjay Saint, *The Saint-Frances Guide to Inpatient Medicine,* 2nd ed. (Lippincott Williams & Wilkins, 2003).

JUSTIN CORFIELD
GEELONG GRAMMAR SCHOOL, AUSTRALIA

Institute for Children's Environmental Health (ICEH)

The Institute for Children's Environmental Health (ICEH), founded in 1999, is a nonprofit educational organization working to ensure a healthy, just, and sustainable future for all children. ICEH's primary goals center around coordinating effective, collab-

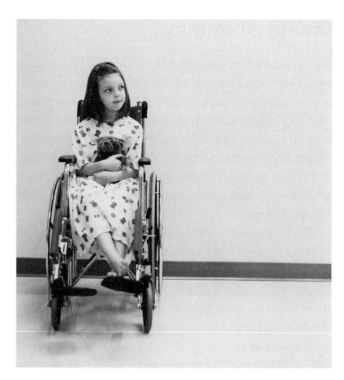

An inpatient is someone staying at a hospital for one or more nights while undergoing medical treatment.

orative strategies among the varied environmental health-focused organizations and institutions in order to mitigate duplicative efforts and diffuse tension over jurisdictional issues, and promoting a project-based environmental health and justice program to be introduced into existing youth forums and schools in order to educate and activate the next generation on environmental health and justice concerns. To support its mission, the ICEH is committed to creating long-term partnerships with other organizations and institutions to build a more effective and collaborative environmental health movement. The Institute also works with health-affected constituencies, in particular learning and developmental disabilities organizations, to educate their members about possible environmental links to various health problems and to nurture their capacity to advocate for policies that protect children from neurotoxicants. Additionally, the ICEH supports policies and actions based on preventive, transparent, democratic, and precautionary practices to ensure that children's unique susceptibilities to environmental exposures are being addressed.

The ICEH has been involved with a number of national programs and initiatives, including the Learning and Developmental Disability Initiative (LDDI), a national network of organizations and individuals interested in collaborating on research, educational and policy initiatives that reduce exposures to pollutants that may undermine healthy brain development. The LDDI is a working group of the Collaborative on Health and the Environment (CHE) and members include researchers, health professionals, learning and developmental disabilities organizations, and environmental health and justice groups. The Partnership for Children's Health and the Environment, a growing coalition of over 270 organizations and leaders in government, academic, and community-based sectors in North America, is committed to sharing information and incubating new collaborative initiatives on children's environmental health issues. The Healthy Futures Project is a project-based program on environmental health and justice for youth in the Pacific Northwest.

This program fosters both scientific thinking and creative expression to inspire youth to serve as change agents for a healthy future, and also focuses on educating students with learning disabilities about environmental health issues. The ICEH also regionally coordinates the Collaborative on Health and the Environment–Washington (CHE-WA), a regional project of national CHE. CHE-WA is a network of over 310 researchers, health-affected groups, healthcare practitioners, environmental health and justice advocates, and other concerned citizens committed to reducing environmental contaminants for a healthier future. The Institute sponsors an annual meeting as well as regional gatherings throughout the country. Its advisory board includes some of the country's leading professionals in the various fields of children's health. The principle funding for the ICEH comes from the Tides Center, a nonprofit foundation dedicated to positive social change, innovation, and environmental sustainability.

SEE ALSO: Environmental Health; Pediatrics.

BIBLIOGRAPHY. American Academy of Pediatrics, www.aap.org (cited September 2006); Ruth Eztel, ed., *Pediatric Environmental Health* (American Academy of Pediatrics, 2004); Natalie Freeman and Dona Schneider, *Children's Environmental Health: Reducing Risk in a Dangerous World* (American Public Health Association, 2000); Institution for Children's Environmental Health, www.iceh.org (cited September 2006); Tides Center, www.tidescenter.org/index_tc.cfm (cited September 2006).

BEN WYNNE, PH.D
GAINESVILLE STATE COLLEGE

Institute of Medicine (IOM)

Founded in 1970 as part of the National Academy of Sciences, the Institute of Medicine (IOM) is a nonprofit organization charged with working as an advisor on ways to improve health. In that capacity, the Institute provides unbiased, evidence-based, and authoritative information and advice concerning health and science policy to legislators, professionals, leaders in every sector of society, and the public at large.

The Institute's work centers principally on committee reports or studies on subjects ranging from the national smallpox vaccination program to protecting the nation's food supply. The IOM's principle concerns are organized into 17 topic areas: mental health, child health, food and nutrition, aging, women's health, education, public policy, healthcare and quality, diseases, global health, workplace, military and veterans, health sciences, environment, treatment, public health and prevention, and minority health. The Institute also convenes roundtables, workshops, and symposia that provide an opportunity for public and private sector experts to discuss contentious issues in an open environment that facilitates evidence-based dialogue. The majority of the Institute's studies and other activities are requested and funded by the federal government. Private industry, foundations, and state and local governments also initiate studies, as does the IOM itself.

The objective in all of the Institute's work is to improve decision making by identifying and synthesizing evidence relative to the deliberative process. The IOM is regularly recognized through its projects as a national resource of judgment and veracity in the analysis of issues relating to human health. Depending on the request, studies by the Institute may be designed to answer very specific and technical questions, or they may be broad-based examinations that span multiple academic disciplines, industries, and international borders.

The IOM is organized into eight oversight boards: Board on African Science Academy Development (joint with the National Research Council [NRC]); Board on Children, Youth, and Families (joint with NRC); Food and Nutrition Board; Board on Global Health; Board on Health Care Services; Board on Population Health and Public Health Practice; Board on Health Sciences Policy; and Board on Military and Veterans Health. In developing a board's membership, the IOM seeks to have expertise in the various relevant disciplines and in subject matter areas that are in the board's portfolio of studies or other activities. In addition, the organization seeks diversity, academic distinction, and geographic balance. The Institute publishes the *IOM News,* a free, bimonthly e-mail newsletter for its members through which it announces new IOM publications, upcoming events, and general information related to the organization's mission. The IOM headquarters is in New York City.

SEE ALSO: National Institute of Health (NIH).

BIBLIOGRAPHY. Board on African Science Academy Development, www7.nationalacademies.org/africa/index.html (cited October 2006); Board on Children, Youth, and Families, www7.nationalacademies.org/bocyf (cited October 2006); Board on Military and Veterans Health, www.iom. edu/CMS/26761.aspx (cited October 2006); Institute of Medicine (IOM), www.iom.edu (cited October 2006); The National Academies, www.nationalacademies.org/nrc (cited October 2006); National Institutes of Health (NIH), www.nih.gov (cited October 2006).

BEN WYNNE, PH.D.
GAINESVILLE STATE COLLEGE

Institutional Review Board (IRB)

Under Food and Drug Administration (FDA) regulations, an institutional review board (IRB) is an appropriately constituted group that has been formally designated to review and monitor biomedical research involving human subjects. In accordance with FDA regulations, an IRB has the authority to approve, require modifications in (to secure approval), or disapprove research. This type of review serves an important role in the protection of the rights and welfare of human research subjects.

The purpose of IRB review is to assure, both in advance and by periodic review, that appropriate steps are taken to protect the rights and welfare of humans participating as subjects in various types of research. To accomplish this mission, IRBs use a group process to review research protocols and related materials such as informed consent documents and investigator brochures. While IRB is a generic term used by the FDA to refer to a group whose function is to review research to assure the protection of the rights and welfare of human subjects, institutions under review may use whatever name they choose.

An IRB is subject to the FDA's IRB regulations when studies of agency-regulated products are reviewed and approved. Although institutions engaged in research involving human subjects will usually have their own IRBs to oversee research conducted within that specific institution or by the staff of the institution, FDA regulations permit an institution without a board to arrange for initial and continuing review through the use of an "outside" IRB. Individuals conducting research in a noninstitutional setting often use established IRBs (either independent or institutional) rather than creating their own. While research that has been reviewed and approved by an IRB may be subject to further review or even disapproval by officials of the institution, those same officials may not approve research if it has been disapproved by the IRB.

Federal policy dictates that IRBs must have at least five members with varying backgrounds to promote a complete review of research activities commonly conducted by an institution. The IRB members must be sufficiently qualified through experience, expertise, and diversity of background, including considerations of racial and cultural heritage and sensitivity to issues related to community attitudes. The United States Department of Health and Human Services, Office of Human Resource Protection (OHRP) sponsors a series of workshop on responsibilities of researchers, IRBs, and institutional officials for the protection of human subjects in research. These conferences are open to everyone with an interest in research involving human subjects.

SEE ALSO: Department of Health and Human Services (DHHS); Food and Drug Administration (FDA).

BIBLIOGRAPHY. The Institutional Review Board—Discussion and News Forum, www.irbforum.org (cited October 2006); Robert J. Levine, *Ethics and Regulation of Clinical Research*, 2d ed. (Urban and Schwarzenberg, 1986); Dennis M. Maloney, *Protection of Human Research Subjects: A Practical Guide to Federal Laws and Regulations* (Plenum, 1984); The Poynter Center for the Study of Ethics and American Institutions, http://poynter.indiana.edu (cited October 2006); United States Department of Health and Human Services, Office of Human Resource Protection, www.hhs.gov/ohrp/irb/irb_guidebook.htm (cited October 2006).

BEN WYNNE, PH.D.
GAINESVILLE STATE COLLEGE

Insurance

Unpredictable illness creates an uncertain need for health services. The institutional response to this uncertainty is to create an insurance mechanism in which participating individuals contribute regularly to a risk-pooling agency that provides reimbursement in the event of an illness. The insuring organization can be public or private, the contribution can be via premiums or taxes, and the reimbursement can be monetary or through direct provision of medical services.

Risk-averse individuals are willing to pay a premium to an insuring agency to avoid taking on risk. This premium is typically far more than the average loss they are likely to confront since the sum of these collected premiums from the insured pool must at least cover the expected benefits the insurance agency expects to pay out, their administrative cost, along with their profit. Three basic challenges to this model have been studied extensively: consumer information issues, moral hazard, and adverse selection.

Consumers in the healthcare market are confronted with the lack of easily available price, paucity of quality information, and the challenge of interpreting complex and technical medical information. These issues can limit the ability of the individual to make rational and informed decisions about medical insurance.

Moral hazard is neither a moral dilemma nor is it necessarily hazardous. Instead, it is a rational consumer's predictable response to a reduction in the price of health services, resulting from participation in an insurance plan. The insurance plan reduces the out-of-pocket cost to the individual for medical services, inducing individuals to consume care that is of less value than the cost of providing that care. In the most extensive controlled experiment on health insurance, the RAND Corporation, a nonprofit research organization, and associated researchers found that being insured increased the likelihood of purchasing medical services and increased the spending amount in the event of an illness.

Insurance companies have introduced deductibles and coinsurance to limit the extent of moral hazard by having the individual feel some level of financial burden. The insurance deductible is a set monetary amount that must be incurred by the insured before the insurance company pays any part of the claim. A policy with coinsurance requires the individual to pay a fixed percentage of every claim, and this cost sharing typically ends after total out-of-pocket spaending reaches some limit. Such solutions allow a balancing between the reduction in financial risk and the effects of increased demand for care.

The third concern is that of adverse selection, whereby the purchasers of insurance have more information about their expected healthcare needs than the insuring organization. Individuals have the ability to conceal their true risk. If enough high-risk individuals conceal themselves as low-risk purchasers, the premiums set by the insurance agency based on actuarial projection will underestimate the expected benefits that will need to be paid out. This will lead to higher-than-average premiums for the pool of individuals and create an incentive for low-risk individuals to drop out of the pool, driving up premiums even more.

These even-higher premiums would drive out more low-risk individuals at the margin, driving premiums even higher. This so-called "death spiral" is prevented by insurance companies by only underwriting prospective risk, and thereby not insuring for preexisting conditions. In addition, they can risk rate prospective customers via having them complete a questionnaire or have a physical exam. In essence, if the insurance agency could identify low- and high-risk individuals, and charge premiums accordingly, then the problem of adverse selection could be averted. Pooling risk through a third-party mechanism such as an employer also serves to mitigate adverse selection. Alternatively, in a national health insurance program, there is no concern for adverse selection because everyone is covered.

SYSTEMS OF HEALTH INSURANCE WORLDWIDE

Countries have taken many different approaches to providing health insurance, and many have been able to successfully provide universal health coverage, that is, insurance to all individuals within a geographic or political entity. This list includes Argentina, Australia, Austria, Belgium, Canada, Cuba, Denmark, Finland, France, Germany, Greece, Ireland, Israel, Italy, Japan, the Netherlands, New Zealand, Norway, Portugal, Russia, Saudi Arabia, South Korea, Spain, Sri Lanka, Sweden, Taiwan, and the United Kingdom. A notable exception from this list is the United States, where over 46 million individuals are uninsured. While each country is unique in its system, below is a brief description of a few countries to provide a flavor of the variety of different mechanisms that have been employed. The type of insurance coverage, the payers, and the nature of the providers are highlighted.

CANADA

National health insurance in Canada, known as Medicare, is a public program administered by the provinces and overseen by the federal government. This single-payer system run by the government is supported by general tax revenues. Federal contributions are linked to population and economic conditions of the provinces, with provinces left to pay the remaining amount. Medicare accounts for 72 percent of total healthcare expenditures, while a majority of Canadians have supplemental private insurance accounting for the remaining 28 percent. A majority of Canadian physicians are in private practice and accept fee-for-service rates set by the government through negotiations with provincial health ministries. More than 95 percent of hospitals are nonprofit, operating under a regional budget with limited fee-for-service payments.

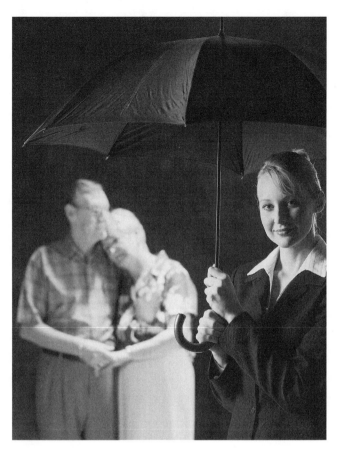

Medicare is a program in the United States providing coverage to people over 65, and is funded by taxes and enrollee premiums.

GERMANY

The national health insurance program of Germany is paid for by Sickness Insurance Funds (SIFs), quasi-governmental groups that serve as insurance companies in terms of collecting premiums, negotiating rates, and paying providers. SIFs are funded by compulsory payroll contributions, an average of 14 percent of wages, equally shared between employers and employees. SIFs cover 92 percent of the population and account for 81 percent of health expenditures. The remaining 8 percent are the affluent self-insured, the self-employed, and civil servants, who are all covered by private insurance based on voluntary, individual contributions. General practitioners do not serve as gatekeepers to specialists, and are paid on a fee-for-service basis.

UNITED KINGDOM

The medical system of the United Kingdom, known as the National Health Service (NHS), handles both healthcare delivery and healthcare financing. In other words, the government is the purchaser and provider of healthcare. The NHS, funded through general taxation, accounts for 88 percent of health expenditures. Complementary private insurance, provided by both for-profit and not-for-profit insurers, covers 12 percent of the population and accounts for four percent of total expenditures. Physicians are paid directly by the government via salary, capitation, and fee-for-service mechanisms. They serve as gatekeepers to specialists. Hospitals are self-governing public trusts that contract with groups of purchasers on a long-term basis.

UNITED STATES

The healthcare system of the United States is a combination of private insurance coverage based primarily on employment, and three major public insurance programs: Medicare, Medicaid, and Veterans Affairs. Medicare is a federal government program providing coverage to people age 65 or older, and is funded by payroll taxes, income taxes, trust fund interest, and enrollee premiums. Ninety percent of this funding comes directly or indirectly from individuals who are younger than 65 years old. Medicaid is a means-tested entitlement program administered by the states, jointly financed with the federal government. U.S. military veterans and current servicemen and servicewomen are provided care directly through a nationwide network of government hospitals organized by the Department of Veterans Affairs. Fifteen percent of the U.S. population is covered by public insurance, 5 percent by private nongroup, and 62 percent by employer-sponsored insurance. This leaves 18 percent uninsured, amounting to more than 46 million individuals without insurance in the United States.

SEE ALSO: World Health Organization (WHO).

BIBLIOGRAPHY. J.W. Henderson, *Health Economics and Policy* (South-Western, 1999); W.G. Manning, et al., "Health Insurance and the Demand for Medical Care: Evidence from a Randomized Experiment," *American Economic Review* (v.77/3, 1987); M.V. Pauly, "The Economics of Moral Hazard," *American Economic Review* (v.58/3, 1968); Thomas Rice, *The Economics of Health Reconsidered* (Health Administration Press, 1998); R.J. Zeckhauser, "Medical Insurance: A Case Study of the Trade-Off between Risk Spreading and Appropriate Incentives," *Journal of Economic Theory* (v.2/1, 1970).

Ashwinkumar Patel
Wharton School of the University
of Pennsylvania

Internal Medicine

Internal medicine is a special branch of conventional medicine that treats diseases of the internal organs of the body. Physicians who become doctors of internal medicine are physicians who train to be doctors for adults. Called internists, "general internists," and "doctors of internal medicine," they are not interns, nor family physician, family practitioners, or general practitioners. General practitioners may have medical training in surgery, obstetrics, pediatrics, or other specialties that are not focused exclusively on adult care.

The practice of internal medicine developed in Germany in the late 1800s when physicians combined laboratory medical science with the care of patients. Americans studying medicine in Germany brought the specialty to the United States.

In the United States at the beginning of the 21st century, primary care for adults is provided by either by physicians engaged in family practice or as general internal medicine physicians. There is some overlap between internists and family practice and pediatricians because all three give care to adolescents.

Physicians who become internists are internal medicine specialists. As internists, they have a specialty in some aspect of medicine affecting the internal systems of the body. They specialize in medicine focused on the diseases experienced from young adult years into old age. Their specialized training is focused on the prevention and treatment of adult medicine.

Internists have either an MD (medical doctor) degree or a DO (Doctor of Osteopathy) degree. Their training is certified by either the American Board of Internal Medicine or by the American Osteopathic Board of Internal Medicine for physicians practicing in the United States. In other countries, other certification agencies are used and the qualifications may differ.

Qualifications needed to be satisfied to become a doctor of internal medicine include a basic medical degree, internist training, and three or more years of study and practice in a internal medicine specialty. Specialties in internal medicine include allergy, cardiology, endocrinology, gastroenterology, genetics, geriatrics, hematology, immunology, infectious diseases, metabolism, molecular medicine, nephrology, neurology, oncology, pulmonology, and rheumatology.

The goal of internal medicine is to prevent adult disease or to cure them. Internists are sometimes called "doctors' doctors" because they may serve as consultants to other physicians in solving diagnostic puzzles. The internist is a personal physician who establishes a long-term relationship with a patient to provide comprehensive care lasting over the lifetime of the patient.

Whether in a routine examination or in a clinical setting that is focused on the management of a chronic disease such as diabetes, the internist provides care that will educate the patient as well as provide treatment for the immediate ailment of the patient.

Internists are trained to deal with any medical problem that a patient brings. It may be that the problem is common or it may be rare. It may be simple or complex, but it is of concern of the internist to solve diagnostic problems that are acute or chronic. In addition they are equipped with the knowledge to also understand and to treat cases where a combination of different diseases strike simultaneously.

Internal medicine is also sufficiently broad in scope to deal not only will illness but also with wellness. Part of their medical advice may be to educate patients in their own self-care that will prevent disease and promote health.

In the modern medical environment, the focus of internists in on caring for patients throughout the adult life cycle. This includes examinations in their office or in a clinic. It also includes care in times of hospitalization, intensive care and in nursing homes in the last stages of life. Care for women, for those with mental health problems, and for those with substance abuse problems are within the realm of internists. Also they are equipped to deal effectively with other problems such as problems of the eyes, ears, skin, nervous system, and the reproductive organs.

If the patient needs the care of other medical specialists such as obstetricians or surgeon, then physicians practicing internal medicine will coordinate with others in dealing with the needs of the patient. They care for and manage all medical problems connected with the care of the patient during the illness, including the hospitalization.

Knowledge of internal medicine is used by internists during physical examination to identify abnormalities that are indicators of disease. Picking up symptoms during the diagnostic process to add to the patient's medical history is used to evaluate the patient's health or diseased conditions. Specifically, internists review the different internal systems of the patient—pulmatory system, digestive system, and the other systems to identify symptoms that are indications of disease. A review of the patient's internal systems that identifies symptoms of disease is more likely to be successful if it follows a structured pattern. Otherwise symptoms may be missed.

For example, in men, prostatitis is a common occurring infection of the prostate gland. It is caused by a bacterial infection most often. It causes inflammation and will be indicated by an abnormal white blood cell count as well as pain in the prostate. In cases of chronic prostatitis, the symptoms will be more severe and require more radical remedies. Generally, a course of antibiotics will eliminate the infection, but the internist in a long-term relationship with the patient will be able to track the symptoms to that the patient's problem is eventually solved.

Urine tests, blood tests, medical imaging, and other tests can be used to rule other possible diseases or confirm their presence. These tests are sometimes called screening tests. They may include X-rays, white blood cell counts, red blood cell counts, electrolyte tests, renal function tests, enzyme test, or blood gas tests. Other tests can be used including biopsies for microbiological cultures. For example, Whipple's disease, which is a malabsorption disease caused by a bacterial infection, can be definitively diagnosed by a biopsy of the jejunum area of the small intestines.

Cancer can be identified by a biopsy taken by an internist who specializes in oncology. The biopsy can read by a pathologist and the specific type of cancer identified. This will allow specific treatment to be made.

Globally, internal medicine is practiced as the primary form of medicine used to treat the majority of diseases. Internists have joined together in a number of organizations to improve the quality of their education, and the quality of the care they deliver. For example, the International Society of Internal Medicine was founded in 1948. It has since become an international association composed of over 60 national societies of internal medicine.

SEE ALSO: Allergy; Cardiology; Endocrinology; Gastroenterology; Genetics; Geriatrics; Hematology; Immunology; Infectious Diseases (General); Nephrology; Neurology; Oncology; Pulmonology.

BIBLIOGRAPHY. Steven S. Agabegi, et al., *Step-up to Internal Medicine* (Lippincott Williams & Wilkins, 2004); Steven A. Haist, Leonard G. Gomella, and John B. Robbins, *Internal Medicine on Call* (McGraw-Hill, 2005); Dennis L. Kasper, et al, *Harrison's Principles of Internal Medicine* (McGraw-Hill, 2004); Raminder Nirula, *Internal Medicine* (Lippincott Williams & Wilkins, 2006); Eugene C. Toy, et al., *Case Files: Internal Medicine 2007* (McGraw-Hill, 2007); James S. Winshall, and Robert Lederman, *Tarascon Internal Medicine & Critical Care Pocketbook* (Tarascon, 2006).

ANDREW J. WASKEY
DALTON STATE COLLEGE

International Agency for Research on Cancer (IARC)

The International Agency for Research on Cancer (IARC) is part of the World Health Organization (WHO), the United Nation's agency dedicated to global health. Located in Lyon, France, the IARC focuses on four goals: monitoring global cancer occurrences; identifying causes of cancer; determining how carcinogens interact with human DNA; and developing scientific strategies to control cancer through prevention and early detection. Although the IARC studies the connection between human cancers and the environment, the agency does not attempt to influence carcinogen-related political legislation.

The IRAC was founded on May 20, 1965, by the governments of Germany, France, Italy, the United Kingdom, and the United States at the Eighteenth World Health Assembly. The initial goal was to promote international collaboration in cancer research; working languages were established as English and French, with speeches in those languages also translated into Russian. Although logistic matters needed a vote, issues considered purely scientific were not subject to a vote and each scientist could express his or her opinion.

Globally, in 2000, there were 10.1 million new cases of cancer diagnosed, 6.2 million deaths and 22.4 million people living with cancer. This represents a 19 percent increase in incidence and an 18 percent increase in mortality since 1990. The IARC works to identify the causes of cancer so that medical researchers can parlay IARC research into studies for cancer prevention, treatments and cures. They believe that 80 percent of all cancers are connected to environmental factors and are therefore preventable; many cancers appear in varying degrees in different geographies and/or populations, and the IARC often focuses its research efforts on uncovering environmental factors that contribute to these patterns and their accompanying mortality rates.

The agency studies environmental risk factors, including exposure to chemicals and biological agents, providing this information to national health agencies attempting to reduce or prevent human exposure to carcinogens. Scientists from a number of disciplines analyze published IARC studies to determine how to rank a particular risk factor. Since 1971, they have reviewed more than 900 such factors, identifying approximately 400 as either carcinogenic or potentially so.

The IARC divides substances under study as Category 1 (carcinogenic to human); Category 2A (probably carcinogenic to humans); Category 2B (possibly carcinogenic to humans); Category 3 (not classifiable as to carcinogenicity in humans); and Category 4 (probably not carcinogenic in humans).

The agency has monitored the "cancer burden" caused by the nuclear leak in the Chernobyl power plant in the Ukraine. IARC scientists project 16,000 cases of thyroid cancer and 25,000 of other types of cancer by 2065 (the 80th anniversary of the nuclear fallout), with an estimated 16,000 deaths from these incidents of cancer.

Three particular forms of cancer that garner IARC focus are breast cancer, cervical cancer, and oral cancer. In many countries, breast cancer is the most common form for women, with increasing incidences in

Africa and Asia. Although, in the United States and other developed countries, mammogram screenings are successfully used as early detection tools, this technology is too expensive and therefore not a feasible strategy in developing countries. The IARC is therefore attempting to institute more practical early detection strategies in these countries.

Similar concerns exist over cervical cancer, a disease that kills more than 288,000 women annually, worldwide, with 80 percent or more of these deaths occurring in poor areas of South Asia, sub-Saharan, and Latin America. The IARC goal is to develop strategies that help women obtain the relatively simple cervical cancer screening tests in vulnerable parts of the world so that prognoses for these women are more favorable.

Oral cancer, which is becoming more prominent in Europe, Japan, and Australia, is also a focus of the IRAC, with early screening a top goal.

Agency scientists also study diet and other lifestyle factors in connection with increased cancer risks. Recent IARC studies have confirmed increased colorectal cancer risk with diets heavy in red meat, and reduced risk with diets of fish. Although increased consumption of fruits and vegetables seems to prevent many cancers and other diseases, no link was found to breast cancer prevention. One specific focus of IARC research is to identify how carcinogens work to mutate human genes that normally suppress tumors. Through this process, researchers learn more about the biology of cancer and they identify optimal points when intervention can prevent cancer development.

The IARC created an online bookstore to disseminate information and they maintain a Cancer Epidemiology Database that lists occurrences of cancer, worldwide. Starting in 1997, the IARC began publishing a series (10 in all) of *IARC Handbooks of Cancer Prevention*, to evaluate the effectiveness of preventative strategies. Topics range from mammograms to the consumption of fruits and vegetables to weight control and physical activity.

The agency has awarded more than 500 fellowships since 1966 to scientists learning cancer research techniques and strategies. They estimate that 85 percent of these scientists return to their home countries to continue their work; approximately 82 percent of the fellows remain active in cancer research efforts. Postdoctoral fellowships are available to scientists who reside in countries with low- or medium-resource levels.

Besides the founding members, the following nations have joined the IARC: Australia (1965), Belgium (1970), Canada (1982), Denmark (1990), Finland (1986), India (2006), Japan (1972), Korea (2006), Netherlands (1987), Norway (1987), Russian Federation (1965), Spain (2003), Sweden (1979), and Switzerland (1990). In 2006, Lars Erik Hanssen of Norway was elected chair of IARC. He lists two priorities: closer study of the hepatitis B vaccine's preventative impact on liver cancer in Gambia and an examination of the links between alcohol consumption and cancer.

SEE ALSO: American Cancer Society (ACS); Cancer (General); National Cancer Institute (NCI); World Health Organization (WHO).

BIBLIOGRAPHY. American Cancer Society (ACS), www.cancer.org (cited December 2006); Vincent James Cogliano, et al., "The Science and Practice of Carcinogen Identification and Evaluation," *Environmental Health Perspectives* (v. 113/12, 2004).

Kelly Boyer Sagert
Independent Scholar

International AIDS Vaccine Initiative (IAVI)

The International AIDS Vaccine Initiative (IAVI) is an international nonprofit organization founded in 1996 to promote HIV vaccine development. While other international coalition groups such as the Global Fund also work to treat and prevent infectious diseases, IAVI is the main international organization that specifically funds HIV vaccine research. The organization strongly believes that, while ongoing treatment for those infected with HIV and suffering from AIDS is vital, as are prevention campaigns aimed at behavior change, a vaccine is essential to stemming the tide of new infections. While HIV is a pressing international health problem, many pharmaceutical companies remain relatively disinterested in funding HIV vaccine research, and thus most funding comes from private donors, foundations, and national governments rather than shareholders. The IAVI serves as a centralized distributing body of funds for HIV vaccine research from a number of nonprofit and governmental organizations, which provide over 90 percent of all funds for HIV vaccine research.

The IAVI also engages in public policy advocacy, encouraging governments to make HIV vaccine development and approval a priority, as well as asserting that any future vaccine should be universally available once it is proven effective. Scientists and research organizations funded by IAVI must pledge to make any future vaccine available in developing countries at cost and in sufficient quantities, regardless of home country intellectual property right laws. The IAVI has also promoted the idea of constructing a quasi-market for vaccines by encouraging G8 countries (United Kingdom, Canada, France, Germany, Italy, Japan, Russia, and United States), among others, to guarantee low-cost loans for developing countries heavily burdened by HIV to purchase vaccines when they become available, loans which can be paid back by future savings on healthcare expenditures.

The IAVI functions by financially supporting the development of promising vaccines from initial stages to human clinical trials through partnerships with private companies, academic institutions, and government research facilities. The IAVI's scientific advisory board selects the most promising vaccine candidates and funds swift acceleration of development and clinical testing. In addition to efficacious promise, one particular concern of the organization is promoting the development of vaccines most effective against the subtypes of HIV that are most prevalent in areas of the world where infection rates are the highest, such as in sub-Saharan Africa. Furthermore, the IAVI is not only concerned with providing an effective vaccine, but also one that is easy to store, administer, and manufacture, so it can be disseminated more quickly and easily in areas with less extensive health infrastructure.

The organization also seeks to build basic scientific research capacity in Asian and African countries by building laboratories and training staff. Recognizing a legacy of mistrust regarding human clinical trials among many nations, regions, and peoples, IAVI also works closely with community and national leaders in areas where clinical vaccine trials are being conducted in an effort to alleviate harm, misunderstanding, and distrust. The IAVI also works to coordinate results of trials from different sites, ensuring that they are scientifically accurate and internationally comparable. As of mid-2006, the IAVI supported over 30 vaccine candidates in small-scale clinical trials worldwide.

SEE ALSO: AIDS; AIDS—Living with AIDS.

BIBLIOGRAPHY. Susan Hunter, *Black Death: AIDS in Africa* (Palgrave Macmillan, 2004); International AIDS Vaccine Initiative, www.iavi.org (cited May 2007).

ANNIE DUDE
UNIVERSITY OF CHICAGO

International Center for Equal Healthcare Access (ICEHA)

Founded by Dr. Marie Charles in 2001, the International Center for Equal Healthcare Access (ICEHA) is a nonprofit organization that engages experienced healthcare professionals to rapidly improve the clinical skills of colleagues in resource-poor countries through the use of innovative methods of mentoring. The Center is based in New York City and is governed by boards of directors in both the United States and the United Kingdom. These boards oversee all activities of the organization and provide strategic, programmatic, legal, and financial direction. The directors on the board comprise an international team of highly qualified and world-renowned experts with expertise in the field of HIV care, developing countries, program design, and legal and financial management.

The ICEHA currently focuses on HIV and infectious diseases, leveraging the wealth of medical expertise in the West for maximum impact on national health systems in developing countries. A consistent, high level of quality of instruction is maintained by requiring volunteers to be trained and certified by ICEHA. After being certified, volunteers are seconded to a clinic in a developing country.

In order to effectively increase access to HIV care and prevention, and to improve overall management of infectious diseases, ICEHA provides technical assistance at two levels: medical expertise and operational delivery systems. The ICEHA's programs are based on the integration of three methods: a locally relevant HIV teaching curriculum, which ensures that the material taught is pertinent to the resource level of each particular country; workshops consisting of formal training sessions using locally relevant teaching curriculum to provide medical expertise to participating physicians and nurses; and on-site coaching using teams of experienced HIV volunteer physicians and nurses to allow the participation of local healthcare providers to translate the theoretical knowledge obtained during the workshop sessions into practical expertise. Focused on the HIV pandemic and infectious diseases, the ICEHA's volunteer clinical mentors equip local health professionals with the skills they need to provide the best care for their patients, enabling developing countries to fight epidemics from within.

The Center's programs have proven the immense impact that individuals can have in the improvement of access to HIV care and AIDS medication for patients in developing countries. The ICEHA provides a defined, structured opportunity through which each clinical mentor's contribution can be maximized, thereby creating access to sustainable HIV/AIDS care throughout a country. Beyond the benefits for patients in the developing world, our volunteer clinical mentors have described their field assignment as "the most extraordinary experience of their professional lives." In addition, by increasing HIV/AIDS knowledge and expertise amongst healthcare providers, the ICEHA helps to set up a system where HIV transmission caused by unsafe medical practices can be eliminated and HIV prevention messages are delivered and reinforced within the healthcare system. This enables healthcare providers to understand that HIV/AIDS can be addressed both in terms of prevention and care.

SEE ALSO: AIDS; International AIDS Vaccine Initiative (IAVI); Preventive Care.

BIBLIOGRAPHY. International Center for Equal Healthcare Access (ICEHA), www.iceha.org/uniquw (cited 2006); The National Centre for HIV/AIDS Dermatology and STDs (NCHADS), http://www.nchads.org/#Top (cited October 2006); United Nations Development Programme, www.undp.org (cited 2006).

BEN WYNNE, PH.D
GAINESVILLE STATE COLLEGE

International Classification of Diseases (ICD)

The International Classification of Diseases (ICD) is the standard diagnostic international classification system for mortality and morbidity data. The ICD is a structured classification system of disease and associated codes that has been designed to promote international compatibility in health data collecting and reporting. During the 1800s, several statisticians started to develop medical-based data reporting systems. The importance of creating a uniform system was realized and several medical statisticians commissioned the completion of this task. The International Statistical Institute adopted the first edition of the ICD in 1893. The first ICD edition was based on the Bertillon Classification of Causes of Death, developed by Jacques Bertillon (the chief of Statistical Services for the City of Paris). In 1898, the American Public Health Association recommended that several countries use this system and revisions be completed once every 10 years. The ICD is an extremely valuable system, allowing for international and national uniform data analysis for tasks such as disease surveillance and mortality analyses.

THE DESIGN

The ICD contains a description of all known diseases and injuries. Each disease is detailed with diagnostic characteristics and given a unique identifier that is used to code mortality data on death certificates and morbidity data from patient and clinical records. The core of the ICD uses one single list of three alphanumeric character codes starting from A00 to Z99. The first letter of the code designates a different chapter; there are 21 in total. Within each chapter, the three character codes are divided so that they specify different classification axes. The ICD has undergone many revisions as the needs of countries change.

CURRENT USE

Every country subscribing to the ICD system uses it in varying degrees. Most countries subscribe to the entirety of the ICD system, while some countries use the ICD in hospitals only, some for morbidity only, and other countries have chosen to implement partial code use. The U.S. Department of Health and Human Services felt that the ICD needed to provide better clinical information and developed a system that is referred to as ICD 9th revision: Clinical Modification (ICD-9-CM). These CM codes are much more precise and allows for stronger analyses. The ICD-9-CM is used by hospitals and other healthcare facilities. The ICD-10, developed in 1992, is the most current version and was adopted for use in 1999. The ICD-10 is currently used to report mortality data, while the ICD-9-CM is still used for reporting morbidity.

THE WORLD HEALTH ORGANIZATION AND INTERNATIONAL STATISTICS

The World Health Organization (WHO) assumed the responsibility of publishing the ICD in 1948 and currently collects all ICD international data for all general epidemiological surveillance and health management purposes. WHO reports international health statistics for those countries that use the ICD system. The ICD is a core classification of the WHO Family of International Classifications (WHO-FIC).

SEE ALSO: Department of Health and Human Services (DHHS); International Epidemiological Association (IEA); World Health Organization (WHO).

BIBLIOGRAPHY. National Center for Health Statistics, "Classifications of Disease and Functioning & Disability," http://www.cdc.gov/nchs/default.htm (cited July 2007); World Health Organization, "History of the Development of the ICD," http://www.who.int/classifications/icd/en/HistoryOfICD.pdf (cited July 2007).

Sudha R. Raminani, M.S.
The Fenway Institute

International Clinical Epidemiology Network (INCLEN)

Created in 1980 as a project of the Rockefeller Foundation, the International Clinical Epidemiology Network (INCLEN) has been an independent nonprofit organization since 1988. The organization is a unique global network of clinical epidemiologists, biostatisticians, health social scientists, health economists, and other health professionals dedicated to improving the health of disadvantaged populations, particularly those in poorer nations, by promoting equitable healthcare based on the best evidence of effectiveness and the efficient use of resources. To accomplish its goals, INCLEN uses the network to conduct collaborative, interdisciplinary research on high-priority health problems, and to train future generations of leaders in health-care research. INCLEN's membership includes medical institutions in more than two dozen countries throughout the world. The multi-disciplinary faculty at member institutions includes clinical epidemiologists, health social scientists, biostatisticians, and clinical economists, each of whom believes that fighting disease in an age of limited financial resources depends on integrating the principles of clinical epidemiology into his or her practice. INCLEN provides a forum for researchers to discuss critical health issues through educational programs, global meetings, and an international communications network.

It supports young researchers and provides network members opportunities to participate in collaborative clinical studies. As a partnership of clinicians and health scientists who are trained to use and produce the best possible evidence in their medical decision making, INCLEN has had a profound impact on healthcare practices globally. The Networks partners include the Child Health Research Project (CHR), COHRED—Collaboration with International Health Research Programmes, the Global Forum for Health Research, The Alliance for Health Policy and Systems Research, Training Programs in Epidemiology and Public Health Interventions Network, and the International Epidemiological Association. Usually held in a different locale annually, INCLEN's Global Meeting is preceded by collaborative research planning meetings and includes continuing education workshops on such topics as Medical Ethics in Research, Pharmacoepidemiology, Reproductive Health, and Environmental Health Issues.

The meeting attracts some 400 attendees annually and is an excellent forum for intellectual exchange and information dissemination. Regional Meetings are held in Latin America, India, China, Africa, and southeast Asia to allow researchers to meet and discuss health issues and present scientific papers. All INCLEN meetings are combined with an ongoing program in continuing education. Faculty members are selected from medical institutions in North America,

Australia, Europe, Africa, Asia, and Latin America. Various educational workshops are held throughout the year by INCLEN faculty at various host member institutions. Published semiannually, the INCLEN newsletter highlights research interests and accomplishments of INCLEN members around the globe, including local, regional, and international collaborative research projects on a wide range of topics. The newsletter also relates news of the network, such as strategic planning at local, regional and global levels; meeting schedules, and funding possibilities.

SEE ALSO: Epidemiologist; Epidemiology.

BIBLIOGRAPHY. Alliance for Health Policy and Systems Research, www.alliance-hpsr.org/jahia/Jahia (cited October 2006); International Clinical Epidemiology Network (INCLEN), www.inclen.org (cited October 2006); David E. Lilienfeld and Paul D. Stolley, *Foundations of Epidemiology* (New York: Oxford University Press; 1994); The International Epidemiological Association (IEA), www.dundee.ac.uk/iea (cited October 2006).

BEN WYNNE, PH.D
GAINESVILLE STATE COLLEGE

International Committee of the Red Cross (ICRC)

With origins dating back to the 1860s, the International Committee of the Red Cross (ICRC) is an impartial, neutral, and independent organization whose exclusively humanitarian mission is to protect the lives and dignity of victims of war and internal violence and to provide them with assistance in times of need. It directs and coordinates international relief activities wherever there is major conflict and endeavors to prevent suffering by promoting and strengthening humanitarian law and universal humanitarian principles.

The Committee's chief tasks revolve around monitoring the compliance of warring nations with regard to the Geneva Convention, organizing care for soldiers wounded on the battlefield, supervising the treatment of prisoners of war, helping with the search for missing person's during time of war, organizing the protec-

tion and care of civilian populations, and arbitration between warring parties during an armed conflict.

In February 1863 in Geneva, Switzerland, the Geneva Public Welfare Society set up a committee of five Swiss citizens to look into the ideas offered by Henri Dunant in his book *Un Souvenir de Solferino* which dealt with the protection of sick and wounded soldiers during combat. The committee had as its members Guillaume Henri Dufour (1787–1875), a general of the Swiss army and a military writer who became the committee's president for its first year and its honorary president thereafter; Gustave Moynier (1826–1910), a lawyer and president of the sponsoring Public Welfare Society who devoted the rest of his life to Red Cross work; Louis Appia (1818–98) and Theodore Maunoir (1806–69), both well-respected medical doctors; and Henri Dunant (1828–1910) himself.

The committee called an international conference that met later in the year which, with 16 nations represented, adopted various resolutions and principles, along with an international emblem, and appealed to all nations to form voluntary units to help the wartime sick and wounded. These units eventually became the National Red Cross Societies, and the Committee of Five eventually became the International Committee of the Red Cross. In 1864, an international diplomatic meeting was held at Geneva at the invitation of the Swiss government. The assembly formulated the Geneva Convention of 1864. This international "Convention for the Amelioration of the Condition of the Wounded and Sick in Armed Forces in the Field" advanced resolutions guaranteeing neutrality for medical personnel and equipment and officially adopting the red cross on a white field as the identifying emblem. A pact was signed on August 22, 1864, by 12 states, and was later accepted by the others. As a result, the work of the Red Cross began. Three other conventions were later added to the first, extending protection to victims of naval warfare, to prisoners of war, and to civilians. Although the Red Cross has always given major service during time of war, it has had an even greater long-term impact through its gradual development and operation of humanitarian programs that serve continuously in both peace and war.

The organization of the ICRC is composed of several elements. The self-governing National Red Cross Societies, including the Red Crescent in Muslim countries and the Red Lion and Sun in Iran, operate on the national level through their volunteer members and also participate in international work. The League of Red Cross Societies is a coordinating world federation that facilitates contact between the individual societies, acts as a clearinghouse for information, assists the societies in setting up new programs and in improving or expanding those already existing, and coordinates international disaster operations. It functions under an executive committee and a board of governors on which every national society has representation. In the modern era, the ICRC itself is private, independent group of Swiss citizens that functions during war or conflict whenever intervention by a neutral body is necessary.

As guardian of the Geneva Conventions and of Red Cross principles, it promotes their acceptance by governments, suggests their revision, works for further development of international humanitarian law, and recognizes new Red Cross Societies. The International Red Cross Conference, which met for the first time in 1867, is the organization's highest legislative body. It is composed of representatives of the National Societies, the International Committee, and those governments that have signed the Geneva Conventions. It meets every four to six years and reviews Red Cross policy and activities, suggests ways that the organization might improve itself, and discusses the adoption of new initiatives.

SEE ALSO: International Federation of Red Cross and Red Crescent Societies; International Red Cross and Red Crescent Movement (RCRC).

BIBLIOGRAPHY. Clyde E. Buckingham, *For Humanity's Sake: The Story of the Early Development of the League of Red Cross Societies* (Public Affairs Press, 1964); Max Huber, *Principles and Foundations of the Work of the International Committee of the Red Cross, 1939–1946* (ICRC, 1947); International Committee of the Red Cross, www.icrc.org (cited October 2006); James Avery Joyce, *Red Cross International and the Strategy of Peace* (Hodder & Stoughton, 1959). Nobelprize.com: International Committee of the Red Cross, nobelprize.org/nobel_prizes/peace/laureates/1963/red-cross-history.html (cited October 2006).

BEN WYNNE, PH.D
GAINESVILLE STATE COLLEGE

International Council of AIDS Service Organizations (ICASO)

A Toronto, Canada-based organization, the International Council of AIDS Service Organizations (ICASO) is a global umbrella organizing body for community-based AIDS service organizations and nongovernmental groups. Founded in 1991, it has secretariats based in five different geographic areas (Africa, Asia/Pacific, Europe, Latin American and the Caribbean, and North America), as well as the main Canadian office. In addition to these official five secretariats, the ICASO is also aligned with several national networks of people living with HIV. Individuals cannot join ICASO directly, although some are appointed based on specific reasons such as past contributions and institutional linkages. A board of 10 advisers is elected annually.

The Council's central focus is promoting dignity, care, services, and human rights for people living with HIV and AIDS. It is a strong international advocate for ending discrimination against HIV-positive persons, harm reduction approaches that enable individuals to make their own choices regarding prevention, and providing universal access to antiretroviral therapy. It does so by lobbying national governments and international agencies directly and by encouraging its nation-level affiliates to do so in their own countries. The Council also lobbies national governments to scale up health systems infrastructure to meet the needs of those living with HIV and AIDS.

The Council also functions by supporting already-existing community-based service organizations, rather than directly providing services. The Council especially tries to channel funding toward communities that are struggling to provide services due to resource constraints, especially populations that shoulder much of the burden of caring for those infected with HIV. The ICASO plays an important role in the governance of the Global Fund, as well as encouraging national governments to implement their commitments under the UNGASS (United Nations General Assembly Special Session) HIV/AIDS resolution.

Like the United States-based National Association of People with AIDS, the Council places a high premium on the participation of HIV-positive people in all of its programs, as well as training people living with HIV/AIDS to become advocates for HIV prevention, research, treatment, and care in their own countries. The Council also encourages communities, however defined, to articulate their own HIV/AIDS prevention and treatment needs, and encourages national governments and international agencies to respect these priorities and values. Recent research initiatives have focused on how communities have been involved in vaccine development, how nations have implemented wide-scale anti-retroviral treatment in their countries, and how community-based groups have increased health literacy in response to HIV/AIDS.

As does the International AIDS Vaccine Initiative, the ICASO strongly believes that the HIV pandemic will be stopped quickest by discovering and disseminating an effective HIV vaccine. Like the International Women's Health Coalition, the ICASO strongly promotes the development of female-based HIV prevention methods, such as vaginal microbicides. The Council receives funding from, among others, the Ford Foundation, the Gates Foundation, the Danish and Canadian governments, UNAIDS, the International AIDS Vaccine Initiative, and several pharmaceutical companies.

SEE ALSO: AIDS; International AIDS Vaccine Initiative (IAVI).

BIBLIOGRAPHY. Michael Pollak, *The Second Plague of Europe: AIDS Prevention and Sexual Transmission among Men in Western Europe* (Haworth Press, 1994); U.S. Department of Health and Human Services, "AIDS info," www.aidsinfo.nih.gov (cited February 2007).

ANNIE DUDE
UNIVERSITY OF CHICAGO

International Epidemiological Association (IEA)

Originally founded in 1954 as the International Corresponding Club, the International Epidemiological Association (IEA) seeks to facilitate communication among those engaged in research and teaching in epidemiology throughout the world, and to engage in the development and use of epidemiological methods in all fields of health including social, community and preventive medicine and health services administration. These aims are accomplished by holding scientific meetings and seminars, by the publication of journals, reports, monographs, transactions or books, by contact among members, and by other activities consistent with these aims.

The founders of the Association were John Pemberton of Great Britain and Harold N. Willard of the United States. Recognizing the importance of the dissemination of current information to healthcare professionals, these men sought to establish an organization "to facilitate the communication between physicians working for the most part in university departments of preventive and social medicine, or in research institutes devoted to these aspects of medicine, throughout the world." This goal was initially achieved by the publication of a bulletin twice a year and by members endeavoring to "ensure a friendly and hospitable welcome for visitors" from other countries. The first issue of the bulletin appeared in January 1955 and contained contributions from 26 correspondents from nine countries. Today, the Association includes more than 1,500 members from over 100 nations.

Every three years, the IEA holds a global scientific meeting at different locations throughout the world, and regional meetings at regular intervals. The Association is governed by a council elected from the IEA's active members and consisting of the president, president-elect, secretary and treasurer, and from seven to 10 other members. Published six times a year, the *International Journal of Epidemiology* is the official, peer-reviewed journal of the Association and an essential requirement for anyone who needs to keep up to date with epidemiological advances and new developments throughout the world.

The Journal encourages communication among those engaged in the research, teaching, and application of epidemiology of both communicable and noncommunicable disease, including research into health services and medical care. Also covered in its pages are new methods, epidemiological and statistical, for the analysis of data used by those who practise social and preventive medicine. As a result of opportunities that the IEA has afforded epidemiologists to meet with colleagues from other countries, several international collaborative studies have been undertaken by Association members. The results of many of these have been published in the Journal. To promote epidemiology as a discipline the IEA works in cooperation with the International Clinical Epidemiology Network (INCLEN), the Field Epidemiology Training Program (FETP) of the United States Centers of Disease Control and Prevention (CDC) and other organizations with similar missions.

SEE ALSO: Epidemiology; International Clinical Epidemiology Network (INCLEN).

BIBLIOGRAPHY. European Epidemiology Federation, www.dundee.ac.uk/iea/euro_Contents.htm (cited October 2006); International Clinical Epidemiology Network (INCLEN), www.inclen.org (cited October 2006); International Epidemiological Association (IEA), www.dundee.ac.uk/iea (cited 2006); International Society for Environmental Epidemiology, www.iseepi.org (cited October 2006), World Health Organization, www.dundee.ac.uk/iea/euro_Contents.htm (cited October 2006).

BEN WYNNE, PH.D
GAINESVILLE STATE COLLEGE

International Federation of Red Cross and Red Crescent Societies (IFRC)

Formed in 1919, the International Federation of Red Cross and Red Crescent Societies (IFRC) exist, to improve the lives of the world's most vulnerable people through the mobilizing of human efforts. Serving as the umbrella organization of 185 Red Cross and Red Crescent societies, this humanitarian society pledges to provide assistance to all, regardless of nationality, race, religious beliefs, class, or political opinions. The Red Crescent replaces the symbol of the Red Cross in Islamic countries.

The IFRC oversees relief operations in four main areas: promoting humanitarian values, disaster response, disaster preparedness, and health and community care. Promoting humanitarian values involves respecting and working with others to solve problems.

Disaster response requires the majority of IFRC time and attention, as they provide assistance to approxi-

mately 30 million people, worldwide, each year. IFRC responds to natural disasters as well as man-made ones such as war and accompanying refugee problems. Although much of their disaster response work involves emergency situations, the IFRC also works on long-term rehab projects.

One longer-term project is the relief efforts following an Iranian earthquake on December 26, 2003, shattered the city of Bam, killing 26,000 people, injuring 30,000 and leaving 75,000 homeless. Eighty-five percent or more of the city's buildings were destroyed, including 131 schools and 119 healthcare facilities. On the third year anniversary of the earthquake, nine schools, two health clinics, an orthopedic center, and a road rescue center, all funded by the IFRC, were dedicated.

Because of the increase in significant natural disasters, the IFRC has increased the funding spent on disaster preparedness, educating people about risks and distributing information about how to respond in a disaster. In health and community care, the IFRC assists communities in providing basic health services and education. The IFRC relies upon volunteer efforts and so the organization spends some resources on volunteer training.

The IFRC Secretariat is located in Geneva, Switzerland. His/her role is to coordinate international disaster relief and elicit cooperation between and among national societies; IFRC societies exist in more than 150 countries. The IFRC also provides training for its societies, including first aid training. It partners with other agencies with compatible goals, from a local level to a global one.

In May 2006, the IFRC published an overview of its first 88 years of service. Out of 2,216 appeals for help, the majority (728) have been from Africa, with 577 coming from Asia and the Pacific region. Overall, 569 of the appeals have been for disaster relief because of floods, storms, and cyclones, with 438 appeals being requests for socioeconomic relief.

The largest donors are Sweden, United Kingdom, European Commission's Humanitarian Aid Office, Norway, Japan, the United States, the Netherlands, Finland, Ireland, Canada, Germany, Switzerland, France, the United Nations High Commissioner for Refugees and Denmark, in that order. From 1997 to 2006, the IFRC has been able to fulfill anywhere from 44 percent to 85 percent of its requests for funding and assistance.

SEE ALSO: American Red Cross (ARC); International Committee of the Red Cross (ICRC); International Red Cross and Red Crescent Movement (RCRC).

BIBLIOGRAPHY. International Federation of Red Cross and Red Crescent Societies, http://www.ifrc.org (cited June 2007).

KELLY BOYER SAGERT
INDEPENDENT SCHOLAR

International Genetic Epidemiology Society (IGES)

The International Genetic Epidemiology Society (IGES) studies the basis for disease, giving significant weight to both genetic factors and the influence of the environment on genetic predispositions toward disease. Society members believe the recently successful mapping of the human genome—the complete set of human genes—will propel research forward in a way that blends together theories of disease as nature (genetics) and disease as nurture (environment) into a cohesive and useful whole.

Members of IGES come from a wide variety of scientific disciplines, ranging from geneticists and biologists to statisticians and mathematicians. The unifying factor is the belief that disease is a complex interaction of predisposed risk factors and inherited conditions that respond in a particular way to environmental triggers and in varying environmental contexts.

Committees include the ELSI committee, and the education, membership, scientific program, and publication committees. ELSI stands for ethical, legal, and social issues; this committee was formed by the National Institutes of Health (NIH) and the United States Department of Energy (DOE) when participating in an international human genome mapping project.

Ethical concerns considered by IGES include the fairness of use of information; who, the researchers must ask, could have access to this private information and how would it be used? Privacy and confidentiality concerns must be addressed and the ownership of genetic information gathered during research must be fairly determined. Researchers must also consider the psychological impact and stigmatization felt by individuals or minority groups whose genetic pattern differs from the norm.

Other ethical issues include reproductive-related questions, such as those surrounding fetal genetic testing; clinical evaluation methods and their accuracy; uncertainties, such as whether minors should be tested for adult-onset diseases; conceptual and philosophical questions regarding genetic determination versus a person's free will; health and environmental issues, especially with genetically modified foods; and commercialization of genetic material, and the accompanying copyright, trade secrets, and patent issues.

IGES publishes *Genetic Epidemiology*, a peer-reviewed journal containing articles sharing research results that analyze the relative weight of genetic and environmental factors in human disease. Specific topics recommended for articles include a review of the natural selection process, dubbed the *ultimate gene by environment interaction* by the journal's editor; and large-scale genetic research projects.

IGES hosts annual scientific meetings featuring lecturers from around the world—often in conjunction with other associations such as the American Society of Human Genetics, the International Congress of Human Genetics, and the Society for Epidemiological Research (SER)—who present the results of their research. The society annually presents two $1,000 awards—the James V. Neel and Roger Williams awards—for the best presentations by a student and by a young scientist, respectively. It also provides continuing education in genetic epidemiology methods and subsidizes travel expenses for students in need. IGES's Web site (http://iges.biostat.wustl.edu/index.htm) is used to post announcements of general interest to those in the field, job openings, and, somewhat surprisingly, humorous audios of songs satirizing genome studies.

SEE ALSO: Gene Mapping; Genetics; Genome; Human Genome Organisation (HUGO); National Human Genome Research Institute (NHGRI).

BIBLIOGRAPHY. International Genetic Epidemiology Society (IGES), http://iges.biostat.wustl.edu/iges.html (cited June 2007); International Society for Environmental Epidemiology, www.iseepi.org (cited June 2007).

KELLY BOYER SAGERT
INDEPENDENT SCHOLAR

International Health Ministries Office (IHMO)

The International Health Ministries Office (IHMO) is a mission-based agency of the Presbyterian Church in the United States (PC USA) that focuses on worldwide health concerns of vulnerable populations. IMHO partners with churches and other collaborative agencies around the world to attempt to prevent, alleviate and treat health concerns in the most impoverished parts of the globe. IMHO serves health needs in over 30 countries, with prevention and treatment for malaria and HIV/AIDS in African nations currently serving as prime foci.

IMHO has chosen "Building Healthy Communities" as a theme for its mission-based activities. Their strategic plan states a holistic health vision and an evolving focus that will place an increasing emphasis on programs that assist global associate churches as they formulate programs to prevent disease. These programs should be community based and should meet local and regional health needs. Some of the programs include immunization clinics in rural locations, HIV/AIDS education, dietary education, and projects that ensure clean drinking water.

Besides providing support and resources to partner churches around the globe, the IMHO guides individual PC USA congregations and presbyteries (regional bodies of Presbyterian churches) in the United States as they develop and participate in overseas health missions. One significant program initiated by IHMO and led by Presbyterian women's groups is The NetWorkers Malaria Prevention Program. This program was developed because of the devastating loss of health, life, and productivity from malaria in African countries; the disease causes more than 1 million deaths in Africa annually. NetWorkers promote the use of insecticide-treated mosquito nets that greatly reduce opportunities for malaria transmission. NetWorkers help purchase nets, insecticide, and educational materials and they also sew nets from kits.

IMHO developed a 10-minute video, the "NetWorkers Safe Motherhood Projects," that shares information about how Presbyterian women in the United States partner with women in Africa to diminish the loss of life and productivity because of malaria. On a broader scale, IMHO developed a plan wherein churches and other philanthropic agencies can effectively work together to combat malaria.

The Presbyterian AIDS Network (PAN) is an international program that responds to the AIDS health crisis in countries hardest hit by the disease, most notable Cameroon, the Democratic Republic of Congo, Ethiopia, and Malawi. Members of PAN share information about the devastating effects of HIV/AIDS in Africa to Presbyterian congregations in the United States and they also raise funds to combat the disease.

Educational components of the PAN program include teaching African women about mother-to-child transmission of HIV/AIDS and encouraging women to be tested for the disease; 90 percent of the children with AIDS in Africa contracted the disease from their mothers. PAN also teaches the A-B-C approach to AIDS prevention: abstinence for youth; be faithful for those with regular sexual partners; and condoms as a way to reduce contact with the AIDS virus for non-abstainers without a regular sexual partner.

SEE ALSO: AIDS; AIDS and Infections; AIDS and Pregnancy; Malaria.

BIBLIOGRAPHY. International Health Ministries Office, www.pcusa.org/health/international/ (cited June 2007); 2005 Fiscal Report of Presbyterian Women/IHMO, www.interchurch.org/resources/uploads/files/77Presbyterian Women.MedicineBoxReport.2005.doc (cited June 2007).

Kelly Boyer Sagert
Independent Scholar

International Red Cross and Red Crescent Movement (RCRC)

The International Red Cross and Red Crescent Movement (RCRC) is the umbrella association of two distinct but interconnected entities: the International Committee of the Red Cross (ICRC) and the International Federation of Red Cross and Red Crescent Societies (IFRC). The RCRC also oversees all of the national Red Cross and Red Crescent societies, located in 186 countries around the globe, as well as the 97 million people volunteering in service to the movement. The ICRC and the IFRC have central offices located in Geneva, Switzerland, while the national societies are located within the countries they represent.

The movement was started by a Swiss businessman named Henry Dunant, who was attempting to meet with Napoleon in 1859 over commerce-related concerns. Heading to Solferino in Italy to meet with him, Dunant found the city to be the site of an intense battle between the French armies and the Austrian armies, with the source of the dispute being the status of Italy's independence. More than 40,000 soldiers were wounded or killed during that battle, and Dunant was stunned at the lack of medical care given to the men and he was shocked by their unrelieved suffering.

Dunant did not pursue his business meeting with Napoleon, instead focusing on finding relief for the wounded soldiers. Afterward, he wrote a book, *A Memory of Solferino*, publishing it with his own money and sending it to military and political leaders throughout Europe. He wanted to publicize his concerns over the suffering of soldiers and advocate for the creation of an international, volunteer-based relief society.

By 1863, his efforts began bearing fruit, with the formation of the International Committee for Relief to the Wounded that had initial support from these countries: Baden, Bavaria, France, Britain, Hanover, Hesse, Italy, the Netherlands, Austria, Prussia, Russia, Saxony, Sweden, and Spain. This was one of the earliest organized attempts to establish methods for treating the wounded on the battlefield and to relieve suffering from combat; the name of this committee was later changed to the International Committee of the Red Cross (ICRC).

In modern times, the ICRC brings aid to victims of war and armed conflict worldwide. The committee directs activities at the sites of international conflict to provide relief, and it works to promote humanitarian principles to prevent future suffering.

The International Federation of the Red Cross (IFRC) was founded in 1919 and it oversees the national societies that carry out humanitarian aid to victims of disasters, whether man-made or natural, such as hurricanes and earthquakes. The IFRC also gives aid to refugees and people in the throes of health emergencies. The IFRC promotes cooperation among its national societies and it works to strengthen their abilities to prepare for disasters and their relief. Member societies also provide health-related programs in their own countries and, during war time, the societies support the military's medical units.

This movement is based on seven principles: humanity, impartiality, neutrality, independence, voluntary service, unity, and universality. To fulfill the principle of humanity, people associated with the movement are committed to protected human health and life, and to promote respect, cooperation, and peace.

Impartiality means no discrimination based on race, religious beliefs, political ideologies, nationality, or any other such category. To maintain neutrality, members of this movement do not participate in divisive debates, whether political, religious, or of any other ideological nature. The movement in each country, although often closely connected to other humanitarian efforts of government agencies, vows to stay independent of political dealings. The movement is voluntary in that participants cannot personally gain from their efforts and all must remain unified, with no more than one society in any country. Finally, each part of the overall movement is equal to every other part, and no one country or society can take precedence over another, except when deemed an initiative leader.

Taken all together, these organizations form the International Red Cross and Red Crescent Movement (RCRC). The Standing Commission of the Red Cross and Red Crescent meets every four years, to determine the strategic direction of the movement, to coordinate efforts, and to assist in the implementation of the Red Cross and Red Crescent resolutions. The Standing Committee does make recommendations for or oversee operational matters.

The symbol of the RCRC, a red cross on a white background, is in fact the Swiss flag in reverse; for countries wherein the Islamic religion is predominant, a red crescent replaces the cross in the flag.

The RCRC movement publishes a quarterly magazine, *Red Cross, Red Crescent*, that shares humanitarian efforts of societies around the world. There is an International Red Cross and Red Crescent Movement Museum located in Geneva, Switzerland, with photos and documents from the past, and information about efforts taking place in the present. Historical figures honored in the museum include founder Henri Dunant; British nurse, Florence Nightingale, and Russian surgeon, Nikolai Pirogov, both of whom nursed the wounded from the Crimean War; and the American nurse, Clara Barton, who nursed the wounded during the U.S. Civil War.

Current initiatives include the introduction of a third icon, the Red Crystal, as a symbol of unity; efforts are now being made to infuse this symbol with the same level of respect now given to the Red Cross and the Red Crescent. Furthermore, the Red Crystal does not have the controversial and potentially divisive connotations of a cross or crescent. Changes in statutes have allowed Israel to join the movement. Other initiatives include a renewed commitment to the protection of women and children during wars.

SEE ALSO: International Committee of the Red Cross (ICRC); International Federation of Red Cross and Red Crescent Societies (IFRC).

BIBLIOGRAPHY. International Committee of the Red Cross (ICRC); http://geneva.usmission.gov/rcrc/RCRCMovement.pdf (cited June 2007); International Red Cross and Red Crescent Movement web site, http://www.redcross.int/en/default.asp (cited June 2007).

KELLY BOYER SAGERT
INDEPENDENT SCHOLAR

International Society for Environmental Epidemiology (ISEE)

The International Society for Environmental Epidemiology (ISEE), founded in 1987, initially provided a U.S.-based forum for epidemiological experts to discuss three topics: clean drinking water technology, air pollution concerns, and the increased risk of cancer in and around nuclear facilities. Since then, ISEE has expanded to an international organization that addresses environmental hazards and adverse health effects connected to exposure to those hazards, the interaction of genetics and environmental influences in causing these health conditions, and ethical questions surrounding these topics.

Membership is open to environmental epidemiologists and other scientists worldwide, and there are now more than 800 members residing in 60 countries. Although approximately 50 percent of members reside in North America, ISEE is committed to continuing the international scope of its society; there are currently ISEE chapters located in Latin America, the Caribbean, the Mediterranean, central and eastern Europe, the Caucasus, south Asia, east Asia, and North America. To further its goal of international participation, ISEE has held annual conferences in the United States, Canada, Mexico, Europe, the Middle East, Asia, Australia, and Africa. The 2007 annual conference, held in Mexico, focused on the theme of "Translating Environmental Epidemiology into Action: Interventions for a Healthy Future."

From the early stages of development, ISEE has fostered an active collaboration with the International Society of Exposure Analysis (ISEA), a society formed in 1989 to further scientific exploration of environmental contaminants and how exposure to them affects humans and their environment. Members of ISEA come from a variety of scientific disciplines and they lobby to have exposure assessment techniques considered while establishing environmental policies. Collectively, ISEE and ISEA work together toward common goals.

Members of ISEE are encouraged to participate in the organization's committees. These include the Nominations Committee, Annual Conference Committee, and Awards Committee, which deal with the ongoing business of ISEE. The Membership Committee and Communications Committee are charged with providing educational and outreach materials to members and prospective members.

The Ethics and Philosophy Committee created one of the first epidemiological codes of ethics, one that addresses obligations to subjects of research, to society, to sponsors, and to colleagues. An ethics-based ISEE award of interest is the ISEE Research Integrity Award, granted to researchers who have withstood significant pressure from special interest groups and continued to act with exceptional integrity to protect public health. Related to this is the ISEE Support for Victimized Colleagues that focuses on the pressures and threats perceived by researchers who identify hazards that adversely affect special interest groups. In these instances, ISEE may write a letter of support and/or otherwise engage ISEE in supporting these researchers, whether they are members of ISEE.

The Capacity Building in Developing Countries Committee encourages collaborations between developed and developing countries and supports training of scientists and researchers in developing countries. ISEE publishes *Epidemiology*, a peer-reviewed journal that publishes original research. The journal welcomes scientific articles that challenge current assumptions.

SEE ALSO: International Genetic Epidemiology Society (IGES); Society for Healthcare Epidemiology of America (SHEA).

BIBLIOGRAPHY. International Genetic Epidemiology Society (IGES), http://iges.biostat.wustl.edu/iges.html; International Society for Environmental Epidemiology, www.iseepi.org/.

KELLY BOYER SAGERT
INDEPENDENT SCHOLAR

International Society for Pharmacoepidemiology (ISPE)

The International Society for Pharmacoepidemiology (ISPE) is a nonprofit organization that provides a global forum for scientific discussions about pharmacoepidemiology, with an ultimate goal of improving public health worldwide. To accomplish that goal, pharmacoepidemiologists study how drugs affect significant numbers of people, using techniques gleaned from pharmacology and epidemiology alike; the field of pharmacoepidemiology has, therefore, been called the bridge between these two scientific disciplines.

Pharmacologists study drugs and those who specialize in clinical pharmacology monitor how drugs affect patients so as to determine the risks and benefits of pharmaceuticals. To determine the probabilities of positive benefits or adverse reactions of a particular pharmaceutical, pharmacoepidemiologists use methodologies typically used in epidemiological studies.

Conversely, the field of epidemiology focuses on the risk factors of disease and the probabilities of diseases appearing in certain populations. There are two branches of epidemiology: descriptive and analytic. Descriptive epidemiology creates a description of diseases, along with the frequency of occurrences. This discipline does not use control groups and, therefore, does not test hypotheses. Analytic epide-

miologists, however, observe disease and record their observations, but they also conduct clinical trials to test their hypotheses. Pharmacoepidemiologists use these methods to study pharmaceuticals.

ISPE has members from 53 countries, with national chapters located in Argentina, Belgium, Denmark, and the Netherlands. Members of ISPE use pharmacoepidemiology studies to develop health-related policies, to educate healthcare professionals about ISPE research results, and to advocate for their field of study and its specialties including the discipline of pharmacovigilance. Researchers conduct ongoing monitoring of adverse affects of pharmaceuticals of already-approved drugs. In practice, this involves healthcare professionals reporting negative reactions to drugs, with pharmacovigilance specialists correlating incoming data to create reports about the level of safety of a particular pharmaceutical, once being used by large numbers of people. This is a much more efficient method of research than basing recommendations on more random reporting of adverse affects.

ISPE recommends increasing the number of patients involved in clinical testing of new pharmaceuticals before they are approved for general use. Moreover, they recommend that physicians fully understand potentially adverse effects of the drugs, and that they receive updated information of adverse affects, which may increase after released at large. ISPE officials also advocate for continuing drug safety testing after pharmaceuticals are approved, which necessitates increased funding for the epidemiological studies required.

Officials of ISPE see a lack of coordination between the pharmaceutical industry and governmental regulatory agencies as another flaw in the drug monitoring process. To ease newly approved pharmaceuticals into use, ISPE recommends limited pharmaceutical to consumer marketing within the first few years of drug approval, thus limiting the potential of harm done by adverse drug affects not noted during its clinical trial stage. Other specialized areas of pharmacoepidemiology study include drug utilization research and therapeutic risk management. Subjects of recent ISPE study include the potential connection between beta-blockers and decreased hip and vertebral fractures; antidepressants and suicide potential in pediatric patients; pulmonary hypertension in newborns; antiepileptic drugs and fractures; and late pregnancy use of serotonin reuptake inhibitors.

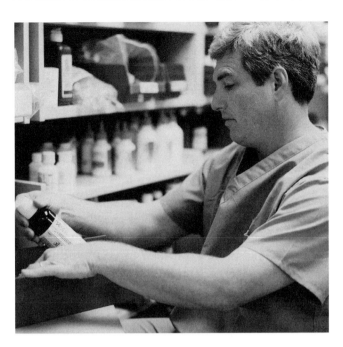

Pharmacoepidemiologists study how drugs affect significant numbers of people.

Members of ISPE may be employed by pharmaceutical companies, government agencies, universities, or private/public nonprofit agencies. Researchers come from a wide variety of scientific disciplines, including epidemiology, biostatistics, medicine, nursing, pharmacology, pharmacy, law, and health economics, while other members have a journalistic background.

ISPE holds conferences and workshops, and publishes a quarterly newsletter along with a journal, *Pharmacoepidemiology and Drug Safety*. Focus of written materials may be on pharmaceuticals still in developmental stages, or a drug's delivery method, use, cost, and/or effects. Other topics include maintaining pharmaceutical databases; the importance of data confidentiality and the difficulties faced in maintaining privacy; and the increasing need for more quality-of-life studies. To ensure timely dissemination of knowledge, the journal contains a "Fast Track Publication" column that provides peer-reviewed overviews of studies as quickly as 15 weeks of receipt by the journal.

SEE ALSO: Epidemiologist; Epidemiology; Pharmacology; Pharmacopeia/Pharmacopoeia.

BIBLIOGRAPHY. "Drug Safety and Risk Management—ISPE Annual Meeting—Medical Media Alert," *PR Newswire* (August 19, 2005), www.highbeam.com/doc/1G1-135276040.html (cited June 2007); International Society for Pharmacoepidemiology, http://www.pharmacoepi.org/; "International Society for Pharmacoepidemiology Raises Concerns about Limitations of Pre-Marketing Drug Trials—Calls for Restrictions on Direct-to-Consumer Advertising," *PR Newswire* (February 22, 2005), www.highbeam.com/doc/1G1-129011578.html (cited June 2007).

KELLY BOYER SAGERT
INDEPENDENT SCHOLAR

International Society of Geographical and Epidemiological Ophthalmology (ISGEO)

The International Society of Geographical and Epidemiological Ophthalmology (ISGEO) promotes research of all aspects of ocular disease with a focus on blindness prevention, sight preservation, and visual therapy. Membership is open to all health professionals who have an interest in epidemiological ophthalmology; the group states a nonpolitical, nonracial, and nonreligious viewpoint.

ISGEO supports epidemiologic research in less economically developed countries and often focuses on diseases affecting third world countries. ISGEO places a special interest in the public health facets of eye disease and the assessment of potentially viable treatments, and it provides partial funding for relevant research projects. Abiding by World Health Organization (WHO) regulations, ISGEO members introduce and debate internationally significant ophthalmologic research, again often focusing on issues relevant to less developed countries.

ISGEO meets every two years to present academic research and members are encouraged to learn about the practices of ophthalmology in these countries and cultures. Meetings have been held in Canada, Israel, Spain, Scotland, Italy, Brazil, the United States, Finland, Tunisia, Kenya, Singapore, Belgium, the Netherlands, and Australia. ISGEO may collaborate with other organizations, such as the International Congress of Ophthalmology or the International Agency for the

Prevention of Blindness, at these international meetings. Members also meet for regional conferences. Conference topics range from presentations on cataracts and glaucoma to macular degeneration, refractive errors, clinical trials in ophthalmology, environmental studies in eye disease, population-based studies of eye disease, and geographic mapping of eye disease.

The 16th ISGEO Congress, held in 2000, focused on trachoma, the leading infectious cause of blindness and a disease that occurs two to four times more frequently in women than men. It frequently occurs in poorer populations in Africa, the Middle East, Asia, and Latin America. Trachoma is caused by *Chlamydia trachomatis*, and researchers continued to explore this topic, post-Congress, publishing their research results in a double issue of the ISGEO journal.

ISGEO publishes *Ophthalmic Epidemiology*, its official journal. The journal contains editorials, articles, books reviews on the subject of ophthalmic epidemiology, public health, and the prevention of blindness. Researchers from around the world have submitted work to this journal, and the *Ophthalmic Epidemiology* has published cost–benefit analyses, results of risk factor studies, and the outcomes of therapies and healthcare treatments.

SEE ALSO: Blindness; Eye Care; Eye Diseases (General); Ophthalmology; Ophthalmologist.

BIBLIOGRAPHY. International Society of Geographical and Epidemiological Ophthalmology, www.interchg.ubc.ca/bceio/isgeo/; *Ophthalmic Epidemiology*, www.tandf.co.uk/journals/titles/09286586.asp; Sheila West, "Contribution of Sex-Linked Biology and Gender Roles to Disparities with Trachoma," *Emerging Infectious Diseases*, www.highbeam.com/doc/1G1-125228849.html (cited June 2007).

KELLY BOYER SAGERT
INDEPENDENT SCHOLAR

International Women's Health Coalition (IWHC)

The International Women's Health Coalition (IWHC) is a New York City-based nongovernmental organization that advocates internationally for women's sexual and reproductive health. The Coalition was initially founded in 1984, partly in response to then-President Reagan's "Mexico City policy" or global "gag rule" that prevented private organizations receiving U. S. government funds for advocating for safe abortion, even if this work was done with non-U.S. funds. Rather than focusing only on population control, the Coalition's main goal is to ensure and enable female reproductive and sexual autonomy, particularly for the estimated 1.2 billion adolescents aged 10–19 throughout the world. The Coalition is particularly adept at shaping the language of international health and population conferences, such as those conducted in Cairo and Beijing in the 1990s, to reflect promoting women's rights and autonomy as a key element of development policy.

The Coalition works mainly by sending monetary support to local partner organizations in Latin America, Asia, and Africa. The Coalition has had particular success working with local researchers, activists, and citizen groups throughout the developing world in addressing reproductive and sexual health issues that were previously considered taboo, such as reproductive tract infections, abortion, and rape. Going beyond providing services, the Coalition has worked with local organizations to promote changes in customs and laws that favor equality for women in other ways as well, such as reforming divorce, child custody, and property inheritance laws.

The organization also has a strong focus on lobbying national governments, international agencies, and international donors in order to direct resource flows toward policies and programs it feels will advance reproductive health and security for women. These programs include comprehensive sexuality education for adolescents and young adults, especially regarding sexually transmitted diseases, violence, unwanted pregnancy, and unsafe abortions. The International Women's Health Coalition also supports full access to a range of contraceptive services, including safe abortions, and has not shied away from fierce political engagement with the United States government, the Vatican, and other governmental and religious authorities. The organization advocates for full sexual rights, including freedom from sexual coercion, violence, assault, and forced marriage. Although the Coalition initially focused solely on women, recently programs have also incorporated men as partners against sexual violence.

Recently, the Coalition has expanded programmatic and policy focus to include promoting sexual equality as a means to help women protect themselves from sexually transmitted diseases, particularly HIV. The Coalition has been a prime supporter of microbicide development, which would allow women to protect themselves against HIV infection using vaginal suppositories that do not require male involvement, as condoms do. Additionally, the Coalition has encouraged programs that recognize and promote sexual responsibility among men, as well as advocating for the rights of women in sexual relationships.

The Coalition receives financing from private foundations, United Nations agencies, European governments, and corporations, and donates $1.5 to $2 million to programs worldwide annually. Because the organization advocates for full access to contraception and safe abortions, it currently receives no funding from the U.S. government.

SEE ALSO: Women's Health.

BIBLIOGRAPHY. Lesley Doyal, *Women and Health Services* (Open University Press, 1998).

ANNIE DUDE
UNIVERSITY OF CHICAGO

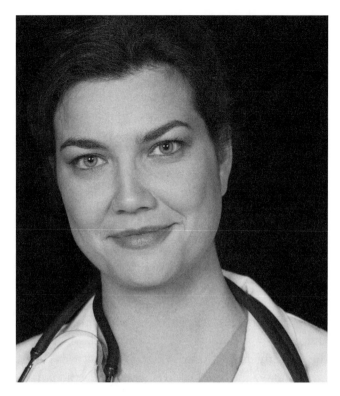

An internist is a medical specialist who focuses his or her medical care on adult medicine.

Internist

An internist, or a practitioner of internal medicine, is a medical specialist who focuses his or her medical care on adult medicine. After the completion of medical school, it takes three to seven years of internal medicine residency to be trained in the fields of preventing, diagnosing, and treating diseases that affect adults. An internist can take the option of specializing in different fields of general medicine, or can take more training to subspecialize (often referred to as a fellowship of one to three years) in one of 13 areas, generally organized by organ system. Specialties range from adolescent medicine to geriatric medicine. Other specialties include specific fields of medicine such as pulmonlogy, hematology/oncology, gastroenterology, and cardiology. For medical practitioners in the United States, there are two main organizations accredited to certify internists within their respective fields: the American Board of Internal Medicine and the American Osteopathic Board of Internal Medicine.

Internists are equipped with the education and knowledge to deal with whatever problem a particular patient suffers from, no matter how common or rare, or how simple or complex. They are specifically trained to solve complicated diagnostic issues and can deal with severe chronic illnesses and situations where several different illnesses may present at the same time. Internists also are trained to help their patients help themselves by maintaining health and wellness. Internists to ensure the best healthcare for their patients follow issues such as disease prevention and the promotion of health, women's health, substance abuse, mental health, as well as regular maintenance treatment of common problems for the eyes, ears, skin, nervous system, and reproductive organs.

In the principles of diagnosis, the essential tools of any physician are the medical history and the physical examination (this is especially true for the internist.) Descriptions of certain diseases or physical signs and symptoms are important in guiding the internist to a diagnostic conclusion. Included in the medical history is a review of systems, which helps to identify conditions experienced by the patient that might not have been mentioned previously but might help to diagnose. Next, the internist will conduct a physical examination, which includes focused exams to a pertaining problem mentioned by the patient as well as a complete checkup. At this point, the internist is most likely able to create a differential diagnosis list, a variety of possible diagnoses that fit the mesh of signs and symptoms. However, this list is often highly specific and exhausting, therefore the internist might narrow down the list by ordering various blood tests, cultures, and medical imaging tests. Often, these tests also serve as screening tests, especially in older patients, to help maintain health maintenance. After this process has been completed, the internist has arrived at a specific diagnosis and is ready to initiate a treatment plan. Most often these treatments include medications; however sometimes they require a more extensive plan, which is addressed and handled at that time.

In today's busy medical environment, most internists will take the time and pride in caring for their patients for life through continuity of care. Whether it is in the office or the clinics, during hospitalizations or intensive care, in nursing homes or assisted living facilities, internists will usually follow through and keep their patients as top priority.

SEE ALSO: Internal Medicine.

BIBLIOGRAPHY. Thomas M. Habermann, *Mayo Clinic Internal Medicine Review*, 7th ed. (Informa Healthcare, 2006); Stephen L. Hauser, Dan L. Longo, and J. Larry Jameson, *Harrison's Principles of Internal Medicine* 15th ed., Eugene Braunwald, Anthony S. Fauci, and Dennis L. Kasper, eds., (McGraw-Hill Professional Publishing, 2001).

ANGELA GARNER
UNIVERSITY OF MISSOURI

Intestinal Parasites

Intestinal parasites are one of the most prevalent, yet overlooked, global health problems. Well over one-third of the population of the world are infected with an intestinal parasite. Many of these 2 billion people are actually infected with more than one type of parasite. Intestinal parasites affect the health of individuals and of populations by contributing significantly to malnutrition, anemia, and other specific disease syndromes.

Intestinal parasites can be divided into two broad groups: single-celled protozoan parasites and complex multicellular worms or helminths. The eggs or cysts of both of these groups are found very commonly in the environment or are associated with animals or foods. While they are found in many different environments, contexts, and across socioeconomic levels, they cause the greatest burden of illness in the developing world where hygiene practices, sanitary infrastructure, nutrition, medical care, and appropriate food preparation may be lacking. Only the most common species and diseases will be discussed here.

WORMS (HELMINTHS)

Intestinal worms range in size from only a few millimeters to several meters in length. The most important clinical and epidemiological differences between the species are related to the nature of their reproductive lifecycle and the way they interact or affect their human hosts. There are three types of helminthes: roundworms (nematodes), tapeworms (cestodes), and flukes (trematodes). Adult roundworms and tapeworms are found in the intestines, whereas adult flukes often live in other tissues such as the liver, blood vessels, or lungs depending on the species. The life cycles, diseases, and treatments associated with trematodes are somewhat more complex than for other helminths and will not be discussed here.

Most intestinal worms (with a few important exceptions) cannot complete their life cycle inside a human host—that is, they cannot multiply and reproduce without exiting the human body and developing further in the soil or another host organism. For this reason, intestinal worms rarely rapidly overwhelm or kill their human hosts. Intestinal parasites are most often transmitted by the fecal-oral route; persons accidentally orally ingest worm eggs present in soil that has been contaminated by human or other feces.

The life cycle of many species involves ingestion as a cyst or egg that hatches in the host stomach or intestines. The larvae then migrate through the body, to the lungs, and back to the intestines. The diseases these parasites cause are usually related to their migration through the lungs, or more often via their effects on the intestines, including preventing absorption of nutrients and obstruction. Most helminths only cause serious disease when they are present in large numbers. These effects may include anemia, retardation of growth and development, malnutrition, decreased work capacity, or increased susceptibility to other diseases. Because they are transmitted by contaminated soil or foods, they are usually more common in children who may be less careful with hygienic practices, may eat or play in contaminated dirt, or be more susceptible to the effects of helminth infections.

Specific types of nematode intestinal worms include the following:

- Ascaris roundworm—the largest worm, which may obstruct the bowels
- Hookworm—a small worm that enters the body through the skin, attaches to the intestinal wall, and lives off of blood, causing anemia
- Pinworm—a small worm common in North America and the rest of the world. It causes an itchy anus and is primarily found in children
- Whipworm—has a whip-like tail and can rarely cause rectal prolapse (rectum falls out through the anus)
- Trichinella—a relatively common worm in North America acquired by eating undercooked pig or game meat. Worm larvae spread throughout the muscles of the body and cause inflammation and illness which is usually treated with steroids

Beef, pork, and fish tapeworms (cestodes) have a very different life cycle than nematodes. Cestodes are usually ingested in cyst form from infected undercooked animals such as beef, pork, and fish. The cysts develop into long worms composed of many reproductive units and a head, which anchors in the intestine. The worms then produce thousands of eggs, which are passed into the stool. Symptoms of tapeworm infections are usually nonspecific and are rarely severe. They include weight loss, malnutrition, nausea, itching, or allergic symptoms. Ingestion of pork tapeworm eggs can result in cysts, rather than adults, in the human tissue causing an entirely different and more dangerous clinical syndrome.

There are several treatments available for intestinal worms. Some medications kill the worms, while others paralyze the worm allowing the body to expel it. Anti-helminth medications must often be taken over two cycles separated by a week to ensure that all worms are killed or expelled. Intestinal worms are so common among children in many parts of the world that deworming is often done in schools at regular intervals.

INTESTINAL PROTOZOA

Protozoa are single-celled eukaryotic (contain a true nucleus) parasites that may infect various human tissues and organs. Malaria, for example, is a protozoal infection of the blood and liver. Intestinal protozoa, as with helminths, are most common in areas with inadequate sanitation and food hygiene, but can be found almost anywhere in the world. There are many different species of protozoa which are often grouped according to their means of locomotion: ciliates—those with small hair-like appendages; flagellates—those with single or multiple whip-like tails; amoeboids—which move using foot-like pseudopods; and sporozoites, which have no means of locomotion but all contain a unique cellular organelle called an apical complex. Protozoa from all of these groups may infect the gastrointestinal tract of humans, as well as that of other mammals. Protozoa have various and complex life cycles which affect the epidemiology and pathological effects of the organisms. Most protozoa can form cysts that allow them to resist harsh environmental conditions until an appropriate host is found. It is the cyst form that is often found on food items or in the environment and accidentally ingested. Intestinal protozoa are not often transmitted directly from person to person; however, they can be transmitted by anal intercourse, with documented outbreaks having occurred among men who have sex with men.

Cryptosporidium is a small organism present in most surface water in the United States. It can cause watery diarrhea for several weeks and is often accompanied by a mild fever, abdominal cramping, and fatigue. It can also lead to chronic diarrhea, but it is usually self-limited in immunocompetent individuals. In immunodeficient patients, particularly those with human immunodeficiency virus (HIV), it can be a severe infection for which few good treatments are available. In 1993, cryptosporidium entered the drinking water supply in Milwaukee and was responsible for making 400,000 people ill and for over 100 deaths.

Cyclospora cayetenensis (cyclosporiasis) may be seasonal or outbreak related. Outbreaks are usually caused by contaminated food items because even thorough washing is not always able to remove all cysts from affected vegetables. Many people who are infected are asymptomatic, but others may have mild to moderate diarrhea. Antibiotic treatments are available if necessary.

Amebiasis is caused by *Entamoeba histolytica* a pathogenic amoeba infecting over 10 percent of the world's population and killing 100,000 people every year. *E. histolytica* is more commonly found in urban areas with up to 90 percent of cases being asymptomatic. Depending on host factors and the number of cysts ingested, its symptoms range from mild to severe diarrhea that may resolve spontaneously or result in severe dehydration or even colitis. Less commonly, *E. histolytica* can also move through the wall of the intestine causing amoebic abscesses in other parts of the body, often the liver. These can be fatal if not appropriately treated.

Giardia lamblia is fairly common in all parts of the world and is seen in North America in returning travelers and in hikers who drink contaminated, unpurified water. About 50 percent of infected persons are asymptomatic with others suffering from watery diarrhea. Medical treatments exist, but the infection may resolve itself.

Other common diarrhea-causing parasites include species from the isospora, microsporidia, and balantidium families.

Both protozoal and helminthic parasitic infections of human intestines are responsible for a very significant burden of disease throughout the world. The majority of these diseases are both treatable and preventable with increased education, awareness, and basic hygiene measures.

SEE ALSO: Parasitic Diseases.

BIBLIOGRAPHY. Stephen L. Hauser, Dan L. Longo, and J. Larry Jameson, *Harrison's Principles of Internal Medicine* 15th ed., Eugene Braunwald, Anthony S. Fauci, and Dennis L. Kasper, eds. (McGraw-Hill Professional Publishing, 2001).

BARRY PAKES M.D., M.P.H.
UNIVERSITY OF TORONTO

Iran

This country in central Asia, known until March 21, 1935 as Persia, remains one of the most powerful countries in its region. It was ruled by the Shah until 1979 when, after the Iranian Revolution, it has been the Islamic Republic of Iran. It has a population of 69,019,000 (2004) and has 85 doctors and 259 nurses per 100,000 people.

There has been a long history of medical research in Persia, with references to medicine in the Stele of Hamurabi from the ancient world. As a great center of learning, many medical doctors worked in the region during the Achaemenian Empire, and in the period of Greek rule that followed. In medieval times, doctors were trained at the university at Ahvaz, and the great Arab medical writer Avicenna (980–1037 C.E.) practiced in Persia. The medical scholar and surgeon, Jorjani (1042–1136) spent much of his life in northeast Iran at what is now Gorgan. During the early modern period, medical specialists such as Hoseini Nourbakhsji, Mozafar Shafai and Hakim Momen made great advances in surgical procedures and medical techniques.

European medical practices were first introduced into Iran with the establishment in 1850 of the Darol Fonoun Polytechnic, with doctors such as the Austrian Dr. Polack, and others such as the Dutchman Dr. Schlimmer and Dr. Albaux also working at the Darol Fonoun Polytechnic. The *Treatise on Small-Pox Vaccination* was one of the first books printed in the city of Tabriz. In the 20th century there were efforts to modernize medical procedures and medical facilities. This saw new hospitals being built throughout the country. The Sanatorium at Sakhtessar in the 1930s was hailed as an example of this modernization process, as was the Nemazi Hospital in Shiraz, opened in March 1956. The Iranian Society of Microbiology was founded in 1940, and an expansion of the university system in the 1960s saw many more doctors trained in the country. The medical congresses of the Iranian Medical Society were held annually from 1951 and the Near and Middle East Medical Congress was held in Iran in October 1962.

The Iranian Revolution led to many doctors leaving Iran to work overseas, but the trend only exacerbated a problem that had faced the country for some years. In March 1976, there were 12,196 physicians in Iran, with about 10,000 others who were practicing overseas. Approximately some 7,000 more left Iran in the first decade after the Revolution, and only 750 new doctors graduated from Iran's medical schools from 1980 until 1986. This has led to a massive shortage of trained doctors in the country, which has partially been addressed during the 1990s and early 2000s, with government and the private sector spending about $300 billion on healthcare in 2006. Nowadays, some 46 percent of doctors in Iran are women. There are now some 730 hospitals and clinics in the country, which have a capacity of 110,797 beds.

The medical problems facing people in the country included typhoid, cholera, tuberculosis, and malaria. The government introduced major malaria eradication measures from 1960, resulting in a very marked decline in the disease. Improvements in sanitation and the provision of fresh water have seen marked declines in typhoid and cholera, with tuberculosis under control. New medical problems include a rising rate of HIV/AIDS, although it is still low compared to many other countries, and also a rise in diseases and conditions associated with greater affluence such as cancer, obesity, and diabetes.

SEE ALSO: AIDS; Obesity; Smallpox; Typhoid.

BIBLIOGRAPHY. Cyril Elgood, *Medicine in Persia* (P.B. Hoeber, 1934); Cyril Elgood, A *Medical History of Persian and the Eastern Caliphate: From the Earliest Times Until the Year AD 1932* (Cambridge University Press, 1951); Cyril Elgood, *Safavid Medical Practice ... Between 1500 AD and 1750 AD,* (B. Luzac, 1970); "History of Medicine in Iran," www.caroun.com/Medicine/IranHistory/After Islam-2.htm (cited August 2007).

JUSTIN CORFIELD
GEELONG GRAMMAR SCHOOL, AUSTRALIA

Iraq

This Middle Eastern country, located across the Tigris and Euphrates Rivers, was formed after World War I, and officially gained its independence from the Ottoman Empire on October 1, 1919, and from Britain on October 3, 1932. It has a population of 25,375,000 (2004) and has 55 doctors and 236 nurses per 100,000 people.

There are descriptions of medical procedures on cuneiform tablets from Babylon, dating from about 2000 B.C.E., and Babylon and later Assyria were centers of great learning. In medieval times, the great Arab surgeon Avicenna (980–1037 C.E.), author of *Canon of Medicine*, was born in Baghdad, which was the center of medical research in the region until 1258 when it was sacked by the Mongols. In 1401, it was again sacked by Tamurlane, and then ruled by the Ottoman Turks, with the city going into decline. In 1920, the Iraqi Medical Society was formed, but it was not until after World War II that the city boomed, with the wealth created from the sale of oil.

Much of the teaching of medicine took place at the University of Baghdad which published the *Journal of the Faculty of Medicine* each quarter, and also the *Journal of the College of Dentistry*. The Mosul branch of the University of Baghdad was founded as a separate university in 1967, and it also has a College of Medicine. The University of Basrah, founded in 1964, has a Faculty of Medicine, and al-Nahrain University (formerly Saddam University), founded in 1993, has a College of Medicine.

The rise to power of the Baath Party in Iraq in 1968 coincided with a period of great wealth for the country, and it was not long before the healthcare system became one of the best in the region. In 1976, the Iraq Cancer Registry was established, being one of the first to be formed in the region. However, the start of the Iran–Iraq War led to a decline in spending on medical care, and the continued rule of Saddam Hussein caused some highly-trained medical personnel to leave Iraq and settle in the West. By 1983, the area around Baghdad known as the Baghdad Governorate, which included about 29 percent of the population, had 37 percent of the hospital beds, 42 percent of the government clinics and 28 percent of the paramedical personnel. This demonstrated that although the focus of the healthcare system was on the capital, as it is in most other countries, the distant parts of the country were not totally neglected.

The health problems faced in Iraq until the 1940s were largely to do with poor sanitation and lack of access to fresh water. With the pollution of irrigation canals by both humans and animals, cholera, typhoid, malaria, and tuberculosis were common, along with trachoma, influenza, measles, and whooping cough. The prevalence of all of these was massively reduced during the 1950s, 1960s, and 1970s. By the 1980s with the decrease in expenditure on medical care, there was a rise in many of these diseases, especially in rural areas. This was exacerbated by the international sanctions imposed on the country after the invasion of Kuwait in August 1990. There have also been problems concerning a large rise in cancer cases which many commentators have associated with the use, by the U.S. military in Desert Storm in 1991, of depleted uranium. The Iraqi government raised this issue, going as far as issuing a postage stamp in 2001 showing two badly scarred children with the caption "DU bombing crime against Iraqi people."

Since the invasion of Iraq in 2002, there has been a major change in the medical services of the country. Even though there has been money spent on the health services by the new government, the insurgency which followed the invasion, and daily bombings throughout the country, has resulted in many more medical personnel leaving Iraq for overseas, and those who remain being overworked dealing with emergency casualties of the fighting, and unable to deal with the health prevention programs, elective surgery, and other medical problems with which they would otherwise have been able to deal.

SEE ALSO: Cancer (General); Typhoid.

BIBLIOGRAPHY. al-Nakshabandi Usama Nasir, *Medical Manuscripts of the Iraq Museums Library* (Dar al-Hurriya, 1981); Hashim al Witry, *Health Services in Iraq* (New Publishers Iraq, 1944); Moses K. der Hagopian, *Public Health in Iraq: The First Half Century* (Ministry of Culture and Information, Republic of Iraq, 1981).

JUSTIN CORFIELD
GEELONG GRAMMAR SCHOOL, AUSTRALIA

Ireland

With a per capita income of $41,100, Ireland is the eighth richest nation in the world. Among European countries, only Luxembourg ($65,900) and Norway ($42,800) report higher per capita incomes. The United Nations Development Programme's (UNDP)Human Development Report ranks Ireland's standard of living as the fourth highest in the world, and healthcare is widely available. Historically, an agricultural economy, Ireland has transformed itself into a major export giant. Between 1995 and 2004, Ireland averaged a seven percent growth rate. Inflation (2.4 percent) and unemployment (4.3 percent) are under control; however, a tenth of the population lives in poverty. Income disparity also exists, and Ireland is rated 35.9 on the gini index of inequality. The poorest ten percent of the population is able to claim only two percent of the country's wealth as opposed to 35.9 percent for the wealthiest 10 percent.

The Irish health system operates through a combination of private insurance and public subsidies. Government spending on health is high, and the government directs an average of 16 percent of the total budget to health programs. Health expenditures comprise 7.3 percent of the Gross Domestic Product (GDP), and the government allots $2,496 per capita for health. Nearly 80 percent of all health spending originates with the government, but only 0.8 percent of that funding is used for social security. Ireland's social insurance and social assistance system covers full-time employees and self-employed and part-time workers whose earnings exceed a base income. Recipients are the elderly, the disabled, and survivors. Cash benefits are paid to the seriously ill, parents on leave for the birth or adoption of a child, the unemployed, and injured workers. Irish residents whose family income is below a certain level are issued a medical card that allows them to receive medical care, medications, hospital services, out-patient care, dental care, medical devices, and maternity and infant care free of charge. Parents are awarded a cash grant upon the birth of each child. Private sources provide just over a fifth of total health expenditures, and 61.90 of that amount is derived from out-of-pocket expenses. There are 2.79 physicians, 15.20 nurses, 4.27 midwives, 0.56 dentists, and 0.07 pharmacists per 1,000 population in Ireland.

The 4,062,235 people of Ireland have a life expectancy of 77.73 years, with females outliving males by an average of six years. Literacy is universal (99 percent), and all Irish in the relevant age groups are enrolled in primary and secondary school. Safe drinking water and improved sanitation are available throughout Ireland. Despite the fact that 88.4 percent of the population identify themselves as Roman Catholic,

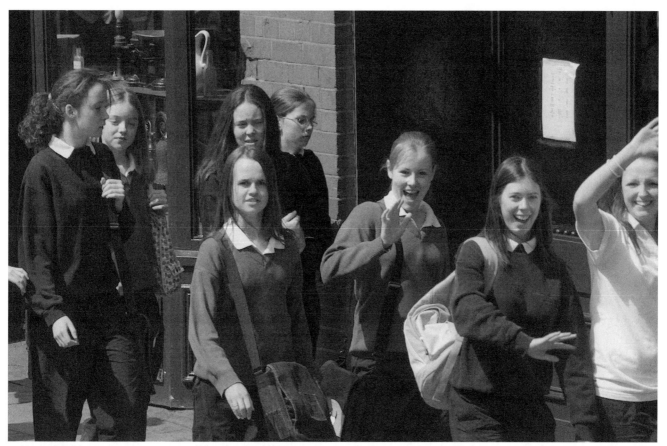

The Irish health system operates through a combination of private insurance and public subsidies. Government spending on health is high, and the government directs an average of 16 percent of the total budget to health programs.

birth control is widely practiced; and the government sponsors a number of family planning programs. On the average, Irish women give birth to 1.86 children each. All births occur in the presence of trained attendants. Natural births are widespread, and Ireland has one of the highest rates in the developed world. The Maternity and Infant Care Scheme has been initiated to provide care to pregnant women and new mothers free of charge. The adjusted maternal mortality rate is low at five deaths per 100,000 live births.

Between 1990 and 2004, infant mortality fell from eight to five deaths per 1,000 live births, and under-five mortality dropped from 10 to six deaths per 1,000 live births. The current infant mortality rate is 5.31 deaths per 1,000 live births. Six percent of infants are underweight at birth. Ninety percent of infants are immunized against tuberculosis. The immunization rate for diphtheria, pertussis, and tetanus (DPT1) is even higher at 96 percent; however, only 89 percent of infants receive the DPT3 vaccination. Rates for other

inoculations range from the low to the high eighties: Polio and *Haemophilus influenzae* type B (89 percent each) and measles (81 percent).

Agricultural runoff has polluted the water of the Emerald Isle, creating a health threat for residents of surrounding areas. HIV/AIDS has also threatened health in Ireland, and the country has a 0.1 percent adult prevalence rate. Some 2,800 people are living with the disease, but less than 100 have died from HIV/AIDS or its complications. Other communicable diseases also present periodic problems in Ireland. In August 2000, an outbreak of measles occurred. Ireland was one of several countries to identify cases of severe acute respiratory syndrome (SARS) in spring 2003. Heart disease is a leading cause of death in Ireland, and the government has made the promotion of healthy lifestyles a major priority, including prevention and early detection of cancer.

SEE ALSO: Healthcare, Europe.

BIBLIOGRAPHY. Spencer Di Scala, *Twentieth Century Europe: Politics, Society, Culture* (McGraw-Hill, 2004); Sandra Halperin, *War and Social Change in Modern Europe: The Great Transformation Revisited* (Cambridge University Press, 2004); Martin A. Levin and Martin Shapiro, eds., *Transatlantic Policymaking in an Age of Austerity: Diversity and Drift* (Georgetown University Press, 2004); Jeremy Rifkin, *The European Dream: How Europe's Vision of the Future Is Quietly Eclipsing the American Dream* (Jeremy P. Tarcher/Penguin, 2004); Peter Taylor-Gooby, *New Risks, New Welfare: The Transformation of the European Welfare State* (Oxford University Press, 2004).

ELIZABETH R. PURDY, PH.D.
INDEPENDENT SCHOLAR

Iridology

Iridology, also sometimes known as iridodiagnosis, is a medical practice with which doctors and others study the eyes of a patient to try to determine major problems in other parts of the human body. As such, it is not a treatment but a form of diagnosis.

The first time that iridological practices were used, although the name was not coined until much later, was in the *Chiromatica Medica*, written by Philippus Meyeus and first published in 1665. It was reprinted five years later, and again in 1691, and mentioned some doctors looking into people's eyes to see whether there are any other problems with the patient.

The idea was more formalized by the Hungarian physician Ignatz von Péczely who used the German word *Augendiagnostik* which translates as "eye diagnosis." The idea apparently came to him after he was treating a person for a broken leg and noticed particular streaks in the eye which were similar to those he had noticed in an owl that had a broken leg many years earlier. However, August von Péczely, the nephew of Ignatz von Péczely, rejected the idea as a myth at the First International Congress of Iridology, held in Brussels, Belgium, in October 2000.

Iridology continued in Germany where Pastor Felke, a homeopathist, established the Felke Institute in Gerlingen. However, many scientists dismissed the idea, although some researchers in recent times have suggested that there might be a number of nonvisual

functions of the eye with Dr. D. A. Waniek, as recently as 1987, postulating that this might well be the case.

During the 1950s, there was increased popularity for iridology in the United States, with Bernard Jensen, an American chiropractor, giving many classes on his method of diagnosis. Jensen had been critical of the exposure of the body to toxins and urged for natural foods to be used as detoxifiers, and claiming to be able to diagnose some aspects of bad diet by observing the eyes of patients. Jensen wrote about his theories in *Iridology Simplified* (2nd ed., 1980).

In 1979, the *Journal of the American Medical Association* allowed three iridologists to study photographs of irises to see whether they could identify kidney disease, and found their diagnoses were in disagreement with each other and inaccurate. This has not stopped the publication of a large number of books on iridology including the *Canadian Journal of the Science and Practice of Iridology*, and there is also the Israeli Center for Advances in Multidimensional Iridology. The 2nd International Congress of Iridology was held at Thessaloniki, Greece, in October 2001, the 4th International Congress of Applied Iridology was held on May 18–21, 2000, and the First Integrated Iridology Conference was held on March 9–11, 2001, in Sydney, Australia.

SEE ALSO: Ophthalmologist; Ophthalmology; Optometrist.

BIBLIOGRAPHY. Stephen Gabriel Allen, *Iris Diagnosis: A Handbook of Iridology* (Goulburn Naturopathic Centre, 2006); E. Ernest, "Iridology: Not Useful and Potentially Harmful," *Archives of Ophthalmology* (v.118/1, 2000); A. Simon, D. M. Worthen, and J. A. Mitas, "An Evaluation of Iridology," *Journal of the American Medical Association* (v.242/13, 1979); John Vriend, *Eyes Talk: Through Iridology to Better Health* (Lothian Books, 1989).

JUSTIN CORFIELD
GEELONG GRAMMAR SCHOOL, AUSTRALIA

Irritable Bowel Syndrome

Irritable bowel syndrome (IBS) is one of the most common gastrointestinal disorders encountered in a clinic. It is a bowel disorder lacking any detectable structural abnormalities in which abdominal discomfort or pain is associated with defecation or a change in bowel habits. Other IBS symptoms include abnormal stool frequency (more than three per day or less than three per week), abnormal stool form (hard or watery), abnormal stool passage (urgency or feeling of incomplete evacuation), passage of mucus, and a heightened sensation of bloating or feeling of abdominal distention. Psychological stresses can influence the onset of IBS. Symptoms of IBS can be alleviated by dietary avoidance of certain food, pharmacological agents, and behavioral-cognitive therapy.

SYMPTOMS

IBS is a disease of no obvious pathological abnormalities. It is a disorder that primarily affects the young. Until recently, IBS was thought to be somatic manifestations of psychological stress. Typically, patients with IBS are young and present symptoms before the age of 45. Symptoms of IBS include abdominal pain, altered bowel habits, gas and flatulence, and upper gastrointestinal symptoms. The most consistent clinical feature of IBS is the alteration in bowel habits. The most common pattern is the alternation of constipation and diarrhea and with one being the dominant symptom.

Initially, constipation occurs on an occasional basis progressing to a steady phase in which laxative treatments are no longer effective. Due to the prolonged retention of the stool in the colon, the stool is dehydrated and is usually hard. The constipation phase of IBS may last for weeks or months interrupted by brief episodes of diarrhea. If diarrhea is the predominating symptom, small, loose stools of volume less than 200 mL is the norm and the patients may also pass large amounts of mucus. Emotional stress and eating can aggravate diarrhea. Blood in the stool is not a feature of IBS unless it comes from hemorrhoids. Even though IBS patients present with constipation and diarrhea, they generally do not present with weight loss as a consequence of malabsorption.

IBS patients also frequently complain of increased passing of gas or belching and complain of distended abdomen. Although some IBS patients may actually have increased production of gas, studies have actually shown that most IBS patients generate normal amount of intestinal gas. Rather, IBS patients have impaired transit and tolerance of intestinal gas leading to indicated symptoms. Up to 50 percent of IBS patients also complain of symptoms in the upper gastrointestinal region. These include heartburn, nausea, dyspepsia, and vomiting. Abdominal pain in IBS patients is highly variable in location and quality. The pain is frequently described as crampy and/or a constant ache.

RISKS

IBS accounts for up to 3.5 million physician visits a year in the United States. It is estimated that up to 50 percent of those with symptoms consistent with a diagnosis of IBS never seek a doctor's care. Those who do seek medical advice often had a major life event prior to seeking help (e.g., death in the family). Although IBS is a global disease, social and cultural factors affect the presentation and the diagnosis of IBS. In the West, it is estimated that up to 20 percent of adults show symptoms consistent with diagnosis of IBS. In the Western hemispheres, women have a higher incidence of the condition and are more likely to consult a physician. In south Asia, men in India have a higher incidence of IBS. In South Africa, IBS symptoms are more prevalent in black, urban dwellers than black, rural dwellers. In the United States, prevalence is equal between blacks and whites.

DIAGNOSIS

The diagnosis of IBS requires the patient to have two of the three following clinical features developed by the Rome Consensus Committee (Rome II Criteria). In order to meet the diagnosis, patients, in the preceding year, have to have at least 12 weeks of abdominal pain or discomfort that is relieved with defecation, experience onset associated with stool frequency, and have onset associated with change in stool appearance and form. The Bristol Stool Form Scale is also utilized to describe the seven types of stool morphology. The scale includes descriptions of stool that ranges from "separate hard lumps like nuts" to "smooth sausage-like" to "watery, no solid pieces."

CAUSES

The pathogenesis for IBS is poorly understood and explanations are numerous. They include abnormal motor and sensory functions in the gut, central nervous dysfunction, psychological disturbances, and stress.

Specifically, the pathology includes or leads to abnormal gut motility due to exaggerated sensory response, heightened and altered sensation to visceral and pain stimulation in the gut or in the central nervous system, and mucosal inflammation. Studies have shown that IBS patients have lower threshold of sensation to pain and gastrointestinal distention.

Studies have also shown that infection may influence the pathogenesis of IBS as up to 30 percent of patients develop symptoms compatible with IBS after episodes of bacterial gastroenteritis. Studies have found that women and patients with increased life stressors at the onset of gastroenteritis are at increased risk for developing "postinfectious" IBS. Increased numbers of inflammatory cells have been found in the gastrointestinal linings and some investigators have suggested that chronic inflammation contributes to alterations in motility or visceral hypersensitivity.

TREATMENT

IBS treatments are broad and include several categories: dietary therapy, pharmacological therapy, and behavior therapy. IBS patients are encouraged to avoid fatty foods and caffeine as they are poorly tolerated. Foods that exacerbate bloating, diarrhea, and pain are to be avoided. These include alcohol, cabbage, cauliflower, raw onions, grapes, plums, and raisins. Studies have shown that a high-fiber diet has little value for IBS patients. Pharmacological interventions include agents that are used to relief the symptoms of spasmodic gut, diarrhea, and constipation. Additionally, agents used to treat intestinal infections have been found to be effective in some IBS patients. Low-dose tricyclic antidepressants and serotonin receptor agonists and antagonists are also found to be helpful in some subsets of IBS patients. Last, because IBS manifestations are aggravated by stress and emotional distress, cognitive-behavioral therapies and relaxation techniques appear to be beneficial in some patients.

SEE ALSO: Constipation; Diarrhea; Digestive Diseases (General); Stress.

BIBLIOGRAPHY. Thomas E. Andreoli, et al., "Irritable Bowel Syndrome," in *Cecil Essentials of Medicine* (Saunders, 2003); Brenda J. Horwitz and Robert S. Fisher, "The Irritable Bowel Syndrome," *New England Journal of Medicine* (v.344/24, 2001); "Irritable Bowel Syndrome," Mayo Clinic, www.mayoclinic.com/health/irritable-bowel-syndrome/DS00106 (cited February 2007).

James S. Yeh
Boston University School of Medicine

Israel

This Middle Eastern country was founded in 1948 from what had been the British mandated territory of Palestine. As the only Jewish state in the world, it has had a policy of encouraging Jewish people from all over the world to settle in the country, resulting in one of the most culturally diverse populations in the world.

Although there are many references to medicine and medical treatment in surviving ancient Jewish texts, the modern history of Israeli medicine effective starts on January 11, 1912, with the establishment of The Hebrew Medicinal Society for Jaffa and the Jaffa District. There were nine doctors present at the meeting, from 32 Jewish physicians living in what became Israel. In 1913, the Hebrew-Speaking Physicians' Society was established and soon accepted membership from Hebrew-speaking doctors who lived outside the Holy Land. By 1914, there were 60 Jewish doctors in the Holy Land, and the two organizations started to cooperate, merging after World War I to become the Hebrew Medical Association in the Land of Israel (HMA). In 1920 the HMA started publishing its quarterly journal *Harefuah*.

One of the major focuses of the medical services in what was then the British mandated territory of Palestine was the improvement of the sanitation in the region. With cholera, typhoid, malaria, and tuberculosis being prevalent, the provision of drinking water to all parts of the territory, as well as diagnosis of problems and money spent to help prevent the spread of these diseases all helped.

By 1939, the HMA had grown significantly in membership and its importance, and with the formation of the State of Israel, the HMA became the Israel Medical Association (IMA). Its initial energies were devoted to protecting doctors working in private hospitals, but with Israel spending considerable funds on establishing a government health sector from 1948 to 1963, the IMA started to help support doctors in public hospitals, as well as help with the formulation of Israeli government policy. From 1965 until 1997 it published the *Israel Journal of Medical Sciences*, which was superseded from 1999 by the *Israel Medical Association Journal.*

It was not long before a number of other medical societies were established in Israel. These included the Israel Society of Allergology, founded in 1949; the Israel Society of Clinical Pediatrics, founded in 1953; the Israel Gerentological Society was founded in 1956; the Israel Society of Internal Medicine, founded in 1958; the Israel Society of Geriatric Medicine, founded in 1963; and the Society for Medicine and Law in Israel, founded in 1972. There are also many medical research institutes in the country, the most well-known being the Rogoff-Wellcome Medical Research Institute, founded in 1955.

Some 70 percent of people in Israel are covered by the Kupat Holim, the sick fund run by Histadrut (the General Federation of Labor in Israel). Another 20 percent covered by insurance from other organizations, with only 10 percent of the population not covered by health insurance. Many of the medical problems now faced by doctors in Israel are connected with a high life expectancy, and affluent lifestyle. These include cancer, obesity, diabetes, and heart disease. There have also been an increasing number of cases of hepatitis and HIV/AIDS The Republic of Israel has a population of 7,047,000 (2006), and has one of the highest doctor to population ratios in the world, with 385 doctors and 613 nurses per 100,000 people.

SEE ALSO: AIDS; Cholera; Malaria.

BIBLIOGRAPHY. James H. Cassedy, "Medical History in Israel," *Bulletin of the History of Medicine* (v.43/4, 1969); A. Michael Davies, *Health and Disease in the Holy Land: Studies in the History and Sociology of Medicine from Ancient Times to the Present* (Edwin Mellen Press, 1996); "Israeli Medical Association: Historical Background," www.ima.org.il/EN; Shifra Shvarts, "Health Reform in Israel: Some Aspects of Seventy Years of Struggle 1925–1995," *Social History of Medicine* (v.11/1, 1988).

JUSTIN CORFIELD
GEELONG GRAMMAR SCHOOL, AUSTRALIA

Italy

The Italian Republic has a per capita income of $28,700, the 28th highest in the world. Aggregate figures are somewhat misleading because the economies of the northern industrial area and the agricultural south are vastly different. Most poverty in Italy is found in the south, which has an unemployment rate of 20 percent as compared to an overall unemployment rate of 7.7 percent. Nearly 66 percent of southern Italians are poor, making them dependent on welfare for survival. Italy is ranked 36 on the Gini index of inequality, and the richest 10 percent of the population claims 26.6 percent of resources while the poorest ten percent hold only 2.1 percent. Evidence exists that as income disparities have expanded, the intensity of poverty has increased.

Economic woes have led the Italian government to privatize social services and create a two-tiered welfare system in which the poorest Italians receive healthcare through government subsidies and more affluent Italians depend on private insurance. As a result of the privatization, funding for health and other social programs was seriously curtailed. No public kindergartens are available, and poor women find it difficult to work because of the paucity of child care. Consequently, these women remain dependent on welfare. Despite the lack of government for education at the lowest and highest levels, literacy rates are high. There is, however, some disparity between male (99 percent) and female (98.3 percent) literacy. All of the relevant population is enrolled in primary and secondary schools. Safe drinking water and improved sanitation are available throughout Italy. According to the United Nations Development Programme's (UNDP) Human Development Report, Italy has the 17th highest standard of living in the world.

An average of 11 percent of the total Italian budget is designated for health. With a spending rate of $2,266 (international dollars) per capita, the government directs 8.4 percent of the Gross Domestic Product (GDP) to healthcare programs. Just over three-fourths of health expenditures in Italy are government generated. Social security accounts for only 0.2 percent of government spending. The private sector is responsible for the remaining fourth of health expenditures, and 83.30 percent of private spending

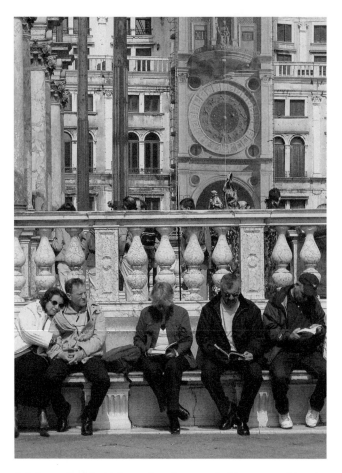

Italy has enjoyed a high pension allowance that is now considered excessive, and reform efforts are underway.

evolves from out-of-pocket expenses. There are 4.20 physicians, 5.44 nurses, 0.29 midwives, 0.58 dentists, and 1.15 pharmacists per 1,000 population in Italy.

The social security program, which covers the elderly, the disabled, and survivors, is funded by employee (8.89 percent of earnings) and employer (23.81 percent of payroll) contributions and government supplements. The program is compulsory for all employed Italians, and special programs cover civil servants and the self-employed. Italy's pension allowances have been considered excessive, and efforts are under way to reform the program. Illness and maternity coverage provides both cash benefits and medical care. New mothers receive 80 percent of their salaries from a month before the expected birth of a child to three to four months after birth. The parental leave policy provides additional leave for either parent at 30 percent salary at any time until a child turns 3 years of age. Special benefits are also provided for those suf-

fering from tuberculosis, with benefits payable for up to two years, plus a Christmas allowance.

Italy's population of 58.133,509 has a life expectancy of 79.81 years, the 14th highest in the world. Females outlive males an average of six years. Italy has the 15th lowest fertility rate among nations of the world, and women give birth to an average of 1.28 children each. Sixty percent of Italian women use some form of birth control even thought 90 percent of the population is Roman Catholic. The adjusted maternal mortality rate is low at five deaths per 100,000 live births.

Between 1990 and 2004, infant mortality plunged from nine to four deaths per 1,000 live births. At the same time, under-5 mortality fell from nine to five deaths per 1,000 live births. Six percent of Italian infants are underweight at birth. Currently, the infant mortality rate is 5.83 deaths per 1,000 live births. Immunization rates are generally high in Italy. Ninety-eight percent of infants are immunized against diphtheria, pertussis, and tetanus (DPT1), 97 against polio, 96 against DPT3, 95 percent against Hepatitis B, 90 percent against Haemophilus influenzae type B, and 84 percent against measles.

There are major environmental health concerns in Italy. Industrial emissions such as sulfur dioxide have polluted the air, and water sources have been tainted by industrial and agricultural effluents. The government needs to address the issue of inadequate waste treatment and disposal. Italy has a 0.5 percent adult prevalence rate of HIV/AIDS. Some 140,000 people are living with the disease, which has proved fatal to less than a thousand people. Italy was one of several nations that experienced outbreaks of severe acute respiratory syndrome (SARS) in spring 2003. That same winter, human influenza A/H3N2 surfaced. The leading causes of death are circulatory diseases, cancer, and transport accidents.

Due to the immigration of around 40,000 females from the sub-Saharan area of Africa, the Italian government has been faced with the health problem of female genital mutilation (FGM). Health officials are forced to walk a tight line between protecting the health of young girls and respecting the cultures of immigrant families. Some hospitals have created special teams trained to deal with caring for girls who have undergone FGM.

SEE ALSO: Healthcare, Europe.

BIBLIOGRAPHY. Spencer Di Scala, *Twentieth Century Europe: Politics, Society, Culture* (McGraw-Hill, 2004); Sandra Halperin, *War and Social Change in Modern Europe: The Great Transformation Revisited* (Cambridge University Press, 2004); Martin A. Levin and Martin Shapiro, eds., *Transatlantic Policymaking in an Age of Austerity: Diversity and Drift* (Georgetown University Press, 2004); Jeremy Rifkin, *The European Dream: How Europe's Vision of the Future Is Quietly Eclipsing the American Dream* (Jeremy P. Tarcher/Penguin, 2004); Peter Taylor-Gooby, *New Risks, New Welfare: The Transformation of the European Welfare State* (Oxford University Press, 2004).

ELIZABETH R. PURDY, PH.D.
INDEPENDENT SCHOLAR

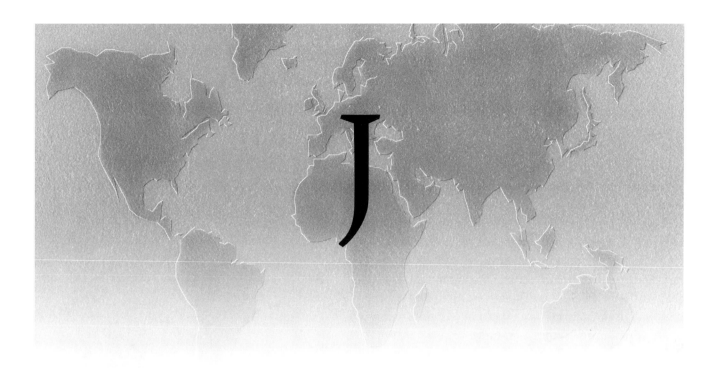

Jamaica

Jamaica is located in the Caribbean Sea, south of Cuba. It is the third largest island and the second largest country in the Caribbean, a tropical land of high, forested mountains that slope down to more than a thousand miles of sandy beaches. Although formally part of the British Commonwealth, Jamaicans are by and large the descendents of African slaves, and they have built a rich heritage and a relaxed culture.

The island has a population of 2.76 million, growing at 0.8 percent annually. The birth rate is 20.82 per 1,000 people and the death rate 6.52 per 1,000 people. The migration rate is negative, with minus 6.27 migrants per 1,000 people. About 1 million Jamaicans have left the island over the past few decades, resettling in other parts of the British Commonwealth or in the United States; this movement is known as the Jamaican diaspora.

The majority of Jamaicans live in the cities along the coast; the urbanization rate is 52 percent and the population density is high at 241 people per square kilometer. The national economy is increasingly based on tourism, but also relies on strong exports in bauxite and agricultural products. Per capita income is $2,900, and less than 2 percent of the population lives on less than $1 a day.

About 93 percent of Jamaicans have access to clean water and 80 percent can access sanitary facilities. Combined with a well-developed monitoring system, this has led to significant decreases in common infectious diseases.

Life expectancy at birth is 71.54 for men and 75.03 for women, with a healthy life expectancy estimated at 64.2 for men and 65.9 for women. The infant mortality rate is fairly low at 15.98 per 1,000 people. Immunization rates for children are high. The fertility rate is 2.41 children per woman, and 66 percent of women use birth control. Maternal mortality is low, with 120 deaths per 100,000 live births. A trained attendant monitors 95 percent of births.

The Ministry of Health oversees a network of 30 hospitals spread out across the island. There are 2,253 doctors working within the country, along with 4,374 nurses. The government allocates about $83 per capita on healthcare.

Jamaicans have a fairly healthy indigenous diet based on root crops, fish, chicken, beans, and rice. Consumption of red meat is low. However, there is a high incidence of cardiovascular disease, leading to about one-third of all deaths. One in seven people smoke. Diabetes is another growing health issue, with 81,000 Jamaicans currently living with the disease. The World Health Organization estimates that that number will grow to 189,000 by 2030 at current rates.

HIV/AIDS affects about 1.2 percent of the population, with an estimated 20,000 Jamaicans infected with the virus. This is low compared to the infection rate elsewhere in the Caribbean but could grow in coming years. In a 2000 survey of risk behavior by the Ministry of Health, one in two respondents said they did not use condoms regularly, one in two men and one in ten women had more than one partner within a year, one in four men and one in eight women had already contracted at least one sexually transmitted disease in their lifetime. One in nine reported regular use of marijuana. The government and other national organizations are working on improving AIDS education within the country.

Young Jamaicans are more likely to die in car crashes or violent crime than any other cause. The country is an active transfer point for guns and drugs traveling between North and South America, and gang violence is common. There are more than 1,000 gang-related homicides per year.

SEE ALSO: AIDS; Diabetes; Marijuana Abuse.

BIBLIOGRAPHY. Arvilla Payne-Jackson and Mervyn C. Alleyne, *Jamaica Folk Medicine: A Source of Healing* (University of West Indies Press, 2004).

HEATHER K. MICHON
INDEPENDENT SCHOLAR

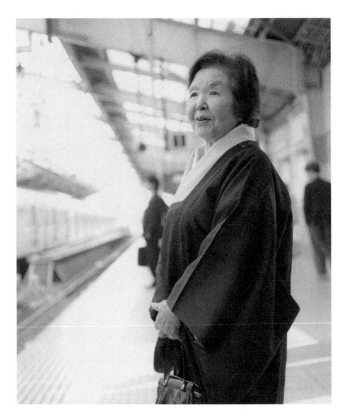

With a life expectancy of 81.25 years among the population of 127,463,611, Japan is ranked sixth in the world in life expectancy.

Japan

The Japanese people are among the healthiest in the world. As the world's second most industrialized nation, Japan enjoys a per capita income of $31,600, ranking as the 20th richest nation. Japan reports no poverty level, and homelessness is virtually nonexistent in this eastern Asian nation. A rating of 37.0 percent on the Gini index of inequality is indicative of Japan's status as the most equal nation in the world. Because the traditional Japanese guarantee of lifetime employment has begun to erode, the current unemployment rate stands at 4.4 percent. Only one percent of the population is considered illiterate, and

100 percent of all children are enrolled in school at the primary level and 99.5 percent at the secondary level. One hundred percent of all Japanese have access to safe drinking water and improved sanitation. The United Nations Development Programme (UNDP) ranks Japan seventh of 177 nations in overall quality-of-life issues.

The first welfare programs in Japan appeared in the late 19th century. Since the end of World War II and the eradication of the huge military sector, the Japanese people have enjoyed expanded benefits of good health combined with substantial government resources. Since 1994, welfare rights have been protected by the Japanese constitution. Health expenditures have remained stable over the last decade. Currently, around two percent of the overall national budget is allocated to healthcare. Some 7.9 percent of the total Gross Domestic Product (GDP) is set aside for health expenditures, an increase from 5.8 percent in 1998. The government allots $2,244 (international dollars) per capita for health costs. Over 80 percent of total health expenditures are provided by government at various levels. Around 90.10 percent of the 19 percent financed by the private sector involves out-of-pocket expenditures. More than 80 percent of all government health expenditures are allocated to finance social security programs. Japan has 1.98 physicians, 7.79 nurses, 0.71 dentists, and 1.21 pharmacists per 1,000 population.

Although Japan has lagged behind other heavily industrialized nations in subsidizing healthcare, a safety net for the neediest people is well established. Known as *Nihongata shakai fukushi shakai*, Japan's welfare system is considered unique because it is based on the notion that family, community, and employers rather than the government share the bulk of responsibility for assisting the needy. The responsibility for public healthcare is shared among the national government, prefectures, and municipalities.

With a life expectancy of 81.25 years among the population of 127,463,611, Japan is ranked sixth in the world in life expectancy. This is chiefly in response to widespread access to healthcare under a national health insurance plan that began in 1938 with a limited target population. In 1961, the public insurance policy was revised to mandate enrollment of all Japanese not otherwise ensured in a community-based healthcare plan. Since 1980, all employers require a 10 percent copayment for employees and 20 percent copayment for family members. Healthcare is also promoted through employer-provided stress-reducing facilities such as spas and leisure resorts. Like other industrialized nations, Japan has a rapidly increasing aging population. It is predicted that by 2015, one in four Japanese will be 65 or older. Modest copayments are required of individuals covered under Social Security insurance. In 1990, the government instituted the Gold Plan, which subsidizes home helps, day care, and short-term nursing home care for the elderly.

In the late 1940s, concern over child and maternal health led to the passage of the Maternal and Child Health Care Law, the Child Welfare Law, and the Childbirth Assistance Program. Maternal mortality is extremely low in Japan with a rate of 8 deaths per 100,000 live births, and all births are attended by skilled personnel. Approximately 59 percent of Japanese women use some method of birth control. In 1994, the Angel Plan was introduced to address the government's ongoing concern about the low fertility rate (1.4 children per woman). The Angel Plan en-

courages women to become more fertile by making life easier for working mothers. Supportive measures include day nurseries, drop-in care for nonworking mothers, special centers for sick children, after-school programs, and counseling. However, the government has been criticized for not providing sufficient local support for the Angel Plan.

Japan has experienced a growing divorce rate over the last several decades, leading to a rise in the incidence of single-parent families. Much criticism has been leveled against the Japanese government for creating welfare benefits designed to assist only those who live in traditional nuclear families. On the other hand, the government has been lauded for its commitment to mothers and children at risk. The Ministry of Health, Labor, and Welfare has been charged with overseeing a number of programs dedicated to maternal and child health that include education, counseling, and healthcare services. These programs support women from the onset of pregnancy and continue until children are enrolled in elementary school. Special care is taken for women experiencing high-risk pregnancies and for newborn infants. Awareness and prevention of breast cancer are also emphasized for all Japanese females.

With an infant mortality rate of 3.24 deaths per 1,000 live births, Japan has the third lowest infant mortality rate in the world. The mortality rate of under-5s was reduced from 6 to 4 per 1,000 live births between 1990 and 2004. The government subsidizes all vaccinations in Japan, and 99 percent of all children under the age of 1 are immunized against measles, diphtheria, pertussis, and tetanus (DPT1 and DPT 3). Some 97 percent of under-1s are immunized against polio.

Japan has only recently acknowledged the inherent problem of child abuse that has been a result of cultural acceptance of inviolable parental rights and which has threatened the health of Japanese children. Educators and the media have banded together to garner support for the children's rights movement. Spousal abuse has also been addressed. In October 2001, the Law for the Prevention of Spousal Violence and the Protection of Victims went into effect, targeting education and prevention of domestic violence. Under the guidance of the Headquarters for the Promotion of Gender Equality, efforts have been made to provide counseling and support for victims, and the police force has been reeducated in proper handling of domestic violence cases.

Despite the escalating HIV/AIDS rate in much of Asia, the Japanese rate remains low at less than 0.1 percent. Attempts to eradicate communicable diseases have also been successful. Between 1990 and 2004, the incidence of tuberculosis in Japan was reduced from 71 cases per 100,000/population to 39. Efforts to prevent the spread of the common cold have led cold sufferers to wear face masks in public to prevent exposure to others. Japan has, however, experienced outbreaks of some preventable diseases. For instance, there was an outbreak of staphylococcal food intoxication in 2000, and in 2004, influenza and severe acute respiratory syndrome (SARS) surfaced in Japan. Concern for disease prevention led to the passage of the Law on Infectious Diseases in 1998, with special attention to the spread of sexually transmitted diseases (STDs). As a result, the Ministry of Education distributes age-appropriate material in Japanese schools to teach children how to avoid exposure to STDs.

SEE ALSO: Healthcare, Asia and Oceania.

BIBLIOGRAPHY. Roger Goodman, *Family and Social Policy in Japan* (Cambridge University Press, 2002); Carlos Gerardo Molina and José Núñez del Arco, eds., *Health Services in Latin America and Asia* (Johns Hopkins University Press, 2001); Leonard J. Schoppa, *Race for the Exits: The Unraveling of Japan's System of Social Protection* (Cornell University Press, 2006).

ELIZABETH PURDY, PH.D.
INDEPENDENT SCHOLAR

Joint FAO/WHO Expert Committee on Food Additives (JECFA)

The Joint FAO/WHO Expert Committee on Food Additives (JECFA) is an international committee comprised of scientific experts who evaluate food additive safety as well as safety levels of contaminants, naturally occurring toxicants, and veterinary drug residues in foods. It formulates standards to determine acceptable food contamination levels and serves as a resource for governments wishing to formulate national food safety programs.

Initially created in 1956 after a joint FAO/WHO Conference on Food Additives in 1955, the JECFA is managed jointly by the Food and Agriculture Organization (FAO) of the United Nations (UN) and the World Health Organization (WHO). The FAO is charged with helping developing countries modernize agriculture and improve nutrition, and generally lead the international initiative to overcome hunger. The WHO is the UN's health agency charged with helping the world's people reach the highest level of physical and mental health and social well-being. JECFA reports to both FAO and WHO, as well as to member countries of each agency and to the Codex Alimentarius Commission (CAC). The CAC is charged with developing and coordinating food standards and guidelines worldwide to protect consumer health.

The JECFA sets food safety levels after conducting risk assessment of additives and contaminants; to make their determinations, they use information from the fields of microbiology, biotechnology, exposure assessment, and food chemistry, including analytical chemistry.

To fulfill their responsibilities, the JECFA relies upon committees of experts. The FAO selects members with chemical expertise for specification development of food additive purity, for the analysis of veterinary drug residue levels in food, and for the assessment of data quality. The WHO selects members for the toxicological evaluation of substances being considered, the establishment of acceptable daily intakes (ADIs), and the providing of measurable health risk estimates. Both organizations select members who are responsible for exposure assessment.

The JECFA establishes ADIs based upon available toxicological data. During this evaluation process, experts focus on standards that will allow for consistently appropriate quality during the manufacturing of commercial food products. For contaminants and naturally occurring toxicants, the JECFA determines provisional maximum tolerable daily intake (PMTDI) or the provisional tolerable weekly intake (PTWI) using a no-observed-effect level. In other words, when a certain consumption of contaminants and natural toxicants cannot be seen to cause an effect on humans, this becomes that substance's PMTDI.

Most humans eat meat, and their food may contain residues of veterinary drugs given to the animal. The JECFA, therefore, determines maximum residue limits (MRLs) that can be found in specific animal tissues, milk, and eggs and still be considered safe for human consumption. These MRLs provide assurance that intake levels of animal product residue likely will not exceed the ADI with proper drug use. The JECFA regularly reviews evaluation processes to ensure up-to-date risk assessments. As a result, the JECFA assumes a key role in worldwide standardization of food chemical hazard assessment.

SEE ALSO: Food and Agriculture Organization of the United Nations (FAO); World Health Organization (WHO).

BIBLIOGRAPHY. Food and Agriculture Organization of the United Nations, http://www.fao.org; Joint FAO/WHO Expert Committee on Food Additives, http://www.who.int/ipcs/food/jecfa/en/; World Health Organization, http://www.who.int/en/.

KELLY BOYER SAGERT
INDEPENDENT SCHOLAR

Joint United Nations Programme on HIV/AIDS

UNAIDS, the Joint United Nations Programme on HIV/AIDS, brings together the efforts and resources of 10 UN system organizations to the global AIDS response. Based in Geneva, the UNAIDS secretariat works on the ground in more than 75 countries worldwide. UNAIDS brings together in the AIDS response the efforts and resources of ten UN system organizations. The 10 UN-AIDS cosponsoring organizations are:

- Office of the United Nations High Commissioner for Refugees (UNHCR)
- United Nations Children's Fund (UNICEF)
- World Food Programme (WFP)
- United Nations Development Programme (UNDP)
- United Nations Population Fund (UNFPA)
- United Nations Office on Drugs and Crime (UNODC)
- International Labour Organization (ILO)
- United Nations Educational, Scientific and Cultural Organization (UNESCO)
- World Health Organization (WHO)
- World Bank

The Cosponsors and the UNAIDS Secretariat comprise the Committee of Cosponsoring Organizations, which meets annually.

UNAIDS has successfully worked with a number of outstanding personalities to strengthen awareness on AIDS. The UNAIDS Special Representatives are prominent individuals from the world of arts, science, literature, entertainment, sport, and other fields of public life who have expressed their desire to contribute to UNAIDS and to move the AIDS response forward. To mark its 10th anniversary, UNAIDS has appointed a number of new Special Representatives.

THE UNIFIED BUDGET AND WORKPLAN

The UNAIDS Unified Budget and Workplan (UBW) is a unique mechanism within the system. It is a two-year program budget and work plan that presents the response to HIV/AIDS of 10 different UN organizations (UNAIDS Cosponsors) and the UNAIDS Secretariat which together constitute UNAIDS. It specifies who does what, where, with how much money and where the resources come from. The UBW also includes a Performance Monitoring and Evaluation Framework so that progress can be measured, accountability ensured, and program adjustments be made. The UBW presents a comprehensive picture, both programmatically and financially, of the joint work on HIV/AIDS of eleven UN entities—ten UNAIDS Cosponsors and the UNAIDS Secretariat—at global and regional level. In addition, the UBW document provides summary information on the estimated country level resources of the Cosponsors and Secretariat.

This revised version of the 2006–2007 Unified Budget and Workplan and its Annex contain the Programme Coordinating Board-approved changes made by the Cosponsors and the Secretariat in the Principal and Key Results in order to align the UBW with the recommendations of the Global Task Team on Improving AIDS Coordination among Multilateral Institutions and International Donors. This document also contains the revised achievement indicators of Principal and Key Results.

This Framework, adopted by the 18th PCB in June 2006, is designed to support results-based management, to promote transparency, strengthen accountability, improve reporting, and reflect links between collective and individual levels of effort. It serves as a framework for monitoring and assessing outcomes of UNAIDS effort, promoting cohesiveness in tracking and reporting, and facilitating access to information on progress across UNAIDS. It is a mechanism for generating information for evidence-based decision-making in the Joint Programme.

SEE ALSO: AIDS; AIDS—Living with AIDS.

BIBLIOGRAPHY. Joint United Nations Programme on HIV/AIDS, *AIDS Epidemic Update* (World Health Organization, 2003); Joint United Nations Programme on HIV/AIDS, *Progress Report on the Global Response to the HIV/Aids Epidemic, 2003: Follow-Up to the 2001 United Nations General Assembly Special Session on HIV/AIDS* (World Health Organization, 2003).

Jose S. Lozada
Case Western Reserve University

Jordan

Since 1999 when King Abdullah II ascended the throne of Jordan after the death of his father King Hussein, the government has been engaged in a series of political reforms designed to raise the standard of living in Jordan. Debt, poverty, and unemployment drain the government of much-needed resources. Some 30 percent of the population live below the poverty line, and around two percent live on less than $1 a day. Poverty eradication is a major element of reforms and is necessary to improve the health of the poorest segment of the population of 5,906,760. The official unemployment rate is 12.5 percent of the labor force, but the unofficial rate is 30 percent. With a per capita income of $4,700, Jordan ranks in the mid-range of world incomes. Income disparity is common, and Jordan ranks 36.4 on the Gini index of human inequality. The poorest 10 percent of the population claim only 3.3 percent of resources, while the richest 10 percent share 29.8 percent. The United Nations Development Programme's (UNDP)

Human Development Report ranks Jordan 86th of 233 countries on general quality-of-life issues.

Healthcare reforms have resulted in free care for those in need, and health insurance for children under the age of 5 is comprehensive. Free premarital exams are free at public health clinics. Throughout the kingdom, 200 health centers provide healthcare services, including perinatal care and family planning. Nongovernmental organizations (NGOs) and international agencies are integral to providing healthcare in Jordan. Commitment to healthcare has resulted in 10 percent of the total budget being earmarked for this purpose. The government spends 9.4 percent of the Gross Domestic Product (GDP) on healthcare, providing $440 (international dollars) per capita to meet healthcare needs. However, less than half (45.2 percent) of total health spending derives from government resources, and only 0.7 percent is targeted for Social Security. The private sector provides 54.8 percent of total healthcare spending, with 74 percent of that amount coming from out-of-pocket expenses. There are 2.03 physicians, 3.24 nurses, 1.29 dentists, and 3.12 pharmacists per 1,000 population in Jordan.

Life expectancy in Jordan is 78.4 years, with women outliving men an average of five years. As is common in many Middle Eastern nations, male literacy (95.9 percent) is considerably higher than female literacy (86.3 percent). Primary school enrollment stands at 91 percent. Some 87 percent of females attend secondary school, as do 85 percent of males. Water supplies are threatened by drought and the lack of adequate natural fresh water resources, and Jordan is one of the 10 countries in the world most threatened by water shortages. Nevertheless, 91 percent of the population have access to safe drinking water. In urban areas, 94 percent of the population have access to improved sanitation, but only 85 percent of rural residents are able to meet this basic need.

Jordan has been successful at reducing fertility rates, and 56 percent of women use birth control of some form. Between 1970 and 1990, the fertility rate dropped from 7.9 to 5.9 births per woman and is currently 2.63. The reduction in fertility is due in part to the work of the Supreme Population Council, which was established in 1973 as the National Population Council. The focus of reproductive health in Jordan is holistic, attempting to bring men and women together to foster reproductive health and to improve the

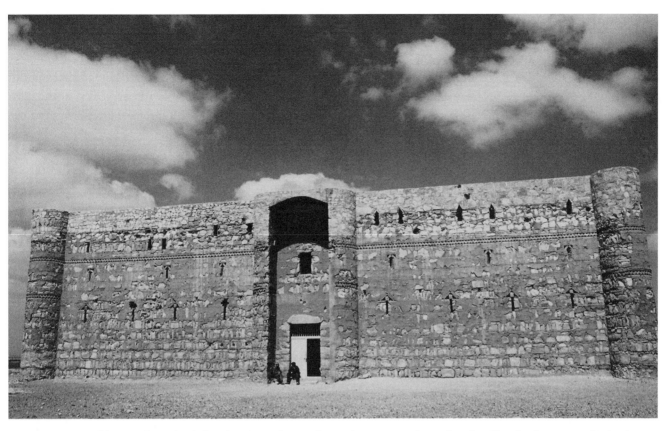

Some 30 percent of the population live below the poverty line, and around two percent live on less than $1 a day. Poverty eradication is a major element of reforms and is necessary to improve the health of the poorest segment of the population of 5,906,760.

health of mothers and children. Skilled professionals attend all births, and 99 percent of women receive prenatal care. The current adjusted maternal mortality rate is 41 deaths per 100,000 live births.

Jordanian infants die at a rate of 16.76 deaths per 1,000 live births, and male infants (20.04) are considerably more vulnerable than female infants (13.28). Between 1990 and 2004, infant mortality declined from 33 to 23 deaths per 1,000 live births, and under-5 mortality dropped from 40 to 27. One-tenth of all infants are underweight at birth, and 4 percent of under-5s fall into this category. Two percent of under-5s suffer from wasting diseases, and 9 percent experience growth stunting. The Jordanian government subsidizes all required infant immunizations; however, vaccination rates for tuberculosis are low (58 percent). Rates in other areas are more in line with what might be expected, and only 1 percent of infants fail to receive measles vaccinations. Some 96 percent receive diphtheria, pertussis, and tetanus (DPT1) immunizations, and 95 percent are vaccinated against

DPT3, polio, hepatitis B, and *Haemophilus influenzae* type B. Only 44 percent of under-5s receive oral rehydration therapy when needed.

HIV/AIDS is under control in Jordan with a 0.1 percent adult prevalence rate. Some 600 people are living with this disease, which has proved fatal to approximately 500 people. The major causes of death in Jordan are cardiovascular diseases (42 percent), cancer (13 percent), and accidents (10.5 percent). The majority of visits to public clinics concern diarrheal diseases, respiratory infections, and hepatitis B and C.

SEE ALSO: Healthcare, Asia and Oceania.

BIBLIOGRAPHY. Michael E. Bonine, ed., *Population, Poverty, and Politics in Middle East Cities* (University Press of Florida, 1997); Helen Chapin Metz, ed., *Jordan: A Country Study* (Federal Research Division, 1991).

ELIZABETH R. PURDY, PH.D.
INDEPENDENT SCHOLAR

Juvenile Rheumatoid Arthritis

Juvenile rheumatoid arthritis (JRA) is the most common form of arthritis occurring in children. Juvenile rheumatoid arthritis does not represent a single disease but a constellation of disease processes which differ in their respective symptoms, treatments, and outcomes. Typically, JRA is clinically diagnosed if a child under the age of 16 has inflammation, limited motion, and swelling in at least one joint that lasts more than six weeks, provided that other diseases have been ruled out. However, in most cases, JRA is not a lifelong condition and symptoms may dissipate in weeks or months.

JRA is not an early-onset form of adult rheumatoid arthritis but a distinctly separate disease. The key difference is that JRA causes chronic inflammation of the synovial membranes lining the joints, but this inflammation is not caused by an autoimmune attack as in adult rheumatoid arthritis. Patients with adult rheumatoid arthritis typically have elevated blood levels of an autoantibody called rheumatoid factor; this is unusual in JRA patients. There are three categories of JRA: pauciarticular, polyarticular, and systemic. The systemic form occurs nearly equally in both sexes, but the first two forms are much more prevalent in females. There is an overall bimodal age distribution, with diagnosis being commonly made between 1 to 3 years or between 8 to 12 years.

Pauciarticular JRA affects approximately 50 percent of all JRA patients. It is defined as arthritis in one to four joints, most commonly involving the knee. A frequent and potentially serious complication of this form of JRA is iridocyclitis, an inflammation of the iris and ciliary body of the eye; all pauciarticular patients should receive regular ophthalmologist exams. Some patients, mostly females, have elevated blood levels of antinuclear antibodies and are at increased risk for iridocyclitis. Another subgroup, mostly males, have the HLA-B27 gene; these patients are at increased risk for developing ankylosing spondylitis, a severe form of arthritis that mainly affects the spine and sacroiliac joints. After several months of symptoms, pauciarticular arthritis patients often enter remission periods lasting years, and thus, this form of JRA carries a relatively good prognosis.

Polyarticular JRA presents with a low-grade fever and at least five arthritic joints. Up to 30 percent of JRA patients have this form of the disease. Typically, the arthritis is symmetrical and affects the same joints on both sides of the body. About 25 percent of these patients actually have elevated levels of rheumatoid factor in their blood, which is typically unusual in JRA. Polyarticular patients, especially those who are positive for rheumatoid factor, often have chronic disease courses.

Systemic JRA, or Still's disease, accounts for about 20 percent of JRA patients. The systemic form is characterized by high fever, rash, arthritic joints, swollen lymph nodes, enlarged liver and spleen, pericarditis, and pleuritis. Also, these patients have markedly elevated white blood cell counts. One in four patients with systemic JRA progresses to long-term severe arthritis.

Early diagnosis and appropriate treatment provide the best chance for a favorable outcome. The goal is to reduce the inflammation, relieve pain, and control joint damage while maximizing function. Antiinflammatory drugs are the mainstays of treatment for all forms of JRA. The pauciarticular form of JRA often responds to nonsteroidal antiinflammatory drugs (NSAIDs) similar to aspirin, particularly naproxen. Injecting steroid drugs into affected joints is another common and effective treatment. For more severe cases, drugs such as methotrexate are used to suppress the proliferation of inflammatory white blood cells that attack the joints. The newer drugs etanercept and infliximab specifically bind to an inflammatory signal molecule, known as tumor necrosis fac-

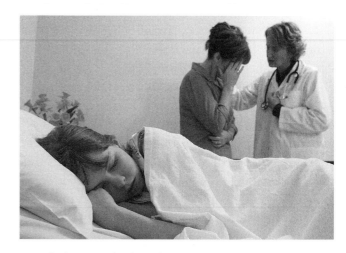

Juvenile rheumatoid arthritis does not represent a single disease but a constellation of disease processes.

tor, preventing its role in sustaining the destructive arthritic process. Regardless of the therapy selected, a multispecialty healthcare team is usually required to provide coordinated care for the patient.

SEE ALSO: Arthritis; National Institute of Arthritis and Musculoskeletal and Skin Diseases (NIAMS); Orthopedics; Orthopedist; Rheumatoid Arthritis.

BIBLIOGRAPHY. Nicholas Athanasou, *Pathological Basis of Orthopaedic and Rheumatic Disease* (Arnold, 2001); Ross Petty, Justine Smith, and James Rosenbaum, "Arthritis and Uveitis in Children: A Pediatric Rheumatology Perspective," *American Journal of Ophthalmology* (v.135, 2003); Emanuel Rubin, et al., *Rubin's Pathology: Clinicopathologic Foundations of Medicine*, 4th ed. (Lippincott Williams & Wilkins, 2005); Harry Skinner, *Current Diagnosis and Treatment in Orthopedics*, 3rd ed. (McGraw-Hill, 2003); Jennifer Weiss and Norman Ilowite, "Juvenile Idiopathic Arthritis," *Pediatric Clinics of North America* (v.52, 2005).

DAVID B. BUMPASS
FRANCIS H. SHEN, M.D.
UNIVERSITY OF VIRGINIA
DINO SAMARTZIS, D.SC., M.SC., DIP. EBHC
HARVARD UNIVERSITY AND ERASMUS UNIVERSITY

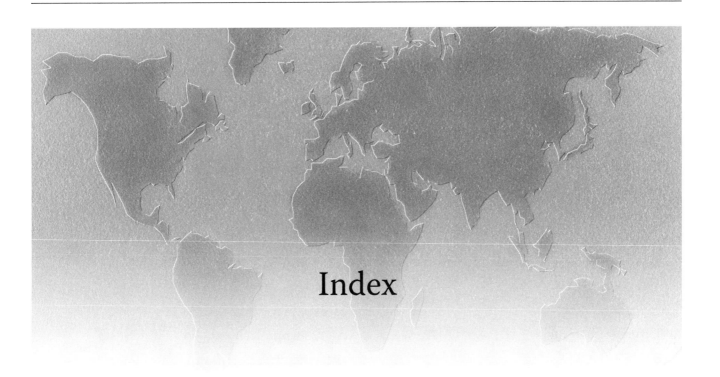

Index

Note: Page numbers in **boldface** refer to volume numbers and major topics. Article titles are in **boldface**.

A

abdominal aortic aneurysms (AAA),
  1:136–137

abdominal pain, **2:**528–529

Abdullah II, **2:**962

Abel, John Jacob, **3:**1368

Abittan, C. S., **3:**1025

ABO blood type system, **1:**60

abortion, 1:1–4, 3:1203, **4:**1480–1481

abscess, anal/rectal, **1:**129

Abse, Dannie, 1:5

abuse:

  alcohol, **1:**55–58

  child, 1:381–383

  drug and substance, **1:**420–422

  of elder populations, 2:591–593

  physical, **1:**381, 382

  sexual, **1:**381, 382

  spousal, **1:**29

Accreditation Council for Continuing Medical
  Education (ACCME), **1:**92, 94, 116

Accutane, **1:**7

acetaminophen, **1:**197

Achenbach, Thomas, **1:**384

achilles tendon, injuries of, **2:**681, **4:**1603

acid-fast stain, **1:**207

acid peptic disease, **4:**1615–1616

acid rain, **1:**49–50

acid reflux, 1:5–6

Ackerman, B. H., **4:**1645

ACL injury, **4:**1602–1603

acne, 1:5–7

acne vulgaris, **1:**6–7

acoustic neuroma, 1:7–8, 290

Acquired Childhood Aphasia, **1:**155

Acquired Immune Deficiency Syndrome (AIDS),
  1:36–41, 209, 210, 212, 253, 286, 334, 364,
  399, 443, 444, 454, **2:**598, 793, 801, 841, 880,

National Institute on Alcohol Abuse and Alcoholism (NIAAA), 1:52, 3:1194–1195

National Institute on Deafness and Other Communication Disorders (NIDCD), 3:1195–1196

National Institute on Drug Abuse (NIDA), 3:1196–1197

National Institute on Mental Health (NIMH), 1:73

National Institute on Nursing Research (NINR), 1:73

National Institutes of Health (NIH), U.S., 1:32, 33, 65, 72, 107, 191, 3:1197–1199

National Library of Medicine (NLM), 3:1199–1200

National Mental Health Association (NMHA), 3:1200–1201

National Network for Immunization Information (NNii), 3:1201–1202

National Network on Aging, 1:17

National Organ Procurement and Transplantation Network (OPTN), 3:1292

National Organ Transplant Act (NOTA), 4:1709

National Osteoporosis Foundation, 1:283

National Program of Cancer Registries (NPCR), 3:1202–1203

National Research Priority, 1:185

National Survey on Drug Use and Health (NSDUH), 3:1069, 1420

National Tuberculosis and Respiratory Disease Association, 1:103

National Women's Health Organization (NWHO), 3:1203–1204

National Women's Law Center, 1:105

Native American health, 2:899–900, 3:1204–1207

natural family planning (NFP), 1:249

natural killer cells, 1:9

natural selection, 2:472, 730

naturopathic medicine/naturopathy, 1:67, 3:1208–1209

Nauru, 3:1210

nausea and vomiting, 2:529, 3:1210–1212

neck and head cancer, 2:779–780

neck disorders and injuries, 3:1212–1214

neglect, 1:383

Neimann-Pick disease, 4:1488

Neisseria gonorrhoeae, 2:746

Neisseria meningitidis, 1:204

nematodes, 3:1083–1084

neonatal intensive care units (NICU), 3:1214, 1418

neonatal nurses, 1:175–176

neonatologists, 3:1214

neonatology, 3:1214–1216

Nepal, 3:1216–1217

nephritis, 3:973

nephrogenic diabetes insipidus (NDI), 2:501

nephrologists, 3:1217–1218

nephrology, 3:1218–1219

nerve agents, 1:233

nerve disorders, peripheral, 3:1354–1356

nervous system:
degenerative nerve disease in, 2:481–483
diabetic neuropathy of, 2:514–515
disabilities, 2:498–499

Netherlands, 3:1219–1221

Neugarten, Bernice, 3:1105

neuralgia, 2:649–650

neural tube defects (NTDs), 1:251, 252, 2:669, 3:1221–1222

neuroblastoma, 1:391, 3:1222–1224

neurodegenerative diseases/disorders, 1:293, 3:1190, 1228–1229

neurodermatitis, 2:498

neuroendocrine tumors, 1:344

neuroendocrinology, 3:1224–1225

Photo Credits